PREVENTIVE NUTRITION

NUTRITION ◊ AND ◊ HEALTH
Adrianne Bendich, Series Editor

Preventive Nutrition: The Comprehensive Guide for Health Professionals,
edited by Adrianne Bendich and Richard J. Deckelbaum

PREVENTIVE NUTRITION

THE COMPREHENSIVE GUIDE
FOR HEALTH PROFESSIONALS

Edited by

ADRIANNE BENDICH, PhD
Hoffmann-La Roche, Paramus, NJ

and

RICHARD J. DECKELBAUM, MD
Columbia University, New York, NY

FOREWORD BY CHARLES H. HENNEKENS, MD, DrPH
AND JOANN E. MANSON, MD

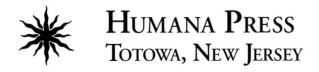

HUMANA PRESS
TOTOWA, NEW JERSEY

© 1997 Humana Press Inc.
999 Riverview Drive, Suite 208
Totowa, New Jersey 07512

For additional copies, pricing for bulk purchases, and/or information about other Humana titles,
contact Humana at the above address or at any of the following numbers: Tel.: 201-256-1699;
Fax: 201-256-8341; E-mail: humana@mindspring.com

Cover design by Patricia F. Cleary.

This publication is printed on acid-free paper. ∞
ANSI Z39.48-1984 (American National Standards Institute) Permanence of Paper for Printed Library Materials.

Printed in the United States of America. 10 9 8 7 6 5 4 3 2

Library of Congress Cataloging-in-Publication Data

Preventive nutrition: the comprehensive guide for health professionals/edited by Adrianne Bendich and Richard J.
  Deckelbaum
      p.   cm.—(Nutrition and health)
    Includes bibliographical references and index.
    ISBN 0-89603-351-1 (alk. paper)
    1. Nutrition. 2. Medicine, Preventive. 3. Nutritionally induced diseases—Prevention. 4. Diet therapy.
  I. Bendich, Adrianne. II. Deckelbaum, Richard J. III. Series: Nutrition and health (Totowa, NJ)
    [DNLM: 1. Nutrition. 2. Nutritional Status. 3. Diet. 4. Primary Prevention.   QU 145 P944 1997]
RM216.P778   1997
615.8'54—dc21
DNLM/DLC
for Library of Congress   96-37937
                                      CIP

FOREWORD

Compelling evidence supports a link between nutrition and numerous acute and chronic diseases. Nutritional science has advanced from a model targeting the prevention of clinical deficiencies of nutrients to the assessment of nutrient intake levels that promote optimal health. Although diet has been implicated in both the prevention and causation of disease, education and training in nutrition among physicians and other health professionals remain inadequate. In this context, *Preventive Nutrition*, edited by Drs. Bendich and Deckelbaum, makes important and timely contributions in summarizing the totality of evidence about nutrition and health.

At present, the chief causes of death in developing countries are malnutrition and infection, and in developed countries are chronic diseases, predominantly cardiovascular disease and cancer. Although improvements in diagnosis and treatment have played a role, major gains have been attributable to prevention. Dietary choices are important determinants of health and longevity. Dietary fat, antioxidant vitamins, folic acid, alcohol, Ω-3 fatty acids, and other nutrients are reviewed in detail, as are the effects of pediatric and adult obesity. The scope of the contributions in *Preventive Nutrition* ranges from malnutrition as a major cause of premature death in developing countries to the role of various nutritional etiologies of premature death in developed countries, including cardiovascular disease and cancer. This book also addresses major nutritional causes of morbidity, including age-related macular degeneration, cataracts, osteoporosis, and birth defects.

Preventive Nutrition also encompasses public health applications, goals, and strategies for developing and developed countries. The implications of clinical nutrition research on public policy issues worldwide are given thoughtful attention. For all these reasons, Drs. Bendich and Deckelbaum are to be commended for *Preventive Nutrition,* which is the most comprehensive and up-to-date textbook in the field.

Charles H. Hennekens
JoAnn E. Manson
Harvard School of Public Health, Boston, MA

v

PREFACE

Preventive nutrition can be defined as dietary practices and interventions directed toward the reduction in disease risk and /or improvement in health outcomes. Preventive nutrition is a critical component of preventive medicine approaches that seek to prevent disease rather than treat the condition after it manifests clinically. Examples of preventive nutrition include current recommendations to reduce fat and saturated fat intakes for cardiovascular disease prevention, the inclusion of iodine in salt for the prevention of iodine deficiency disease, and the inclusion of certain B vitamins, vitamins A and D, iron, and calcium in staple foods, such as grain products, milk, and cereals, for the prevention of other essential nutrient-related deficiencies. These preventive nutrition strategies have been underway as part of public health policy for more than a generation and have been shown to be extremely effective.

Within the past 20 years, further nutrient-based research has demonstrated the potential for essential micronutrients to reduce the risk of many common chronic diseases. Thus, the overall goal of this volume, *Preventive Nutrition*, is to assess and describe these recent nutritional approaches for promoting health and preventing, delaying, or modifying disease processes. The new research on dietary components that are not considered to have traditional "nutritional value," but have been shown to have important health consequences, such as fiber, specific long-chain fatty acids, nonprovitamin A carotenoids, and other phytochemicals, are placed in perspective with regard to the available knowledge to date.

The first objective of this volume is to provide practicing health professionals, including physicians, nutritionists, dentists, pharmacists, dieticians, health educators, policy makers, and research investigators, with the new and up-to-date research indicating that the risk of many of the major diseases affecting middle-aged adults can be prevented, or at least delayed, with simple nutritional approaches. Many health professionals are asked daily about the new studies with vitamins or other nutrients in their local newspaper or on the evening news. As examples, patients want advice from their health care providers about β-carotene, antioxidants, fiber, and the myriad of bioactive phytochemicals, such as those found in garlic and other foods.

This volume attempts to provide answers based on the totality of evidence, rather than on the findings of any single study. Major disease categories are included, such as the leading two causes of mortality in the United States and elsewhere, cardiovascular disease and cancer, as well as such progressively debilitating conditions as diabetes, cataracts, and osteoporosis. The potential of nutrients to affect immunocompetence, which may be an underlying factor in many of the abovementioned and other conditions, is examined.

The second objective is to examine key research linking nutritional status with the prevention of birth defects and optimization of birth outcomes. Recent evidence that micronutrient status can also improve the potential for the health, vision, and intellectual capacity of children is discussed. The need for physicians and nutritional care providers as well as both potential parents to strongly advocate a new paradigm of long-range planning for pregnancy is underscored. Research clearly shows that the periconceptional period, about three months before conception through the third month of pregnancy, is the time when many serious birth defects occur; thus, the old paradigm that women can wait for prenatal care until weeks or months after conception is no longer valid.

A unique feature of this volume is the section that examines the successes and consequent public health implications of national preventive nutrition strategies, not only in the United States and Europe, but also in "Westernizing" nations and developing countries. As the demographics of US and European populations change and become more multicultural, it is increasingly important for health professionals to understand the nutritional backgrounds and diversities of their patients. As important, there may be significant national dietary initiatives that provide roadmaps for effective implementation of preventive nutrition within an overall strategy of health improvement, especially for vulnerable members of the population, such as the poor.

The evaluation of the totality of the evidence will be critical in leading to recommendations that can lower risk of disease, morbidity, and mortality and at the same time reduce the burden of health care costs for all. The economic consequences of preventive nutrition cannot be easily overlooked. Based on the annual costs associated with hospitalizations alone, documented in the 1992 National Hospital Discharge Survey, the estimated savings associated with reducing chronic disease risk has been shown to be substantial. For coronary heart disease, the chronic disease responsible for the largest number of hospitalizations per year in the United States, the total for hospitalization charges, excluding physician fees, was approx $57.6 billion in 1995 dollars. Using the recent epidemiologic literature examining the reduction in risk of heart disease associated with the highest antioxidant status, it can be estimated that $22 billion per year could be saved in this disease category alone once preventive nutrition measures were fully implemented (Chapter 9).

The costs associated with hospitalizations resulting from cancer are also substantial. The average annual hospitalization charges for stomach cancer are about $1 billion; breast cancer costs about $1.8 billion; for head and neck cancers, which are more rare than the two other cancers discussed, the hospitalization costs are still high, although under $1 billion per year. It is estimated that hospitalization costs associated with stomach and breast cancer could each be reduced by one-third; head and neck cancers could be halved based on projections that use published esimates of risk reduction associated with the highest intakes of antioxidant micronutrients (Chapters 3–5).

Cataract surgery is the most common single operation performed in the United States. Epidemiologic studies in the United States and Europe have consistently found a reduced risk of cataract incidence and need for surgery in those individuals who use a multivitamin and have the highest intakes of vitamins C, E, and β-carotene (Chapter 14). The cost savings for hospitalizations alone could reach $2 million per year. Most cataract surgeries are done on outpatients and therefore this cost estimate is lower than might be expected.

Cardiovascular disease, cancer, and cataracts are examples of chronic diseases with long durations of onset; thus, long-term preventive nutritional strategies are needed. Therefore, the economic benefits that are projected would not be realized in a short period of time, and it may take years before the economic as well as personal and national health benefits can be seen. There are, however, other adverse health conditions that are more acute in time frame, and the economic consequences could be measured in a shorter time period than required for prevention of chronic diseases. For example, the effects of preventive nutrition strategies on the hospitalization costs involved in adverse pregnancy outcomes could be documented in a relatively short period of time.

Table 1
Potential Economic Consequences of Preventive Nutrition

Disease	Reductions based on only hospitalization costs/yr, $
Cardiovascular disease	22 billion
Cancer	1 billion
Cardiovascular birth defects	800 million
Low birth weight	500 million
Neural tube birth defects	70 million
Cataract	2 million

Birth defects are the number one cause of hospitalizations associated with birth-related disorders. Low birth weight accounts for the second largest number of hospitalizations. Birth defects and low birth weight are also the two major causes of infant mortality in the United States. Thus, the potential to reduce both infant morbidity and mortality through nutritional interventions provides a real possibility of verifying the economic and consequent health benefits of relatively short-term dietary changes.

As a specific example, within the past decade, significant research has documented that women who take a folic acid-containing multivitamin daily for at least one month before conception and during their pregnancies have approximately a 50% decrease in neural tube defect (NTD) outcomes (Chapter 19). The expected annual savings associated with lowered NTD-related outcomes is about $70 million. By far the greatest savings would be seen in the reduction of cardiovascular birth defects, which are the greatest cause of birth-related hospitalizations. Based on intervention and epidemiologic studies, it is estimated that the annual savings could reach $800 million. In addition to NTD and cardiovascular birth defects, there are also significant reductions in renal defects, cleft lip/palate, and limb reductions seen in women who use multivitamin supplements before and during pregnancy (Chapter 19).

Low-birth-weight infants include those from premature births as well as small for gestational age term infants. In both cases, hospitalization costs are projected to be over $2 billion annually. There are studies that indicate that reduction in iron deficiency anemia, as well as improved zinc and/or folic acid status, can significantly reduce the risk of low-birth-weight pregnancy outcomes (Chapter 21). The estimated hospital-associated savings would be many millions of dollars per year (Table 1).

Economic estimates have not been made for all of the areas covered in the chapters in this book. However, it seems logical that the improvement seen in the immune responses of the elderly who took a multivitamin supplement (Chapter 17) would result in lowered hospitalizations associated with respiratory infections, for instance. Likewise, improved immune status via vitamin A supplementation in children could prevent infection-associated morbidity and mortality (Chapter 18).

Although the economic analysis is limited to US hospitalization data, the chapters that describe the major health benefits seen with national nutrition strategies, for example in Chile (Chapter 27) and Norway (Chapter 25), provide further evidence that preventive measures have real economic benefits and improve the quality of life for the populations that benefit from enlightened governmental preventive medicine strategies, including nutritional components.

It should be realized that many of the nutrient recommendations provided in this volume that appear to be related to one specific health factor or disease in fact "cross over" and appear

Table 2
Dietary Factors Linked to Health Outcome Improvements[a]

	Decrease total and/or saturated fat	Increase antioxidants	Increase folic acid	Increase calcium	Increase complex CHO, fiber	Increase omega–3 fatty acids
Cardiovascular disease	+	+	+	+	+	+
Cancer	+	+	+	+	+	+
Diabetes	+	+			+	+
Cataract/AMD	+	+				
Obesity	+				+	
Osteoporosis				+		
Birth outcomes		+	+		+	+
Immune function	+	+	+		+	+

[a]+ = Positive impact on health outcomes.

valid for many of the health areas discussed (Table 2; Chapters 1 and 23). Importantly, there are many more commonalities in the recommendations provided for disease risk reduction than there are differences. For example, lowering fat intake and increasing antioxidants, fiber, and calcium intake are suggested for reducing cardiovascular and cancer risks and at the same time may lower the risk of osteoporosis and cataracts. Increased intake of folic acid would likely lead to decreases in NTDs as well as cardiovascular disease. Of critical importance, no single recommendation provided in this volume targeted to a single condition will lead to adverse effects in another health area. Thus, overall, the guidelines suggested in the individual chapters have the potential to not only reduce individual morbidity and health care costs, but can also contribute positively to the national health care debate.

As editors, we are very excited about the contents of this book. Generally, each chapter is organized to provide an overview of the field, the author's own research, and how those findings fit with the overview. Extensive summary tables and figures illustrate the depth of knowledge in the area and recommendations for various patient groups. There is an extensive index. Also included is a list of journals that specialize in publishing clinical studies in preventive nutrition and a bibliography of recent, relevant books. By addressing the nutrition questions most often raised, and by examining the issues based on disease as well as age, it is hoped that this volume will serve as the critical resource for health professionals interested in enhancing their ability to utilize nutrition to improve health outcomes of individuals, and assist in the planning of national disease prevention programs for enhancing the health status of populations.

Adrianne Bendich
Richard J. Deckelbaum

DEDICATION

A. B. dedicates this book to Tyler James Schiff, her first grandchild, with the hope that preventive nutrition becomes an accepted component of medical practice in his lifetime.

R. J. D. thanks his wife, Kaya, and children Ariel, Dan, Mikael, and Leona for their understanding and support.

The authors acknowledge the technical assistance of Paul Brock, Diane Russo, and Mayra Pabon. In addition, the authors express their sincere appreciation to Paul Dolgert, Editorial Director, Humana Press.

CONTENTS

Foreword, by Charles H. Hennekens and JoAnn E. Manson v

Preface vii

Contributors.. xvii

PART I   PUBLIC HEALTH IMPLICATIONS OF PREVENTIVE NUTRITION

   A   CANCER PREVENTION

     1   Public Health Implications of Preventive Nutrition...................... *1*
       Jeffrey B. Blumberg

     2   Diet and Childhood Cancer: *Preliminary Evidence*...................... 17
       Greta R. Bunin and Joan M. Cary

     3   Prevention of Upper Gastrointestinal Tract Cancers *33*
       Elizabeth T. H. Fontham

     4   Diet and Nutrition in the Etiology and Primary Prevention
        of Colon Cancer *57*
       Roberd M. Bostick

     5   Nutrition and Breast Cancer *97*
       Geoffrey R. Howe

     6   Preventive Nutrition and Lung Cancer...................................... *109*
       George W. Comstock and Kathy J. Helzlsouer

     7   Nonnutritive Components in Foods as Modifiers
        of the Cancer Process *135*
       John A. Milner

   B   CARDIOVASCULAR DISEASE

     8   Dietary Fat and Coronary Heart Disease.................................. *153*
       K. C. Hayes

     9   Antioxidant Vitamins and Cardiovascular Disease *171*
       Julie E. Buring and J. Michael Gaziano

    10   Iron and Heart Disease: *A Review of the Epidemiologic Data* *181*
       Christopher T. Sempos, Richard F. Gillum,
         and Anne Condon Looker

    11   Homocysteine, Folic Acid, and Cardiovascular Disease Risk *193*
       Shirley A. A. Beresford and Carol J. Boushey

    12   Omega-3 Fatty Acids from Fish: *Primary and Secondary*
        Prevention of Cardiovascular Disease *225*
       William E. Connor and Sonja L. Connor

PART II   PREVENTION OF MAJOR DISABILITIES

    A   CATARACTS AND MACULAR DEGENERATION

        13   The Relationship Between Nutritional Factors
             and Age-Related Macular Degeneration 245
             Shirley Hung and Johanna M. Seddon

        14   Antioxidant Status and Risk for Cataract 267
             Allen Taylor and Paul F. Jacques

    B   OSTEOPOROSIS

        15   Osteoporosis: *Vitamins, Minerals, and Other Micronutrients* 285
             Robert P. Heaney

    C   IMMUNE FUNCTION

        16   Antioxidant Nutrients and Prevention of Oxidant-Mediated,
             Smoking-Related Diseases 303
             Ronald Anderson

        17   Micronutrients and Immunity in Older People 317
             John D. Bogden and Donald B. Louria

        18   Impact of Vitamin A on Immunity and Infection
             in Developing Countries 337
             Richard D. Semba

PART III   OPTIMAL BIRTH OUTCOMES

        19   Folic Acid-Containing Multivitamins and Primary Prevention
             of Birth Defects 351
             Andrew E. Czeizel

        20   Nutritional Prevention of DNA Damage to Sperm
             and Consequent Risk Reduction in Birth Defects
             and Cancer in Offspring 373
             Alan A. Woodall and Bruce N. Ames

        21   Maternal Nutrition and Preterm Delivery 387
             Theresa O. Scholl and Mary L. Hediger

        22   Dietary Polyunsaturated Fatty Acids for Optimal
             Neurodevelopment: *Recommendations for Perinatal
             Nutrition* 405
             Ricardo Uauy-Dagach, Patricia Mena, and Patricio Peirano

PART IV   BENEFITS OF PREVENTIVE NUTRITION IN THE UNITED STATES AND EUROPE

        23   Potential Benefits of Preventive Nutrition Strategies:
             Lessons for the United States 423
             Walter C. Willett

        24   Nutrient Addition to Foods: *The Public Health Impact
             in Countries with Rapidly Westernizing Diets* 441
             Paul A. Lachance

25 Nutrition and Food Policy in Norway: *Effects on Reduction of Coronary Heart Disease* *455*
Kaare R. Norum, Lars Johansson, Grete Botten, Gunn-Elin Aa. Bjørneboe, and Arne Oshaug

26 Prevention of Pediatric Obesity: *Examining the Issues and Forecasting Research Directions* *471*
Myles S. Faith, Angelo Pietrobelli, David B. Allison, and Steven B. Heymsfield

PART V   IMPLICATIONS OF PREVENTIVE NUTRITION FOR THE FAR EAST, SOUTH AMERICA, AND DEVELOPING AREAS

27 Effect of Westernization of Nutritional Habits on Obesity in Latin America: *Recommendations for the Region* *487*
S. Jaime Rozowski and Manuel Moreno

28 Prevention of Malnutrition in Chile *505*
Fernando Mönckeberg

29 Effects of Western Diet on Risk Factors of Chronic Diseases in Asia *523*
Kaichi Kida, Takuo Ito, Sei Won Yang, and Vichai Tanphaichitr

30 Goals for Preventive Nutrition in Developing Countries *535*
Osman M. Galal and Gail G. Harrison

PART VI   NUTRITION-RELATED RESOURCES

A   BOOKS RELATED TO PREVENTIVE NUTRITION *549*

B   NUTRITION-RELATED JOURNALS AND NEWSLETTERS *551*

Index *559*

CONTRIBUTORS

DAVID B. ALLISON • *Obesity Research Center, St. Luke's-Roosevelt Hospital Center, Columbia University College of Physicians and Surgeons, New York, NY*

BRUCE N. AMES • *Department of Biochemistry and Molecular Biology, University of California, Berkely, CA*

RONALD ANDERSON • *Medical Research Council Unit, Department of Immunology, Institute for Pathology, University of Pretoria, Pretoria, South Africa*

SHIRLEY A. A. BERESFORD • *Department of Epidemiology, University of Washington, Seattle, WA*

GUNN-ELIN AA. BJØRNBOE • *Institute for Nutrition Research, University of Oslo, and National Nutrition Council, Oslo, Norway*

JEFFERY B. BLUMBERG • *USDA Human Nutrition Research Center on Aging, School of Nutrition, Tufts University, Boston, MA*

JOHN D. BOGDEN • *Department of Preventive Medicine and Community Health, UMDNJ-New Jersey Medical School, Newark, NJ*

ROBERD M. BOSTICK • *Department of Public Health Science, Bowman Gray School of Medicine, Wake Forest University, Winston-Salem, NC*

GRETE BOTTEN • *Institute for Nutrition Research, University of Oslo, and National Nutrition Council, Oslo, Norway*

CAROL J. BOUSHEY • *Department of Animal Science, Food, and Nutrition, Southern Illinois University, Carbondale, IL*

GRETA R. BUNIN • *Division of Oncology, Children's Hospital; Department of Pediatrics, University of Pennsylvania School of Medicine, Philadelphia, PA*

JULIE E. BURING • *Department of Medicine, Division of Preventive Medicine, Brigham and Women's Hospital, Harvard Medical School, Boston, MA*

JOAN M. CARY • *Medical College of Pennsylvania, Hahnemann University, Philadelphia, PA*

GEORGE W. COMSTOCK • *School of Hygiene and Public Health, Training Center for Public Health Research, Johns Hopkins University, Hagerstown, MD*

SONJA L. CONNOR • *Department of Medicine, Oregon Health Sciences University, Portland, OR*

WILLIAM E. CONNOR • *Department of Medicine, Oregon Health Sciences University, Portland, OR*

ANDREW E. CZEIZEL • *Department of Human Genetics and Teratology, National Institute of Hygeine, Gyali, Hungary*

MYLES S. FAITH • *Obesity Research Center, St. Lukes-Roosevelt Hospital, Columbia University College of Physicians and Surgeons, New York, NY*

ELIZABETH T. H. FONTHAM • *Department of Pathology, Louisiana State University Medical Center, New Orleans, LA*

OSMAN M. GALAL • *Department of Community Health Sciences, UCLA School of Public Health, Los Angeles, CA*

J. MICHAEL GAZIANO • *Department of Medicine, Division of Preventive Medicine, Brigham and Women's Hospital, Boston, MA*

RICHARD F. GILLUM • *National Center for Health Statistics, Centers for Disease Control and Prevention, Hyattsville, MD*

GAIL G. HARRISON • *Department of Community Health Sciences, UCLA School of Public Health, Los Angeles, CA*

K. C. HAYES • *Foster Biomedical Research Laboratory, Brandeis University, Waltham, MA*

ROBERT P. HEANY • *John A. Creighton University Professor, Creighton University, Omaha, NE*

MARY L. HEDIGER • *Department of Obstetrics and Gynecology, UMDNJ-NJ School of Medicine, Stratford, NJ*

KATHY J. HELZLSOUER • *Department of Epidemiology, School of Hygiene and Public Health, Johns Hopkins University, Baltimore, MD*

STEVEN B. HEYMSFIELD • *Obesity Research Center, St. Lukes-Roosevelt Hospital Center, Columbia University College of Physicians and Surgeons, New York, NY*

GEOFFREY R. HOWE • *Division of Epidemiology, School of Public Health, Columbia University, New York, NY*

SHIRLEY HUNG • *Epidemiology Unit, Massachusetts Eye and Ear Infirmary, Boston, MA*

TAKUO ITO • *Department of Pediatrics, Ehime University School of Medicine, Ehime, Japan*

PAUL F. JACQUES • *USDA, HNRC on Aging, Tufts University, Boston, MA*

LARS JOHANSSON • *Institute for Nutrition Research, University of Oslo, and National Nutrition Council, Oslo, Norway*

KAICHI KIDA • *Department of Pediatrics, Ehime University School of Medicine, Ehime, Japan*

PAUL A. LACHANCE • *Department of Food Science, Rutgers, The State University of New Jersey, New Brunswick, NJ*

ANNE CONDON LOOKER • *National Center for Health Statistics, Centers for Disease Control and Prevention, Hyattsville, MD*

DONALD B. LOURIA • *Department of Preventive Medicine, UMDNJ-New Jersey Medical School, Newark, NJ*

PATRICIA MENA • *Institute of Nutrition and Food Technology, University of Chile, Santaigo, Chile*

JOHN A. MILNER • *Department of Nutrition, The Pennsylvania State University, University Park, PA*

FERNANDO MÖNCKEBERG • *Universidad Santo Tomas, Santiago, Chile*

MANUEL MORENO • *Faculty of Medicine, Department of Endocrinology, Metabolism, and Nutrition, Catholic University of Chile, Santiago, Chile*

KAARE R. NORUM • *Institute for Nutrition Research, University of Oslo, and National Nutrition Council, Oslo, Norway*

ARNE OSHAUG • *Institute for Nutrition Research, University of Oslo, and National Nutrition Council, Oslo, Norway*

PATRICIO PEIRANO • *Institute of Nutrition and Food Technology, University of Chile, Santiago, Chile*

ANGELO PIETROBELLI • *Obesity Research Center, St. Luke's-Roosevelt Hospital Center, Columbia University College of Physicians and Surgeons, New York, NY*

S. JAIME ROZOWSKI • *Department of Endocrinology, Metabolism, and Nutrition, Faculty of Medicine, Catholic University of Chile, Santiago, Chile*

THERESA O. SCHOLL • *Department of Obstetrics and Gynecology, UMDNJ-NJ School of Medicine, Stratford, NJ*

JOHANNA M. SEDDON • *Epidemiology Unit, Massachusetts Eye and Ear Infirmary, Boston, MA*

RICHARD D. SEMBA • *Ocular Immunology Service, Johns Hopkins University, Baltimore, MD*

CHRISTOPHER T. SEMPOS • *Department of Medicine, College of Medicine, University of Illinois at Urbana-Champaign, Urbana, IL. Present Address: Epidemiology and Biometry Program, Division of Epidemiology and Clinical Applications, National Heart, Lung, and Blood Institute, Bethesda, MD*

VICHAI TANPHAICHITR • *Research Center, Ramathibodi Hospital, Bangkok, Thailand*

ALLEN TAYLOR • *Laboratory of Nutrition and Vision Research, USDA Human Nutrition Research on Aging, Tufts University, Boston, MA*

RICARDO UAUY-DAGACH • *Institute of Nutrition and Food Technology, University of Chile, Santiago, Chile*

WALTER C. WILLETT • *Department of Nutrition and Medicine, School of Public Health, Harvard Medical School, Boston, MA*

ALAN A. WOODALL • *Division of Biochemistry and Molecular Biology, University of California, Berkeley, CA*

SEI WON YANG • *Department of Pediatrics, Seoul National University Children's Hospital, Seoul, Korea*

PART I
PUBLIC HEALTH IMPLICATIONS
OF PREVENTIVE NUTRITION

1

Public Health Implications of Preventive Nutrition

Jeffrey B. Blumberg

1. INTRODUCTION

The recent debate about health care reform has focused largely on issues of equal access, cost containment, and delivery of primary care with some minor appreciation of the need for continued support for research and development. The central paradigm of this discussion is universal coverage and ways to finance it. Largely absent from consideration is the recognition that public health policies must drastically reduce the current disease-oriented treatment approach by encouraging significant changes in provider and consumer attitudes toward health promotion and health maintenance. Abundant evidence indicates that a health care system with a goal of promoting health and preventing illness will cost less than the present system, which basically operates to respond to the presence of illness with expensive diagnostic and therapeutic interventions. Consensus reports, like those from the US Surgeon General and National Research Council, clearly support the notion of preventive nutrition: that the most important choice people can make to influence their long-term health prospects is the choice of diet *(1–3)*. Importantly, the modalities of this choice extend beyond a knowledgeable selection of food items and include nutrient enrichment, fortification, supplementation, and most recently, the potential of functional foods *(4)*.

The accumulating evidence of a link between diet and disease, particularly the chronic degenerative diseases, has led to an expansion in the focus of nutrition recommendations. The first major sources of nutrition guidance in North America, the US Recommended Dietary Allowances (RDA) and the Canadian Recommended Nutrient Intakes, were developed to recommend amounts of essential nutrients principally according to age and sex *(3,5)*. More recent nutrition recommendations, such as the USDA/DHHS Dietary Guidelines for Americans *(6)* and those promulgated by the National Cancer Institute *(7)*, go well beyond standards for the prevention of nutrient deficiencies and target the reduction in risk of such conditions as heart disease, hypertension, stroke, diabetes, and some forms of cancer. Recently, the Institute of Medicine's Food and Nutrition Board has questioned whether the RDA should be revised to accommodate this link and include the concept of chronic disease prevention in the development of nutrient allowances *(8)*.

Translating nutritional recommendations to public health policy will also require going beyond judgments based on the relative strength of the associations between diet and disease, and also take into account the current patterns of morbidity and mortality.

From: *Preventive Nutrition: The Comprehensive Guide for Health Professionals*
Edited by A. Bendich and R. J. Deckelbaum Humana Press Inc., Totowa, NJ

For example, a weak association between a dietary component and a disease having a major impact on the health of a population should merit greater consideration than evidence suggesting a stronger alteration in risk for a rare condition. Although nutritional guidelines for public health should always be conservative, with the potential benefits and efficacy of changes defined in the near absence of risk, there is little evidence to suggest any adverse consequence to such recommendations. Importantly, the recommendations must be developed such that people will accept the changes proffered and try, if only with partial success, to incorporate them into their lives. Of course, certain preventive nutrition approaches, e.g., fortification of the food supply, largely circumvent this obstacle to compliance.

There are subtle but important differences between health and the absence of disease and between health promotion and disease prevention. The Constitution of the World Health Organization states in its preamble that "health is a state of complete physical, mental, and social well-being and not merely the absence of disease or infirmity." Definitions of health promotion and disease prevention promulgated by the US Department of Health and Human Services differ in terms of personal behavior, level of prevention, and sense of well-being (2). Health promotion is defined as personal, environmental, or social interventions that facilitate behavioral adaptations conducive to improved health, level of function, and sense of well-being. Disease prevention is defined as personal, environmental, or social interventions that impede the occurrence of disease, injury, disability, or death, or the progression of detectable but asymptomatic disease.

The historical goal of nutrition recommendations has been directed to diets that provide all the essential nutrients and just enough energy to meet individual requirements (5). This objective represented a reasonable approach to the major causes of morbidity and death through the midpart of this century. Public health measures, such as the creation of a safe water supply and the medical contribution of vaccines and antibiotic therapies, have done much to eliminate or reduce the threats of smallpox, tuberculosis, and other virulent infectious diseases of the past. In the nutrition arena, public health measures, such as enriching grains with B vitamins and iron, iodizing salt, fortifying margarine with vitamin A and milk with vitamins A and D, and adding vitamin C to fruit juices, have helped to eliminate the previously common risks of beri-beri, pellagra, goiter, rickets, and scurvy. Despite the success of these efforts, it is important to recognize that risks of nutritional deficiencies have not been totally eliminated, e.g., the marked prevalence of inadequate intakes of calcium, iron, vitamin D, and folate among women. Indeed, the National Health Promotion and Disease Prevention Objectives, Healthy People 2000, continues to target increased intakes of calcium and iron as high priority public health issues (9), and the Public Health Service has promulgated recommendations for folic acid to reduce the incidence of neural tube birth defects among women of childbearing age (10). Some health authorities suggest that supplementation may be the most practical way for women to increase their folic acid intake (11,12), particularly because plans to fortify the food supply with the vitamin have not yet been implemented. Without any intent to minimize the critical contribution to be made by folic acid in protecting against birth defects, this chapter will focus on the impact of preventive nutrition on chronic diseases.

Prevention can occur at various times during the natural history of a disease (13). Primary prevention involves risk factor modification to prevent the occurrence of disease, such as increasing dietary fiber intake to reduce the incidence of colorectal cancer *(14)*. Secondary prevention involves screening for a disease before it is symptomatic, such as the routine use of serum cholesterol testing to assess risk of coronary heart disease (CHD), with an appropriate follow-up intervention, such as decreasing dietary fat, niacin therapy, and so forth *(15)*. Tertiary prevention involves treating and minimizing the complications of a disease once it has occurred, an apparent example being the use of antioxidant supplements to minimize coronary artery lesion progression in patients with coronary artery bypass grafts *(16)*. Within the context of tertiary preventive nutrition, it important to also note that nearly 17 million Americans are treated for illnesses or injuries that place them at high risk of being malnourished *(17)*. Thus, dietary changes and other nutritional interventions appear capable of playing a significant role in each facet of prevention strategies.

2. PATTERNS OF MORBIDITY AND MORTALITY AND THE INFLUENCE OF NUTRITION

The illness burden has shifted during this century from acute to chronic illness and from younger to older individuals. About 75% of deaths in people over the age of 65 are now from heart disease, cancer, and cerebrovascular disease (Table 1) *(18,19)*. In contrast, at the turn of the century infectious disease was responsible for 50% of deaths whereas heart disease, cancer, and stroke combined contributed 35%. Preventive measures apparently have had major positive effects in increasing life expectancy *(20)*. A significant portion of the decline in the mortality rate observed since 1960 has been the postponement of death from chronic diseases. Nonetheless, the wider spread knowledge and more successful implementation of preventive measures related to these diseases could further decrease premature deaths. It is worthwhile to briefly consider some of the leading causes of morbidity and mortality in the context of preventive nutrition.

2.1. Coronary Heart Disease

The incidence of CHD increases with age and is responsible for approx 24% of total deaths in the United States. CHD had become a major cause of death by 1920 and increased by 1–2% / yr to 300 deaths / 100,000 population in the mid 1960s; CHD mortality rates began to decrease around 1968, and today are about 30% lower *(21)*. This decline follows a pattern that is compatible with a drop in incidence caused by the adoption of preventive health practices *(20)*. Although an increased awareness of some of the risk factors associated with CHD with subsequent nutritional and other behavioral modifications must be partly responsible for the improvement, some reports argue that empirical proof is lacking to indicate this trend has resulted from risk factor modification *(22,23)*. Although some of the decrease in mortality rates may be secondary to improved long-term survival after a myocardial infarction, most studies do not support this contention or otherwise suggest that advances in medical treatment account for a significant proportion of the change *(24,25)*. The annual economic cost of CHD is currently estimated at greater than $80 billion, with total cardiovascular disease costs exceeding $138 billion.

Dietary changes, particularly a reduction in total and saturated fat and an increase in soluble fiber, is considered the cornerstone of therapy to reduce borderline and high-risk serum cholesterol levels whether or not drug therapy is eventually added to the regimen

Table 1
Estimated Total Deaths and Percent of Total Deaths for the 10 Leading Causes of Death
in the United States (19)

Rank	Cause of death	Number	Percent of total deaths
1[a]	Heart diseases	759,400	35.7
	Coronary heart disease	511,700	24.1
	Other heart disease	247,700	11.6
2[a]	Cancers	476,700	22.4
3[a]	Strokes	148,700	7.0
4[b]	Unintentional injuries	92,500	4.4
	Motor vehicle	46,800	2.2
	All others	45,700	2.2
5	Chronic obstructive lung diseases	78,00	3.7
6	Pneumonia and influenza	68,600	3.2
7[a]	Diabetes mellitus	37,800	1.8
8[b]	Suicide	29,600	1.4
9[b]	Chronic liver disease and cirrhosis	26,000	1.2
10[a]	Atherosclerosis	23,100	1.1
All causes		2,125,100	100.0

[a]Causes of death in which diet plays a part.
[b]Causes of death in which excessive alcohol consumption plays a part.

(15). Recent research has substantially expanded the classic cholesterol-heart disease relationship by indicating a significant protective impact and a potential therapeutic role for vitamins C, E, and β-carotene and other antioxidant phytochemicals (26) and vitamins B6, B12, and folate (27) (Figs. 1 and 2).

2.2. Cancer

Cancer is the cause of death in 22% of Americans. It has been estimated that at least a third of cancer mortality is related to dietary factors. Unlike heart disease, mortality rates for cancer continue to rise. Overall, cancer mortality is increasing at a rate of 0.5% / yr for men with no change for women; the total cancer incidence each year is increasing by 1.8% for men and 0.8% for women (28,29). The complete figures are complex, since the incidence of cancer at some sites associated with diet (e.g., breast, colon, prostate) has increased, whereas at other sites (most notably the stomach), it has decreased. However, these figures are revealing, because it is particularly changes in incidence rates that are indicative of disease prevention. Although a decline in the mortality rate may suggest some success with a preventive strategy, it may also be a consequence of improved treatment leading to increased survival times following diagnosis. The annual economic cost of cancer is currently estimated at greater than $104 billion.

Efforts to decrease the incidence of lung cancer, potentially one of the most preventable cancers, and the most common cause of cancer deaths for both men and women, has proven difficult. Although tobacco use and environmental exposures are the most important risk factors, sufficient progress has not been made in either the behavioral or the political aspects of controlling these elements to affect the subsequent

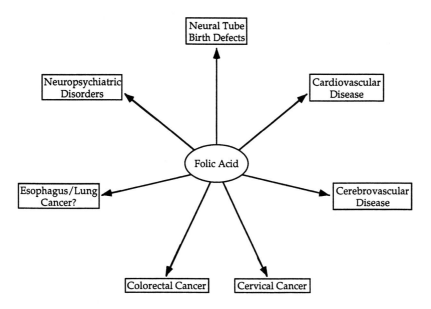

Fig. 1. The divergent capacity of folic acid for disease prevention.

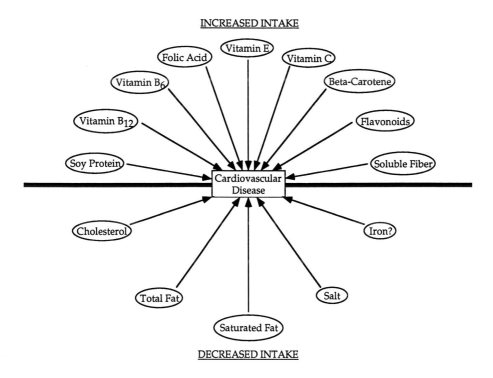

Fig. 2. The convergent capacity of nutrients to affect cardiovascular disease.

morbidity and mortality. Interestingly, screening for lung cancer, a secondary prevention step, is not recommended because it is ineffective *(30)*. An attempt to reverse the risk of lung cancer in life-long smokers with β-carotene and vitamin E supplementation proved ineffective, although this method may work in nonsmokers *(31,32)*.

Various studies indicate that a high intake of total fat increases the risk of some types of cancer, notably cancer of the breast and colon, but also of the prostate, rectum, and ovaries. Other dietary factors, including smoked, salt-cured, and nitrate-cured foods, alcohol, and naturally occurring contaminants, such as aflatoxins and N-nitroso compounds, also pose a potential cancer risk. Dietary patterns emphasizing foods high in fiber are associated with low rates of certain cancers, especially breast and colon cancer. Fruits and green and yellow vegetables, important sources of the antioxidant vitamins, putative chemopreventive phytochemicals like phenols and indoles, as well as fiber, are also associated with reduced risk of several forms of cancer. For example, high intakes of β-carotene appear to reduce the incidence of lung, breast, oral mucosa, bladder, and esophageal cancers *(33)*. Vitamin C appears to have a protective effect against esophageal, stomach, cervical, breast, and lung cancers *(34)*. Low intakes of vitamin E are strongly correlated with risk of cancer in several organs *(35)*. Evidence also suggests that calcium and selenium have protective effects against cancer *(36)*.

2.3. Stroke

Stroke is the third leading cause of death among older adults, with the rate increasing with the age of the population. However, a trend of decreasing incidence of stroke has been observed over the last few decades *(37)*. Since short-term fatality and survival rates for hospitalized stroke patients have not changed appreciably during this period, this decline in incidence suggests an effect of such preventive measures as hypertension control, although modification of this risk factor does not explain all of the observed change *(38,39)*. The prevalence of stroke approximates 2 million cases, with about 15% as short-term case fatalities, 16% requiring institutional care, and 50% of survivors permanently disabled *(38)*. The annual economic cost of stroke is currently estimated at greater than $30 billion.

Animal fat, saturated fatty acids, and total fat have been positively related to the risk of cerebral infarct, but inversely correlated with the incidence of cerebral hemorrhage in some but not all studies *(40–42)*. Recently, a poor nutritional status of folate and vitamin B6 and high plasma homocysteine concentrations have been strongly correlated with an increased risk of extracranial carotid-artery stenosis in older adults, suggesting an important role for these two vitamins in stroke prevention *(43)*. Vitamin E has been associated with a reduced risk of ischemic stroke but an increased risk of hemorrhagic stroke *(31)*.

2.4. Type II Diabetes Mellitus

Type II (noninsulin-dependent) diabetes mellitus has been diagnosed in approx 2.4% of the total population, with almost 9% of those 65 and older presenting with this condition and an estimated 4–5 million individuals believed to have undiagnosed diabetes *(44)*. The complications of this disease, particularly nephropathy, neuropathy, retinopathy, and cardiovascular disease, have a major impact on the diabetic's functional status and active life expectancy. These complications are a major reason why diabetes consumes one of every seven health care dollars, almost $100 billion annually.

Relative body weight is the only factor consistently related to the prevalence of type II diabetes, but diet, weight loss, and exercise can normalize blood sugars in most patients and appear to serve to delay the onset of the diabetic sequela. Diabetics are generally counseled to substitute carbohydrates from fruits and vegetables for fats in the diet, increase intake of soluble fiber, and avoid high protein consumption. Micronutrient intake may be a factor in primary and secondary prevention, since supplemental chromium *(45)* and vitamin E *(46)* have been noted to improve glucose tolerance, insulin action, and the nonoxidative metabolism of glucose in hyperglycemic and nondiabetic individuals.

2.5. Osteoporosis

Osteoporosis occurs most frequently in postmenopausal white women and in the elderly of both sexes. Approximately 20% of American women suffer one or more osteoporotic fractures before age 65, and as many as 40% sustain fractures later in life *(47)*. Osteoporosis is not frequently observed in men and black women until after age 60, after which fracture rates progressively increase in these groups. Importantly, those persons who sustain a hip fracture have an excess of 12–20% age-adjusted 1 yr mortality. Almost 50% of those who sustain a fracture need long-term care services. The annual cost of caring for osteoporosis patients in the United States has been estimated at $10 billion and, without intervention, these costs are projected to rise during the next 25 yr to $30–60 billion.

Substantial evidence supports a role for calcium and vitamin D as protective agents against osteoporosis *(36)*. High calcium intake during early years contributes to greater peak bone mass and during later years, together with vitamin D, prevents negative calcium balance and reduces the rate of bone loss *(48)*. Although there is a lack of concordance in epidemiologic studies associating calcium and vitamin D intake and fracture risk, because of the limitations of observational research, clinical trials with daily supplements of these nutrients clearly demonstrate a significant reduction in the rate of age-related bone loss and secondary hyperparathyroidism and the incidence of fractures, especially of the hip *(49–51)*. In addition to calcium, other minerals, including boron, copper, magnesium, manganese, and zinc, appear to contribute to the maintenance of bone density with age *(52–54)*. Although not well established, dietary risk factors for osteoporosis include excess consumption of caffeine, protein, and/or alcohol.

2.6. Other Chronic Conditions

A growing body of evidence suggests that preventive nutrition strategies may also play a significant role in other chronic conditions that are not necessarily directly associated with risk of fatality, but that do impair independence and the quality of life and affect national health care expenditures. For example, studies have demonstrated that supplementation with antioxidant vitamins, vitamin B6, and/or multivitamin/mineral formulations can enhance immune responses in older people. This action appears to be associated with reduced risk and duration of infectious disease episodes in older adults *(55–57)*. Evidence has accumulated suggesting an important relationship between the incidence of age-related cataract and nutritional status, particularly of the antioxidants *(58)*. In two prospective, randomized clinical trials conducted in China, supplementation with a multivitamin preparation or a riboflavin/niacin formula was found to significantly reduce the prevalence of nuclear cataract in older subjects relative to placebo controls *(59)*. Recently, epidemiologic studies have indicated an inverse association between generous intakes of dietary carotenoids and vitamins C and E with the incidence of age-related macular degeneration, the leading cause of irreversible blindness among older adults *(60,61)*. Several studies have suggested that mild or subclinical vitamin deficiency in free-living populations play a role in the pathogenesis of declining neurocognitive function with age. Healthy older adults with low blood levels of some vitamins, particularly folate, vitamin B12, vitamin C, and riboflavin, have been found to score poorly on tests of memory and nonverbal abstract thinking *(62)*. Significant correlations have also been reported between poor indices of thiamin, riboflavin, and iron nutriture and impaired cognitive performance and electroencephalographic indices of neuropsychological function *(63)*. As mentioned above, the inverse correlation between plasma homocysteine levels and carotid artery stenosis suggests that low B vitamin status may be related to the risk of cerebrovascular disease with its associated changes in cognitive function (Fig. 1) *(43)*.

3. ASSESSMENT OF NUTRITION-DISEASE RELATIONSHIPS

When reviewing the value of preventive nutrition interventions, it is worthwhile discussing the basis for the association between dietary factors and risk of chronic disease. A risk factor is an attribute or exposure that is associated with an increased probability of disease. A nutritional risk factor can be established as a major contributor to pathogenesis or prevention if a difference in intake between groups is significantly associated with a change in the incidence of the disease under study. The complexity that arises in identifying which nutrients or other dietary components influence disease etiology becomes clear when the issues that must be addressed are considered. In studies of chronic degenerative conditions it is difficult to identify a specific component of the diet and conclude with confidence that an inadequate or a generous intake directly influenced the incidence of the disease. Some risk factors are readily amenable to comparison or intervention, e.g., cigarette smoking, where there are populations with varying degrees of exposure and others with none, and at least some of the former can be engaged to stop the behavior. The no-exposure situation obviously does not exist with diet, and assessing the precise intake of nutrients is seriously limited by the accuracy of self-reports, the extent of the nutrient databases, and the long latent period associated with chronic diseases.

Clinical signs and symptoms of chronic disease are not generally apparent until middle age, although they are a consequence of pathogenic events occurring in early adulthood or even in adolescence. Thus, age at onset of disease is almost impossible to determine. This situation makes it difficult to ascertain whether exposure to the suspected "cause" actually preceded the disease. Chronic diseases also have several other environmental and heritable risk factors that influence their pathogenesis, so research efforts must be directed at identifying the characteristics of individuals who are susceptible; further, there are often interrelationships between the risk factors *(64)*.

Several criteria must be met to establish a causative relationship between a dietary factor and a chronic disease *(65)*. Whereas the strength of the association is usually indicated by the magnitude of the relative risk, particularly in linking cause and effect, the attributable risk (the size of the difference in risk) may often be a more important measure of the impact of the relationship on public health. The association should also be consistently observed in different studies with different populations, even though variations in the magnitude of the relative risk are to be expected, to provide confidence in the observation. The temporal relationship of the association must also be logical, with exposure of the suspected causal factor preceding the onset of the disease and usually accompanying the entire pathogenic process. Although specificity of the association is a usual criterion for determining causality, the known risk factors for chronic diseases seldom have a single effect, so lack of specificity should not rule out a contributing causal effect by a nutrient. Finally, there must be a biological plausibility in support of the association.

It is necessary to appreciate that in most cases increases in disease risk associated with a particular dietary factor are not dramatic in their magnitude, often being only twice or less that of the group with the lowest (or highest) intake. In contrast, risk of lung cancer is 32 times greater for people who smoke more than 25 cigarettes/d compared to nonsmokers (66). It is unlikely that any diet-disease relationship will approach this magnitude. Nonetheless, as noted above, a weak association between a dietary component and a disease having a major impact on the health of a population could have a significant impact on health promotion and disease prevention. One reason for the reported more modest impact of dietary factors on chronic disease is that levels of intake, particularly within a national population or culture, are simply not large enough to allow for strong associations. For example, some of the more compelling evidence about the relationship between dietary fat and disease has been derived from crosscultural, international studies where intakes cover a much broader range than found within a single country (67). Studies of micronutrient intake offer an advantage in that the use of vitamin and mineral supplements can create substantial differences in intake between users and nonusers. For example, an examination of the Health Professionals Follow-up Study revealed median intakes of vitamin E from 6–420 IU/d among quintiles and significant trends for reduced CHD risk across all quintiles, but only the suggestion of an inverse relationship between dietary vitamin E consumption and CHD (68). Additionally, micronutrient supplementation allows for relatively short-term human studies examining intermediary biomarkers or other proxy measures of chronic disease that can help provide the biologic plausibility necessary to strengthen epidemiologic observations, e.g., the dose-dependent inhibition of the oxidative modification of low-density lipoprotein cholesterol by vitamin E (69). As a consensus about the validity of specific biomarkers for chronic disease is developed, the use of these measures will substantially decrease the time and cost associated with translating new knowledge derived from clinical trials to recommendations for public health.

4. PREVENTIVE NUTRITION AND THE HEALTH SPAN

It is not unreasonable to suggest that the most efficient way to reduce health care costs is to institute prevention to avoid the premature diseases common among older adults (70–73). This change might also result in further gains in life expectancy, although such an effect is likely to be modest (74). Although simply prolonging life does not imply better health, evidence suggests that effective prevention does not trade longer life for an extended period of frailty and dependency. Thus, preventive nutritional interventions offer the potential for maintaining physiological function and preserving the independence of older people (75).

Increasing life expectancy has been a traditional measure of the success of a health care system. Indeed, life expectancy is a standard yardstick used to compare the quality of medical care in one country with that in another. However, a more relevant goal for a health care system should be assisting individuals to remain in vigorous good health for the length of their biologic life-span. Use of recently developed and validated measures of functional well-being could assist greatly in more appropriately defining health status *(76)*. Leaf *(73)* has suggested that just establishing criteria for optimal health would focus medical and public attention on what interventions are likely to promote it, and help clarify which measures are the responsibility of the individual and which depend on the medical care system. Such an effort would help balance the current preoccupation of the medical care system with "curative" (more often palliative) measures with an involvement in health promotion and disease prevention. It is worth noting that the impressive, albeit usually expensive, achievements of the technologically advanced treatments for chronic diseases, e.g., drugs, surgeries, and devices like cardiac pacemakers, are palliative and not curative. Thus, these interventions, even when efficacious, do nothing about the underlying cause of the disease and thus will have no impact on the next generation of 30-, 40-, or 50-year olds.

One of the compelling and cost-effective aspects of preventive nutrition is the convergence of nutritional recommendations for so many diseases with very similar dietary guidelines proffered by the American Heart Association, National Cancer Institute, the US Surgeon General, the Department of Agriculture, and others (Fig. 3). The convergent capacity of several nutrients to reduce disease risk similarly underscores the broad potential of benefits for preventive nutrition—this is not a "one nutrient, one disease" situation. For example, generous intakes of calcium and vitamin D have been associated with decreased risk of osteoporosis, hypertension, colon cancer, and lead poisoning. Dietary antioxidants, including vitamins C and E and β-carotene, have been associated with decreased risk of some cancers, cataract, hypertension, infectious disease, and heart disease, as well as injury from pro-oxidant environmental pollutants. Vitamins B6, B12, and folic acid are associated with reduced risk of some cancers, cognitive impairments, and heart disease, as well as neural tube birth defects (Fig. 1). A reduction in total and saturated dietary fats is inversely associated with atherosclerosis and cardiovascular disease, hypertension, gallbladder disease, obesity, and cancer. It is important to recognize the public health implications of the divergent capacity of single nutrients, e.g., the potential benefits associated with folic acid intake, when considering such interventions as fortification and supplementation (Fig. 1).

Fries *(75,77–79)* has proposed that, because our life-span is finite and the onset of chronic disease is relatively easily delayed, the period between the onset of chronic infirmity and illness to death can be greatly shortened. Implicit in this "compression of morbidity" paradigm is the need to emphasize preventive approaches to health. In contrast, some reports present an opposite "increasing misery" scenario in which life is seen as longer but health worse *(81–84)*. However, evidence is available that prevention is effective in reducing morbidity, more so than mortality *(20,84,85)*. Interestingly, it is in middle-aged and older adults rather than young people that the greatest leverage from health promotion practices can be obtained, because the targeted conditions for prevention are more likely to occur, appear sooner, and cost more to treat in this group *(86–88)*. As noted above, even small changes in these populations would yield substantial and rapid differences in health and economic endpoints. A 5-yr delay in the onset of cardio-

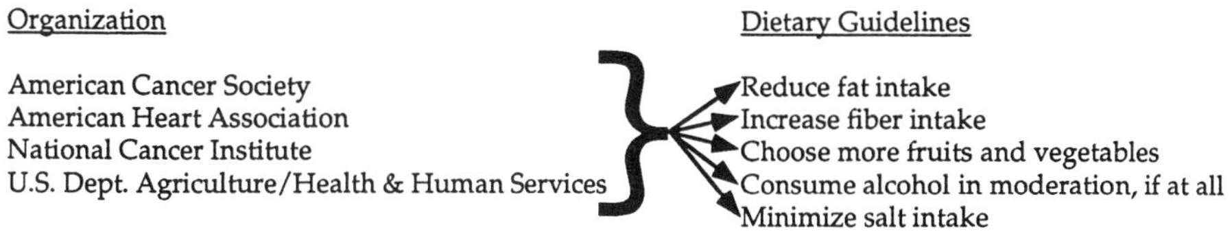

Organization   Dietary Guidelines

American Cancer Society   Reduce fat intake
American Heart Association   Increase fiber intake
National Cancer Institute   Choose more fruits and vegetables
U.S. Dept. Agriculture/Health & Human Services   Consume alcohol in moderation, if at all
                                                                  Minimize salt intake

Fig. 3. The convergence of nutritional recommendations by health organizations.

vascular disease could save about $69 billion annually. A delay in the onset of strokes by 5 yr would be associated with annual savings of $15 billion. A 5-yr delay in the occurrence of hip fracture annually could cut the number of events by 140,000 each year and save an estimated $5 billion annually. The annual cost of lens extractions is almost $5 billion, but if the rate of cataract development could be delayed 10 yr, 50% of these operations could be avoided and $2.5 billion could be saved annually.

5. THE CHALLENGE OF PREVENTIVE NUTRITION FOR THE HEALTH CARE SYSTEM

Each year the United States devotes more of its resources to health care. In 1960, health care expenditures were 5.2% of the gross national product (GNP); by 1990, health care expenditures reached 12.2% of the GNP, almost $700 billion. These costs are not divided evenly among the population: 1992 per capita health care expenditures for people 65 and older ($9125) was nearly four times that of younger people ($2350) with 38% of the year's $800 billion national health care bill directed to older adults. Total health care costs in the United States are projected to surpass $1 trillion in 1995.

It has been estimated that approx 0.25% of health care expenditures are invested in prevention *(72)*. Establishing a new balance between the "curative" and preventive approach to public health will require substantial cultural changes on the part of health care providers and the public. Health care providers will have to avoid perpetuating the concept that when illness strikes medicine will make available a pill or operation to erase the adverse health effects of a lifetime of self-abuse. Practitioners will have to learn how to counsel both patients and the public at large on preventing disease. The public will also have to accept more responsibility individually for their own health through choices they make and the lifestyles they pursue.

At least some signs suggest a growing consumer interest in nutrition and new labeling of foods and supplements have further served to heighten the public's interest in products with claims of specific health benefits. Another force acting to increase consumer interest in nutrition-related health issues is the frequent association of nutritional interventions with the perceived efficacy of alternative medical therapies. Eisenberg et al. *(89)* included the use of nutrition products in their survey of unconventional medicine in the United States and noted that respondents who used commercial diet supplements and megavitamins reported out-of-pocket expenditures averaging $228 and $203 per person per year (yielding national projections of approx $1.2 and $0.8 billion), respectively. Although this pattern does not necessarily reflect rational use of such products, it does indicate an interest and willingness of people to adopt nutritional strategies in health promotion.

It has been suggested that too many physicians are trained in the medical specialties and that an increase in the number of primary general physicians would better serve the national need to establish preventive medical practices. Unfortunately, nutrition education for physicians and other health care providers remains an orphan discipline and little improvement has occurred since the recognition of this situation more than two decades ago *(90,91)*. However, the failure to shift the public health paradigm from treatment to prevention is not solely the fault of medical education. A significant basis of the problem lies in the current reimbursement system for health care providers. Leaf *(73)* has suggested that as long as procedure-oriented physicians are reimbursed, often at several-fold the rate of general practitioners, internists, and pediatricians, the ranks of the former specialties will swell at the expense of the latter. This situation would be readily corrected if government and third-party medical insurers made the necessary changes in remuneration policies. It is worth noting that Blue Cross/Blue Shield and Medicare will pay $30,000 for coronary bypass graft operations and more than $100,000 for heart transplant surgery, but not for a $1000 cardiac rehabilitation program. Medicare specifically eschews reimbursement for preventive measures. Because there is virtually no reimbursement available for preventive medicine or nutrition, it is not surprising that beneficial and effective health promotion measures receive short shrift in medical education and practice.

Shifting the health care system from its current emphasis on treatment to prevention will take time. Even as such changes are implemented, more time will be required before its impact on chronic disease mortality will become apparent because of long latency periods, although a delay in the onset of clinical symptoms will be detected earlier. The dividends of prevention in reducing the population illness burden and enhancing of the quality of life can be substantial. Efforts must be strengthened to encourage all segments of the population to adopt preventive nutrition strategies, not just those who are high risk. Food habits develop early in life, and this is a useful time to adopt preventive nutrition behaviors, although an emphasis on older adults appears more critical at this juncture, since by 2004 the cost of health care for those over 65 is projected to constitute 50% of the total national health care bill. Together with an increase in physical activity and the cessation of tobacco use, dietary modification and improvements in nutritional status present us with the greatest potential for reducing the incidence of chronic disease, improving public health, and limiting the growth of health care expenditures.

6. REFERENCES

1. US Surgeon General. Report on nutrition and health. Washington, DC: US Department of Health and Human Services, 1988.
2. National Research Council. Diet and health: implications for reducing chronic disease risk. Washington, DC: National Academy Press, 1989.
3. Health and Welfare Canada. Nutrition recommendations: the report of the Scientific Review Committee. Ottawa: Minister of Supply and Services, 1990.
4. Goldberg I. Functional foods: designer foods, pharmafoods, nutraceuticals. New York: Chapman & Hall, 1994.
5. National Research Council. Recommended dietary allowances. Washington, DC: National Academy Press, 1989.
6. US Department of Agriculture, Department of Health and Human Services. Nutrition and your health: Dietary guidelines for Americans. 3rd ed, 1990. [Home and Garden Bulletin No. 232.]

7. US Department of Health and Human Services, National Cancer Institute, National Institutes of Health. Diet, nutrition and cancer prevention: a guide to food choices. Washington, DC: US Government Printing Office, 1984. [NIH publication no. 85-2711.]

8. Food and Nutrition Board, Institute of Medicine. How should the Recommended Dietary Allowances be revised? Washington, DC: National Academy Press, 1994.

9. National Center for Health Statistics. Healthy People 2000 Review, 1994. Hyattsville MD: Public Health Service, 1995. [DHHS Publication No. 95-125-61.]

10. US Public Health Service. Recommendation for the use of folic acid to reduce the number of cases of spina bifida and other neural tube defects. Morb Mortal Wkly Rep 1992; 41:RR–14.

11. Canadian Task Force on the Periodic Health Examination. 1994 update: 3. Primary and secondary prevention of neural tube defects. Can Med Assoc J 1994; 151:159–166.

12. Elwood M. Prevention of neural tube defects: clinical and public health policy. NZ Med J 1993; 106:517–518.

13. Hennekens CH, Buring JE. Epidemiology in Medicine. Boston: Little, Brown, 1987.

14. Kune S, Kune GA, Watson LF. Case-control study of dietary etiological factors: The Melbourne Colorectal Cancer Study. Nutr Cancer 1987; 9:21–42.

15. Expert Panel on Detection, Evaluation, and Treatment of High Blood Cholesterol in Adults. Summary of the second report of the National Cholesterol Education Program expert panel on detection, evaluation, and treatment of high blood cholesterol in adults (adult treatment panel II). JAMA 1993; 269:3015–3023.

16. Hodis HN, Mack WJ, LaBree L, Cashin-Hemphill L, Sevanian A, Johnson R, Azen SP. Serial coronary angiographic evidence that antioxidant vitamin intake reduces progress of coronary artery atherosclerosis. JAMA 1995; 273:1849–1854.

17. Nielson GJ. Technical report: analysis of costs associated with the clinical use of nutritional supplements. Columbus, OH: Abbott Laboratories, 1993.

18. Cassel CK, Brody JA. Demograph, epidemiology, and aging. In: Geriatric Medicine, 2nd ed. Cassel CK, Riesenberg DE, Sorensen LB, Walsh JA, eds. New York: Springer Verlag, 1990; 16–27.

19. National Center for Health Statistics. Monthly Vital Statistics Report 1988; 37:April 25.

20. Fries JF, Green LW, Levine S. Health promotion and the compression of morbidity. Lancet 1989; 4:481–483.

21. Havlick RJ, Feinleib M, eds. Proceedings of the conference on the decline in coronary heart disease mortality. Bethesda, MD: Public Health Service. [DHEW Publication No. (NIH). 1979:79–161].

22. Rose G. Strategy of prevention: lessons from cardiovascular disease. Br Med J 1981; 282:1847–1851.

23. Beaglehole R. Medical management and the decline in mortality from coronary heart disease. Br Med J 1986; 292:33–35.

24. Gomez-Marin O, Folsom AR, Kottke TE, Wu SC, Jacobs DR Jr, Gillum RF, Edlavitch SA, Blackburn H. Improvement in long-term survival among patients hospitalized with acute myocardial infarction: 1970 to 1980. New Engl J Med 1987; 316:1353–1359.

25. Goldberg RJ, Gore JM, Alpert JS, Dalen JE. Recent changes in attack and survival among patients hospitalized with acute myocardial infarction (1975 through 1981). JAMA 1986; 255:2774–2779.

26. Keaney JF, Frei B. Antioxidant protection of low-density lipoprotein and its role in the prevention of atherosclerotic vascular disease. In: Natural Antioxidants in Human Health and Disease. Frei B, ed. San Diego: Academic Press, 1994; 303–352.

27. Ueland PM, Refsum H, Brattström L. Plasma homocysteine and cardiovascular disease. In: Atherosclerotic Cardiovascular Disease, Hemostasis, and Endothelial Function. Francis RB Jr, ed. New York: Marcel Dekker, 1992; 183–236.

28. Rose G. Sick individuals and sick populations. Int J Epidemiol 1985; 14:32–38.

29. Ballar JC, Smith EM. Progress against cancer. New Engl J Med 1986; 314:1226–1232.

30. Eddy DM. Screening for lung cancer. Ann Intern Med 1989; 111:232–237.

31. The Alpha-Tocopherol, Beta-Carotene Cancer Prevention Study Group. The effect of vitamin E and beta-carotene on the incidence of lung cancer and other cancers in male smokers. New Engl J Med 1994; 330:1029–1035.

32. Mayne ST, Janerich DT, Greenwald P, Chorost S, Tucci C, Zaman MB. Dietary beta carotene and lung cancer risk in U.S. nonsmokers. J Natl Cancer Inst 1994; 86:33–38.

33. Ziegler R. A review of epidemiologic evidence that carotenoids reduce the risk of cancer. J Nutr 1989; 119:116–122.

34. Block G. Vitamin C and cancer prevention: the epidemiologic evidence. Am J Clin Nutr 1991; 54:270S–282S.

35. Knekt P. Epidemiology of vitamin E: evidence for anticancer effects in humans. In: Vitamin E in Health and Disease. Packer L, Fuchs J, eds. New York: Marcel Dekker, 1993; 513–527.
36. Optimal calcium intake. NIH Consensus Statement 1994. Jun 6–8; 12(4):1–31.
37. Klag MJ, Whelton PK, Whelton AA. Decline in U.S. stroke mortality: demographic trends and antihypertensive treatment. Stroke 1989; 20:14–21.
38. Kannel WB, Wolf PA. Epidemiology of cerebrovascular disease. In: Vascular Disease of the Central Nervous System. Russell RWR, ed. Edinburgh: Churchill Livingstone, 1983:1–24.
39. Bonita R, Beaglehole R. Does treatment of hypertension explain the decline in mortality from stroke? Br Med J 1986; 292:191, 192.
40. Reed D, Yano K, Kagan A. Lipid and lipoproteins as predictors of coronary heart disease, stroke, and cancer in the Honolulu Heart Program. Am J Med 1986; 80:871–878.
41. Tanaka H, Hayashi M, Date C, Imai K, Asada M, Shoji H, Okazake K, Yamamoto H, Yoshikawa K, Shimada T, Lee SI. Epidemiologic studies of stroke in Shibata, a Japanese provincial city: preliminary report on risk factors for cerebral infarction. Stroke 1985; 16:773–780.
42. Snowden DA. Animal product consumption and mortality because of all causes combined, coronary heart disease, stroke, diabetes, and cancer in Seventh-Day Adventists. Am J Clin Nutr 1988; 48:739–748.
43. Selhub J, Jacques PF, Bostom AG, D'Agostino RB, Wilson PWF, Belanger AJ, O'Leary AH, Wolf PA, Schaefer EJ, Rosenberg IH. Association between plasma homocysteine concentrations and extracranial carotid-artery stenosis. New Engl J Med 1995; 332:286–291.
44. US Department of Health and Human Services, National Diabetes Data Group. National Institute of Health. Public Health Service Diabetes in America: Diabetes data compiled 1984. National Institute of Arthritis, Diabetes and Digestive and Kidney Diseases, 1985. [NIH Publ. No 85-1468].
45. Anderson RA. Chromium metabolism and its role in disease processes in man. Chem Physiol Biochem 1986; 4:31–41.
46. Paolisso G, Di Maro G, Galzerano D, Cacciapuotti F, Varricchio G, Varrichio M, D'onofrio F. Pharmacological doses of vitamin E and insulin action in elderly subjects. Am J Clin Nutr 1994; 59:1291–1296.
47. Cummings SR, Kelsey JL, Nevitt MC, O'Dowd KJ. Epidemiology of osteoporosis and osteoporotic fractures. Epidemiol Rev 1985; 7:178–208.
48. Dawson-Hughes B, Krall EA, Harris S. Risk factors for bone loss in healthy postmenopausal women. Osteoporosis Intl 1993; 3:S27–S31.
49. Chapuy MC, Arlot ME, Duboeuf F, Brun J, Crouzet B, Arnaud S, Delmas PD, Meunier, PJ. Vitamin D$_3$ and calcium to prevent hip fractures in elderly women. New Engl J Med 1992; 327:1637–1642.
50. Heikinheimo RJ, Inkovaara JA, Harju EJ, Haavisto MV, Kaarela RH, Kataja JM, Hokko AM, Kolho LA, Rajala SA. Annual injection of vitamin D and fractures of aged bones. Calcif Tissue Int 1992; 51:105–110.
51. Aloia JF, Vaswani A, Yeh JK, Ross PL, Flaster E, Dilmanian FA. Calcium supplementation with and without hormone replacement therapy to prevent postmenopausal bone loss. Ann Int Med 1994; 120:97–103.
52. Saltman PD, Strause LG. The role of trace minerals in osteoporosis. J Am Coll Nutr, 1993; 12:384–389.
53. Strause L, Saltman P, Smith KT, Bracker M, Andon MB. Spinal bone loss in postmenopausal women supplemented with calcium and trace minerals. J Nutr 1994; 124:1060–1064.
54. Nielsen FH. Studies on the relationship between boron and magnesium which possibly affects the formation and maintenance of bones. Magnesium Trace Elements, 1990; 9:61–69.
55. Blumberg JB. Vitamins. In: Diet, Nutrition, and Immunity. Forse RA, ed. Boca Raton, FL: CRC, 1994; 237–246.
56. Chandra RK. Effect of vitamin and trace-element supplementation on immune responses and infection in elderly subjects. Lancet 1992; 340:1124–1127.
57. Bogden JD, Bendich A, Kemp FW, Bruening KS, Skurnick JH, Denny T, Baker H, Louria DB. Daily micronutrient supplements enhance delayed hypersensitivity skin test responses in older people. Am J Clin Nutr 1994; 60:437–447.
58. Jacques PF, Chylack LT Jr, Taylor A. Relationships between natural antioxidants and cataract formation. In: Natural Antioxidants in Human Health and Disease. Frei B, ed. San Diego: Academic, 1994; 515–533.
59. Sperduto RD, Hu T-S, Milton RC, Zhao JL, Everett DF, Cheng Q-F, Blot WJ, Bing L, Taylor PR, Jun-Yao L, Guo W-D. The Linxian Cataract Studies: two nutrition intervention trials. Arch Ophthalmol 1993; 111:1246–1253.
60. West S, Vitale S, Hallfrisch J, Muñoz B, Muller D, Bressler S, Bressler NM. Are antioxidants or supplements protective for age-related macular degeneration? Arch Ophthalmol 1994; 112:222–227.
61. Seddon JM, Ajani UA, Sperduto RD, Hiller R, Blair HN, Burton TC, Farber MD, Gragoudas ES, Haller J, Miller DT, Yannuzzi LA, Willett W. Dietary carotenoids, vitamins A, C, and E, and advanced age-related macular degeneration. JAMA 1994; 272:1413–1420.

62. Goodwin JS, Goodwin JM, Garry, PJ. Association between nutritional status and cognitive functioning in a healthy elderly population. JAMA 1983; 249:2917–2921.
63. Tucker DM, Penland JG, Sandstead HH, Milne DB, Heck DG, Klevay LM. Nutrition status and brain function in aging. Am J Clin Nutr 1990; 52:93–102.
64. Rose G. Sick individuals and sick populations. Int J Epidemiol 1985; 14:32–38.
65. Stehbens WE. The concept of cause in disease. J Chron Dis 1985; 38:947–950.
66. Doll R, Hill AB. Mortality in relation to smoking: ten years' observations of British doctors. Br Med J 1964; 1:1399–1410.
67. Rose G. Incubation period of coronary heart disease. Br Med J 1982; 284:1600–1601.
68. Rimm EB, Stampfer MJ, Ascherio A, Giovannucci E, Colditz GA, Willett WC. Vitamin E consumption and the risk of coronary heart disease in men. New Engl J Med 1993; 328:1450–1456.
69. Jialal I, Fuller CJ, Huet BA. The effect of α-tocopherol supplementation on LDL oxidation. Arteriosclerosis Thromb Vasc Biol 1995; 15:190–198.
70. Gori G, Richter BS. Macroeconomics of disease prevention in the United States. Science 1978; 200:1124–1129.
71. Schneider EL, Guralnik JM. The aging of America: impact on health care costs. JAMA 1990; 263:2335–2340.
72. Fries JF. Aging, illness, and health policy: implication of the compression of morbidity. Perspect Biol Med 1988; 31:407–428.
73. Leaf A. Preventive medicine for our ailing health care system. JAMA 1993; 269:616–618.
74. Olshansky SJ, Carnes BA, Cassel C. In search of Methuselah: estimating the upper limits to human longevity. Science 1990; 250:634–639.
75. Fries JF. Reduction of the national morbidity. Gerontol Perspect 1987; 1:54–65.
76. Tarlov AR, Ware JE, Greenfield D, Nelson EC, Perin E, Zubkoff N. The Medical Outcomes Study: an application of methods for monitoring the results of medical care. JAMA 1989; 262:925–930.
77. Fries JF. Aging, natural death, and the compression of morbidity. New Engl J Med 1980; 303:130–136.
78. Fries JF, Crapo LM. Vitality and Aging. New York: Freeman, 1981.
79. Fries JF. The compression of morbidity: miscellaneous comments about a heme. Gerontologist 1984; 24:354–359.
80. Tornstam L. The quo vadis of gerontology: on the scientific paradigm of gerontology. Gerontologist 1992; 32:318–326.
81. Olshandsky SJ, Rudberg MA, Carnes BA, Cassell CK, Brody JA. Trading off longer life for worsening health: the expansion of morbidity hypothesis. J Aging Health 1991; 3:194–216.
82. Guralnick JM, LaCroix AZ, Branch LG, Kasi SV, Wallace RB. Morbidity and disability in older persons in the years prior to death. Am J Public Health 1991; 81:443–447.
83. Rudberg MA, Cassel CK. Are death and disability in old age preventable? Fact Res Gerontol 1993; 7:191–201.
84. Multiple Risk Factor Intervention Trial Research Group. Coronary heart disease death, non-fatal acute myocardial infarction and other clinical outcomes in the multiple risk factor intervention trial. Am J Cardiol 1986; 58:1–13.
85. Tsevat J, Weinstein MC, Williams LW, Tosteson AN, Goldman L. Expected gains in life expectancy from various coronary heart disease risk modifications. Circulation 1991; 83:1194–1201.
86. Fries JF, Tilton-Fries S, Parcell CL, Harrington H. Health risk changes with a low-cost individualized health promotion program: effects at up to 30 months. Am J Health Promotion 1992; 6:364–371.
87. Leigh JP, Richardson N, Beck R, Kerr C, Harrington H, Parcell CL, Fries JF. Randomized controlled study of a retiree health promotion program: the Bank of America study. Arch Intern Med 1992; 152:1201–1206.
88. Pelletier KR. A review and analysis of the health and cost-effective outcome studies of comprehensive health promotion and disease prevention program. Am J Health Promotion 1991; 5:311–313.
89. Eisenberg DM, Kessler RC, Foster C, Norlack FE, Calkins DR, Delbanco TL. Unconventional medicine in the United States: prevalence, costs, and patterns of use. New Engl J Med 1993; 328:246–252.
90. National Academy of Sciences. Nutrition education in U.S. medical schools. Washington DC: National Academy Press, 1985.
91. Feldman EB. Networks for medical nutrition education—a review of the U.S. experience and future prospects. Am J Clin Nutr 1995; 62:512–517.

2   Diet and Childhood Cancer

Preliminary Evidence

Greta R. Bunin and Joan M. Cary

1. BACKGROUND

Cancer is the most common fatal disease of childhood in the United States. Between ages 1 and 15, only accidents kill more children. Approximately 14/100,000 children develop cancer each year, or about 7500 children in the United States *(1,2)*. This incidence rate indicates that about 1 in 500 children develop cancer before the age of 15. The common cancers of childhood are not those of later life; leukemia accounts for about one-third of childhood cancers and brain tumors about one-fifth. The other major cancers, in order of frequency, are lymphoma, neuroblastoma, Wilms' tumor, soft tissue sarcoma, osteogenic sarcoma, and retinoblastoma *(2)*. Since the early 1970s, the incidence of childhood cancer appears to be increasing slowly *(1)*, but whether the observed increase reflects better diagnosis or real change is not known. The same time period has also seen a dramatic improvement in the survival of children with cancer, with approx 70% of these children now alive 5 yr after diagnosis *(2)*. However, some are left with long-term medical and cognitive problems.

Little is known about the etiology of cancers in children. The medical literature contained few epidemiologic studies of childhood cancer before the 1970s, but the extent of interest and investigation has increased dramatically since then. Many risk factors have been investigated, including genetic abnormalities and parental occupational exposures, in addition to aspects of diet that are the focus of this chapter.

The relationship between diet and childhood cancer has not been widely studied. In fact, nearly all the data discussed here come from ten studies *(see* Table 1) *(3–13)*. The possibility that a child's diet or the mother's diet during pregnancy can raise or diminish the risk of these rare cancers at first seems unlikely. The adult cancers most strongly linked with diet, such as stomach and colon, are believed to have latency periods of several decades. In contrast, cancers in children by definition have latencies of no more than 15 yr and often less < 5 yr. Furthermore, cancers of the digestive tract and of other sites linked to diet in adults rarely occur in children. Therefore, researchers first focused their search for causes on genetic predisposition and exposure to environmental toxins rather than diet.

The cancers of childhood, mainly leukemia, brain tumor, lymphoma, and sarcoma, occur relatively rarely in adulthood and the etiologic hypotheses about these cancers have generally not been dietary. Therefore, the literature on adult cancers adds only a limited amount to the discussion, but is considered where relevant.

From: *Preventive Nutrition: The Comprehensive Guide for Health Professionals*
Edited by A. Bendich and R. J. Deckelbaum Humana Press Inc., Totowa, NJ

17

Table 1
Studies of Childhood Cancer and Diet[a]

Authors and reference	Sample size	Age	Cancer type	Paternal cured meat consumption
Preston-Martin et al., 1982 (3)	209 Cases 209 Controls	0–14	Tumors of brain or cranial meninges	
Howe et al., 1989 (4)	74 Cases 138 Controls	0–19	Tumors of brain and cranial meninges	
Kuijten et al., 1990 (5)	163 Cases 163 Controls	0–14	Astrocytic glioma	
Bunin et al., 1993 (6)	166 Cases 166 Controls	0–6	Medulloblastoma/primitive neuroectodermal tumor of brain	
Bunin et al., 1994 (7)	155 Cases 155 Controls	0–6	Astrocytic glioma	
McCredie et al., 1994 (8,9)	82 Cases 164 Controls	0–14	Tumor of brain or cranial nerves	
Sarasua and Savitz, 1994 (10)[d]	45 Cases 206 Controls	0–14	Brain tumors	
Cordier et al., 1994 (11)	75 Cases 113 Controls	0–15	Brain tumors	
Peters et al., 1994 (12)	232 Cases 232 Controls	0–10	Leukemia	Hot dogs, OR = 5.1[c] Other individual cured meats, OR = 1.0 ORs = 1.0–1.7[c]
Sarasua and Savitz, 1994 (10)[d]	56 Cases 205 Controls	0–14	Acute lymphocytic leukemia	
Shu et al., 1988 (13)	309 Cases 618 Controls	0–14	Total leukemia, acute lymphocytic leukemia, acute nonlymphocytic leukemia	

18

Authors and reference	Maternal cured meat consumption	Maternal fruit and vegetable consumption	Maternal vitamin supplement use
Preston-Martin et al., 1982 (3)	All cured meats, OR[b] = 2.3[c] Individual cured meats, ORs = 1.1–1.9[b] Hot dogs, OR = 1.7	Nitrate-rich vegetables, no association	Vitamin supplement, OR = 0.6
Howe et al., 1989 (4) Kuijten et al., 1990 (5) Bunin et al., 1993 (6)	All cured meats, OR = 2.0[c] All cured meats, OR 1.1 Bacon, OR = 1.7[c] Hot dogs, OR = 1.0	Vegetables, OR = 0.4[c] Fruit, OR = 0.3[c] Green salad, spinach, sweet potatoes, citrus fruit, peaches, ORs = 0.3–0.5[c]	Multivitamin, no association Multivitamin in first six weeks of pregnancy, OR = 0.6[c] Vitamin C, OR = 0.3[c]
Bunin et al., 1994 (7)	All cured meats, OR = 1.7 (p = 0.10) Hot dogs, OR = 1.9[b]	Vegetables, OR = 0.6 Fruit, OR = 0.7	Multivitamin, OR = 0.6[c]
McCredie et al., 1994 (8,9)	All cured meats, OR = 2.5[c]	Vegetables, OR = 0.4 (p = 0.06) Fruit, OR = 1.5	
Sarasua and Savitz, 1994 (10)[d]	Hot dogs, OR = 2.3[c] Other individual cured meats, ORs = 0.4 and 1.0		Vitamin supplement, OR = 0.7[e]
Cordier et al., 1994 (11)	Individual cured meats, ORs = 0.5–0.8	Carrots, leeks, green peppers, ORs = 0.3–0.4[c]	
Peters et al., 1994 (12)	Hot dogs, OR = 2.4 Other individual cured meats, ORs = 1.0–1.3	Oranges, OR = 0.4 Grapefruit, OR = 0.6 Oranges or orange juice, OR = 0.8 Grapefruit or grapefruit juice, OR = 1.1 Apple juice, OR = 0.9	
Sarasua and Savitz, 1994 (10)[d]	Hot dogs, OR = 0.9 Other individual cured meats, ORs = 1.0 and 1.5		Vitamin supplement, OR = 0.5[e] (p = 0.09)
Shu et al., 1988 (13)			

(Continued)

19

Table 1 (*Continued*)

Authors and reference	Child's cured meat consumption	Infant's/child's fruit consumption	Infant's/child's vitamin supplement use
Preston-Martin et al., 1982 (3)	All cured meats, OR = 2.3[c]		
Howe et al., 1989 (4)	All cured meats, OR = 1.1	Fruit juice, OR = 0.2[c]	Vitamin supplement, no association; Vitamin C, OR = 0.9
Kuijten et al., 1990 (5)			
Bunin et al., 1993 (6)		No fruit as infant, OR = 4.3[c]; Orange juice, apple juice, other fruit juice as infant, no association	Multivitamin as infant, OR = 0.7
Bunin et al., 1994 (7)		Fruit, individual fruit juices as infant, no association	Multivitamin as infant, no association
McCredie et al., 1994 (8,9)		Fruit as infant, OR = 0.4; Orange juice as infant, OR = 1.8	Vitamin supplement as infant, OR = 0.9; Vitamin syrup as infant, OR = 0.5; Apple juice as infant, OR = 0.3; Vitamin supplement, OR = 0.4[c]
Sarasua and Savitz, 1994 (10)[d]	Hot dogs, OR = 2.1; Other individual cured meats, ORs = 0.6 and 1.4; Individual cured meats in absence of vitamin supplements, ORs = 3.2–6.8[c]; All cured meats, OR = 0.7		
Cordier et al., 1994 (11)		Fresh fruit, OR = 0.6; Orange juice, OR = 0.5; Oranges or orange juice, OR = 1.1; Grapefruit or grapefruit juice, OR = 1.0; Apple juice, OR = 1.6	Vitamin supplement, OR = 0.2[c]
Peters et al., 1994 (12)	Hot dogs, OR = 5.8[c]; Other individual cured meats, ORs = 1.6–2.7[c]		
Sarasua and Savitz, 1994 (10)[d]	Hot dogs, OR = 1.3; Other individual cured meats, ORs = 1.1 and 1.2; Individual cured meats in absence of vitamin supplements, ORs = 2.9[c]		Vitamin supplement, OR = 0.6
Shu et al., 1988 (13)			Cod-liver oil, OR = 0.3

[a]For all foods, odds ratio presented is that for highest level of consumption.
[b]OR: odds ratio.
[c]Statistically significant.
[d]Listed as two studies because separate analyses presented for brain tumors and acute lymphocytic leukemia.

Diet might act to alter cancer risk in children by mechanisms similar to and different from those proposed for adult cancers. Antioxidants, such as vitamin C and β-carotene, may protect against various cancers by their ability to neutralize free radicals and thus prevent oxidative damage to DNA *(14)*. Folic acid deficiency may encourage malignant transformation of normal cells by altering gene expression and weakening chromosomal structure *(15)*. Exposure to *N*-nitroso compounds (NOC) may initiate cancer through direct acting or metabolically activated carcinogens in this class of substances. Antioxidants and folic acid may act in fetuses and children through the same mechanisms as they are hypothesized to act in adults. Carcinogens may also act through the same mechanisms at all ages, but fetuses may be more susceptible to carcinogens, as suggested by animal studies of some NOCs. Some substances might actually have the opposite effect in fetuses as in adults, as proposed for topoisomerase II inhibitors (*see* Leukemia). Mechanisms unique to the embryo or fetus may also exist. An excess or deficiency of a dietary component could result in malformation of an organ or more subtle cellular changes that increases the organ's susceptibility to cancer. This type of altered development has been proposed as a mechanism leading to cancer in young women after prenatal DES exposure *(16–18)*.

2. N-NITROSO COMPOUNDS

Most of the data on childhood cancer and diet come from studies of exposure to NOCs and risk of brain tumors. The overall category of NOCs can be broken down into subgroups that include nitrosamines, nitrosamides, and nitrosoureas. NOCs occur in our environment, as do substances that can combine to form these compounds. Nitrite, nitrogen oxides, and other nitrosating agents can react with nitrogen-containing compounds, such as amines, amides, and ureas, to form NOCs. Particularly relevant to the discussion of the relationship between diet and cancer are preformed NOCs, nitrite, and nitrate, which can be reduced to nitrite in saliva.

Many NOCs are potent mutagens and animal carcinogens. NOCs have been found to be carcinogenic in a variety of tissues and organs in 40 animal species. Some NOCs when administered to pregnant animals induce tumors in the offspring. Of particular relevance to childhood cancer is the fact that some nitrosoureas are potent nervous system carcinogens when given transplacentally *(19)*.

Not only are NOCs potent carcinogens, but exposure to these compounds is widespread. Humans are exposed to NOCs directly and to precursor compounds that can combine to form NOCs in the body. NOCs have been detected in many common products, including cigarette smoke, rubber, cured meats, cosmetics, alcoholic beverages, medications, pesticides, and automobile interiors, and in water, air, and some industrial settings *(19–21)*. Almost all the data on the sources of NOCs are on the occurrence of nitrosamines. Less is known about the distribution of other NOCs, including the nitrosoureas that are transplacental nervous system carcinogens in animals.

Although NOCs occur in the environment, most human exposure is thought to occur via endogenous synthesis. There is evidence that NOCs can be synthesized in the stomach and elsewhere in the body *(19)*. Cured meats, baked goods, and cereal contribute most of the nitrite (a NOC precursor) in the diet *(20,22)*. For nitrates, which can be converted to nitrites, vegetables are the main dietary source *(20,22)*.

The endogenous formation of NOCs induces tumors in animals. When animals are fed *N*-nitroso precursors, for example, nitrite and an amine, the expected compound, in this case a nitrosamine, is produced in the stomach and tumors result as they do from feeding the preformed nitrosamine *(19)*. There are substances that inhibit the formation of NOCs from precursors in vivo, including vitamin C, vitamin E, selenium, and glutathione *(19)*. In animals, these substances inhibit the formation of NOCs from precursors and reduce the proportion of animals that develop tumors *(23)*. In some studies, very large doses of vitamin C prevented 100% of tumors *(23)*. In addition to inhibitors, accelerators of the nitrosation reaction are also known and include metal ions, thiocyanate, and certain carbonyl compounds *(19)*.

Based on the animal data, particularly those concerning transplacental carcinogenesis, Preston-Martin et al. hypothesized that exposure to NOCs during gestation increases the risk of brain tumors in children *(3)*. Children whose mothers frequently ate foods containing NOCs or nitrite were hypothesized to be at increased risk. The effect of nitrate-rich foods was more difficult to predict; vegetables contribute the majority of nitrates in the diet but also contain vitamin C, an inhibitor of nitrosation. High intakes of vitamins C and E were hypothesized to decrease the risk because of their action as inhibitors of nitrosation reactions.

3. BRAIN TUMORS

Brain tumors are the second most common type of cancer among children in the United States, accounting for about 20% of these cancers. The annual incidence is approx 3/million children under the age of 15 and has increased substantially since the early 1970s *(1)*. Whether the trend reflects a genuine increase or improved diagnosis is not known. Some brain tumors occurring in children can be cured surgically, but others require a combination of surgery, radiation, and chemotherapy. With the use of multimodality therapy, survival from childhood brain tumors has improved to almost 50% *(2)*, but survivors are often left with neurologic, cognitive, or endocrinologic problems.

Many different histologic types of brain tumor occur in childhood. The major categories are astrocytic glioma and medulloblastoma (sometimes referred to as primitive neuroectodermal tumor), which account for approx 50 and 20% of childhood brain tumors, respectively *(24)*. Other types of glioma, ependymoma and oligodendroglioma, comprise another 10% of the total *(24)*. The remaining brain tumors are soft tissue sarcomas, germ cell tumors, and tumors of unspecified type *(24)*.

The patterns of incidence with age and gender differ among the histologic types *(25)*. For example, astrocytic glioma affects boys and girls with equal frequency, but boys have a higher risk of medulloblastoma. The incidence of astrocytic glioma peaks between 4 and 8 yr of age compared to a peak before age 3 for medulloblastoma. These differences in demographic pattern suggest that the two major categories of childhood brain tumors might differ etiologically. On the other hand, the fact that all tumor types arise in the brain and, thus, share that environment, might imply a common etiology. Perhaps, some etiologic factors are common among different histologic types of brain tumors and others are specific to particular types.

In most epidemiologic investigations, childhood brain tumors have been studied together as a single entity. If risk factors differed by type of brain tumor, one would expect the studies of all types combined to mostly reflect risk factors for astrocytic glioma, the most common type. For this reason, studies of all types and astrocytic glioma are discussed together and the single study of medulloblastoma is considered separately.

3.1. Maternal Diet

Epidemiologists have conducted seven case-control studies of childhood brain tumors that considered a possible role of pregnancy diet (Table 1) *(3,5–11)*. Four of the studies considered all brain tumors combined *(3,8–11)*, two considered astrocytic gliomas *(5,7)*, and one medulloblastoma *(6)*. In the earlier studies, the mothers answered questions about their frequency of consumption of a small number of foods relevant to the *N*-nitroso hypothesis. In later studies, investigators aimed to calculate total intake of food components related to the same hypothesis, which required collecting data on many more foods, usually between 50 and 60. None of the studies have investigated overall diet, which is usually assessed by data on 100 or more foods, and thus, no data are available on macronutrients, such as fat and protein, and most micronutrients, such as B vitamins and zinc.

Six of the seven studies investigated maternal diet during pregnancy in relation to all brain tumors or astrocytic gliomas with fairly consistent results for nitrite-cured meat consumption. In the three largest studies and one small study, frequent consumption of cured meats was associated with about a doubling of risk *(3,5,7,9)*. The two studies in which an association with cured meats as a group was not seen had small numbers of cases and therefore lower statistical power *(10,11)*. Although one of these studies found no effect of cured meats as a group, it did observe an association with hot dogs *(10)*. The remaining study was completely negative *(11)*. In all three studies that appeared to collect information on hot dogs as an individual item, odds ratios of about 2 were observed *(3,7,10)*. The study of medulloblastoma did not observe an association with cured meats as a group, although the odds ratio for bacon consumption was significantly elevated *(6)*. In summary, frequent maternal consumption of nitrite-cured meats in general, and hot dogs in particular, has been fairly consistently associated with elevated risk of all brain tumors and astrocytic glioma. The results for medulloblastoma appear different, although not totally inconsistent with those for the other groups of brain tumors.

The evidence on the effect of fruit and vegetable consumption during pregnancy is quite limited (*see* Table 1). Statistically significant effects of maternal fruit consumption were not observed in the three studies of all brain tumors or astrocytic glioma *(7,9,11)*. The only suggestion of a protective effect of fruit comes from nonsignificant findings in two of the studies. In one, investigators observed decreased risk with frequent consumption of fruit *(7)*, although no individual fruit, including citrus, had a significant effect. In the other study *(11)*, oranges and orange juice were associated with a decrease in risk that was not statistically significant. In contrast to the findings for all brain tumors and astrocytic glioma, fruit overall, citrus fruit, and peaches were associated with lower risk of medulloblastoma *(6)*. The limited data on fruit eaten during pregnancy suggest a stronger association with medulloblastoma than with astrocytic glioma.

The evidence linking vegetables with lower risk of brain tumors is stronger than that for fruit. McCredie et al. observed a trend of decreasing risk with increasing consumption of vegetables *(9)*. In another study *(11)*, frequent consumption of carrots, leeks, and green peppers was associated with decreased risk; results were not presented for all vegetables combined. The study of astrocytic glioma observed a risk that was lower but not significantly so for vegetable consumption *(7)*. For medulloblastoma, a strong, significant effect for vegetables was observed with individually significant effects of green salad, spinach, and sweet potatoes (6). The evidence, although limited, suggests a possible protective effect of vegetable consumption for all types of childhood brain tumors.

Vitamin supplements are also sources of vitamin C and other nitrosation inhibitors. Several studies (3,7,10) observed decreased risk with multivitamin use during pregnancy, although the results have been nonsignificant generally. In the study of medulloblastoma, use of multivitamins at any time during pregnancy did not affect risk, but use in the first 6 wk of pregnancy appeared to lower the risk significantly (6).

In three studies, the investigators calculated the mother's intake of selected vitamins and other food components from the information on the foods she ate and the frequency with which she ate them (6,7,11). Intake from supplements was not included. The food components selected were generally those relevant to the N-nitroso hypothesis, because this hypothesis motivated the choice of food items. Only in the study of medulloblastoma were any of the food components studied significantly related to risk. In that study, intakes of vitamin C and nitrate were associated with lower risk (6). The association with nitrate reflects that with vegetable consumption because vegetables are the major source of nitrate. Bunin et al. (7) and Cordier et al. (11) observed nonsignificant decreases in risk with higher vitamin C intake for astrocytic glioma and all brain tumors, respectively. The N-nitroso precursors, nitrite or nitrate, and dimethylnitrosamine were not associated with increased risk (6,7).

Although the studies of maternal diet focused on the N-nitroso hypothesis, a few unrelated foods were included. Caffeinated beverages did not appear to affect risk of either astrocytic glioma or medulloblastoma (6,7). No effect of charcoal-broiled foods on risk of brain tumors overall was noted (10). In the study of medulloblastoma, intake of folic acid appeared to decrease the risk (6), but the original hypotheses were unrelated to folate and therefore the assessment of folic acid intake was incomplete. As cited above, risk of medulloblastoma also appeared to decrease with maternal use of multivitamins early in pregnancy. Intriguingly, the findings for folate and multivitamins are similar to those for neural tube defects and other congenital anomalies (26–31).

The studies discussed above were motivated mainly by the N-nitroso hypothesis. The N-nitroso hypothesis predicts that cured meat is associated with higher risk and fruit, especially those types rich in vitamin C, with lower risk. Vegetables, which contain nitrates and vitamin C, might either raise or lower the risk. Vitamin supplements, most of which contain vitamin C and other inhibitors of NOC formation, would also be expected to lower the risk. The finding of an association with maternal cured meat consumption in most studies of all brain tumors or astrocytic glioma supports the hypothesis. The evidence linking fruit consumption to lower risk of the same groups of brain tumors is weak, because there were no statistically significant findings. The evidence for vegetables is stronger, with significant associations observed for all vegetables combined or some individual vegetables in two of the three relevant studies. For vitamin supplements, no significant protective effects were observed. In summary, current evidence on maternal diet and risk of childhood brain tumors as a group or of astrocytic glioma supports the N-nitroso hypothesis to some extent, but important inconsistencies exist.

The findings from the single study of medulloblastoma differed from those for all tumors or astrocytic glioma. Strong, protective associations were observed between fruit and vegetable consumption and risk of medulloblastoma. However, cured meats as a group did not appear to affect risk. For the other groups of tumors, the strongest support for the N-nitroso hypothesis was from the findings for cured meat. For medulloblastoma, the observations regarding cured meat do not support the hypothesis, but those regarding fruit and vegetables do. Like those for the other groups of tumors, the results of the medulloblastoma study are somewhat consistent with the N-nitroso hypothesis.

In some instances, inconsistencies with the hypothesis can be explained by limitations of the data. For example, calculated intake of dimethylnitrosamine has not been associated with higher risk. This nitrosamine was used as a marker for all N-nitroso compounds because data on the concentration of other compounds in foods are extremely limited. However, in animal studies, nitrosoureas rather than nitrosamines induce brain tumors. Another example concerns the fact that vitamin supplements are predicted to decrease risk but have not been observed to do so in a statistically significant way. In the populations studied, however, nearly all women took supplements, making it unlikely that a real effect could be observed. Furthermore, the animal data predict that the timing of intake of supplements and foods rich in an inhibitor of nitrosation, such as vitamin C, may play a role. Eating such foods or taking supplements with cured meat would inhibit the formation of N-nitroso compounds and therefore lower the risk. If the cured meat was eaten at one time and the inhibiting supplement or food later, the risk would not be as low.

Although limitations of the data collected may explain the inconsistencies with the N-nitroso hypothesis, other possibilities must also be considered. For example, the association of maternal cured meat consumption with increased risk of childhood brain tumors is compatible with causal exposures other than N-nitroso compounds. Perhaps a dietary characteristic correlated with frequent cured meat consumption is the causal exposure. For example, high fat or low β-carotene intake may explain the observed association with cured meat consumption. Inconsistencies between the data and the hypothesis might also have occurred by chance as a result of the few studies, most of which had relatively small sample sizes. Similarly, the apparent differences in dietary findings between astrocytic glioma and medulloblastoma might reflect chance variation rather than distinct etiologies. Future research should examine maternal diet during pregnancy in a comprehensive way, collecting data on macronutrients, such as fat, and micronutrients, such as folate, as well as on food components relevant to the N-nitroso hypothesis. With these data, epidemiologists will be able to further test the hypothesis as well as more extensively investigate the role of maternal diet in general.

3.2. Child's Diet

Seven studies have investigated some aspects of the child's diet as possible risk factors *(3,4,6–8,10,11)*. As for maternal diet, the interest in the child's diet is motivated by the N-nitroso hypothesis. In all studies, the information collected on the child's diet was limited to vitamin supplements and no more than 15 food items. Researchers considered the child's diet in the first year of life in three of the studies and the child's usual diet before diagnosis in the other four studies

Little evidence on infant diet supports the N-nitroso hypothesis. The N-nitroso hypothesis predicts a protective effect of vitamin C and therefore of fruit, especially citrus, and vitamin supplements (*see* Table 1). The only statistically significant finding that supports the hypothesis comes from the study of medulloblastoma *(6)*, in which eating fruit in the first year of life was associated with decreased risk compared to eating no fruit at all. In a study that included all types of brain tumors, McCredie et al. also observed a decreased risk associated with fruit consumption, although it was not statistically significant *(8)*. An effect of fruit was not seen in the study of astrocytic glioma *(7)*. None of the three studies observed a decreased risk associated with orange juice or vitamin supplements, although a few odds ratios of <1.0 were noted for the latter. In addition, Cordier et al. noted an apparent protective effect of supplemented powdered milk *(11)*. The studies collected data on consumption of cured meats, but few infants eat these products and no significant associations were observed. Although no strong findings resulted, more comprehensive examination of infant diet may be a fruitful area of research.

Four studies investigated the child's usual diet before diagnosis and could better address the cured meat question *(3,4,10,11)*. Only one of the four observed a significant association with cured meat consumption *(3)* and in that study, when child and maternal consumption were analyzed simultaneously, the child's cured meat consumption was not associated with risk. The evidence, then, does not strongly suggest a role for cured meat consumption by the child. However, Sarasua and Savitz found evidence of a possible synergistic effect between cured meats and vitamin supplements *(10)*. They observed odds ratios of 3.2–6.8 for the joint effect of high cured meat consumption and lack of vitamin supplement use. The possible synergistic effect is consistent with the *N*-nitroso hypothesis. Animals fed a *N*-nitroso precursor and a nitrosating agent along with vitamin C produced smaller amounts of NOCs and developed fewer tumors than those not given vitamin C *(19,23)*. Of the two other studies that investigated vitamin supplement use, one observed an apparent protective effect *(4,11)*. The studies of childhood diet illustrate the need to analyze multiple aspects of diet simultaneously and to analyze the mother's and the child's diet simultaneously.

To our knowledge, only one study has investigated serum micronutrient levels in children in relation to cancer risk. Malvy et al. compared serum levels of antioxidant micronutrients in children with cancer to those in controls *(32)* and observed that children with brain tumors had lower levels of β-carotene and vitamin E compared to controls. Whether these differences reflect a protective effect of antioxidants or metabolic and nutritional disturbances of the brain tumor itself is not known.

3.3. Comparison with Adult Brain Tumor Studies

Researchers have conducted a number of studies that investigated dietary factors relevant to the *N*-nitroso hypothesis in relation to brain tumors in adults. The six studies of glioma are discussed below. This category of tumors includes the astrocytic gliomas, which are the most common brain tumor at all ages *(33–38)*. Some of these researchers have also studied meningiomas but these studies are not discussed here because these tumors are very rare in childhood. Three studies observed an increased risk associated with cured meat consumption overall and/or individual products *(35,36,38)* and three did not *(33,34,37)*. Even in the studies that observed associations, the evidence is not strong. In one study, for example, men but not women appeared to incur increased risk from frequent eating of cured meats *(38)*. The results for fruit are similarly inconsistent. Although one study observed protective effects of several types of fruit *(34)*, other studies have generally not replicated these results. The results for citrus fruit do not suggest a protective effect. Although one study observed an association of oranges with decreased risk *(33)*, there was no association with orange juice in the same study and no association with citrus in four other studies *(33,36–38)*. The evidence on vitamin supplements is not more convincing. Two studies observed no effect *(37,38)*, one observed a protective effect of any vitamin supplement *(33)*, and one a protective effect of vitamin C and vitamin E supplements *(34)*. In adults, the results on cured meat and supplements are conflicting and the evidence on citrus fruit suggests a lack of association. The evidence from studies of adult glioma seems less consistent with the *N*-nitroso hypothesis than that for childhood brain tumors.

4. LEUKEMIA

Leukemia accounts for about one-third of all cancer in children under age 15. In the United States, the annual incidence rate of leukemia in children is 4/100,000, with about 70% surviving at least 5 yr *(1,2)*. Three-quarters of leukemias in children are classified as acute lymphocytic leukemia and 15% as acute myeloid leukemia. Other types of leukemia and leukemias not categorized as a specific type make up the remaining 10%. Similarly to the different types of brain tumors, different types of leukemia vary in patterns of incidence *(39)*. Acute lymphocytic leukemia in children is more common in males than females and in whites than blacks, and peaks in incidence between ages 3 and 5. The incidence patterns for acute myelocytic leukemia are quite different; male-female and white-black differences are slight and incidence is fairly constant throughout childhood.

A specific hypothesis regarding diet has been put forth for leukemia, particularly in infants *(39)*. In the great majority of infant leukemias, the leukemia cells have abnormalities in band q23 of chromosome 11. Leukemias that occur after cancer treatment with epipodophyllotoxins, a class of chemotherapeutic agents, also have 11q23 abnormalities. Epipodophyllotoxins inhibit an enzyme called topoisomerase II, which is necessary for DNA replication. If epipodophyllotoxins inhibit topoisomerase II and increase the risk of leukemias with 11q23 abnormalities, perhaps other inhibitors of this enzyme also increase the risk of the same leukemias. Other inhibitors of topoisomerase II exist in nature, including certain flavonoids and medications *(40,41)*. Flavonoids, substances found in plants, occur in the diet in fruits, vegetables, herbs, beans, wine, beer, and other plant-derived foods *(42)*. Medications that inhibit topoisomerase II include quinolones, which are used to treat urinary tract infections *(43)*.

The specific hypothesis of Ross et al. regarding leukemia is that maternal exposure to topoisomerase II inhibitors during pregnancy increases the risk of leukemias with 11q23 abnormalities in infants *(39)*. According to the hypothesis, children of mothers who frequently ate fruits, vegetables, beans, and other plant-derived foods would be at higher risk of leukemia. Paradoxically, these foods and flavonoids themselves have been associated with a decreased risk of some cancers *(44)*. Perhaps, as Ross et al. speculate, flavonoids affect fetuses and adults differently. Fetuses are rapidly growing and have high rates of cell division and thus high levels of topoisomerase II, whereas adults have much lower rates of cell division and topoisomerase II activity. Ross et al. suggest that topoisomerase II inhibition may be detrimental in a rapidly growing fetus.

No data are available on exposure to natural inhibitors of topoisomerase II and risk of infant leukemia. In fact, very few data exist on any aspect of diet in relation to childhood leukemia. Two groups of investigators have examined the effects of a small number of dietary factors related to the *N*-nitroso hypothesis *(10,12)*. Although animal data have not linked *N*-nitroso compounds with leukemia, the potency of these carcinogens and the possibility of enhanced potency through transplacental exposure suggested investigation. Peters et al. conducted a study in California of 232 children ages 0–10 with leukemia and the same number of controls *(12)*. Sarasua and Savitz included all types of cancer before age 15 in their study and present analyses that compare the 56 cases of acute lymphocytic leukemia to the 206 controls *(10)*. In neither study was diet the major focus and thus, the amount of information collected on diet is limited. Peters et al. collected data on 11 food items and Sarasua and Savitz on five food items and on vitamin supplements.

The study by Peters et al. observed an increased risk associated with frequent consumption of hot dogs by the mother, father, and child. The risks were high, with relative risks of about 5, which were significant for the father and child. The investigators also observed elevated risks for eating of other cured meats by the child, but not by the parents. When the diet and other factors were considered simultaneously, the father's and the child's frequent hot dog consumption remained strongly and significantly associated with increased risk.

In contrast to the findings of Peters et al., Sarasua and Savitz did not observe increased risk associated with the mother's or child's eating of hot dogs. However, for the child, when the effect of frequent cured meat consumption and not using vitamin supplements was analyzed, a threefold increased risk was observed for each of the cured meats, including hot dogs.

Peters et al. investigated another dietary item, citrus fruit, relevant to the *N*-nitroso hypothesis because of its concentration of vitamin C. Consumption of citrus fruit or juice by the child or the mother did not appear to influence risk.

A few foods not related to the *N*-nitroso hypothesis were also studied. Both studies included hamburgers among the food items in the questionnaire. In the larger study of Peters et al., no effect was observed, although Sarasua and Savitz's smaller study observed a doubling of risk. Charbroiled meats did not affect risk of leukemia in either study. The increased risk associated with the child's cola drinking *(12)* disappeared when adjusted for hot dog eating and other variables.

Another study with data relevant to the question of childhood leukemia and diet was conducted in Shanghai, China *(13)*. In a case-control study with 309 cases and twice as many controls, use of cod liver oil for more than a year appeared to decrease the risk of both acute lymphocytic leukemia and acute nonlymphocytic leukemia. Cod liver oil contains vitamins A and D.

The study of serum antioxidant levels cited in the brain tumor section also presented data on leukemia *(32)*. Compared to controls, children with leukemia had lower serum levels of β-carotene, retinol, selenium, and zinc. The interpretation is difficult, because the differences may reflect the effects of the leukemia itself rather than etiologic influences.

Knowledge of adult leukemia does not add much to this discussion. A case-control study of acute leukemia in Poland included questions on frequency of consumption of about 40 food items *(45)* and observed frequent drinking of milk and consumption of poultry to be associated with higher risk and frequent eating of vegetables with lower risk. To our knowledge, no other case-control or cohort study has investigated the relationship between diet and leukemia in adults. In a ecological study of data from 24 countries, total and lymphocytic leukemia incidence was significantly correlated with total calorie intake *(46)*. Countries with high caloric intake tended to have high leukemia incidence and those with low caloric intake had lower incidence. Findings from ecological studies can provide only indirect evidence, but the international correlation fits well with animal data that calorie or protein restriction reduces the incidence of leukemia *(47)*.

The data on diet and childhood leukemia, although limited, suggest that further study may be productive. Any observed dietary association with childhood leukemia is worthy of pursuit, because we still know very little about the etiology of this disease. The findings concerning hot dogs and vitamins are consistent with the *N*-nitroso hypothesis, although the findings on citrus fruit do not fit. The association with hot dog consumption might also be consistent with risk factors of fat intake, total calories, infrequent vegetable consumption, and weight. Clearly, comprehensive studies of diet and childhood leukemia are required.

5. VITAMIN K

The role of vitamin K has been studied in relation to its administration to newborns rather than as a component of diet. In many industrialized countries, newborns are routinely given vitamin K to prevent hemorrhagic disease, unexpected bleeding in previously healthy neonates. In 1990, Golding et al. reported an association between receiving vitamin K as a newborn and development of cancer before age 10 *(48)*. The finding of an approximate doubling of risk arose unexpectedly in a nested case-control study of children born in 1970 in Great Britain. The results of a second study in Great Britain observed an increase in risk of similar magnitude for vitamin K administered intramuscularly but not orally *(49)*. The finding corroborated the first study since in 1970, the year of birth of the children in that study, vitamin K was almost always given intramuscularly. These two studies raised concern, because newborns in many industrialized countries receive vitamin K routinely by intramuscular injection. Oral vitamin K can be given, but is less effective at preventing hemorrhagic disease. Swedish researchers studied 1.3 million infants born full-term after uncomplicated delivery between 1973 and 1989 *(50)*. By record linkage, these children were followed until 1992; approx 2350 children in the cohort developed cancer. No increase in risk of cancer overall or of leukemia was observed with exposure to intramuscular vitamin K. Similarly, a US study did not observe cancer risk to be associated with vitamin K given to neonates *(51)*. When the four studies are considered together, it seems unlikely that vitamin K given neonatally is a major cause of cancer during childhood.

6. OTHER CANCERS

A few studies of other childhood cancers have reported isolated findings related to diet. A small study of rhabdomyosarcoma observed an increased risk associated with the child's eating of organ meats *(52)*. In a much larger study designed to follow-up on this and other findings, investigators were unable to confirm the observation (S. Grufferman, personal communication). A decreased risk of retinoblastoma was observed in relation to use of multivitamins by the mother during pregnancy *(53)*.

7. CONCLUSION

Studies of the relationship between diet and risk of childhood cancer are few and have focused on one hypothesis. Only the two most common cancers of childhood, leukemia and brain tumor, have been studied in any detail. Our knowledge of the role of diet in the etiologies of these cancers is meager. Nonetheless, the findings of the few studies suggest that diet does play a role in at least some childhood cancers. Future research will elucidate the particulars and extent of the role.

8. RECOMMENDATIONS

Maternal cured meat consumption has been fairly consistently associated with brain tumor risk in children, but whether the association is causal is unclear. Also, the frequency of cured meat consumption that was associated with higher risk varied greatly among the studies. For these reasons, a specific recommendation is not possible or appropriate. However, since cured meats are high in salt and fat, nutritional concerns other than the child's cancer risk, such as keeping one's fat and salt intake within recommendations, require that cured meats be eaten in no more than moderate quantities. Women eating cured meats several times a week or more might wish to reduce their intake during pregnancy.

REFERENCES

1. Ries LAG, Miller BA, Hankey BF, et al. eds. SEER Cancer Statistics Review, 1973–1991: Tables and Graphs, National Cancer Institute NIH Pub. No. 94-2789. Bethesda, MD, 1994.
2. Bleyer A. The impact of childhood cancer on the United States and the world. CA Cancer J Clin 1990; 40:355–367.
3. Preston-Martin S, Yu MC, Benton B, Henderson BE. N-nitroso compounds and childhood brain tumors: a case-control study. Cancer Res 1982; 42:5240–5245.
4. Howe GR, Burch JD, Chiarelli AM, Risch HA, Choi BCK. An exploratory case-control study of brain tumors in children. Cancer Res 1989; 49:4349–4352.
5. Kuijten RR, Bunin GR, Nass CC, Meadows AT. Gestational and familial risk factors for childhood astrocytoma: results of a case-control study. Cancer Res 1990; 50:2608–2612.
6. Bunin GR, Kuijten RR, Buckley JD, Rorke LB, Meadows AT. Relation between maternal diet and subsequent primitive neuroectodermal brain tumors in young children. New Engl J Med 1993; 329:536–541.
7. Bunin GR, Kuijten RR, Boesel CP, Buckley JD, Meadows AT. Maternal diet and risk of astrocytic glioma in children: a report from the Children's Cancer Group. Cancer Causes Control 1994; 5:177–187.
8. McCredie M, Maisonneuve P, Boyle P. Perinatal and early postnatal risk factors for malignant brain tumours in New South Wales children. Int J Cancer 1994; 56:11–15.
9. McCredie M, Maisonneuve P, Boyle P. Antenatal risk factors for malignant brain tumours in New South Wales children. Int J Cancer 1994; 56:6–10.
10. Sarasua S, Savitz DA. Cured and broiled meat consumption in relation to childhood cancer. Cancer Causes Control 1994; 5:141–148.
11. Cordier S, Iglesias M-J, Goaster CL, Guyot M-M, Mandereau L, Hemon D. Incidence and risk factors for childhood brain tumors in the Ile de France. Int J Cancer 1994; 59:776–782.
12. Peters JM, Preston-Martin S, London SJ, Bowman JD, Buckley JD, Thomas DC. Processed meats and risk of childhood leukemia. Cancer Causes Control 1994; 5:195–202.
13. Shu XO, Gao YT, Brinton LA, Linet MS, Tu JT, Zheng W, Fraumeni JF. A population-based case-control study of childhood leukemia in Shanghai. Cancer 1988; 62:635–644.
14. Frei B, Stocker R, Ames BN. Antioxidant defenses and lipid peroxidation in human blood plasma. Proc Natl Acad Sci USA 1988; 85:9748–9752.
15. Butterworth CE. Folate deficiency and cancer. In: Micronutrients in Health and in Disease Prevention. Bendich A, Butterworth CE Jr., eds. New York: Marcel Dekker, 1991; 165–183.

16. Mittendorf R. Teratogen update: carcinogenesis and teratogenesis associated with exposure to diethylstilbe-strol (DES) in utero. Teratol 1995; 51:435–445.

17. Nelson KG, Sakai Y, Eitzman B, Steed T, McLachlan J. Exposure to diethylstilbestrol during a critical developmental period of the mouse reproductive tract leads to persistent induction of two estrogen-regulated genes. Cell Growth Differ 1994; 5:595–606.

18. McLachlan JA, Newbold RR. Estrogens and development. Environ Health Perspect 1987; 75:25–27.

19. Lijinsky W. Chemistry and biology of N-nitroso compounds. New York: Cambridge University Press, 1992.

20. National Academy of Sciences. The health effects of nitrate, nitrite and N-nitroso compounds. Washington: National Academy Press, 1981.

21. Bartsch H, Castegnaro M, O'Neill IK, Okada M (eds.) N-nitroso compounds: occurrence and biological effects. Lyon: International Agency for Research on Cancer, 1982.

22. Howe GR, Harrison L, Jain M. A short diet history for assessing dietary exposure to N-nitrosamines in epidemiologic studies. Am J Epidemiol 1986; 124:595–602.

23. Mirvish SS. Experimental evidence for inhibition of N-nitroso compound formation as a factor in the negative correlation between vitamin C consumption and the incidence of certain cancers. Cancer Res 1994; 54:1948s–1951s.

24. Young JL, Ries LG, Silverbert E, Horm JW, Miller RW. Cancer incidence, survival, and mortality for children younger than 15 years. Cancer 1986; 58:598–602.

25. Gurney JF, Severson RK, Davis S, Robision LL. Incidence of cancer in children in the United States. Cancer 1995; 75:2186–2195.

26. MRC Vitamin Study Group. Prevention of neural tube defects: results of the Medical Research Council Vitamin Study. Lancet 1991; 338:131–137.

27. Mulinare J, Cordero JF, Erickson JD, Berry RJ. Periconceptional use of multivitamins and the occurrence of neural tube defects. JAMA 1988; 260:3141–3145.

28. Bower C, Stanley FJ. Dietary folate as a risk factor for neural-tube defects: evidence from a case-control study in Western Australia. Med J Aust 1989; 150:613–619.

29. Shaw GM, Lammer EJ, Wasserman CR, O'Malley CD, Tolarova MM. Risks of orofacial clefts in children born to women using multivitamins containing folic acid periconceptionally. Lancet 1995; 346:393–396.

30. Czeizel AE. Prevention of congenital abnormalities by periconceptional multivitamin supplementation. Br Med J 1993; 306:1645–1648.

31. Li De-Kun, Daling JR, Mueller BA, Hickok DE, Fantel AG, Weiss NS. Periconceptional multivitamin use in relation to the risk of congenital urinary tract anomalies. Epidemiology 1995; 6:212–218.

32. Malvy DJ-M, Burtschy B, Arnaud J, Sommelet D, Leverger G, Dostalova L, Drucker J, Amedee-Manesme O, and the Cancer in Children and Antioxidant Micronutrients French Study Group. Serum beta-carotene and antioxidant micronutrients in children with cancer. Int J Epidemiol 1993; 22:761–771.

33. Preston-Martin S, Mack W, Henderson BE. Risk factors for gliomas and meningiomas in males in Los Angeles County. Cancer Res 1989; 49:6137–6143.

34. Burch JD, Craib KJP, Choi BCK, Miller AB, Risch HA, Howe GR. An exploratory case-control study of brain tumors in adults. J Natl Cancer Inst 1987; 78:601–609.

35. Ahlbom A, Navier IL, Norell S, Olin R, Spannare B. Nonoccupational risk indicators for astrocytomas in adults. Am J Epidemiol 1986; 124:334–337.

36. Boeing H, Schlehofer B, Blettner M, Wahrendorf J. Dietary carcinogens and the risk for glioma and meningioma in Germany. Int J Cancer 1993; 53:561–565.

37. Ryan P, Lee MW, North JB. Risk factors for tumors of the brain and meninges: results from the Adelaide Adult Brain Tumor Study. Int J Cancer 1992; 51:20–27.

38. Giles GG, McNeil JJ, Donnan G, Webley C, Staples MP, Ireland P, Hurley SF, Salzberg M. Dietary factors and the risk of glioma in adults: results of a case-control study in Melbourne, Australia. Int J Cancer 1994; 59:357–362.

39. Ross JA, Davies SM, Potter JD, Robison LL. Epidemiology of childhood leukemia, with a focus on infants. Epidemiol Rev 1994; 16:243–272.

40. Austin CA, Patel S, Ono K, Nakane H, Fisher LM. Site-specific DNA cleavage by mammalian DNA topoisomerase II induced by novel flavone and catechin derivatives. Biochem J 1992; 282:883–889.

41. Yamashita Y, Kawada S-Z, Nakano H. Induction of mammalian topoisomerase II dependent DNA cleavage by nonintercalative flavonoids, genistein and orobol. Biochem Pharmacol 1990; 39:737–744.

42. Pierpoint WS. Flavonoids in the human diet. In: Plant Flavonoids in Biology and Medicine: Biochemical, Pharmacological, and Structure-Activity Relationships. Cody V, Middleton E, eds. New York: Alan R. Liss, Inc., 1986:125–140.

43. Epstein RJ. Topoisomerases in human disease. Lancet 1988; 1:521–524.

44. Steinmetz KA, Potter JD. Vegetables, fruit, and cancer. II. Mechanisms. Cancer Causes Control 1991; 2:327–342.

45. Kwiatkowski A. Dietary and other environmental risk factors in acute leukaemias: A case-control study of 119 patients. Eur J Cancer Prev 1993; 2:139–146.

46. Hursting SD, Margolin BH, Switzer BR. Diet and human leukemia: an analysis of international data. Prev Med 1993; 22:409–422.

47. Gross L. Inhibition of the development of leukemia in mice and rats after reduction in food intake. Cancer 1988; 62:1463–1465.

48. Golding J, Paterson M, Kinlen LJ. Factors associated with childhood cancer in a national cohort study. Br J Cancer 1990; 62:304–308.

49. Golding J, Greenwood R, Birmingham K, mott M. Childhood cancer, intramuscular vitamin K, and pethidine given during labour. Br Med J 1992; 305:341–346.

50. Ekelund H, Finnstrom O, Gunnarskog J, Kallen B, Larsson Y. Administration of vitamin K to newborn infants and childhood cancer. Br Med J 1993; 307:89–91.

51. Klebanoff MA, Read JS, Mills JL, Shiono PH. The risk of childhood cancer after neonatal exposure to vitamin K. New Engl J Med 1993; 329:905–908.

52. Grufferman S, Wang HH, Delong ER, Kimm SYS, Delzell ES, Falletta JM. Environmental factors in the etiology of rhabdomyosarcoma in childhood. J Natl Cancer Inst 1982; 68:107–113.

53. Bunin GR, Meadows AT, Emanuel BS, Buckley JD, Woods WG, Hammond GD. Pre- and post-conception factors associated with heritable and non-heritable retinoblastoma. Cancer Res 1989; 49:5730–5735.

3   Prevention of Upper Gastrointestinal Tract Cancers

Elizabeth T. H. Fontham

1. INTRODUCTION

This chapter will focus on lifestyle factors associated with cancers of the esophagus and stomach. Unlike such major cancers as prostate and breast, whose etiologies remain obscure at the present time, hindering primary prevention, cancers of the upper gastrointestinal tract offer well-defined intervention opportunities. Epidemiologic studies have clearly established the important role of alcohol, tobacco, and diet, and recent findings have documented the relation between infection with *Helicobacter pylori* and cancer of the stomach. These factors and their interactions will be discussed for cancers of each of these two sites, which together account for approx 35,000 new cases and 25,000 deaths annually in the United States *(1)*.

2. CANCER OF THE ESOPHAGUS

For many years, cancer of the esophagus in the United States and in most areas throughout the world was virtually synonymous with squamous cell carcinoma *(2)*. Hence, most of the established risk factors for esophageal cancer are specific to this cell type, which comprised the vast majority of cases in studies of this cancer. Recent shifts in the histopathologic cell type have given rise to a rapid increase in the incidence of adenocarcinoma of the esophagus in the United States, particularly among white males *(3)*. Because of the increasing importance of esophageal adenocarcinoma, a separate section will consider this entity, which may differ in etiology from squamous cell carcinoma.

2.1. Squamous Cell Carcinoma

2.1.1. TOBACCO AND ALCOHOL CONSUMPTION

Both tobacco and heavy alcohol consumption are well-established risk factors for esophageal carcinoma. In the United States and other Western countries, over 90% of the risk can be attributed to the individual and joint effects of tobacco and alcohol *(4)*.

An early study by Wynder and Bross *(5)* graphically examined the interaction between alcohol and tobacco and the data suggest a multiplicative effect. Tuyns et al. *(6)* evaluated this relation more formally in data from a case-control study in Brittany. At the highest level of consumption of both alcohol (≥ 121 g ethanol/d) and tobacco (≥ 30 g/d) the risk of esophageal cancer was over 150 times greater than in non- or light con-

From: *Preventive Nutrition: The Comprehensive Guide for Health Professionals*
Edited by A. Bendich and R. J. Deckelbaum Humana Press Inc., Totowa, NJ

Table 1
Adjusted Odds Ratios[a] for Cancer of the Esophagus
by Alcohol and Tobacco Consumption[b]

Smoking status	Alcohol (drinks per week)		
	< 35	35–59	≥ 60
Nonsmoker	1.0[c]	2.2	2.6
Light	2.1	4.4	5.5
Moderate	4.4	9.7	11.4
Heavy	8.4	18.5	21.8

[a]Adjusted for age, residence, education and profession
[b]Adapted from Barón et al. (8)
[c]Reference category

sumers. The increased risk associated with alcohol consumption appears exponential whereas increased tobacco smoking appears to yield a more linear increase. Saracci (7) estimates that the excess risk of esophageal cancer as a result of the interaction of alcohol and tobacco is about 25-fold.

Data from a recent case-control study in Italy are presented in Table 1 (8). Study subjects included 271 male cases and 1754 male controls with acute illnesses unrelated to tobacco and alcohol consumption. Even with a reference category that included moderate alcohol consumption (< 35 drinks/wk) by nonsmokers, the estimated relative risk of esophageal cancer among heavy smokers (≥ 25 cigarettes/d, ≥ 40 yr) and very heavy drinkers (≥ 60 drinks/wk) is 22. This report was updated in 1994 to include women (9). Among alcohol drinkers (any vs none), similar risks were observed for women and men, 3.0 and 4.7, respectively; however, male abstainers had a twofold increased risk whereas female nondrinkers had a reduced risk, 0.7, compared with light to moderate drinkers. This study of esophageal cancer fails to support the hypothesis posed by Blume (10) that women may be more susceptible to the effects of alcohol, at least for this particular cancer site.

Whether the increased risk of esophageal cancer attributed to alcohol use is a function of the dose of ethanol or whether the type of alcoholic beverage and its other constituents play a role has also been examined, most recently in a Japanese study by Hanaoka et al. (11). Their findings confirm those of others that indicate that the amount of alcohol consumed, rather than any particular type, is the primary determinant of risk.

2.1.2. THERMAL IRRITATION

Thermal injury as a result of drinking very hot liquids has been suggested to increase risk of esophageal cancer by increasing susceptibility to other carcinogenic exposures (12,13). This hypothesis has some support in both ecologic and analytic studies. Persons living in regions of the world with high rates of esophageal cancer, such as northern Iran and Siberia, are reported to drink excessively hot tea (14,15).

Martinez (16) found that more cases than controls reported drinking hot, rather than warm or cold, coffee in Puerto Rico. Both Segi (17) and Hirayama (18) found an increased risk of esophageal cancer in persons consuming hot tea gruel. In Latin America, several studies have examined the role of maté drinking. DeStefani et al. found a strong association between hot maté consumption and risk of esophageal cancer in Uruguay

(19). An earlier case-control study in Brazil found no such association *(20)*. In 1994 Castelletto et al. examined the role of maté in an Argentinean case-control study *(21)*. They found alcohol, tobacco and barbecued meat, but not hot maté, to be the primary risks factors.

A study of chronic esophagitis, a precursor lesion for esophageal cancer, in a high risk region in China lends support to an etiologic role of thermal injury *(22)*. A greater than fourfold excess of mild and moderate esophagitis was found in young persons 15–26 yr of age consuming burning hot beverages (odds ratio 4.39, confidence interval [CI] 95%: 1.72–11.3). This study design minimizes recall/response bias because case-control status is not known at the time of interview, and suggests that this factor may be important at a relatively early stage in the development of this cancer.

2.1.3. NUTRITION

2.1.3.1. DIETARY STUDIES

Fruits and fresh vegetables are consistently associated in studies throughout the world with decreased risk of esophageal cancer, even after controlling for tobacco and alcohol use. Deficiencies of vitamin C, one of several micronutrients contained in fruits and vegetables, have been reported in several areas of the world with exceptionally high rates of esophageal cancer. These include northern Iran *(14)*, Linxian County, China *(23)*, and northern and eastern Siberia *(15)*, among others. Other dietary deficiencies are also strongly associated with esophageal cancer risk; these include iron, riboflavin, niacin, molydenium, zinc, and other trace elements *(24)*.

The 1961 report by Wynder and Bross noted significantly lower consumption levels of green and yellow vegetables among male cases compared to controls, and a non-significantly lower consumption level of fruit *(5)*. Potatoes (RR=0.4, $p < 0.05$) and bananas (RR=0.3, $p < 0.01$) were determined to be protective in a case-control study in Singapore *(25)*. Frequent consumption of 16 different fruits and vegetables was associated with decreased risk of esophageal cancer in Iran *(26)*. Relative risks for high vs low consumption levels ranged from 0.4–0.9 and findings for 10 of the 16 foods were significantly protective.

A significant inverse trend ($p < 0.001$) was reported between monthly vitamin C consumption and esophageal cancer in white males in New York state *(27)*. A weaker but significant inverse association was observed for vitamin A intake ($p=0.03$). A fivefold reduction in risk in the highest tertile of fruit and vegetable consumption (> 81 times/mo) was also found. A more recent report from New York found no association with vitamin C derived from vegetables *(28)*. However, in this study only 24% of the eligible cases were included and they may not be representative of the total series of cases.

Ziegler et al. *(29)* found significant inverse associations between relative risk of esophageal cancer and five indicators of general nutritional status, including total fruit and vegetable consumption (RR=0.5, p-trend < 0.05). This case-control study focused on high-risk black males in Washington, DC. An index of vitamin C intake yielded an estimated relative risk of 0.55 (p-trend < 0.05) for the highest tertile of consumption. The only other micronutrient significantly inversely associated with risk was riboflavin.

Two case-control studies conducted in the high-risk region of Calvados, France, found a protective effect of vitamin C on esophageal cancer risk *(30,31)*. Approximately threefold significant reductions in risk were observed at the highest level of intake of citrus fruits and of dietary vitamin C. Similarly, DeCarli et al. *(32)* reported a relative risk of 0.3 (0.1–0.6) for high-level fruit consumption and nonsignificant reductions in risk for high-level vegetable intake. In India, Notani and Jayant *(33)* found a more modest reduction from high-level fruit intake (RR=0.8, 0.5–1.3), but a significant risk reduction among daily consumers of vegetables (RR=0.4, 0.2–0.7).

Two 1988 reports support the findings of others indicative of protection from high intake of dietary vitamin C and fresh fruits *(34,35)*. Brown et al. *(34)* found a significant halving in risk in the highest tertile of consumption of citrus, fruit, all fruits combined, and dietary vitamin C ($p < 0.05$). A relative risk of 0.4 (0.2–0.8) for high-level consumption of raw vegetables and fresh fruit was found in the California study of Yu and colleagues *(35)*. Li et al. *(36)* found no reduction in esophageal cancer risk associated with fruit consumption in a high-risk region of China, but a homogeneously low level of intake of fruit in this population makes it a poor one in which to evaluate the association *(37)*. Strong protective effects (*p*-trend < 0.001) associated with consumption of citrus fruits and other fruits were reported by Cheng et al. *(38)*, who conducted a large case-control study in Hong Kong. The proportion of esophageal cancer cases attributable to low consumption levels of citrus fruits in this population was estimated to be 26%. A retrospective cohort study of esophageal cancer in Linxian, China, reported a significant reduction in risk associated with regular consumption of fresh vegetables, (RR= 0.66 [0.44–0.99] *(39)*.

A large Italian study of esophageal cancer in lifelong nonsmokers afforded the opportunity to evaluate other risk factors in the absence of residual confounding by tobacco use *(40)*. Although the major risk factor was not unexpectedly alcohol, green vegetables and fresh fruit were associated with significantly reduced relative risks of 0.6 and 0.3, respectively. Similar reductions in risk were associated with β-carotene intake. The estimated relative risk for the combination of high alcohol and low β-carotene was 8.6, with an attributable risk of approx 45%.

Several dietary factors in addition to fruits and vegetables and their constituent micronutrients have been proposed as candidate protective factors, although the epidemiologic evidence to date is considerably more limited. One such factor is green tea, *Camellia sinensis*. Experimental studies have demonstrated antimutagenic and anticarcinogenic effects, especially in the esophagus *(41–44)*. Findings in a recent population-based case-control study in China provide some support to this hypothesis *(45)*. After adjustment for confounders, including tobacco and alcohol, a significant halving of risk was observed in women drinking green tea (OR=0.50, CI 95%: 0.30–0.83) and an inverse dose-response was observed. The findings in men were not statistically significant; however, a significant protective effect was observed in both men and women who did not smoke or drink alcohol. Since green tea, as well as other drinks, can be consumed at hot temperatures and since excessively hot fluids have been associated with increased risk of this cancer, the relation between drinking burning-hot fluids was also evaluated. The protective effect of green tea was limited to tea taken at normal temperatures.

Ginseng, which may be taken as a tea, powder, or as a slice of the root, has also been proposed as a potential anticarcinogen. Unlike the polyphenols in green tea, no specific component or mechanism has been elaborated *(46,47)*. Yun and Choi *(48)* reported a case-control study in Korea where ginseng is commonly used. The relative risk of esophageal cancer associated with ginseng intake was 0.20 (CI 95%: 0.09–0.38) after adjustment for tobacco, alcohol, and other confounders. This large reduction in risk was observed in both smokers and nonsmokers. Additional studies are obviously necessary to confirm this preliminary finding.

2.1.3.2. Biochemical Studies

A number of studies have examined biochemical nutritional indicators in blood or tissue, with particular focus on antioxidants. Chen et al. *(49)* collected blood samples from a sample of the population in 65 different counties in China and correlated the concentration of over 10 different antioxidants with county-specific mortality rates for several cancers, including esophageal. A highly significant inverse relation was found between esophageal cancer rates and both plasma ascorbic acid and selenium in men and selenium in women. Another study in a high-risk region of China found low levels of zinc *(50)*. A recent population-based, case-control study conducted in Washington state *(51)* found no significant difference in nail zinc concentrations in esophageal cancer cases and controls, but a large and significant reduction in risk associated with dietary intake of zinc from foods and supplements: odds ratios of 0.5 and 0.1 for the middle and upper tertile of consumption respectively, p-trend < 0.001. Other elements in nail tissue associated with esophageal cancer were iron (OR=2.9 high vs low levels), calcium (OR=2.6), and cobalt (OR=1.9). Although this study suggests a number of differences in mineral levels of cases and controls reflecting differences in intake, metabolism or both, additional investigation is warranted to determine which, if any, of these findings is etiologically meaningful.

2.1.3.3. Chemoprevention Studies

Chemoprevention as defined by Sporn and Newton *(52)* is prevention of cancer with pharmacological agents used to inhibit or reverse the process of carcinogenesis. In this relatively new field, which has grown in acceptance in the 1980s and 1990s, esophageal cancer is one of the few cancer sites for which results from completed trials are available.

Muñoz et al. *(53)* reported findings from the first short-term intervention trial in 1985. A total of 610 subjects ages 35–64 in the high-risk region of Huixian, China, were randomized to receive 15 mg (50,000 IU) retinol, 200 mg riboflavin, and 50 mg zinc or placebo once per week for 13.5 mo. Five hundred sixty-seven participants completed the trial and underwent endoscopy for histological diagnosis of premalignant lesions of the esophagus (esophagitis, atrophy, dysplasia). The combined treatment had no effect on the prevalence of precancerous lesions of the esophagus. It should be noted, however, that the dose was relatively small and the intervention period short. Micronuclei in exfoliated cells of buccal and esophageal mucosa were evaluated in 170 study subjects from this same trial as an indicator of chromosomal damage *(54)*. No reduction in micronuclei was found in subjects after treatment, but a significant reduction in the percentage of micronucleated cells were observed in treated subjects (0.19%) compared to the placebo group (0.31%), $p=0.04$. In a third report from this same trial, Wahrendorf et al. *(55)* reanalyzed data by blood levels of retinol, riboflavin, and zinc at the beginning and end of the trial because improvement in blood retinol and zinc levels had been observed in the placebo group as well as the actively treated group. Individuals who had large increases in retinol, riboflavin, and zinc blood levels were more likely to have a histologically normal esophagus at the end of the trial regardless of treatment group.

Two large intervention studies conducted in the high-risk population of Linxian, China, were recently reported *(56,57)*. A six-year randomized trial of daily vitamin/mineral supplementation vs placebo found no significant reductions in cancer incidence or mortality among adults with pre-existing precancerous lesions of the esophagus *(56)*. The larger trial in this same area included 29,584 subjects from the general population randomly allocated to placebo or combinations of retinol and zinc, riboflavin and niacin, vitamin C and molybdenum, and/or β-carotene, vitamin E, and selenium in doses of one to two times US Recommended Daily Allowances. Significantly reduced total mortality (RR=0.91, 0.84–0.99) and stomach cancer mortality (RR=0.79, 0.64–0.99) were observed in those taking β-carotene, vitamin E, and selenium. No significant effects on mortality or cancer incidence, including esophageal cancer, were observed for any of the other vitamin/mineral combinations.

Wang et al. *(58)* evaluated whether any of the vitamin/mineral supplement combinations affected the prevalence of clinically silent precancerous lesions and early invasive cancers of the esophagus and stomach as determined by endoscopy and biopsy in this same trial. No significant reductions in risk of dysplasia or cancer were observed for any of the supplements, although retinol and zinc were suggestively associated with a lower risk of gastric cancer, OR=0.38, $p=0.09$. Similarly, Dawsey et al. *(59)* evaluated the effect of the single vitamin/mineral supplement used in the trial of persons with esophageal dysplasia to see if treatment reduced the prevalence of histological dysplasia or early cancer of the esophagus or gastric cardia. Modest, nonsignificant risk reductions were observed compared to placebo (OR=0.86, 0.54–1.38). The authors conclude that longer interventions with larger numbers of subjects are required to adequately evaluate the effectiveness of micronutrient supplementation in this high-risk population. In subjects from this same trial, Rao et al. *(60)* evaluated whether epithelial proliferation, an early step in carcinogenesis, was reduced by treatment after 30 mo of intervention. The results were similarly inconclusive.

2.2. Adenocarcinoma

2.2.1. BARRETT'S ESOPHAGUS AND MEDICATIONS

Barrett's esophagus is characterized by the replacement of the lower esophagus, which is normally stratified squamous epithelium, by metaplastic columnar epithelium *(61)*. This condition, attributed to chronic esophageal reflux, is believed to be premalignant lesion for esophageal adenocarcinoma *(62)*.

Barrett's esophagus displays a similar age, race, and gender distribution as does esophageal adenocarcinoma: it is most common in white males over age 40 *(3,63)*. The reported incidence of esophageal adenocarcinoma in patients with Barrett's is from 30 to over 100 times greater than the rate observed in the general population *(63–66)*.

There also appears to be a familial form of this disease, inherited as an autosomal dominant trait *(67–69)*. Two recent reports of families with the inherited form of Barrett's provide additional support for Barrett's as a precursor lesion *(67,69)*.

A related hypothesis has proposed that the use of medications that relax the esophageal sphincter, and thereby promote reflux, may increase risk of adenocarcinomas of the esophagus and gastric cardia *(70)*. Histamine H_2 receptor antagonists used routinely for treatment of peptic ulcer and gastroesophageal reflux disease have also been proposed as an etiologic factor *(71)*. In a 1995 report, Chow et al. *(72)* examined the relation between reflux disease and its treatment to risk of adenocarcinomas of the esophagus and gastric cardia. Significant increased risks of adenocarcinoma were associated with esophageal reflux (OR=2.1, 1.2–3.6); hiatal hernia (OR=3.8, 1.9–7.6); and esophagitis/esophageal ulcer (5.0, 1.5–16.4). Although a fourfold increased risk was associated with four or more prescriptions for H_2 antagonists, the odds ratio was reduced to 1.5 (0.4–5.4) after adjusting for predisposing conditions. The relation with use of anticholinergics adjusted for number of conditions was actually inverse: Risk decreased with increasing number of prescriptions (p-trend=0.08). The study findings support the elevated risk of adenocarcinoma conferred by reflux disease, but indicate that the mechanism is not strongly related to treatment of reflux.

2.2.2. TOBACCO AND ALCOHOL

Two population-based studies of cancers of the esophagus and gastric cardia conducted in western Washington state 1983–1990 were analyzed to evaluate risk factors for adenocarcinoma compared to squamous cell *(73)*. Use of alcohol and cigarettes was significantly associated with increased risk of both histologic types, but the odds ratios were markedly higher for squamous cell carcinoma. For current smokers of 80+ pack-yr compared to nonsmokers, the odds ratios were 16.9 (4.1–6.91) for squamous cell carcinoma and 3.4 (1.4–8.0) for adenocarcinoma. Similarly, for persons who reported drinking 21 or more drinks per week compared to <7/wk, the respective odds ratios were 9.5 (4.1–22.3) and 1.8 (1.1–3.1). Population-attributable risk estimates found that cigarette smoking and alcohol together accounted for 87% of the squamous cell carcinomas, whereas for adenocarcinoma the estimate for cigarettes was 34% and 10% for alcohol consumption of seven or more drinks per week.

Estimates of esophageal adenocarcinoma risk for alcohol and tobacco use by Kabat et al. *(74)* were similar: current smokers, 2.3 (1.4–3.9); 4+ oz of whiskey-equivalents per week, 1.9 (1.3–4.3). Brown et al. *(75)* also report that tobacco and alcohol are likely etiologic factors, but conferring lower magnitude risk than that associated with squamous cell cancers. The odds ratios at the highest level of smoking (≥ 40 cigarettes/d) and drinking (≥ 29 drinks/wk) were 2.6 (p-trend < 0.01) and 2.8 (p-trend < 0.05), respectively. Their study included white men from Atlanta, Detroit, and New Jersey. Significantly increased risks were also found associated with history of ulcer, especially duodenal, and with low social class. The authors note that alcohol and tobacco use, although associated with esophageal adenocarcinoma, does not explain the rapid increase in these tumors.

2.2.3. OBESITY AND DIET

Two 1995 reports have linked obesity to adenocarcinoma of the esophagus *(73,75)*. A threefold increased risk ($p < 0.01$) was observed at the highest level of body mass index (>26.6 kg/m^2) compared to the lowest in white men *(75)*. No significant associations were found for dietary fat, total calories, meals eaten per day, or consumption of coffee and tea. A protective effect of high intake of raw fruit (OR=0.4, $p < 0.05$) and vegetables (OR=0.4, $p < 0.05$) was observed. Vaughan et al. *(73)* report divergent associations for squamous cell and adenocarcinoma with body mass index. A significantly increased risk of adenocarcinoma was found at the highest decile of body mass index (OR=1.9, 1.1–3.2), whereas body mass was inversely associated with squamous cell carcinoma. The population-attributable risk for body mass index above the 50th percentile was 18% for adenocarcinoma. These observations are consistent with esophageal reflux associated with obesity.

3. CANCER OF THE STOMACH

A steady decline in gastric cancer has been apparent in many countries for the past several decades. The declining rates were first noted in the United States as early as 1930 *(76)* and have persisted throughout this century *(1)*. Survival rates have not appreciably changed *(1,77)*; therefore, the decline in deaths cannot be attributed to better treatment and prolonged survival but to actual declines in incidence that are now well documented *(78)*. This decline, believed to reflect changes in environmental factors, has been referred to an "unplanned triumph" since the shifts did not result from active medical or public health intervention and are believed to result from large shifts in food processing and consumption *(79)*. It should be noted that the increase in esophageal adenocarcinoma documented in the previous section does include an increase in adenocarcinomas of the gastroesophageal junction and gastric cardia.

3.1. Histologic Types

Adenocarcinomas account for more than 97% of gastric cancers, and studies of etiology are generally limited to this histologic type *(80)*. Building on an earlier observation that gastric carcinomas were often accompanied by features found in intestinal epithelium *(81)*, Laurén *(82)* proposed a classification of adenocarcinomas into two subtypes, "intestinal" and "diffuse." Many, but not all tumors, can be thus classified because some tumors contain characteristics of both types and others neither. Diffuse carcinomas, sometimes referred to as "endemic," tend to occur with similar frequency throughout the world, whereas the distribution of intestinal or "epidemic" type tends to parallel the distribution of overall gastric cancer rates, i.e., this type is relatively more common in areas with high rates and lower where gastric cancer rates are low *(83)*.

3.2. Risk Factors

3.2.1. HELICOBACTER PYLORI

Spiral-shaped bacteria in contact with gastric mucosa were first reported about 100 years ago by Pel *(84)* and ignored for the next 90 years. In 1983, Marshall *(85)* and Warren *(86)* reported isolating these bacteria in cultures of biopsies taken from patients with gastritis and peptic ulcers undergoing endoscopy. By 1994, the International Agency for Research on Cancer, World Health Organization, had determined that infection with *Helicobacter pylori* is carcinogenic to humans, and declared it a Group 1 carcinogen based on the large body of research developed during the 11-yr period *(87)*.

H. pylori infection is one of the most prevalent infections worldwide, ranging from 20–40% in developed countries and as high as 70–90% in some developing countries *(88,89)*. Prevalence increases with age and no difference in seroprevalence has been found between males and females *(90)*. Socioeconomic status, including poor housing conditions, large family size, and low education attainment, is a predictor of prevalence of infection as well as of gastric cancer *(91, 92)*.

The role of *H. pylori* in gastric carcinogenesis has been explored in correlation and case-control studies, but this approach has yielded equivocal results, largely because of difficulties in determining temporality *(87)*. Three different cohort studies provided material for nested case-control analyses that resolved the issue of temporality. *H. pylori* infection was determined by IgG antibodies in serum collected at the time of cohort enrollment 6–14 yr earlier. Forman et al. *(93)* found an approximate threefold increased risk of subsequent gastric cancer in cohort of Welsh men; Parsonnet et al. *(94)* reported a relative risk of 3.6 (1.8–7.3) in a cohort of men and women in California; and Nomura et al. *(95)* a sixfold significantly increased risk in Japanese-American men living in Hawaii.

The mechanisms by which *H. pylori* infection increases gastric cancer risk are not well-established and are the focus of ongoing investigation. *H. pylori* infection, the main cause of chronic gastritis, has been demonstrated to decrease the concentration of ascorbic acid in gastric juice *(96–99)*. *H. pylori* infection is also associated with varying degrees of inflammation *(100)*. In inflammatory states, nitric oxide may be generated and interact with reactive oxygen species forming new cytotoxic compounds *(101,102)*. Thus, *H. pylori* infection has the potential to increase oxidative stress and decrease antioxidant capacity.

3.2.2. TOBACCO AND ALCOHOL

Although both tobacco and alcohol use are weakly associated with increased risk of gastric cancer, the strength and magnitude of the association is much less clear than that for esophageal cancer.

Early case-control studies of gastric cancer and alcohol intake were equivocal, with some reporting positive associations *(103,104)* and others none *(105,106)*. Continued study has yielded similar mixed results. Correa et al. *(107)* found twofold elevations in risk of gastric cancer at the highest level of alcohol intake for both whites and blacks in Louisiana. After controlling for other risk factors, wine (OR=2.10, 1.13–3.89) and hard liquor (OR=1.95, 1.14–3.34) were significantly associated with risk in whites, but not in blacks. A 1990 report of stomach cancer in Los Angeles males also found an increased risk (OR=3.0, 1.1–8.7) at the highest level of total ethanol intake and significant risks for daily consumption of beer *(108)*. The effect of alcohol was stronger for cancer of the gastric cardia than at other sites.

A twofold increased risk of stomach cancer was found for beer consumption in a German study, but wine and hard liquor were associated with decreased risk *(109)*. This is in contrast to a French study that reported a very large relative risk (RR=6.9, 3.3–14.3) associated with heavy use of red wine *(110)*.

Two cohort studies, however, suggest that alcohol is not an independent risk factor for gastric cancer. Nomura et al. *(111)* found no increased risk of gastric cancer associated with consumption of beer, wine, or hard liquor in Japanese-American men living in Hawaii. Kneller et al. *(112)* likewise found no association for total alcohol or for any specific type.

More consistent findings link smoking to a 1.5- to threefold increased risk of gastric cancer *(107–112)*; however, the overall increased risk has often failed to demonstrate a dose-response *(103,111,113)*. The cohort study by Kneller et al. did find significant increases in risk with both increasing number of cigarettes smoked per day and pack-years of smoking *(112)*. At the highest number of pack-yr the relation of risk was 2.3 (1.23–4.33) and for current use of 30 or more cigarettes/d the relative risk was 5.8 compared to nonsmokers. Although age at death did not significantly modify risk, the association with smoking was stronger for younger cases. The authors suggest that this finding may reflect a higher proportion of adenocarcinomas of the gastric cardia at younger ages and a stronger relation between smoking and cancers of the cardia than with cancers of other sites in the stomach.

3.2.3. SALTED, PICKLED, AND SMOKED FOODS

Salt has been demonstrated in animal studies to enhance gastric carcinogenesis *(114–117)*. It has been suggested that the action of salt as a gastric mucosal irritant facilitates the action of carcinogens and thus salt acts as a cocarcinogen *(118)*.

Epidemiologic studies also suggest an increased risk of gastric cancer associated with high salt intake when salted and pickled foods are included in total intake. Death rates throughout regions of Japan *(119)* were found to be correlated with consumption of salted fish and salted vegetables. A geographic correlation has also been demonstrated in China *(120)*. Consumption of salt-cured meats, salted fish, and other salt-preserved foods have been associated with increased risk in case-control studies throughout the world *(121–123)*. Several studies have also reported associations with the addition of salt to foods *(121,124)* or a reported "heavy intake" *(125,126)*.

Many of the strongest findings have been noted in areas of the world where there is a wide range of intake, including very high levels, such as in Korea *(123)*. A recent nested case-control analysis reported by Friedman and Parsonnet *(127)* failed to find evidence that routine salting led to increased risk in a California study population. "Heavy" salt intake in US populations may be quantitatively less than "heavy" intake in other areas of the world and may not be sufficient to demonstrate an increased risk. For example, salted fish and salted vegetables in Japan may contain up to 30% NaCl, compared to isotonic saline, which is 0.8% *(118,119)*.

Numerous N-nitroso compounds have demonstrated carcinogenicity *(128)*. Based on studies of premalignant lesions of the stomach, it has been hypothesized that intragastric synthesis of N-nitroso compounds is a factor in the gastric carcinogenic process *(129)*.

Two recently reported studies evaluated factors associated with in vivo nitrosamine formation in humans using the test developed by Ohshima and Bartsch *(130)*, which measures urinary excretion of noncarcinogenic N-nitrosoproline after ingesting a given dose of proline. Mirvish et al. *(131)* found that men in rural Nebraska who drank water from private wells with a high nitrate content excreted significantly higher N-nitroso proline than men drinking water with a low nitrate content. Their findings parallel those of a study in Denmark *(132)*. Sierra et al. *(133)* used the nitrosoproline test in children living in high- and low-risk areas for stomach cancer in Costa Rica. They found the concentration excreted by children in the high-risk area significantly greater ($p < 0.04$) compared to children from the low-risk area. They also found that excretion was markedly reduced when ascorbic acid, an inhibitor of nitrosation reactions, was given with the proline.

Associations between gastric cancer and dietary intake of nitrate, nitrite, and preformed nitroso compounds are suggestive *(134–139)*, but the validity of such indexes is not well established given the multiple sources, including food, water, and endogenous formation.

3.2.4. FRUITS AND VEGETABLES

Table 2 presents an extensive compendium of dietary studies of gastric cancer *(105,111,112,123,125,134–158)*. The strong, consistent inverse association between consumption of fruits and vegetables is abundantly clear. Of the 26 studies described that specifically examined foods and food groups, 24 found a decreased risk of stomach cancer associated with high intake of one or more fruits and vegetables, and the vast majority were statistically significant with up to twofold reductions in risk. Only two studies reported an increased risk of gastric cancer associated with fruits *(112)* or vegetables *(122)*, and their findings do little to cast doubt on the apparent protective effect of fruits and vegetables. The findings of Tajima and Tominaga *(122)* stand in contrast to many case-control studies in Japan and elsewhere, and the study by Kneller et al. *(112)* was based on a very limited dietary questionnaire that increases the likelihood of misclassification.

3.2.5. MICRONUTRIENTS

Consumption of fruits and vegetables serves as a dietary source of a plethora of vitamins, minerals, fiber, and less well-studied trace compounds. Many of these are highly correlated with one another, particularly when exposure is based on dietary assessment; therefore, a finding attributed to one may actually reflect the effect of another constituent from the same foods. The strongest findings, therefore, are based on biochemical studies, e.g., blood levels prior to cancer onset and chemoprevention trials, which actually test the efficacy of specific micronutrients in prevention. The micronutrients believed to be most strongly associated with reduced gastric cancer risk based on studies to date are vitamin C, β-carotene, and vitamin E/selenium.

Findings from dietary estimates of intake are also included in Table 2. Relatively high consumption of vitamin C and β-carotene is consistently associated with reduced risk of gastric cancer *(125,134,136–138,140,143,147,148,150,153,156)*. Serological assessment also supports a role. Prospective studies which have evaluated vitamin C are scant because vitamin C deteriorates quickly unless specimens are acid stabilized prior to freezing *(159)*. A large well-conducted cohort study, the Basel study *(160)*, did have such material available. Mean plasma vitamin C was significantly lower in persons who died of cancer than in survivors: 47.61 ± 1.78 μmol/L vs 52.76 ± 0.44 μmol/L, respectively, $p < 0.01$. The findings were also significant ($p < 0.05$) for persons who subsequently died of stomach cancer and their blood levels were even lower, 42.86 ± 4.88. Low plasma levels of vitamin C were associated with a relative risk of 2.38 for gastric cancer. Low plasma levels of carotene were similarly associated with significantly increased risk of overall mortality from cancer ($p < 0.01$) and cancer of the stomach ($p < 0.01$), with a relative risk of 2.95. No association was observed between plasma levels of vitamin A or E and gastric cancer.

Haenszel et al. *(161)* measured serum micronutrient levels in persons with various premalignant gastric lesions. Carotene levels in both men and women and vitamin E levels in men were significantly lower in subjects with gastric dysplasia than in subjects with normal mucosa or less advanced lesions.

A recent report from Japan *(162)* evaluated prediagnostic serum selenium and zinc levels and found no excess risk of stomach cancer in those with the lowest levels of selenium (OR=1.0) or zinc (OR=1.2).

The most compelling evidence to date for specific micronutrients in chemoprevention of gastric cancer comes from the previously described population trial in China *(57)* that found a significant reduction in stomach cancer mortality among persons taking a combination of β-carotene, vitamin E, and selenium. No reduction in risk was observed among persons taking vitamin C; however, there was no attempt in this trial to

Table 2
Selected Epidemiological Studies of Diet and Stomach Cancer Risk

Study (reference)	Population	Number of cases/ controls or cohort size	Food or nutrient	Relative risk, high vs low intake
Case-Control				
Meinsma (140)	Holland	340/1060	Vitamin C	Inverse association
				$p=.01$ males
			Citrus fruit	$p=.001$ females
Higginson (141)	United States	93/279	Dairy foods	0.6
			Fresh fruits	Inverse association
			Raw vegetables	Inverse association
Haenszel et al. (142)	Japanese in Hawaii	220/440	Tomatoes	0.4 ($p < .05$)
			Celery	0.4 ($p < .05$)
			Corn	0.5 ($p < .05$)
			Onion	0.5 ($p < .05$)
			Lettuce	0.8 (NS)
			Western vegetables combined	0.4 ($p < .05$)
Graham et al. (105)	United States	276/2200	Lettuce	0.64 (trend < 0.01)
Bjelke (143)	Norway and United States	162/1394 (Norway)	Vegetable index (Norway)	Inverse association (Norway & United) States
		259/1657 (United States)	Vitamin C	Inverse association (Norway & United States)
			Fruits & vegetables (United States)	Inverse association (Norway & United States)
Haenszel et al. (144)	Japan	783/1566	Fruit	0.7 ($p < 0.05$)
			Plum and pineapple	0.7 ($p < 0.01$)
			Celery	0.6 ($p < 0.01$)
			Lettuce	0.7 ($p < 0.01$)
Correa et al. (125)	United States	391/391	Vitamin C	0.50 (trend $p < 0.05$) whites
				0.33 (trend $p < 0.001$) blacks
			Fruit index	0.47 (trend $p < 0.005$) whites
				0.33 (trend $p < 0.001$) blacks
			Vegetable index	0.50 (trend $p < 0.05$) blacks
			Smoked foods	1.98 (trend $p < 0.025$) blacks

44

(continued)

Reference	Country	Cases/Controls	Factor	OR (CI / p)
Risch et al. (134)	Canada	246/246	Vitamin C	0.43 (trend $p = 0.099$)
			Citrus fruit	0.75 (trend $p = 0.006$)
			Nitrite	2.61 (1.61–4.22)
			Carbohydrates	1.53 (1.07–2.18)
Trichopoulos et al. 145	Greece	110/100	Lemons	0.24 (trend $p < 0.01$)
			Oranges	0.33 (trend $p < 0.01$)
			Pasta	3.42 (trend $p < 0.001$)
			Brown bread	0.79 (trend $p < 0.01$)
			Onions	0.68 (trend $p < 0.001$)
Tajima and Tominaja (122)	Japan	93/186	Oranges	0.9 (NS)
			Other fruit	1.4 (NS)
			Spinach	2.5 ($p < 0.05$)
			Cabbage	2.2 ($p < 0.01$)
			Green pepper	2.0 ($p < 0.01$)
Jedrychowski et al. (146)	Poland	110/110	Fruit	0.3 (0.1–0.6)
			Vegetables	0.6 (0.3–1.4)
LaVecchia et al. (147)	Italy	206/474	Vitamin C	0.46 ($p < 0.001$)
			Fruits, index	0.53 (trend $p < 0.01$)
			Citrus fruit	0.58 (trend $p < 0.01$)
			Green vegetables index	0.33 (trend $p < 0.01$)
			Ham	1.6 ($p = 0.04$)
			Polenta	2.32 ($p = 0.007$)
			β-Carotene	0.39 ($p < 0.001$)
You et al. (148)	China	564/1131	Vitamin C	0.5 (0.3–0.6)
			Fresh fruit	0.4 (0.3–0.6)
			Fresh vegetables	0.6 (0.4–0.8)
Buiatti et al. (149)	Italy	1016/1159	Raw vegetables	0.6 (trend $p < 0.001$)
			Citrus fruits	0.6 (trend $p < 0.001$)
			Other fresh fruits	0.4 (trend $p < 0.001$)
Graham et al. (150)	United States	293/293	Raw vegetables	0.43 (0.23–0.78)
			Fruits	No association
			Vitamin C	No association
			Carotene	0.79 (0.63–0.98)
			Sodium	1.51 (1.20–1.91)
			Retinol	1.47 (1.17–1.85)

Table 2
Continued

Study (reference)	Population	Number of cases/ controls or cohort size	Food or nutrient	Relative risk, high vs low intake
Chyou et al. (135)	Japanese in Hawaii	111/361	Fat	1.37 (1.08–1.74)
			Vegetable index	0.7 (p-trend < 0.001)
			Fruit index	0.8 (p-trend = 0.20)
			Nitrite	No association
Buiatti et al. (136)	Italy	1016/1159	vitamin C	0.5 (p-trend < 0.001)
			α-Tocopherol	0.6 (p-trend < 0.01)
			β-Carotene	0.6 (p-trend < 0.01)
			Protein	2.6 (p-trend < 0.001)
			Nitrites	1.9 (p-trend < 0.001)
Wu-Williams et al. (151)	United States	137/137	Fruit index	0.7 (N.S.)
			Beef	1.6 (1.0–2.6)
Buiatti et al. (137)	Italy	923/1159	Vitamin C	0.5 (0.3–0.6) intestinal type
				0.5 (0.3–0.7) diffuse type
			Citrus fruits	0.5 (0.4–0.7) intestinal type
				0.6 (0.4–0.9) diffuse type
			Other fresh fruits	0.5 (0.4–0.7) intestinal type
				0.4 (0.3–0.6) diffuse type
			Raw vegetables	0.6 (0.4–0.8) intestinal type
				0.6 (0.4–0.9) diffuse type
			α-Tocopherol	0.5 (0.3–0.8) intestinal type
				0.5 (0.2–0.8) diffuse type
			β-Carotene	0.7 (0.5–0.8) intestinal type
				0.6 (0.4–0.7) diffuse type
			Nitrites	1.8 (1.2–2.8) intestinal type
				2.8 (1.5–5.0) diffuse type
			Protein	2.4 (1.02–5.6) intestinal type
				5.8 1.8–1.84) diffuse type
Negri et al. (152)	Italy	564/6147	Green vegetables	0.4 (0.3–0.6) (p-trend < 0.001)
			Fruit	0.4 (0.3–0.5) (p-trend < 0.001)

Reference	Country	Cases/Controls	Food/nutrient	Result
Boeing et al. (153)	Germany	143/579	Vitamin C	0.37 (p-trend < 0.01)
			Citrus fruit	0.46 (p-trend < 0.01)
			Cheese	0.44 (p-trend < 0.01)
			Processed meat	1.74 (p-trend < 0.01)
			Whole wheat bread	0.37 (p-trend < 0.001)
Gonzalez et al. (154)	Spain	354/354	Cooked vegetables	0.5 (p-trend = 0.02)
			Noncitrus fresh fruits	0.6 (p-trend = 0.006)
			Dried fruits	0.4 (0.2–0.8)
Hoshiyama and Sasaba (155)	Japan	251/483	Meat	0.6 (p-trend = 0.02)
			Fruits	Inverse association
			Raw vegetables	Inverse association
			Pickled vegetables	Increased risk
LaVecchia et al. (156)	Italy	723/2024	β-Carotene	0.38 (p-trend < 0.001)
			Vitamin C	0.53 (p-trend < 0.001)
			Methionine	2.40 (p-trend < 0.001)
Lee et al. (123)	Korea	213/213		
Hansson et al. (157)	Sweden		Total vegetables	0.58 (0.37–0.89) (p-trend = 0.01)
			Citrus fruits	0.49 (0.29–0.81) (p-trend = 0.004)
Hansson et al. (138)	Sweden		Vitamin C	0.47 (0.30–0.76) (p-trend = 0.003)
			β-Carotene	0.73 (0.45–1.18) (p-trend = 0.10)
			Nitrates	0.97 (0.60–1.59) (p-trend = 0.99)
Lopez-Carrillo et al. (158)	Mexico	220/752	Chili peppers (ever, never)	5.49 (2.72–11.06)
			Chili peppers (high vs none)	17.11 (7.78–37.59)
Gonzales et al. (139)	Spain	354/354	Nitrosomines	2.1 (p-trend = 0.007)
			Fiber	0.35 (p-trend < 0.001)
			Folate	0.50 (p-trend = 0.008)
			Vitamin C	0.58 (p-trend = 0.017)
Cohort				
Nomura et al. (111)	Japanese in Hawaii	150/7990	Fruit index	0.8 (0.5–1.3)
			Fried vegetables	0.8 (0.4–1.6)
Kneller et al. (112)	United States	75/17,633	Fruit index	1.5 (p-trend, NS)
			Vegetable index	0.9 (p-trend, NS)
			Carbohydrates	1.6 (p-trend < 0.05)

Table 3
Dietary Recommendations of Selected Health Agencies

Agency	Obesity	Fat	Fruits and vegetables	Dietary fiber	Alcohol	Sodium/cured foods
American Cancer Society, 1990	Avoid obesity	Cut down on total fat intake	Include a variety of vegetables and fruits in the daily diet	Eat more high fiber foods, such as whole grain cereals, vegetables, and fruits	Limit consumption of alcoholic beverages, if you drink at all	Limit consumption of salt-cured, smoked, and nitrite-cured food
National Cancer Institute, 1987	Avoid obesity	Reduced fat intake to no more than 30% of total calories	Include a variety of fruits and vetetables in the daily diet	Increase fiber intake to 20–30 g, not to exceed 35 g daily	Consume alcoholic beverages in moderation, if at all	Minimize consumption of salt-cured, salt-pickled, and smoked foods
American Heart Association, 1988	Achieve and maintain desirable weight	Reduce fat to no more than 30% of total calories; polyunsaturated and saturated fat each provide no more than 10% of total calories; up to 300 mg of cholesterol daily	At least 50% of total calories should be provided by carbohydrates, especially complex carbohydrates		No more than 1–2 oz daily	Up to 3000 mg of sodium daily

eradicate *H. pylori*, which is known to decrease the concentration of ascorbic acid in gastric juice, either by increased oxidation, impaired secretion from blood into the gastric cavity, or both *(96–99)*.

4. RECOMMENDATIONS

Primary prevention of esophageal cancer obviously begins with prevention of tobacco use by teenagers and cessation among addicted adults. Use of nicotine patches and gum in conjunction with behavioral modification may improve the success rate for smokers attempting to quit. A reduction in tobacco use by teenagers has proven a persistent challenge because education programs are offset by well-funded, effective, targeted marketing by tobacco companies. Limiting alcohol consumption to moderate levels is particularly important in smokers, and physicians should actively counsel patients accordingly. Physician prompting and participation in smoking cessation efforts has proven effective.

Intake of fresh fruits and vegetables in the United States continues to fall short of the recommended "5-A-Day" *(163)*. Increased consumption should continue to be promoted, and benefits are expected to accrue in reduced rates of both of these upper digestive tract cancers as well as other epithelial tumors. Effective population-based approaches are important, and since dietary patterns are often established in childhood, promotion of healthy choices in school-based food service programs is an opportunity that should not be missed.

The current dietary recommendations of the American Cancer Society, the American Heart Association, and the National Cancer Institute are remarkably similar in direction, but differ in specificity. They are included for reference in Table 3.

The efficacy of vitamin/mineral supplements has not yet been established in clinical trials; however, in case-control and cohort studies the individuals in the highest level of intake of specific micronutrients often combine high dietary intake with supplements. With the obvious caution to avoid excessive intake, a multivitamin/mineral supplement or specific antioxidant supplement may complement dietary intake, particularly among persons with excessive oxidative stress, such as smokers.

Treatment and eradication of *H. pylori* is currently recommended only for persons with gastric and duodenal ulcers, but not for persons with nonulcer dyspepsia *(164)*. Although the spectrum of clinical outcomes associated with *H. pylori* infection is wide-ranging, from asymptomatic to gastric cancer, treatment and eradication of infection when possible seems prudent because the cofactors that predispose an infected individual to gastric cancer have not yet been established.

REFERENCES

1. Cancer Facts and Figures. American Cancer Society, Atlanta, GA; 1995, p. 6.
2. Moses FM. Squamous cell carcinoma of the esophagus. Natural history, incidence, etiology and complications. Gastroenterol Clin North Am 1991; 20:703–716, 1991.
3. Blot WJ, Devesa SS, Kneller RW, Fraumeni JF Jr. Rising incidence of adenocarcinoma of the esophagus and gastric cardia. JAMA 1991; 265:1287–1289.
4. Day NE, Muñoz N. Oesophagus. In: Cancer Epidemiology and Prevention. Schottenfeld D, Fraumeni JF, eds. Philadelphia: WB Saunders Co, 1982, 596–623.
5. Wynder EL, Bross IJ. A study of etiologic factors in cancer of the esophagus. Cancer 1961; 14:389–413.
6. Tuyns AJ, Pequinot G, Jenson OM. Le cancer de l'oesophage en Ille et Vilaine en fonction des niveaux de consommation d'alcool et de tabac. Des risques qui se multiplient. Bull Cancer 1977; 64:45–60.

7. Saracci R. The interactions of tobacco smoking and other agents in cancer etiology. Epid Rev 1987; 9:175–193.
8. Barón AE, Franceschi S, Barra S, Talamini R, LaVecchia C. A comparison of the joint effects of alcohol and smoking on the risk of cancer across sites in the upper aerodigestive tract. Cancer Epi Biomarkers Prev 1993; 2:519–523.
9. Franceschi S, Bidoli E, Negri E, Barbone F, LaVecchia C. Alcohol and cancers of the upper aerodigestive tract in men and women. Cancer Epid Biomarkers Prev 1994; 3:299–304.
10. Blume SB. Women and alcohol. A review. JAMA 1986; 256:1467–1470.
11. Hanaoka T, Tsugane S, Ando N, Ishida K, Kakegawa T, Isono K, et al. Alcohol consumption and risk of esophageal cancer in Japan: a case-control study in seven hospitals. Jpn J Clin Oncol 1994; 24(5):241–246.
12. Watson WL. Carcinoma of oesophagus. Surg Gynecol Obstet 1993; 56:884–897.
13. Kwan KW. Carcinoma of the esophagus, a statistical study. Chin Med J 1937; 52:237–254.
14. Iran—IARC Study Group. Esophageal cancer studies in the Caspian littoral of Iran: results of populations studies. A prodrome. J Natl Cancer Inst. 1977; 59:1127–1138.
15. Kolicheva NI. Epidemiology of esophagus cancer in the USSR. In: Levin D, ed. Joint USA/USSR Monograph on Cancer Epidemiology in the USA and USSR; 1980.
16. Martinez I. Factors associated with cancer of the esophagus, mouth and pharynx in Puerto Rico. J Natl Cancer Inst 1969; 42:1069–1094.
17. Segi M. Tea-gruel as a possible factor for cancer of the esophagus. Gann 1975; 66:199–202.
18. Hirayama T. An epidemiological study of cancer of the esophagus in Japan, with special reference to the combined effect of selected environmental factors. In: Monograph No. 1, Seminar on Epidemiology of Oesophageal Cancer, Bangalore, India, November 1971, pp. 45–60.
19. DeStefani E, Muñoz N, Esteve J, Vasallo A, Victora CG, Teuchmann S. Maté drinking, alcohol, tobacco, diet and esophageal cancer in Uruguay. Cancer Res 1990; 50:426–431.
20. Victora CG, Muñoz N, Day NE, Barcelos LB, Peccin DA, Braga NM. Hot beverages and esophageal cancer in southern Brazil: a case-control study. Int J Cancer 1987; 39:710–716.
21. Castelletto R, Catellsague X, Muñoz N, Iscovich J, Chopita N, Jmelnitsky A. Alcohol, tobacco, diet, maté drinking and esophageal cancer in Argentina. Cancer Epid Biomarkers Prev 1994; 3:557–564.
22. Wahrendorf J, Chang-Claude J, Liang QS, Rei YG, Muñoz N, Crespi M, Raedsch R, Thurnham D, Correa P. Precursor lesions of oesophageal cancer in young people in a high-risk population in China. Lancet 1989; 2(8674):1239–1241.
23. Miller RW. Epidemiology. In: Cancer in China. Kaplan HS and Tschitani PJ, eds. New York: Liss, 1978; 38–57.
24. Mettlin C, Graham S. Dietary risk factors in human bladder cancer. Am J Epidemiol 1979; 11:255–263.
25. De Jong UW, Breslow N, Goh Ewe Hong J, Sridhara M, Shanmugaratnan K. Aetiological factors in oesophageal cancer in Singapore Chinese. Int J Cancer 1974; 13:291–303.
26. Cook-Mozaffari PJ, Azordegan F, Day NE, Ressicaud A, Sabai C, Aramesh B. Oesophageal cancer studies in the Caspian Littoral in Iran: results of a case-control study. Br J Cancer 1979; 39:293–309.
27. Mettlin C, Graham S, Priore R, Marshall J, Swanson M. Diet and cancer of the esophagus. Nutr Cancer 1979; 2:143–147.
28. Graham S, Marshall J, Haughey B, Brasure J, Freudenheim J, Zielezny M, Wilkenson G, Nolan J. Nutritional epidemiology of cancer of the esophagus. Am J Epidemiol 1990; 131:454–467.
29. Ziegler RG, Morris LE, Blot WJ, Pottern LM, Hoover R, Fraumeni JF Jr. Esophageal cancer among black men in Washington, D.C: II. Role of nutrition. J Nat Cancer Inst 1981; 67:1199–1206.
30. Tuyns AJ. Protective effect of citrus fruit on esophageal cancer. Nutr Cancer 1983; 5:195–200.
31. Tuyns AJ, Riboli E, Doombos G, Pequignot G. Diet and esophageal cancer in Calvados (France). Nutr Cancer 1987; 9:81–92.
32. De Carli A, Liati P, Negri E, Franceschi S, LaVechhia C. Vitamin A and other dietary factors in the etiology of esophageal cancer. Nutr Cancer 1987; 10:29–37.
33. Notani PN, Jayant K. Role of diet in upper aerodigestive tract cancer. Nutr Cancer 1987; 10:29–37.
34. Brown LM, Blot WJ, Schuman SH, Smith VM, Ershow AG, Marks RD, Fraumeni JF Jr. Environmental factors and a high risk of esophageal cancer among men in coastal South Carolina. J Natl Cancer Inst 1988; 80:1620–1625.
35. Yu MC, Garabrant DH, Peters JM, Mack T. Tobacco, alcohol, diet, occupation, and carcinoma of the esophagus. Cancer Res 1988; 48:3843–3848.

36. Li JY, Ershow AG, Chen ZJ, Wacholder S, Li GY, Guo W, Li B, Blot WJ. A case-control study of cancer of the esophagus and gastric cardia in Linxian. Int J Cancer 1989; 43:755–761.
37. Block G. Vitamin C and cancer prevention: the epidemiologic evidence. Am J Clin Nutr 1991; 53:270S–282S.
38. Cheng KK, Day NE, Duffy SW, Lam TH, Fok M, Wong J. Pickled vegetables in the aetiology of oesophageal cancer in Hong Kong Chinese. Lancet 1992; 339:1314–1318.
39. Yu Y, Taylor PR, Li J-Y, Dawsey SM, Wang G-Q, Guo W-D, Wang W, Liu B-Q, Blor WJ, Shen Q, Li B. Retrospective sohort study of risk factors for esophageal cancer in Linxian, People's Republic of China. Cancer Causes Control 1993; 4:195–202.
40. Tavani A, Negri E, Franceschi S, LaVecchia C. Risk factors for esophageal cancer in lifelong nonsmokers. Cancer Epidemiol Biomarkers Prev 1994; 3:387–392.
41. Jain AK, Shimoi K, Nakamura Y, Kada T, Hara Y, Tomita I. Crude tea extracts decrease the mutagenic activity of N-methyl-N'-nitrosoguanidine in vitro and in intragastric tract of rats. Mutat Res 1989; 210:1–8.
42. Ito Y, Ohnishi S, Fujie K. Chromosome aberrations induced by aflatoxin B in rat bone marrow cells in vivo and their suppresion by green tea. Mutat Res 1989; 222:253–261.
43. Sasaki YF, Imanishi H, Ohta T, Watanabe M, Matsumoto K, Shirasu Y. Supressing effect of tannic acid on the frequencies of mutagen-induced sister-chromatid exchanges in mammalian cells. Mutat Res 1989; 213:195–203.
44. Stich HF, Rosin MP. Naturally occurring phenolics as antimutagenic and anticarcinogenic agents. Ad Exp Med Biol 1984; 177:1–29.
45. Gao YT, McLaughlin JK, Blot WJ, Ji BT, Dai Q, Fraumeni JF Jr. Reduced risk of esophageal cancer associated with green tea consumption. J Natl Cancer Inst 1994; 86(11):855–858.
46. Yun T-K, Yun Y-S, Han H-H. Anticarcinogenetic effect of long-term oral administration of red ginseng on newborn mice exposed to various chemical carcinogens. Cancer Detect Prev 1983; 6:515–525.
47. Yun T-K, Kim S-H, Lee Y-S. Trial of a new medium-term model using benzo(a)pyrene induced lung tumor in newborn mice. Anticancer Res 1995; 15 (No. 3):839–845.
48. Yun T-K, Choi S-Y. Protective effect of ginseng intake against various human cancers: a case-control study on 1987 pairs. Cancer Epid Biomarkers Prev 1995; 4:401–408.
49. Chen J, Geissler C, Parpia B, Li J, Campbell TC. Antioxidant status and cancer mortality in China. Int J Epidemiol 1992; 21:625–635.
50. Thurnham DI, Rathakette P, Hambidge KM, Muñoz N, Crespi M. Riboflavin, vitamin A, and zinc status in Chinese subjects in a high-risk area for oesophageal cancer. Hum Nutr Clin Nutr 1982; 36C:337–349.
51. Rogers MAM, Thomas DB, Davis S, Vaughan TL, Nevissi AE. A case-control study of element levels and cancer of the upper aerodigestive tract. Cancer Epid Biomarkers Prev 1993; 2:305–312.
52. Sporn M, Newton DL. Chemoprevention of cancer with reinoids. Fed Proc 1979; 38:2528–2534.
53. Muñoz N, Wahrendorf J, Fian-Bang L, Crespi M, Thurnham DI, Day NE, Jiz H, Grassi A, Yan LW, Lin LG, Quan LY, Yun ZC, Fang ZS, Yao LJ, Correa P, O'Connor GT, Bosch X. No effect of riboflavine, retinol and zinc on prevalence of precancerous lesions of esophagus. Lancet 1985; 2:111–114.
54. Muñoz N, Hayashi M, Jian-Bang L, Wahrendorf J, Crespi M, Boxch FX. Effect of riboflavine, retinol and zinc on micronuclei of buccal mucosa and esophagus: a randomized double-blind intervention study in China. J Natl Cancer Inst 1987; 79:687–691.
55. Wahrendorf J, Muñoz N, Jiang-Bang L, Thurnham DI, Crespi M, Bosch FX. Blood, retinol and zinc riboflavine status in relation to precancerous lesions of the esophagus: findings from a vitamin intervention trial in the People's Republic of China. Cancer Res 1988; 48:2280–2283.
56. Li J-Y, Taylor PR, Li B, Dawsey S, Wang GQ, Ershaw AG, Guo W, Liu S-F, Yang CS, Shen Q, Wang W, Mark SD, Zuo X-N, Greenwald P, Wu Y-P, Blot WJ. Nutrition intervention trials in Linxian, China: multiple vitamin/mineral supplementation, cancer incidence, and disease specific mortality among adults with esophageal dysplasia. J Natl Cancer Inst 1993; 85:1492–1498.
57. Blot WJ, Li J-Y, Talor PR, Guo W, Daysey S, Wang G-Q, Yang CS, Zheng SE, Gail M, Li G-Y, Yu Y, Lui B, Tangrea J, Sun Y, Liu F, Fraumeni JF Jr, Zhang Y-H, Li B. Nutrition intervention trials in Linxian, China. Supplementation with specific vitamin/mineral combinations, cancer incidence and disease specific mortality in the general population. J Natl Cancer Inst 1993; 85:1483–1492.
58. Wang G-Q, Dawsey SM, Li J-Y, Taylor PR, Li B, Blot WJ, Weinstein WM, Liu F-S, Lewin KJ, Wang H, Wiggett S, Gail MH, Yang CS. Effects of vitamin/mineral supplementation on the prevalence of histological dysplasia and early cancer of the esophagus and stomach: results from the general population trial in Linxian, China. Cancer Epid Biomarkers Prev 1994; 3:161–166.

59. Dawsey SM, Wang G-Q, Taylor PR, Li J-Y, Blot WJ, Li B, Lewin KJ, Liu F-S, Weinstein WM, Wiggett S, Wang H, Mark SD, Yu Y, Yang CS. Effects of vitamin/mineral supplementation on the prevalence of histological dysplasia and early cancer of the esophagus and stomach: results from the dysplasia trial in Linxian, China. Cancer Epid Biomarkers Prev 1994; 3:167–172.

60. Rao M, Liu F-S, Dawsey SM, Yang K, Lipkin M, Li J-Y, Taylor PR, Li B, Blot WJ, Wang G-Q, Lewin KJ, Yu Y, Yang CS. Effect of vitamin/mineral supplementation on the proliferation of esophagus squamous epithelium in Linxian, China. Cancer Epid Biomarkers Prev 1994; 3:277–279.

61. Barrett NR. Chronic peptic ulcer of the esophagus and "esophagitis." Br J Surg 1950; 38:178–182.

62. Garewal HS, Sampliner R. Barrett's esophagus: a model premalignant lesion for adenocarcinoma. Prev Med 1989; 18:749–756.

63. Sjogren RW, Johnson LF. Barrett's esophagus: a review. Am J Med 1983; 74:313–321.

64. Spechler SJ, Robbins AH, Rubins HB, Vincent ME, Heeren T, Doos WG, Colton T, Schimmel EM. Adenocarcinoma and Barrett's esophagus:an overrated risk? Gastroenterology 1984; 87:927–933.

65. Spechler SJ, Goyal RK. Barrett's esophagus. New Engl J Med 1986; 315:362–271.

66. Hameeteman W, Tytgat GN, Houthoff J, Van den Tweel JG. Barrett's esophagus: development of dysplasia and adenocarcinoma. Gastroenterology 1989; 96:1249–1256.

67. Eng C, Spechler SJ, Ruben R, Li FP. Familial Barrett's esophagus and adenocarcinoma of the gastroesophageal junction. Cancer Epid Biomarkers & Prev 1993; 2:397–399.

68. Crabb DW, Berk MA, Hall TR, Conneally PM, Biegel AA, Lehman GA. Familial gastroesophageal reflux and development of Barrett's esophagus. Am Intern Med 1985; 103:52–54.

69. Joachem VJ, Fuerst PA, Fromkes JJ. Familial Barrett's esophagus associated with adenocarcinoma. Gastroenterology 1992; 102:1400–1402.

70. Wang HH, Hsieh C, Antonioli DA. Rising incidence rate of esophageal adenocarcinoma and use of pharmaceutical agents that relax the lower esophageal sphincter. Cancer Causes Control 1994; 5:573–578.

71. Elder JB, Ganguli PC, Gillespie IE. Cimetidine and gastric cancer. Lancet 1979; 1:1005,1006.

72. Chow W-H, Finkle WD, McLaughlin JK, Frankl H, Ziel HK, Fraumeni J. The relation of esophageal reflux disease and its treatment. JAMA 1995; 274:474–477.

73. Vaughan TL, Davis S, Kristal A, Thomas DB. Obesity, alcohol and tobacco as risk factors for cancers of the esophagus and gastric cardia: adenocarcinoma versus squamous cell carcinoma. Cancer Epid Biomarkers Prev 1995; 4:85–92.

74. Kabat GC, Ng SK, Wynder EL. Tobacco, alcohol intake and diet in relation to adenocarcinoma of the esophagus and gastric cardia. Cancer Causes Control 1993; 4:123–132.

75. Brown LM, Silverman DT, Pottern LM, Schoenberg JB, Greenberg RS, Swanson GM, Liff JM, Schwartz AG, Hayes RB, Blot WJ, Hoover RN. Adenocarcinoma of the esophagus and esophagogastric junction in white men in the United States: alcohol, tobacco and socioeconomic factors. Cancer Causes Control 1994; 5:333–340.

76. Haenszel W. Variation in incidence and mortality from stomach cancer with particular reference to the United States. J Natl Cancer Inst 1958; 21:231–262.

77. Levin DL, Devesa SS, Godwin JD, Silverman DT. Cancer Rates and Risks, 2nd edition, USDHEW, 1974.

78. Devesa SS, Silverman DT. Cancer incidence and mortality trends in the United States: 1935–1974. J Natl Cancer Inst 1978; 60:545–571.

79. Howson CP, Hiyama T, Wynder EL. The decline in gastric cancer: epidemiology of an unplanned triumph. Epidemiol Review 1986; 8:1–27.

80. Nomura A. Stomach. In Cancer Epidemiology and Prevention. Schottenfeld D, Fraumeni JF, eds. Philadelphia: Saunders, 1982; 624–637.

81. Järvi O, Laurén P. On the role of heterotopias of intestinal epithelium in pathogenesis of gastric cancer. Acta Path Microbiol Scand 1951; 29:26–44.

82. Laurén P. The two histological main types of gastric carcinoma: diffuse and so-called intestinal-type carcinoma. An attempt at a histoclinical classification. Acta Pathol Microbiol Scand 1965; 64:31–49.

83. Muñoz N, Correa P, Cuello C, Duque E. Histologic types of gastric cancer in high- and low-risk areas. Int J Cancer 1968; 3:809–818.

84. Pel PK. Ziekten van de Maag (Diseases of the Stomach). Amsterdam: De Erven F Bohn; 1899.

85. Marshall BJ. Unidentified curved bacilli on gastric epithelium in active chronic gastritis. Lancet 1983; 1:1273–1275.

86. Warren JR. Unidentified curved bacilli on gastric epithelium in active chronic gastritis. Lancet 1983; 1:1273.

87. IARC Monographs in the Evaluation of Carcinogenic Risks to Humans. Schistosomes, Liver Flukes and *Helicobacter pylori*. vol 61, World Health Organization, Lyons, France, 1994.
88. Mégraud F. Epidemiology of *Helicobacter pylori* infection. Gastroenterology Clinics of North America 1993; 22:73–88.
89. Parsonnet J. The epidemiology of *C. pylori*. In: *Campylobacter pylori* in Gastritis and Peptic Ulcer Disease. Blaser MJ, ed. New York: Igaku-Shoin, 1989; 51–60.
90. The EuroGast Study Group. An international association between *Helicobacter pylori* infection and gastric cancer. Lancet 1993; 341:1359–1362.
91. The EuroGast Study Group. Epidemiology of, and risk factors for, *Helicobacter pylori* infection among 3194 asymptomatic subjects in 17 populations.
92. Sitas F, Forman D, Yarnell JWG, Burr ML, Elwood PC, Pedley S, Marks KJ. *Helicobacter pylori* infection rates in relation to age and social class in a population of Welsh men. Gut 1991; 32:25–28.
93. Forman D, Newell DG, Fullerton F, Yarnell JWG, Stacey AR, Wald N, Sitas F. Association between infection with *Helicobacter pylori* and risk of gastric cancer: evidence from a prospective investigation. Br Med J 1991; 302:1302–1305.
94. Parsonnet J, Friedman GD, Vandersteen DP, Chang Y, Vogelman JH, Orentreich N, Sibley RK. *Helicobacter pylori* infection and the risk of gastric carcinoma. New Engl J Med 1991; 325:1127–1131.
95. Nomura A, Stemmermann GN, Chyou P-H, Kato I, Pérez-Pérez GI, Blaser MJ. *Helicobacter pylori* infection and gastric carcinoma among Japanese-Americans in Hawaii. New Engl J Med 1991; 325:1132–1136.
96. Sobala GM, Schorah CJ, Sanderson M, Dixon MF, Tompkins DS, Godwin P, Axon ATR. Ascorbic acid in the human stomach. Gastroenterol 1989; 97:357–363.
97. Rathbone BJ, Johnson AW, Wyatt JI, Kelleher J, Heatley RV, Losowsky MS. Ascorbic acid: a factor concentrated in human gastric juice. Clin Sci 1989; 76:237–241.
98. Sobala GM, Pignatelli B, Schorah CJ, Bartsch H, Sanderson M. Levels of nitrite, nitrate, N-nitroso compounds, ascorbic acid and total bile acids in gastric juice of patients with and without precancerous conditions of the stomach. Carcinogenesis 1991; 12:193–198.
99. Ruiz B, Rood JC, Fontham ETH, Malcom GT, Hunter FM, Sobhan M, Johnson WD, Correa P. Vitamin C concentration in gastric juice before and after anti-*Helicobacter pylori* treatment. Am J Gastroenterol 1994; 89:533–539.
100. Wyatt JJ, Rathbone BS. Immune response of the gastric mucosa to *Campylobacter pylori*. Scand J Gastroenterol (Suppl 42) 1988; 23:44–49.
101. Routledge MN, Wink DA, Keefer LK, Dipple A. Mutations induced by saturated acqesus nitric oxide in the pSPI 89 sup F gene in human Ad 293 and E. coli MBM 7070 cells. Carcinogenesis 1993; 14:1251–1254.
102. Rodi R, Beckman JS, Bush KM, Freeman BA. Peroxynitrite oxidation of sulfhydryl. The cytotoxic potential of superoxide and nitric oxide. J Biol Chem 1991; 266:4244–4250.
103. Hirayama T. Epidemiology of stomach cancer. GANN Monogr Cancer Res 1971; 11:3–19.
104. Wynder EL, Kmet J, Dungal N, Segi M. An epidemiologic investigation of gastric cancer. Cancer 1963; 16:1461–1496.
105. Graham S, Schotz W, Martino P. Alimentary factors in the epidemiology of gastric cancer. Cancer 1972; 30:927–938.
106. Acheson ED, Doll R. Dietary factors in carcinoma of the stomach: a study of 100 cases and 200 controls. Gut 1964; 5:126–131.
107. Correa P, Fontham E, Pickle LW, Chen V, Lin Y, Haenszel W. Dietary determinants of gatric cancer in south Louisiana inhabitants. J Natl Cancer Inst 1985; 75:645–654.
108. Wu-Williams AH, Yu MC, Mack TM. Lifestyle, workplace and stomach cancer by subsite in young men of Los Angeles county. Cancer Res 1990; 50:2569–2576.
109. Boeing H, Frentzel-Beyme R, Berger M, Berndt V, Göres W, Körner M, Lohmeier R, Menarcher A, Mänal HFK, Meinhardt M, Müller R, Ostermeier H, Paul F, Schwemmle K, Wagner KH, Wahrendorf J. A case-control study on stomach cancer in Germany. Int J Cancer 1991; 47:858–864.
110. Hoey J, Montvernay C, Lambert R. Wine and tobacco risk factors for stomach cancer in France. Am J Epidemiol 1981; 113:668–674.
111. Nomura A, Grove JS, Stemmermann GN, Severson RK. A prospective study of stomach cancer and its relation to diet, cigarettes and alcohol consumption. Cancer Res 1990; 50:627–631.
112. Kneller RW, McLaughlin JK, Bjelke E, Schuman LM, Blot WJ, Wacholder S, Gridley G, CoChien HT, Fraumeni JF Jr. A cohort study of stomach cancer in a high risk population. Cancer 1991; 68:672–678.

113. Kahn HA. The Dorn study of smoking and mortality among U.S. Veterans: report of 8 1/2 years of observation. Natl Cancer Inst Mongr 1966; 19:1–126.

114. Kinosita R. Studies on factors affecting chemical carcinogenesis of mouse stomach. Gann Monogr 1969; 8:263–268.

115. Tatematsu M, Takahashi M, Fukushima S, Hananouchi M, Shirai T. Effects in rats of sodium chloride on experimental gastric cancer induced by N-methyl-N-nitro-N-nitrosoguanidine or 4-nitroquinoline-1-oxide. J Natl Cancer Inst 1975; 55:101–106.

116. Takahashi M, Kokubo T, Furukawa F. Effects of sodium chloride, saccharin, phenobarbitol and aspirin on gastric carcinogenesis in rats after irritation with N-methyl-N-nitrosoguanidine. Gann 1984; 75:494–501.

117. Kodama M, Kodama T, Suzuki H. Effect of rice and salty rice diets on the structure of mouse stomach. Nutr Cancer 1984; 6:135–147.

118. Mirvish SS. The etiology of gastric cancer: intragastric nitrosamine formation and other theories. J Natl Cancer Inst 1983; 71:631–647.

119. Sato T, Fukuyama T, Suzuki T. Studies of the causation of gastric cancer. The relation between gastric cancer mortality rate and salted food intake in several places in Japan. Bull Inst Publ Health (Jpn) 1959; 8:187–198.

120. Lu J-B, Qin Y-M. Correlation between high salt intake and mortality rates for esophageal and gastric cancers in Henan province, China. Int J Epidemiol 1987; 16:171–176.

121. Buiatti E, Palli D, DeCarli A, Amadori D, Avellini C, Bianchi S, Biserni R, Cipriani F, Cocco P, Giacosa A, Marubini E, Puntoni R, Vindigni C, Fraumeni J Jr, Blot W. Italian multicenter case-control study on gastric cancer and diet. 1. Frequencies of food consumption. Int J Cancer 1989; 44:611–616.

122. Tajima K, Tominaga S. Dietary habits and gastro-intestinal cancers: a comparative case-control study of stomach and large intestinal cancers in Nagoya, Japan. Jpn J Cancer Rest (Gann) 1985; 76:705–716.

123. Lee J-K, Park B-Y, Yoo K-Y, Ahn Y-O. Dietary factors and stomach cancer: a case-control study in Korea. Int J Epidemiol 1995; 24:33–41.

124. Tuyns AJ. Salt and gatrointestinal cancer. Nutr Cancer 1988; 11:229–232.

125. Correa P, Fontham E, Pickle LW, Chen V, Lin Y, Haenszel W. Dietary determinants of gastric cancer in South Louisiana inhabitants. J Natl Cancer Inst 1985; 75:645–654.

126. La Vecchia C, Negri E, DeCarli A, D'Avanzo B, Franceschi S. A case-control study of diet and gastric cancer in northern Italy. Int J Cancer 1987; 40:484–489.

127. Friedman GD, Parsonnet J. Salt intake and stomach cancer: some contrary evidence. Cancer Epid Biomarkers Prev 1992; 1:607–608.

128. Bogovski P, Bogovski S. Animal species in which N-nitroso compounds induce cancer. Int J Cancer 1981; 27:471–474.

129. Correa P, Haenszel W, Cuello C, Tannenbaum S, Archer M. A model for gastric cancer epidemiology. Lancet 1975; 11:58–60.

130. Ohshima H, Bartsch H. Quantitative estimation of endogenous nitrosation in humans by monitoring N-nitroproline excreted in the urine. Cancer Res 1981; 41:3658–3662.

131. Mirvish SS, Gandjean AC, Moller H, Fiki S, Mayard T, Jones L, Rosensky S, Nie G. N-nitrosoproline excretion by rural Nebraskans drinking water of varied nitrate content. Cancer Epid Biomarkers Prev 1992; 1:455–461.

132. Moller H, Landt J, Pederson E, Jenson P, Autrup H, Jenson OM. Endogenous nitrosation in relation to nitrate exposure from drinking water and diet in a Danish rural population. Cancer Res 1989; 49:3117–3121.

133. Sierra R, Chinnock A, Ohshima H, Pignatelli B, Malaveille C, Gamboa C, Teuchmann S, Muñoz N, Bartsh H. In vivo nitrosoproline formation and other risk factors in Costa Rican children from high- and low-risk areas for gastric cancer. Cancer Epid Biomarkers Prev 1993; 2:563–568.

134. Risch HA, Jain M, Choi N, Fodor JG, Pfeiffer CJ, Howe GR, Harrison LW, Craib KJP, Miller AB. Dietary factors and the incidence of cancer of the stomach. Am J Epidemiol 1985; 122:947–959.

135. Chyou PH, Nomura AMY, Hankin J, Stemmermann GN. A case-control study of diet and stomach cancer. Cancer Res 1990; 50:7501–7504.

136. Buiatti E, Palli D, DeCarli A, Amadori D, Avellini C, Bianchi S, Bonaguri C, Cipriani F, Cocco P, Giacosa A, Marubini E, Minacci C, Puntoni R, Russo A, Vindigni C, Fraumeni JF Jr, Blot WJ. A case-control study of gastric cancer and diet in Italy II. Association with nutrients. Int J Cancer 1990; 45:896–901.

137. Buiatti E, Palli D, Bianchi S, DeCarli A, Amadori D, Avellini C, Cipriani F, Cocco P, Giacosa A, Lorenzini L. A case-control study of gastric cancer and diet in Italy III. Risk patterns by histologic type. Int J Cancer 1991; 48:369–374.

138. Hansson L-E, Nyren O, Bergström R, Wolk A, Lindgren A, Baron J, Adami H-O. Nutrients and gastric cancer risk. A population-based case-control study in Sweden. Int J Cancer 1994; 57:638–644.
139. Gonzales CA, Riboli E, Badosa J, Batiste E, Cardona T, Pita S, Sanz JM, Torrent M, Agudo A. Nutritional factors and gastric cancer in Spain. Am J Epidemiol 1994; 139:466–473.
140. Meinsma I. Nutrition and cancer. Voeding 1964; (Cited in Bjelke, 1974) 25:357–365.
141. Higginson J. Etiological factors in gastrointestinal cancer in man. J Natl Cancer Inst 1966; 37:527–545.
142. Haenszel W, Kurihara M, Segi M, Lee RK. Stomach cancer among Japanese in Hawaii. J Natr Cancer Inst 1972; 49:969–988.
143. Bjelke E. Epidemiologic studies of cancer of the stomach, colon and rectum. Scand J Gatroenterol 1974; 9 (Suppl 31):1–235.
144. Haenszel W, Kurihara M, Locke FB, Shimuzu K, Segi M. Stomach cancer in Japan. J Natl Cancer Inst 1976; 56:265–274.
145. Trichopoulos D, Ouranos G, Day NE, Tzonou A, Manousos O, Papadimitriou CH, Trichopoulo A. Diet and cancer of the stomach: a case-control study in Greece. Int J Cancer 1985; 36:291–297.
146. Jedrychowski W, Wahrendorf J, Popiela T, Rachtan J. A case-control study of dietary factors and stomach cancer risk in Poland. Int J Cancer 1986; 37:837–842.
147. La Vecchia C, Negri E, DeCarli A, D'Avanzo B, Franceschi S. A case-control study of diet and gastric cancer in northern Italy. Int J Cancer 1987; 40:484–489.
148. You WC, Blot WJ, Chang YS, Ershow AG, Yang ZT, An Q, Henderson B, Xu GW, Fraumeni JF Jr, Wang TG. Diet and high risk of stomach cancer in Shandong, China. Cancer Res 1988; 48:3518–3523.
149. Buiatti E, Palli D, DeCarli A, Amadori D, Avellini C, Biserni R, Cipriani F, Cocco P, Giacosa A, Marubini E, Puntoni R, Vindigni C, Fraumeni J Jr, Blot WC. A case-control study of gastric cancer and diet in Italy. Int J Cancer 1989; 44:611–616.
150. Graham S, Haughey B, Marshall J, Brasure J, Zielezny M, Freudenheim J, West D, Nolan J, Wilkenson G. Diet in the epidemiology of gastric cancer. Nutr Cancer 1990; 13:19–34.
151. Wu-Williams AH, Yu MC, Mack TM. Life-style, workplace, and stomach cancer by subsite in young men of Los Angeles County. Cancer Res 1990; 50:2569–2576.
152. Negri E, LaVecchia C, D'Avanzo B, Gentile A, Boyle P, Parazzini F. Vegetable and fruit consumption and cancer risk. Int J Cancer 1991; 48:350–354.
153. Boeing H, Frentzel-Beyne R, Berger M, Berndt V, Gores W, Korner M, Lohmeier R, Menarcher A, Mannl H, Meinhardt M, Muller R, Ostermeier H, Paul F, Schwemmle K, Wagner K, Wahrendorf J. Case-control study on stomach cancer in Germany. Int J Cancer 1991; 47:858–864.
154. Gonzalez CA, Sanz JM, Marcos G, Pita S, Brullet E, Saigi E, Badia A, Riboli E. Dietary factors and stomach cancer in Spain: a multicenter case-control study. Int J Cancer 1991; 49:513–519.
155. Hoshiyama Y, Sasabe T. A case-control study of single and multiple stomach cancers in Saitama Prefecture, Japan. Jpn J Cancer Res 1992; 83:937–943.
156. LaVecchia C, Ferreroni M, D'Avanzo B, Di Carli A, Francheschi S. Selected micronutrient intake and the risk of gastric cancer. Cancer Epid Biomarkers Prev 1994; 3:393–398.
157. Hansson L-E, Nyren O, Bergström R, Wolk A, Lindgren A, Baron J, Adami H-O. Diet and risk of gastric cancer. A population-based case-control study in Sweden. Int J Cancer 1993; 55:181–189.
158. Lopez-Carillo L, Avila MH, Dubrow R. Chili pepper consumption and gastric cancer in Mexico: a case-control study. Am J Epidemiol 1994; 139:263–271.
159. Basu TK, Schorah CJ. Vitamin C reserves and requirements in health and disease. In Vitamin C in Health and Disease. West Port, CT. AVI 1982, 62–92.
160. Stähelin HB, Gey KF, Eichholzer M, Lüdin E, Bernasconi F, Thurneysen J, Brubacher G. Plasma antioxidant vitamin and subsequent cancer mortality in the 12-year follow-up of the prospective Basel Study. Am J Epidemiol 1991; 133:766–775.
161. Haenszel W, Corra P, López A, Cuello C, Zarama G, Zavala D, Fontham E. Serum micronutrient levels in relation to gastric pathology. Int J Cancer 1985; 36:43–48.
162. Kabuto M, Imai H, Yonezawa C, Nerüshi K, Akiba S, Kato H, Suzuki T, Land CE, Blot WJ. Prediagnostic serum selenium and zinc levels and subsequent risk of lung and stomach cancer in Japan. Cancer Epidemiol Biomarkers Prev 1994; 3:465–469.
163. Serdula MK, Coates RJ, Byers T, Simoes E, Mokdad AH, Subar AF. Fruit and vegetable intake among adults in 16 states: results of a brief telephone survey. Am J Public Health 1995; 85:236–239.
164. *Helicobacter pylori* in peptic ulcer disease. NIH Consensus Statement 1994; 12(1):1–22.

4 Diet and Nutrition in the Etiology and Primary Prevention of Colon Cancer

Roberd M. Bostick

1. INTRODUCTION

In the United States, cancer is the second leading cause of death, and cancer of the colon and rectum is the second most common cause of cancer mortality *(1)*. It is estimated that most cancers may be preventable, and that 35% of all cancers may be related to diet *(2)*. Ecologic and migration studies indicate the importance of environmental factors in colon cancer *(3)*. Diet appears to have a particularly strong association with occurrence of this cancer *(4,5)* and thus offers promise for intervention. Furthermore, mortality from colon cancer in the United States has not changed substantially over the past 50 years *(6)*, suggesting that prevention may offer the best opportunity to control the disease.

In this chapter on diet and nutrition in the etiology of prevention of colon cancer, factors associated with either increased or decreased risk of this disease are reviewed. Both older, well-established (fat, meat, fiber, vegetables, and fruit) and newer, intriguing, but less well-established (sucrose, calcium, vitamin D, milk products, antioxidants and antioxidant-enzyme associated micronutrients, and folate) hypothesized associations are addressed. The former are covered first, but because they are reviewed extensively elsewhere, are summarized in less detail than the latter. That the newer hypotheses receive more space in the review should not be construed as a suggestion that they are thought more likely to be causal. Alcohol is not reviewed except in context with the folate-colon cancer association.

2. FAT AND MEAT

The hypothesis that dietary meat and/or fat increases risk of colon cancer has been one of the dominant hypotheses related to colon carcinogenesis for the past generation. The observation that higher colon cancer mortality rates occurred in countries where fat and meat consumption was higher led to the hypothesis that these food items contributed to an individual's risk of developing colon cancer and was a stimulus for the current intense interest in dietary intake in most analytic studies of the etiology of colon cancer *(4,5,7,8)*.

Highly plausible explanatory hypotheses have been developed in support of a causal relationship between meat and fat intake and colon cancer (*see* Table 1) and the sup-

From: *Preventive Nutrition: The Comprehensive Guide for Health Professionals*
Edited by A. Bendich and R. J. Deckelbaum Humana Press Inc., Totowa, NJ

Table 1
Potential Mechanisms of Increased Risk of Colon Cancer with High Intakes
of Meat or Fat[a]

Fat increases bile acid production
    Bile acids damage DNA
    Bile acids are toxic to colon cells resulting in compensatory colonic epithelial cell proliferation
    Bile acids in meat eaters vs in vegetarians more readily transformed into potential carcinogens
High fat intake associated with increased oxidative damage
Meat increases fecal iron, which catalyzes oxidative reactions, leading to increased oxidative
    damage
Meat cooked at high temperatures contains higher amounts of carcinogenic heterocyclic amines

---

[a]Potential mechanisms may not be mutually exclusive, and may be additive or synergistic.

portive data from animal and metabolic studies in support of these hypotheses have
been substantial. The oldest hypothesis asserts that fat intake increases bile acid production, ultimately increasing the exposure of the bowel mucosa to the toxic,
trophic, and tumor- or cancer-promoting effects of bile acids (5). High-fat diets increase excretion of bile acids in both animals (9,10) and humans (9,11). Bile acids
have been shown to damage DNA (12). In animals, bile acids have toxic effects on
colon epithelial cells, resulting in compensatory colonic epithelial cell proliferation
(13) and promotion of tumorigenesis (14,15). Also in animals, a high intake of saturated (16,17) and unsaturated fat (17,18) has increased the incidence of chemically
induced colon cancer (although not entirely consistently [19]). In metabolic epidemiologic studies, increased fecal concentrations of bile acids have been found in
populations with higher rates of colon cancer (9,20) as well as in patients with colon
polyps (21) or colon cancer (22,23) (again, not entirely consistently [24]). In animals, the tumor-enhancing effects of bile acids are increased after enzymatic modification by intestinal bacteria (25). Among humans, the capacity of colonic flora
to transform bile acids into potential carcinogens has been found to be greater in
populations with high rates of colon cancer and among meat-eating populations than in
vegetarian populations (9,26). Furthermore, this capacity is reduced when the intake of
beef fat is reduced (26,27).

A more recent hypothesis is the cooked food hypothesis (28), which proposes that the
association with fat is misleading, at least in part. High-fat diets contain greater amounts
of carcinogenic heterocyclic amines (from meat proteins) (29) and promoters as a consequence of cooking at high temperature (cooking in fat produces higher temperatures
than cooking in water) (28). Thus, the argument goes, the meat hypothesis is really the
high temperature: high carcinogens and promoters/low temperature: low carcinogens
and promoters hypothesis. The two explanatory hypotheses are not incompatible and, if
anything, enhance the plausibility of the meat/fat colon cancer association.

A third and very recent hypothesis is that a high consumption of meat, particularly
red meat, may increase fecal concentrations of iron, which catalyzes oxidative reactions, leading to increased lipid peroxidation and oxidative DNA damage, and, as described in more detail in Section 9, to increased risk for colon cancer (30). Also, as discussed in Section 9, a high fat consumption has been associated with increased levels of
oxidative damage.

As reviewed elsewhere *(31)* of 24 analytic epidemiologic studies investigating the meat/colon cancer association (for example, refs. *32–42*), 13 found a direct association (for example, refs. *33,34,37–39*), one an inverse association *(40)* and 11 no definite association (for example, refs. *35,41,42*). The only study to find an inverse association was a prospective mortality study in Japan *(40)*, a society generally at low risk for colon cancer. Only three other prospective studies have examined the association; one, a mortality study in Seventh Day Adventists, reported a null association *(41)*, the second, the Nurses' Health Study *(39)*, reported a direct association, and the third, the Iowa Womens' Health Study, reported a null association *(42)*.

As reviewed elsewhere *(31)*, of 18 studies investigating the fat/colon cancer association 10 found a direct association (for example, refs. *33,34,37–39*), one an inverse association *(43)*, and seven no definite association (for example, refs. *35,42*). The only study to find an inverse association *(43)* was a prospective study of Hawaiians of Japanese descent, another population that has been at low risk for colon cancer. Only two other prospective studies have examined the association; one, the Nurses' Health Study, reported a direct association *(39)* and the second, the Iowa Womens' Health Study, reported a null association *(42)*.

Of interest is that the Nurses' Health Study *(39)*, the Iowa Womens' Health Study *(42)*, and one case-control study *(38)* used essentially the same dietary assessment instrument. The Nurses' Health Study and the Iowa Womens' Health Study are both extant large prospective studies limited to women that used similar statistical techniques in their reported analyses. The Nurses' Health Study, however, was limited to women who were 30- to 55-yr-old registered nurses living in 11 large US states, whereas the Iowa Womens' Health Study was limited to 55- to 69-yr-old women living in a single state but of any employment status or occupation. The case-control study, a 1989 population-based study in Los Angeles, CA limited to 45- to 69-yr-old men and women, found null associations for meat and fat (as did the Iowa Womens' Health Study). Although these three studies differed on statistical significance, directions of associations with meat, types of meat, and fat were fairly consistent across studies. Of further note is that the Iowa Womens' Health Study, the Nurses' Health Study, and several (for example, refs. *34,36*), but not all (for example, ref. *35*) other studies that have investigated different types of meats in relation to colon cancer reported associations that involved higher-fat meats (red meats, processed meats, and so forth) were consistent with increased risk whereas associations that involved fish and/or other seafoods were consistent with decreased risk.

Although associations between fat and meat and colon cancer have now been investigated in over 30 analytic epidemiologic studies *(31,42)*, and although direct associations were found in approximately two-thirds of these studies, findings are too inconsistent to establish causal relationships. Furthermore, as pointed out by Willett et al. *(39,44)* the interpretation of many studies is hampered by the common finding of a direct association between total energy intake and colon cancer risk (for examples, *see* refs. *45–49*), thus raising uncertainty whether it is the total amount of food consumed or the fat or meat components of the diet that is etiologically important. Differences in the findings of the many studies may be because of differences in study designs, populations (for a good illustration, *see* Whittemore et al. *[50]*), different ranges of dietary intake across populations, dietary assessment methodologies, and analysis procedures (including energy adjustment techniques and groupings of meat and fat). Null associations in many studies may be related to dietary homogeneity within populations and the lack of accuracy of currently available dietary assessment instruments. Another possibility related to population differences and the inconsistent findings regarding the meat/colon cancer association is that yet unidentified high-risk subgroups may be driving the association, and these subgroups may be differentially proportionately represented across study populations. For example, perhaps only subpopulations with a specific genetic susceptibility to colon cancer (51) and/or those with the fast acetylator genotype (52), are sufficiently susceptible to colon cancer to suffer a higher incidence of the disease with consumption of higher intakes of meats that have been cooked at high temperatures.

Opposite findings within many studies for higher-fat meats (increased risk) vs fish or seafoods (decreased risk) may have etiologic implications and suggest the need to investigate more vigorously various meat groupings. For example, if the mechanism of the hypothesized meat/colon cancer relationship is more a matter of low-fat meats vs high-fat meats, then the bile acid explanatory hypothesis may be more tenable than the cooked-meat hypothesis. Alternative explanations, however, include other unidentified or accounted for healthy behaviors associated with low-fat meat consumption, potential protective effects of omega-3 fatty acids in seafoods (for example, omega-3 fatty acids have reduced colonic epithelial cell proliferation in a small clinical trial in humans [53]), and different cooking methods associated with red meats vs seafoods.

3. FIBER

The hypothesis that fiber decreases the risk of colon cancer, has, in addition to the fat hypothesis, been one of the dominant hypotheses related to colon carcinogenesis for over a quarter of a century. The idea was first proposed by Burkitt in 1969 based on his clinical observations that colon cancer appeared to be rare in Africans whose diets were high in unrefined foods (54). As reviewed elsewhere (55), mechanistic hypotheses (see Table 2) include that fiber, which comes primarily from plant foods:

1. increases stool bulk, diluting the opportunity for fecal mutagens to contact the colon mucosa;
2. decreases stool transit time, thus providing less time for fecal mutagens to contact the colon mucosa;
3. binds or dilutes bile acids, thereby reducing their toxic, trophic, and promoting effects (see discussion of bile acids in Section 2);
4. ferments to volatile fatty acids that may be anticarcinogenic;
5. ferments to volatile fatty acids that decrease pH, thereby reducing the conversion of primary to secondary bile acids and reducing the solubility of free bile acids, thus decreasing their availability for cocarcinogenic activity;
6. ferments, thus leading to the release of bound calcium (see implications for this in Section 6);
7. binds carcinogens; and
8. induces different patterns of colonic bacteria, thus influencing types and degrees of metabolic reactions.

It is becoming more apparent, however, that looking at dietary fiber as a single entity may be misleading and oversimplifying the fiber-colon cancer association. Fiber classifications that may be important etiologically include nonstarch polysaccharides (cellulose, hemicelluloses, pectin, gums, mucilages) vs nonpolysaccharides (lignin), water-

Table 2
Potential Colon Anticarcinogenic Mechanisms of Dietary Fiber[a]

Increases stool bulk, diluting fecal mutagens
Decreases stool transit time, decreasing fecal mutagen contact time
Binds or dilutes bile acids
Binds or dilutes carcinogens
Ferments
   to volatile fatty acids that are potentially anticarcinogenic
   to volatile fatty acids that decrease pH that reduces conversion of primary to secondary bile
     acids and reduces solubility, thus carcinogenic activity, of free bile acids
   leading to release of bound calcium, which may bind bile acids
Induces different patterns of colonic bacteria

  [a]Potential mechanisms may not be mutually exclusive, and may be additive or synergistic.

soluble (pectin, gums, mucilages, and some hemicelluloses) vs water-insoluble (cellulose, lignin, and most hemicelluloses), fermentable vs nonfermentable, cereal vs vegetable, and so forth. For example, cellulose and wheat bran have been shown to decrease fecal bile acid concentrations, whereas oat and corn bran have been shown to increase concentrations. Insoluble fiber tends to increase fecal bulk and decrease transit time, whereas soluble fiber has less effect. (Cellulose is found primarily in root and leafy green vegetables and legumes; hemicellulose primarily in cereal brans; pectin in fruit, and gums in legumes and oats.)

Furthermore, results of animal studies involving fiber feeding and colon cancer have been mixed *(55–57)*. Part of the inconsistency may be caused by feeding different types of fiber. Wheat bran, although not in every study, has been the fiber most consistently providing an apparent protective effect. Results of studies of oat bran, corn bran, and pectin have been more mixed.

The results of observational epidemiologic studies of fiber and colon cancer have been mixed *(55,58,59)*, but generally supportive of the fiber-colon cancer hypothesis. Of 13 case-control studies assessing fiber intake as a specific dietary constituent, five provided strong support for a protective effect, four provided moderate support, two no support, and two suggested an increased risk with increased fiber intake. However, in a recent meta-analysis of 13 case-control studies (using original data) *(60)*, an approximate halving of risk was found for those in the highest quintile of fiber intake compared to those in the lowest quintile (p for trend < 0.0001). The results of two prospective cohort studies in women *(39,61)* have not provided strong support for dietary fiber, on the whole, as being protective against colon cancer. In the Nurses Health Study *(39)*, total dietary fiber, vegetable fiber, and cereal fiber were not associated with risk. However, decreasing risk with increasing intake of fruit fiber was observed with an odds ratio of 0.6 (confidence interval [CI] 95% 0.4–1.1) for the highest compared to the lowest quintile of intake. In the Iowa Women's Health Study *(61)*, total dietary fiber was not associated with risk, although the relative risk for cancer of the distal colon was 0.66 (CI 95%: 0.34–1.29) for the highest quartile compared to the lowest, but there was no suggestion of a dose-response.

On the whole, then, the idea that at least some types of dietary fiber may afford protection against colon cancer is highly plausible, and the animal experimental and human observational literature is generally supportive of the hypothesis. Much work needs to be done to sort out which type(s) of fiber, if any, are protective in animals; and to include valid estimates of intake of different fiber types in observational epidemiologic studies.

4. VEGETABLES AND FRUIT

As reviewed more extensively elsewhere *(55)*, vegetables and fruit contain a myriad of potentially anticarcinogenic compounds, and as a food group have been more consistently associated with risk (a reduced risk) of colon cancer than any other dietary factor. Potential anticarcinogenic agents in plants *(see* Table 3) include fiber (reviewed in Section 3.), antioxidants and antioxidant enzyme-associated micronutrients (reviewed further in Section 9.), and folate (reviewed in Section 10.). Other potential anticarcinogenic compounds (reviewed briefly in this section) for which there has of yet been little study (including no clinical trials) in humans include: dithiolthiones, glucosinolates and indoles, isothiocyanates and thiocyanates, coumarins, flavonoids, phenols, protease inhibitors, plant sterols, isoflavones, saponins, inositol hexaphosphate, allium compounds, and limonene.

Plant potential anticarcinogenic compounds, including the lesser studied ones, have both complementary and overlapping mechanisms of action, including the induction of detoxification enzymes, inhibition of nitrosamine formation, provision of substrate for formation of antineoplastic agents, dilution and binding of carcinogens in the digestive tract, alteration of hormone metabolism, antioxidant effects, and others. Dithiolthiones are present in cruciferous vegetables; when administered to animals increase levels of glutathione and increase activities of glutathione reductase, glutathione transferase, quinone reductase, glucose-6-phosphate dehydrogenase, and 6-phosphogluconate dehydrogenase; and are thought to protect against cancer by blocking the reaction of electrophilic carcinogens with cellular macromolecules (the mechanism probably depends on the induction of glutathione and the related conjugation enzymes) *(55,62,63)*. Glucosinolates and indoles are both present in cruciferous vegetables and some of these compounds increase microsomal mixed-function oxidase activity, which can lead to either activation or detoxification of carcinogenic compounds, the aggregate effect of which appears to be anticarcinogenic *(55,64)*. Indoles have been found to protect against a variety of tumors in animals *(55)*. Isothiocyanates and thiocyanates are present in cruciferous vegetables, inhibit DNA methylation, induce Phase II xenobiotic-metabolizing enzymes such as glutathione S-transferase, and have been shown to be inhibitors of both early and late stages of carcinogenesis in animals *(55,63)*. Coumarins are found in vegetables and citrus fruits, induce glutathione S-transferase activity, and have inhibited tumor formation in animals *(55,63)*. Flavonoids (for example, quercetin and others) are found in most vegetables and fruits; have antioxidant properties (see more on antioxidants in Section 9.), influence mixed-function oxidase activity, and have produced mixed results in animal anticarcinogenesis experiments *(55)*. Phenols are found in a variety of vegetables and fruits; some are also classified as antioxidants, flavonoids, or coumarins (others are not) and induce detoxification enzymes (Phase II conjugation reactions), whereas others inhibit *N*-nitrosation reactions and have been found to decrease tumors in animals. Protease inhibitors are widely distributed in plants, but are particularly abundant in seeds, legumes, potatoes, and sweet corn; they competitively inhibit proteases by forming complexes that block or otherwise affect their cat-

Table 3
Potentially Anticarcinogenic Constituents of Vegetables and Fruit[a]

Constituents	Common plant sources	Potential anticarcinogenic mechanisms
Fiber	All plants	See Table 2
Antioxidants	All plants	Protect against oxidative damage
Folate	Leafy green vegetables	Protects against DNA hypomethylation
Dithiolthiones	Cruciferous vegetables	Increase glutathione
		Increase glutathione reductase
		Increase glutathione transferase
		Increase quinone reductase
		Increase glucose-6-phosphate dehydrogenase
		Increase 6-phosphogluconate dehydrogenase
		Block reaction of electrophilic carcinogens with cellular macromolecules
Glucosinolates	Cruciferous vegetables	Increase mixed-function oxidase activity
Indoles	Cruciferous vegetables	Increase mixed-function oxidase activity
Isothiocyanates	Cruciferous vegetables	Inhibit DNA methylation
		Induce Phase II xenobiotic metabolizing enzymes
Thiocyanates	Cruciferous vegetables	Inhibit DNA methylation
		Induce Phase II xenobiotic metabolizing enzymes
Coumarins	Vegetables, citrus fruit	Induce glutathione S-transferase activity
Flavonoids	Most vegetables, fruit	Antioxidant properties
		Influence mixed-function oxidase activity
Phenols	Variety of vegetables, fruit	Some are antioxidants, flavonoids, coumarins
		Induce detoxification enzymes
		Some inhibit N-nitrosation reactions
Protease inhibitors	Most plants, especially in seeds, legumes, potatoes, sweet corn	Competitively inhibit proteases
Plant sterols	Most plants	Possible beneficial effects on cell membranes
Isoflavones	Variety of plants, especially soybeans	Weak estrogenic activity
		Inhibit tyrosine kinase
		Inhibit certain P450 enzymes
Saponins	Variety of plants, especially soybeans	Bind bile acids
		Reduce colonic epithelial cell proliferation
Inositol hexaphosphate	Variety of plants, especially soybeans and cereals	Decrease lipid peroxidation
Allium compounds	Allium vegetables (e.g., onions, garlic)	Induce glutathione S-transferase
		Induce microsomal monooxygenase
		Inhibit bacterial conversion of nitrate to nitrite
Limonene	Citrus fruit	Induces glutathione S-transferase

[a]Potential mechanisms may not be mutually exclusive, and may be additive or synergistic.

alytic sites and reduce the occurrence of tumors in animals *(55,63,66)*. Plant sterols are found in vegetables, pass through the gastrointestinal tract almost completely unabsorbed, and were found to decrease occurrence of chemical carcinogen-induced tumors in rats *(55,67)*. The possible mechanism of action is unclear, but, because their structure is similar to cholesterol, may involve affecting cellular membranes. Isoflavones are found in a variety of plants, but genistein, daidzein, and equol are particularly abundant in soybeans; they have weak estrogenic activity (may bind to estrogen receptors, thus blocking more potent estrogens but without eliciting a major estrogenic response). Some inhibit tyrosine kinases and other enzymes that are associated with the transmission of signals from cellular growth factor receptors and expressed at high levels in transformed cells, may inhibit certain P450 enzymes, and have been shown to reduce tumors in rodents *(68–70)*. A high intake of soy products has been associated with a reduced risk of cancer *(55)*. Saponins are found in a variety of plants, but are found in particularly high amounts in soybeans; they bind bile acids and cholesterol and have been shown to reduce colonic epithelial cell proliferation and decrease the growth and rate of DNA synthesis of various types of tumor cells *(55,68)*. Inositol hexaphosphate is found in a variety of plant foods, but is particularly high in soybeans and cereals; it is associated with decreased lipid peroxidation (perhaps by binding the oxidation catalyst, iron) and decreased colon cancer in animals *(68)*. Ecologic studies have found a strong inverse association of inositol hexaphosphate with colon cancer that is stronger than the one between fiber and colon cancer *(68)*. Allium compounds are found in the allium vegetable family, such as onions and garlic, induce detoxification enzymes, such as glutathione S-transferase and microsomal mono-oxygenase, inhibit bacterial conversion of nitrate to nitrite, and have been shown to reduce occurrence of tumors in animals *(55,71)*. Increased consumption of garlic has been found to be associated with a decreased risk of colon cancer in a prospective study of women *(61)*. Limonene is found in citrus fruits and induces glutathione S-transferase activity in animals *(55)* (*See* Chapter 7).

Potter *(72)* postulates that a diet regularly high in plant foods is the one to which humans are most adapted. This diet, then, provides regular high amounts of substances to which human metabolism is dependent for optimum health, some of which have not been identified as essential nutrients. Many of these substances can serve to keep inducible enzyme systems "tuned" to handle occasional high intakes of carcinogens; inhibit the formation of other carcinogens, reduce the capacity of transformed cells to proliferate, and act as antioxidants, and so forth. Thus, abandonment of the vegetable and fruit anticarcinogen "cocktail" to which we are adapted increases the risk of colon cancer.

The analytic epidemiologic literature on the association of vegetables and fruit and colon cancer is very consistent. As reviewed more extensively elsewhere *(61,73)*, of 22 analytic epidemiologic studies (20 case-control studies and two cohort studies) that investigated the possible association of vegetables and fruit and incidence of colon cancer, 20 were in an inverse direction (15 were statistically significant) and two were in the direction of increased risk. A meta-analysis of six case-control studies found a combined odds ratio of 0.48 (CI 95%: 0.41–0.57) *(59)*. The only prospective study to report combined vegetable and fruit findings in relation to colon cancer incidence was the Iowa Women's Health Study, which found a relative risk of 0.73 (CI 95%: 0.47–1.13) *(61)*. In the latter study, a relative risk of 0.68 (CI 95%: 0.46–1.02) was found for garlic intake. Among the case-control studies, analyses for specific categories of vegetables revealed inverse associations with cruciferous vegetables in five of seven studies examining this category; carrots in three of five; cabbage in two of six; and green vegetables in

Table 4
Potential Colon Carcinogenic Mechanisms of Sucrose[a]

When cooked, contains compounds that are genotoxic
Increases colon transit time
Increases fecal concentration of total and secondary bile acids
Increases colorectal epithelial cell proliferation
May increase aberrant crypt foci formation

[a]Potential mechanisms may not be mutually exclusive, and may be additive or synergistic.

two of four *(73)*. Intake of fruit was inversely related in two of seven, and intake of legumes was positively associated in two of three studies *(73)*. Of the four case-control studies that found no significant or a positive association with overall vegetable and fruit consumption, all were among the first few ever conducted, and the two finding the positive associations were conducted in Japanese populations *(73)*. There are no reported clinical trials of vegetable and fruit consumption and risk of colon cancer.

In summary, a decreased risk of colon cancer with an increased consumption of vegetables and fruit is biologically plausible and supported by the most consistent analytic observational epidemiologic literature of any diet-colon cancer association; however, more prospective data are needed. The multiplicity of potential mechanisms, rather than detracting from the plausibility of a protective effect of vegetables and fruit, make a strong case for the potential of increased vegetables and fruit in the primary prevention of colon cancer.

5. SUCROSE

It has long been known that a high intake of sucrose is a prominent distinguishing feature of the high-risk Western-style diet *(74–76)*. Little attention, however, has been paid to the possibility that this historically recent prominent dietary constituent might be etiologically linked to colon carcinogenesis. It has now been shown (*see* Table 4) that:

1. Uncooked sucrose increases colonic epithelial cell proliferation and aberrant crypt foci formation in rodents *(77)*;
2. Cooked sucrose contains compounds that are genotoxic under in vitro conditions *(78,79)*;
3. Cooked sucrose increases microadenoma formation in rodents *(28)*;
4. Cooked sucrose contains the thermolysis product 5-hydroxymethyl-2-furaldehyde, a compound that has also increased microadenoma formation in rodents initiated with a colon carcinogen *(80)*; and
5. In humans, a high sucrose diet increases mouth-to-anus transit time despite decreasing the mouth-to-cecum time; it also increases the fecal concentration of both total and secondary bile acids *(81)*.

Few epidemiologic studies have investigated the sucrose/colon cancer association *(32–38,42,82–86)*, only one of which has been prospective *(42)*.

Table 5
Comparisons of Selected Characteristics of Analytic Epidemiologic Studies Reporting Investigating Sucrose[a] Intake in Relation to Colorectal Cancer

Study	Study type	Population	Endpoint	No. of cases	OR/RR[b]	Comments
Phillips (32)	Cohort	Seventh-Day Adventists/ California	Colon cancer mortality	41	2.0	Exposure = cake or pie
Manousos et al. (33)	Case-control	Hospital-based/Greece	Incident colorectal cancer	100	0.7	Exposure = sucrose-containing foods
Miller et al. (82)	Case-control	Hospital cases and neighborhood controls/ Canada	Incident colorectal cancer	348	1.40 (men) 1.13 (women)	Exposure = sugar
Pickle et al. (34)	Case-control	Hospital-based/Nebraska	Incident colon cancer	58	1.4	
Bristol et al. (84)	Case-control	Hospital-based/United Kingdom	Incident colorectal cancer	50	3.6[c]	Unadjusted, and total energy intake was directly associated
Macquart-Moulin et al. (35)	Case-control	Hospital-based/France	Incident colorectal cancer	399	1.28	
Macquart-Moulin et al. (85)	Case-control	Hospital-based/France	Incident colorectal adenoma	252	2.17[c]	
LaVecchia et al. (36)	Case-control	Hospital-based/Italy	Incident colorectal cancer	575	1.22	
Tuyns et al. (83)	Case-control	Population-based/Belgium	Incident colon cancer	453	2.31[c]	Exposure = sugar
Benito et al. (37)	Case-control	Population-based/ Majorca, Spain	Incident colorectal cancer	286	1.64	Nearly significant at $p \leq 0.05$
Bidoli et al. (86)	Case-control	Hospital-based/Italy	Incident colon cancer	123	1.6	Nearly significant at $p \leq 0.05$
Peters et al. (38)	Case-control	Population-based, white/ Los Angeles, CA	Incident colorectal cancer	746	1.0	Per 100 Kcal
Bostick et al. (42)	Cohort	General population, women/Iowa	Incident colon cancer	212	2.00[c]	Exposure = sucrose-containing foods

[a]Exposure is sucrose as a macronutrient score unless otherwise specified in comments column of table.
[b]Odds ratio or relative risk, highest quantile of intake vs lowest.
[c]95% CI does not include 1.0.

To date, 13 analytic epidemiologic studies (*see* Table 5) have reported investigating the association of sucrose and colon neoplasia *(32–38,42,82–86)*; of these, eleven *(32,34–37,42,82–86)* reported an association in the direction of increased risk (findings were significant in four *[36,42,84,85]*; however, in one of these there was no adjustment for total energy intake despite a significant direct association of energy intake and colon cancer *[84]*), one reported an odds ratio (OR) of exactly 1.0 *(38)*, and one reported a statistically nonsignificant inverse association *(33)*. Among the three studies that found a significantly increased risk with higher sucrose intakes and also reported adjusted measures of association, the prospective Iowa Womens' Health Study *(42)* reported a relative risk (RR) of 2.0, a Belgian case-control study of incident colon cancer reported a similar risk estimate, but with more evidence of a dose-response relationship *(83)*, and a French case-control study of incident colorectal adenoma also reported a similar risk estimate, but with more evidence for a limitation to the highest intake grouping *(85)*. A Spanish case-control study *(37)* and an Italian case-control study *(86)* also reported risk estimates similar to these three studies but narrowly missed statistical significance at the $p < 0.05$ level. Another of the studies that suggested a direct association (RR = 2.0, also similar in magnitude to the Iowa Womens' Health Study) was the only previous prospective study to investigate the sucrose-colon cancer association; however, the study endpoint was colon cancer mortality, the number of cases was small ($n = 41$), and the sucrose exposure measurement was limited to consumption of cake or pie *(32)*. The study that reported the OR of 1.0, a 1989 population-based incident colon cancer case-control study of 45–69-year old men and women in Los Angeles, CA, used the same semiquantitative food frequency questionnaire as the Iowa Womens' Health Study *(38)*. The only study to suggest an inverse association was a small hospital-based case-control study in Greece *(33)*.

The Iowa Womens' Health Study, the only prospective study to address sucrose intake and colon cancer incidence *(42)*, found a nearly twofold increased risk of colon cancer in women associated with high intakes of sucrose and sucrose-containing foods. Among the sucrose-containing foods, no individual foods or groupings of foods appeared to contribute disproportionately to the overall association, and the association for sucrose was approximately the same as for the total sucrose-containing food grouping. No multiplicative interactions were seen between meat and sucrose-containing foods or between fat and sucrose. These observations suggest that it is increased sucrose consumption *per se* that is associated with increased risk of colon cancer, rather than the consumption of sucrose in combination with something else or sucrose that has been used in a certain way (e.g., cooked vs uncooked). There was a suggestion, however, that the association involving a grouping of all sucrose-containing foods was stronger after removing the calcium-rich food items (ice cream and ice milk). This suggests a hypothesis that a protective effect of calcium may have been partially negating a risk-enhancing effect of sucrose.

The sucrose findings of the several studies, then, in relation to incident colon cancer are fairly consistent, and several are not only statistically significant, but are relatively strong for diet-disease associations. Taken as a whole, the findings of the analytic epidemiologic studies are generally supportive of the possibility of a causal relationship, and as discussed above, are biologically plausible.

6. CALCIUM

6.1. Calcium and Colorectal Epithelial Cell Proliferation

6.1.1. COLORECTAL EPITHELIAL CELL PROLIFERATION AS AN INTERMEDIATE ENDPOINT FOR THE STUDY OF COLON CANCER PREVENTION

It has been hypothesized that calcium may reduce the risk of colon cancer by normalizing colonic crypt cell proliferation kinetics (87). Several studies (88–102) have reported that, compared to patients at low risk for colon cancer, patients with colon cancer (87–97) and patients in every category known to be at higher risk for colon cancer (those with a history of sporadic adenoma [88–91,93–97], familial polyposis [92,98] ulcerative colitis [88,99,100] or a family history of colon cancer [92,93,101] and the elderly [89,102]), on average, exhibit in their normal-appearing mucosa both an increased colonic epithelial cell proliferation rate and an extension of the colon crypt proliferative zone from the lower (basal) 60% of the crypt to include the upper (luminal) 40% of the crypt. In patients with previous colon cancer or sporadic adenomas, these changes also predict adenoma recurrence (103,104). In large bowel tumors in humans, an upward shift in the proliferative zone is found in colon cancers and adenomas, but not in hyperplastic polyps (105). As reviewed elsewhere (106–108), proliferative changes in normal-appearing mucosa have been shown to be a consequence of both cancer-initiating and cancer-promoting agents: Proliferative changes both precede and accompany colonic neoplasms in rodents given chemical carcinogens and a high fat diet produces proliferative changes in both rodents and humans. Animal experimental evidence and preliminary evidence in humans strongly suggest that these two proliferation abnormalities (hyperproliferation and upward shift of the proliferation zone) are reversible biomarkers or precursors for colon neoplasia (106–109). In humans, the two proliferation abnormalities appear to be independent variables (95,110) and rectal biopsy findings on both measures reflect those throughout the colon (97,111).

6.1.2. CALCIUM AND COLORECTAL EPITHELIAL CELL PROLIFERATION INTERVENTIONS IN ANIMALS AND HUMANS

Calcium administration has ameliorated the proliferative changes in rodents (112–114), and the findings in several (115–119), but not all (108,120) small preliminary clinical trials and a recently completed full-scale clinical trial (121) suggest similar effects in humans. Some preliminary clinical trial evidence suggested, and the recently completed full-scale trial confirmed, that calcium normalizes the distribution of proliferating cells within the colon crypts without affecting the proliferation rate (118,121). Hypothesized mechanisms have included the binding of calcium with bile acids (thought to be promoters) to form inert soaps (87), and the direct induction by calcium of terminal differentiation of the colonic epithelial cells (106–109).

The only full-scale randomized clinical trial to assess the efficacy of higher calcium consumption in normalizing cell proliferation kinetics in humans (121) was a randomized, double-blind, placebo-controlled, three-armed (two doses of calcium: 1.0 and 2.0 g), parallel group clinical trial (n = 193) to determine whether calcium supplementation can reduce the colorectal epithelial cell proliferation rate and normalize the distribution of proliferating cells within colorectal crypts (i.e., shift the zone of proliferation from one that includes the entire crypt to one that is confined to the lower 60%, or normal proliferative zone, of the crypt). Data from this trial provided evidence for a relative downward shift of the proliferative zone in colorectal crypts of sporadic adenoma patients in response to calcium supplementation, and thus were consistent with the hypothesis that a higher consumption of calcium may reduce the risk of colorectal cancer. The data provided no evidence that the overall colorectal epithelial cell proliferation rate can be reduced by calcium supplementation.

As a result of these data, the mechanistic hypotheses for how calcium affects cell proliferation in vivo and may reduce colon cancer needs to be re-examined. The first and most cited hypothesis for how calcium might reduce colorectal cancer risk has been that calcium binds intraluminal bile acids, thus preventing their toxic effects with their resultant promotion of compensatory hyperproliferation *(87)*. However, the data from this trial provide little evidence for this explanatory hypothesis. First, there was no evidence for an effect on the overall cell proliferation rate. Second, the hypothesis would predict that for a person consuming a level of fat and calcium in the Western-style diet range, the 1.0 g calcium dose (resulting in a total calcium intake of 1.5–2.0 g daily) would have provided as great an effect as the 2.0 g dose. The data, however, were consistent with a greater effect provided by the higher dose. Further, recent reports of studies that have examined the effects of calcium supplementation on stool bile acids in humans are inconsistent *(122–125)*. These lines of evidence do not rule out a beneficial effect of calcium via bile acid-binding, but do suggest that, if this is involved, that the mechanism is more complex than previously thought.

Based on in vitro data showing that calcium directly affects the cell cycle, modulating cell proliferation and inducing terminal differentiation, it has also been hypothesized that calcium may exert a similar influence in vivo in the cells of the colon mucosa *(106,108,126)*. The data from the full-scale calcium and colorectal epithelial cell proliferation trial *(121)* are consistent with this hypothesis. Even when proliferation rates are fast, if differentiation occurs rapidly as cells migrate up the crypt, they are more likely to have completed proliferation lower in the crypt. A consequence of this may be that since the DNA of a cell undergoing replication is more vulnerable to damage by various agents, and since cells proliferating lower in the crypt may be less likely to be exposed to injurious intraluminal agents, such cells may be less likely to be involved in colorectal carcinogenesis.

The mechanisms by which calcium affects cell cycle are not clear; however, several lines of research indicate that calcium may exert such effects by interacting with cyclic AMP *(127)*, calmodulin *(107,128)*, tyrosine kinase *(129)*, and ornithine decarboxylase *(106,129)*. In addition, calcium may influence other mechanisms; for example, cell adhesion mechanisms involving E-cadherin, a calcium-dependent cell adhesion molecule that interacts in complex fashion with the APC (Adenomatous Polyposis Coli) gene product *(130,131)*. (Also, calcium administration has reduced k-*ras* G to A mutations in colorectal neoplasms in rats *[132]*.)

All calcium and colorectal epithelial cell proliferation trials except the recent full-scale trial were small and most were uncontrolled *(108,115–120)*. Most examined only the overall cell proliferation rate. The uncontrolled trials each suggested that calcium would reduce the overall cell proliferation rate *(115–118)*; however, two *(108,120)* of the three *(108,119,120)* preliminary controlled trials did not. The data of the full-scale trial indicate that the findings of uncontrolled trials of calcium and the overall cell proliferation rate (termed the labeling index, or LI) were likely the result of regression to the mean and/or the Hawthorne effect (i.e., participants under the intense scrutiny characteristic of the clinical trial setting unconsciously change their behavior). Alternatively, based on the results of one uncontrolled trial, the authors speculated that patients with relatively high proliferation rates may be calcium responsive and that those with relatively low rates may be unresponsive *(118)*. However, in the full-scale trial, relative changes (calcium vs placebo) in the LI were similar in both those with high and low proliferation at baseline, thus indicating that the findings of the uncontrolled trial were likely the result of regression to the mean. Previous studies *(95,110)* have shown that the LI and $\emptyset_h$ (an indicator of distribution of proliferating cells in the crypt; defined as the proportion of labeled cells in the entire crypt that fall in the upper 40% of the crypt) are statistically independent variables, and other preliminary controlled trials testing other agents hypothesized to normalize colorectal proliferative kinetics and to reduce risk of colon cancer have found reductions in the $\emptyset_h$ without reductions in the LI *(53,133)*.

Although studies in humans have found that cell proliferation kinetics found on rectal biopsies reflect those found throughout the colon *(97,111)*, and studies in rodents have found that calcium affects cell proliferation kinetics throughout the colon *(112–114)*, there is no direct evidence from this or any other study that calcium affects cell proliferation throughout the colon in humans. This remains an important question, especially since the epidemiology of rectal cancer appears different in several respects from that of colon cancer *(31)*. In addition, colorectal epithelial cell proliferation kinetics remain unproven but logical and well-supported intermediate endpoints for colon cancer. The existing cell proliferation studies in humans, therefore, cannot prove that because calcium normalizes one of the cell proliferation endpoints in the rectum it can reduce the risk of colon cancer; they do, however, provide justification for further study of the calcium-colon cancer association.

6.2. Epidemiology of Calcium and Colorectal Cancer

The analytic observational epidemiologic literature on the association of calcium and colon cancer is somewhat inconsistent, but inverse associations have more frequently been found (*see* Table 6). Of 15 analytic epidemiologic studies (nine case-control studies *[35,38,48,136–138,140–142]* and six cohort studies *[39,134,135,139,143,144]*) that investigated the possible association of calcium and colon cancer, 10 suggested inverse associations *(35,38,134–139,143,144)* and three positive associations *(140–142)* (no direction of association was reported in two studies *[39,48]*). None of these studies found a statistically significant increased risk associated with higher calcium intake. Statistically significant decreased risk associated with higher calcium intake was found in three of the case-control studies *(136,137)* and in two of the cohort studies *(134,135)* (limited to the sigmoid colon in one of the latter *[135]*). Statistically significant associations were not found in the remaining studies; however, of the studies that reported strength of association, five were in the direction of decreased risk *(35,138,139,143,144)* and three were in the direction of increased risk *(140–142)*. One of the studies that reported no association (but did not report the actual strength of association) was the prospective cohort Nurses' Health Study, which used a food frequency questionnaire virtually identical to that used in the Iowa Womens' Health Study *(39)*. Most of the studies that reported significant inverse associations *(38,134,135,137)* focused on delineating the association of calcium, vitamin D, and/or milk products with colon cancer. The strongest associations were reported by Garland et al. *(134)*; Slattery et al. *(137)*; and Peters et al. *(38)*. Data reported by Garland et al. *(134)*, from the West-

Table 6
Comparisons of Selected Characteristics of Analytic Epidemiologic Studies Reporting Investigating Dietary Calcium Intake in Relation to Colorectal Cancer Incidence

Study	Study type	Population	Endpoint	No. of cases	OR/RR[a]
Garland et al. (134)	Cohort	Western Electric Study/Chicago, IL	Colorectal	49	0.32[b]
Macquart-Moulin et al. (35)	Case-control	Hospital-based/France	Colorectal	399	0.71
Wu et al. (139)	Cohort	Retirement community/Los Angeles, CA	Colorectal	126	0.86 (men)[d,e] 0.89 (women)[d,e]
Kune et al. (136)	Case-control	Community-based/Australia	Colorectal	715	0.56 (women)[b] 0.79 (sexes combined)
Tuyns et al. (141)	Case-control	Population-based/Belgium	Colon	453	1.34
Slattery et al. (137)	Case-control	Population-based/Utah	Colon	231	0.41 (men)[b] 0.50 (women)[b]
Graham et al. (48)	Case-control	Hospital and neighborhood-based/Western New York state	Colon	428	NS/not given
Lee et al. (138)	Case-control	Hospital-based/Chinese in Singapore	Colon	132	0.88
Stemmerman et al. (135)	Cohort	Japanese descent Hawaiians	Colon	189	0.77 (total) 0.59 (sigmoid)[b]
Negri et al. (142)	Case-control	Hospital-based/Italy	Colon	558	1.1
Willett et al. (39)	Cohort	Nurses/11 US states	Colon	150	NS/not given
Benito et al. (140)	Case-control	Population/hospital-based/Majorca, Spain	Colorectal	286	1.48[g]
Peters et al. (38)	Case-control	Population-based, white/Los Angeles, CA	Colon	746	0.42[b,c]
Bostick et al. (143)	Cohort	General population, women/Iowa	Colon	212	0.68
Kampman et al. (144)	Cohort	General population/Netherlands	Colorectal	326	0.92

[a]Odds ratio or relative risk, highest quantile of intake vs lowest.
[b]95% CI does not include 1.0.
[c]Estimates by sex approximately the same. Stronger associations distally than proximally.
[d]Calcium only from dairy sources.
[e]Excluding rectum (n = 20) did not change results.
[f]Not statistically significant, i.e., 95% CI includes 1.0.
[g]Univariate estimate.

71

ern Electric Study indicated a relative risk of 0.32 (my calculations from the published quartile-specific incidence rates) for colon cancer for those in the highest quartile group of calcium intake compared to those in the lowest quartile group. This study is important because of its 19-yr prospective design and the careful dietary methodology (two 28-d dietary histories 1 yr apart). Slattery et al. *(137)*, using an extensive food frequency questionnaire in a population-based case-control study in Utah, reported a halving of colon cancer risk (adjusted-odds ratios of 0.41 for men and 0.50 for women) for those in the highest quartile group of calcium intake compared to the lowest quartile group of intake. Peters et al. *(38)*, in a large population-based case-control study in California using essentially the same food frequency questionnaire as in the Nurses' Health Study and the Iowa Womens' Health Study, also reported a more than halving of colon cancer risk for both men and women (adjusted odds ratio OR=0.42 for men and women combined). Of the three studies suggesting positive associations of calcium intake with risk of colon cancer *(140–142)* one reported only univariate results even though total energy intake was positively associated with colon cancer *(140)*. In a second, for men and women combined, the reported odds ratio was 1.1, a figure not meaningfully different from 1.0 *(142)*. Otherwise, when these 13 analytic epidemiologic studies were compared across study type, location, endpoint (colon cancer vs colorectal cancer), size, number of cases, population age and sex, other population characteristics, and dietary methodology, no pattern distinguishing studies reporting inverse associations vs positive associations was found.

Several factors make it difficult to draw strong conclusions from these reported analytic epidemiologic studies investigating the association of calcium with colon cancer. In general, observational studies are hampered by the relative homogeneity of diets within populations, the multitude of dietary variables, the problem of unmeasured nutrient-nutrient interactions, and the lack of precision in current dietary measures used in large population studies. Although the majority of the studies reviewed here reported associations suggesting decreased risk of colon cancer with relatively high intakes of calcium, reporting and publication biases cannot be ruled out. Residual confounding in the reviewed studies also cannot be ruled out. Although the epidemiologic appearance of colon cancer is different from that of rectal cancer, many of these studies combined the two for reported analyses, possibly attenuating observed associations. Furthermore, few of the studies reported taking into account supplement intake—a factor that is especially important given the homogeneity of diets within most populations. Most of the studies were reported before the emergence of strong theoretical and experimental support for calcium as a potential protective factor against colon cancer and did not focus specifically on calcium intake; consequently, they did not fully address all confounding and interaction issues related to current hypotheses regarding this dietary constituent. In only a few studies were associations with colon subsite investigated. Overall, however, despite these limitations, the epidemiologic literature can be considered weakly supportive of the hypothesis that a relatively high intake of calcium protects against colon cancer.

6.3. Summary

In summary, biologically plausible mechanisms of action for protective effects of calcium against colon cancer exist. Currently, animal experimental data are strongly supportive. Epidemiologic data are inconsistent but overall, are weakly supportive as well. A full-scale intermediate endpoint chemoprevention trial found that calcium supplementation, without affecting the proliferation rate, normalizes the distribution of proliferating cells in the rectal mucosa of sporadic adenoma patients. The results of this trial support the hypothesis that higher calcium consumption may reduce the risk of colon cancer. They also support the hypothesis that the possible chemoprotective action of calcium may not be by simply binding bile acids and thereby reducing compensatory hyperproliferation, but they are consistent with the hypothesis that calcium exerts its possible chemoprotective effect by directly affecting cell cycle and increasing rates of cell differentiation. The mechanism(s) by which calcium affects colorectal epithelial cell proliferation in humans remain(s) to be resolved and a causal relationship between calcium intake and colorectal cancer incidence, although increasingly supported, cannot be considered established.

7. VITAMIN D

Compared to calcium, similar but less extensive evidence exists to support a role for vitamin D in lowering colorectal cancer risk. Vitamin D is intimately related to calcium metabolism *(145)*, has reduced cell proliferation in human colon cell lines in vitro *(146)*, has reduced colonic epithelial cell proliferation in rodents *(147)*, was a necessary cofactor in reducing k-*ras* G to A mutations in colorectal neoplasms in rats *(132)*, and has reduced tumorigenesis in rats *(148,149)*.

Of six analytic epidemiologic studies (four cohort studies *[39,134,143,150]* and two case-control studies *[38,140]*) that investigated the possible association of vitamin D and colon cancer (*see* Table 7), four suggested an inverse association *(134,140,143,150)*. One reported a null association *(38)*. The sixth, the prospective cohort Nurses' Health Study, showed no significant association, and, as with calcium, did not report the direction of the association *(39)*. The inverse associations reported in the other two cohort studies were statistically significant. In one, the 19-yr prospective Western Electric Study, the data indicated a relative risk of 0.55 (my calculations from the published quartile-specific incidence rates) for colon cancer for those in the highest quartile group of intake as opposed to those in the lowest quartile group of intake of vitamin D *(134)*. In the second, the Washington County, MD, prospective cohort study, a nested case-control analysis showed an odds ratio of 0.3 for colon cancer for those with a 25-hydroxyvitamin D serum level of ≥ 20 ng/mL compared to those with a serum level < 20 ng/mL *(150)*. Both of these analyses were focused on vitamin D. A case-control study from the island of Majorca, Spain that did not focus on vitamin D and combined colon and rectal cancers in the analysis showed no significant association but the direction was toward a reduced risk for those in the highest quartile group of intake compared to those in the lowest quartile group (OR=0.74) *(140)*.

8. MILK PRODUCTS

Although milk products have received little attention in laboratory experiments related to colon cancer, they are major sources of calcium and vitamin D in the American diet. Of 15 analytic epidemiologic studies (11 case-control studies *[33–35,37,38,82, 136–138,142,151]* and four cohort studies *[41,143,144,152]*) that investigated the possible association of milk and colon cancer (*see* Table 8), 11 suggested an inverse association *(34,35,38,41,136–138,143,144,151,152)*; three a positive association *(33,37,82)*;

Table 7
Comparisons of Selected Characteristics of Analytic Epidemiologic Studies Investigating Vitamin D in Relation to Colorectal Cancer Incidence

Study	Study type	Population	Endpoint	No. of cases	OR/RR[a]
Willett et al. (39)	Cohort	Nurses/11 US states	Colon	150	NS[d]/not given
Garland et al. (134)	Cohort	Western Electric Study/Chicago, IL	Colorectal	49	0.55[b]
Garland et al. (150)	Cohort/nested case control	Washington County, MD	Colon	34	0.3[b,c]
Benito et al. (140)	Case-control	Population and hospital-based/Majorca, Spain	Colorectal	286	0.74
Peters et al. (38)	Case-control	Population-based, white/Los Angeles, CA	Colon	746	NS[d]/not given[e]
Bostick et al. (143)	Cohort	General population, women/Iowa	Colon	212	0.73

[a]Odds ratio or relative risk, highest quantile of intake vs lowest.
[b]95% CI does not include 1.0.
[c]Exposure was serum 25-hydroxyvitamin D rather than dietary vitamin D.
[d]Not statistically significant, i.e., 95% CI includes 1.0.
[e]In protective direction without calcium in model, null with calcium in model.

Table 8
Comparisons of Selected Characteristics of Analytic Epidemiologic Studies Reporting Milk Product Intake in Relation to Colorectal Cancer

Study	Study type	Population	Endpoint	No. of cases	OR/RR[a]
Miller et al. (82)	Case-control	Hospital and neighborhood-based/Canada	Incident colon	348	1.2 (men) 1.3 (women)
Manousos et al. (33)	Case-control	Hospital-based/Greece	Incident colorectal	100	1.17
Pickle et al. (34)	Case-control	Hospital-based/Nebraska	Incident colon	58	0.74
Phillips et al. (41)	Cohort	Seventh-Day Adventists/California	Colon mortality	147	0.5 (men) 1.1 (women)
Takuma and Tominaga (151)	Case-control	Hospital-based/Japan	Incident colon	50	0.69
Macquart-Moulin et al. (35)	Case-control	Hospital-based/France	Incident colorectal	399	0.66[b]
Kune et al. (136)	Case-control	Community-based/Australia	Incident colorectal	715	0.59 (women)[b] 0.89 (sexes combined)
Slattery et al. (137)	Case-control	Population-based/Utah	Incident colon	231	0.44 (men)[b] 0.55 (women)[b]
Lee et al. (138)	Case-control	Hospital-based/Chinese in Singapore	Incident colon	132	0.81
Ursin et al. (152)	Cohort	Norway	Incident colon	92	0.85
Benito et al. (37)	Case-control	Population and hospital-based/Majorca, Spain	Incident colon	148	1.07
Negri et al. (142)	Case-control	Hospital-based/Italy	Incident colon	558	1.0
Peters et al. (38)	Case-control	Population-based/Utah	Incident colon	746	0.83[c]
Bostick et al. (143)	Cohort	General population, women/Iowa	Incident colon	212	0.72
Kampman et al. (144)	Cohort	General population/Netherlands	Incident colorectal	326	0.86[d]

[a]Odds ratio or relative risk, highest quantile of intake vs lowest.
[b]95% CI does not include 1.0.
[c]Per 10 servings/mo of yogurt. For milk was 0.97[b] without calcium in model, null with calcium in model.
[d]For unfermented milk. Not given for total milk products. RR for fermented milk was 0.89 and for hard cheese, 0.88.

75

and one no association (OR=1.0) *(142)*. None of these studies showed a statistically significant positive association. The inverse associations were statistically significant in four case-control studies *(35,38,136,137)*. Observed associations were not statistically significant in the remaining studies; however, of the studies that reported strength of association, seven *(34,41,82,138,143,144,151,152)* (including the four cohort studies *[41,143,144,152]*) were in the direction of decreased risk and three *(33,37,82)* were in the direction of increased risk. None of the four cohort studies reported positive associations *(41,143,144,152)* and all studies reporting positive associations were hospital-based case-control studies *(33,37,82)*. The only study that reported a strong association was the population-based Utah case-control study *(137)*, which focused specifically on calcium and milk in relation to colon cancer. Relatively high milk intake was significantly associated with a reduced risk of colon cancer in both men (multivariate-adjusted OR=0.44) and women (multivariate-adjusted OR=0.53). Otherwise, as with calcium, no strong patterns distinguishing studies that reported inverse associations vs positive associations were found.

9. ANTIOXIDANTS AND ANTIOXIDANT ENZYME-ASSOCIATED MICRONUTRIENTS

9.1. *Biological Plausibility of Antioxidants Protecting Against Colon Cancer*

9.1.1. OXIDATIVE DAMAGE AND CANCER

The plausibility of a role in carcinogenesis for reactive oxygen molecules and oxygen-derived free radicals (*see* Fig. 1) is undergirded by a massive basic science literature, the subject of several recent reviews *(153–164)*. Briefly, these compounds apparently act as both initiators and promoters of carcinogenesis: they are known to:

1. Alter nucleic acids, leading to mutations, sister chromatid exchanges, and chromosome aberrations that can lead to propagated initiated cells or to cell death (the latter leading to the promoting effects of compensatory cell hyperproliferation);
2. Damage cells by reacting with unsaturated bonds in membrane lipids and by denaturing proteins, which can lead to cell death, thereby increasing compensatory cell proliferation (Also, both the breakdown of cell membrane barriers and increased cell division may in turn expose DNA to easier damage, and thus to initiation or to further promotion from cell death-induced compensatory cell proliferation. Furthermore, some of the cell membrane breakdown products are themselves mutagenic.);
3. Modulate gene expression of initiated cells by affecting genes that regulate cell differentiation and growth.

Sources of reactive oxygen molecules and oxygen-derived free radicals include endogenous production from normal metabolic reactions as well as exogenous sources. These compounds may also be important in aging and in the pathogenesis of coronary heart disease and other chronic diseases.

Oxidative damage may be of particular relevance to colon cancer (*see* Fig. 2). It has been recently discovered that feces contain large quantities of oxygen-derived free radicals and that the rate of formation corresponds to that which would be produced by over 10,000 rads of γ radiation per day *(30)*. As reviewed elsewhere *(30)*, the respiratory activity of fecal bacteria is an abundant source of oxygen-derived free radicals. Another source in the colon is the lipoxygenase activity of normal or sloughed colon epithelial

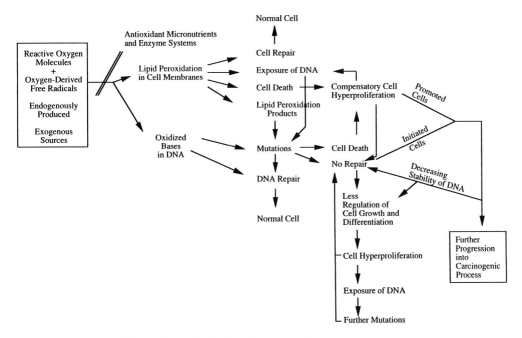

Fig. 1. The role of oxidative damage in carcinogenesis.

cells. Iron, which is present in relatively high concentrations in feces, facilitates the production of oxygen-derived free radicals (the Fenton reaction); furthermore, bile pigments, also present in feces, keep iron soluble, thereby enhancing iron's availability for the Fenton reaction. Radicals formed in the colon can cause oxidative DNA damage, can initiate lipid peroxidation leading to formation of substances shown to stimulate DNA synthesis and cell proliferation in colonic epithelium, can be involved in free radical oxidations that mimic those produced by the cytochrome P450 system of the liver (which is known to convert procarcinogens to active carcinogens), and can participate in aromatic hydroxylation reactions (involving ingested organic compounds) to form carcinogenic products. These observations are consistent with the high incidence of cancer of the colon and rectum compared to other regions of the gastrointestinal tract. They are also consistent with the association of a higher incidence of colon cancer with a high intake of red meat (which increases stool iron), and with a high intake of fat (which has been associated with increased levels of oxidative damage in humans *(165)*, and that may increase the fecal content of bile pigments and fecal procarcinogens *[30]*).

9.1.2. ANTIOXIDANTS AND CANCER

As reviewed elsewhere *(162,166)*, vitamin E, vitamin C, and the carotenoids are micronutrients that act as antioxidants, trapping reactive oxygen molecules and oxygen-derived free radicals, and as such are a prominent part of the body's primary defenses against these damaging agents. The micronutrients selenium, riboflavin, niacin, zinc, and manganese are essential components of various important antioxidant enzymes. Vitamin E is the major lipid-soluble antioxidant found in all cellular membranes, where it protects against lipid peroxidation (i.e., oxidative cell membrane damage). Vitamin E acts directly with oxygen-derived free radicals as well as with reactive oxygen mole-

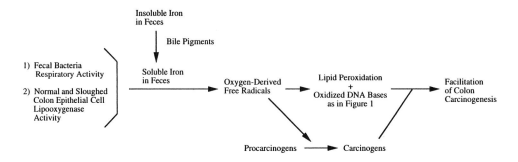

Fig. 2. Enhanced production of oxygen-derived free radicals in the colon and their role in colon carcinogenesis.

cules. β-carotene, the major carotenoid precursor of vitamin A, is also fat-soluble and present in cell membranes, and is one of the most effective quenchers of reactive oxygen molecules known in nature. (Vitamin A has minimal antioxidant properties.) Vitamin C is water-soluble and can quench both reactive oxygen molecules and oxygen-derived free radicals. Selenium is an essential component of the enzyme glutathione peroxidase, which reduces oxygen-derived free radicals and thus prevents damage to intracellular membranes. Riboflavin, niacin, zinc, and manganese are also essential constituents of various intracellular antioxidant enzyme systems (as are iron, copper, and molybdenum, which, however, also have pro-oxidant properties). Of particular importance is that various antioxidant micronutrients have been shown to enhance or even be essential to the antioxidant effects of one another *(162,167–178)*. Vitamin E, the carotenoids, vitamin C, and selenium can also stimulate the immune system and may protect against the development of cancer by enhancing immune surveillance *(166,179,180)*. Vitamins E and C can also reduce nitrite, inhibiting the production of nitrosamines and nitrosamides *(180)*, compounds that induce tumors in experimental animals and possibly in humans. β-Carotene *(181)* and selenium *(182,183)* may also inhibit cell proliferation by effects independent of their antioxidant activities.

9.2. Antioxidants and Cancer in Animal Experiments

Specific antioxidant micronutrients have been shown to protect against various cancers, including colon cancer in animals. Vitamin E has been shown to reduce tumorigenesis in five different cancer sites, carotenoids reduced it in five, vitamin C in six, and selenium in five; all four agents reduced tumorigenesis in colon *(166,184,185)*. Furthermore, in several studies, antioxidant micronutrients enhanced the effects of one another *(169,170,172,177,178)*, emphasizing their interdependence.

9.3. Epidemiology of Antioxidants and Colon Cancer

There is also epidemiologic support for a protective effect of antioxidant micronutrients against a variety of cancers, including colon cancer in humans. First, in analytic epidemiologic studies, vegetables and fruit, the predominant sources of antioxidant micronutrients, were statistically significantly associated with various cancers in 128 of 156 studies that reported measures of risk *(186)*. Twenty-three of 28 such studies investigating colon cancer reported an inverse association, a higher level of consistency than that seen for fiber intake *(31)*.

Second, in analytic epidemiologic studies, intakes of specific antioxidant micronutrients have also been shown to be inversely associated with various cancers, including colon cancer. Furthermore, some studies have found interactions involving some of the antioxidants *(167,168)*, again emphasizing their interdependence. Vitamin E, which has received relatively little attention in epidemiologic studies, was inversely associated with cancer in several studies. Of eight larger analytic epidemiologic studies since 1987 of diet and cancer, six found associations in the direction of decreased risk (relative risk or odds ratio [RR/OR] range 0.4–0.8, median 0.6) and two found associations in the direction of increased risk (RR/OR 1.2) *(166,185)*. Vitamin E intake was inversely associated with cancers of six different sites, including colon *(166,185)*. In the prospective Iowa Women's Health Study (n=35,215) *(187)*, an adjusted RR of 0.32 (CI 95%: 0.19–0.54) was found for those in the highest quintile of intake of total vitamin E (primarily resulting from supplemental intake) compared to those in the lowest quintile of intake. The association was even more striking in the youngest age group (55–59 yr old) for which the RR was 0.16 (CI 95%: 0.04–0.70). Prediagnostic serum levels of vitamin E in prospective cohort studies have been inversely associated with all cancers combined (RRs=0.6, 0.8) and with five different cancer sites, including colon *(166,185)*. Of note is that findings in five prospective studies suggested that the level of α-tocopherol was lower in subjects who subsequently developed colorectal cancer than in noncases *(188)*. Differences were not statistically significant in any one of the five studies, but when the original data from the five studies were pooled and analyzed *(188)*, the OR for the highest quartile of serum α-tocopherol concentration compared to the lowest was 0.6 (CI 95%: 0.4–1.0). Adjustment for serum cholesterol level attenuated the odds ratio to 0.7 (CI 95%: 0.4–1.1).

Carotenoids have been found to be inversely associated with cancer of eleven different sites, including colon *(166,185)*. Of 34 larger, analytic epidemiologic studies since 1987 of diet and cancer, 28 found associations in the direction of decreased risk (RR/OR range 0.2–0.9, median 0.7), four found a relative risk of 1.0, and two found associations in the direction of increased risk (RR/OR 1.1, 1.2). Furthermore, in the relatively few prospective cohort studies that measured them, prediagnostic serum levels of carotene were inversely associated with all cancers combined (RRs 0.6, 0.7) and with cancers of the lung (RRs 0.4, 0.5, 0.5, 0.6) and colon (RR 0.8) *(166,185)*.

Vitamin C has been found to be inversely associated with cancers of eight different sites, including colon *(166,185)*. Of 18 larger analytic epidemiologic studies of diet and cancer since 1987, 15 found associations in the direction of decreased risk (RR/OR range 0.2–0.9, median 0.5), and three found associations in the direction of increased risk (RR/ORs 1.1, 1.1, 1.2) *(166,185)*.

Selenium has also been found to be inversely associated with various cancers, including colon cancer. Dietary intake of selenium cannot be measured accurately in larger, analytic epidemiologic studies: Selenium content of food varies with soil and growing conditions, rendering dietary values meaningless in such studies. In ecologic studies *(189,190)*, both in the United States and internationally, dietary selenium, local plant selenium levels, and blood selenium concentrations were significantly inversely correlated with age-adjusted mortality from cancers of all sites combined as well as from nine different cancer sites, including colon and rectum. Low blood selenium levels

were associated with an increased risk of cancer of all sites in six of nine cohort studies
(166). In three cohort studies that measured serum selenium levels and documented
colon cancer incidence *(166)*, a marginal association was observed in one, lower mean
levels of selenium were found in individuals who developed colon cancer in a second,
and a null association was found in the third. In another prospective cohort study, toenail selenium levels were marginally, but not statistically, associated with risk of colon
cancer *(191)*. In the prospective Iowa Women's Health Study, the adjusted relative risk
of colon cancer for those taking selenium supplements compared to those who were not
was 0.6 (CI 95%: 0.27–1.32) *(187)*.

Despite the strong plausibility for a protective effect against cancer, riboflavin,
niacin, zinc, and manganese have not been as extensively studied as the other antioxidant-related micronutrients in experimental animal or in human observational or randomized studies; however, the limited data are generally *(192,193)*, but not entirely
(194), supportive for a protective effect for them too.

9.4. Antioxidants and Oxidative Damage: Experiments in Animals and Humans

In a randomized clinical trial, levels of oxidized DNA were reduced in seminal fluid
by ascorbic acid *(195)*, and in a small clinical study, levels in urine were reduced with
increased vegetable and fruit intake *(196)*. A higher fat diet increased lipid peroxidation
in both laboratory animals *(197–199)* and humans *(200,201)*, but this increase was
blocked by higher vitamin E intake in both laboratory animals *(198,199)* and humans
(200,201). Lipid peroxidation was increased in the skin of mice after topical administration of cancer-initiating and promoting compounds, but the increases in lipid peroxidation and skin tumor incidence were both reduced if an antioxidant micronutrient combination (vitamin C, vitamin E, and selenium) was applied *(202)*. In small human trials,
levels of lipid peroxidation products in both exhaled air and in serum were reduced in a
dose-response manner by β-carotene in a controlled trial in young healthy adults
(203,204); they were reduced in serum by an antioxidant micronutrient combination in
a randomized placebo-controlled trial in geriatric patients *(205)*, and by selenium in a
controlled trial in top athletes *(206)*. Levels of release of lipid peroxidation products
from platelets were reduced by vitamin E in diabetics in a small randomized, placebo-
controlled clinical trial *(207)*.

9.5. Colon Cancer Intermediate Endpoint Trials

9.5.1. ANTIOXIDANTS AND HUMAN TRIALS OF MARKERS OF RISK FOR COLON CANCER

In humans given 400 mg supplemental vitamin E plus 400 mg ascorbic acid daily,
fecal mutagenicity was reduced by 26% ($p < 0.01$) *(208)*.

9.5.2. ANTIOXIDANTS AND CELL PROLIFERATION EXPERIMENTS IN VITRO AND IN ANIMALS

Several animal and in vitro studies of the effects of antioxidants on cell proliferation, including colorectal epithelial cell proliferation, have now been reported. An antioxidant mixture primarily containing α-tocopherol reduced cell proliferation in the
colon, rectum, and mammary glands of mice *(209)*. Both organic and inorganic selenium reduced colonic epithelial cell proliferation while concomitantly reducing the in-

cidence and multiplicity of colon adenocarcinomas in rats given chemical carcinogens *(210)*. Colorectal epithelial cell proliferation was reduced in rats given chemical carcinogens when given a diet low in fat and protein and high in vitamin E, selenium, vitamin A, and fiber *(211)*. Carotene reduced epidermal cell proliferation while reducing skin and intestinal carcinogenesis in mice *(181)*. Increased cell proliferation in the skin of mice was found in the presence of low antioxidant concentrations in the skin *(212)*. In cell culture, ascorbic acid alone did not have an antiproliferative effect, but it did enhance the antiproliferative effect of other antioxidants *(176)*, again emphasizing their interdependence.

9.5.3. ANTIOXIDANTS AND COLORECTAL EPITHELIAL CELL PROLIFERATION: CLINICAL TRIALS

Four small trials in humans also suggest that antioxidants can reduce colorectal epithelial cell proliferation. In a small randomized, placebo-controlled clinical trial in adenoma patients ($n = 41$), those given 70 mg α-tocopherol plus 1000 mg ascorbic acid plus 30,000 IU vitamin A had a 45% greater reduction than those given placebo in the labeling index (LI) of the upper 40% of the colonic crypts *(133)*. In an uncontrolled trial ($n = 10$), the labeling index dropped 33% in sporadic adenoma patients given 200 µg of selenium for 1 mo *(213)*. In a 1-mo randomized placebo-controlled four-armed parallel group trial in sporadic adenoma patients ($n = 48$), those given 750 mg vitamin C had a 54% drop in LI, those given 9 mg β-carotene had a 41% drop, and those given 160 mg α-tocopherol or placebo had no change *(214)*. Finally, in a trial in familial polyposis patients ($n = 17$), those given 3.0 g ascorbic acid daily had a 19% greater reduction in the labeling index than those on placebo *(215)*.

9.5.4. ANTIOXIDANTS AND COLON POLYP RECURRENCE: CLINICAL TRIALS

Antioxidant micronutrients have reduced polyp formation in small trials in humans, but not in a larger full-scale trial. In the most striking small trial, a randomized, placebo-controlled clinical trial of polyp recurrence, sporadic adenoma patients ($n = 209$) treated with 70 mg vitamin E plus 1.0 g vitamin C plus 30,000 IU vitamin A daily over 18 mo had a polyp recurrence rate of 5.7% vs 35.9% for those on placebo ($p < 0.001$) *(216)*. In a pilot randomized, placebo-controlled trial, sporadic adenoma patients ($n = 129$) treated with 400 mg vitamin E plus 400 mg ascorbic acid daily over 2 yr had a polyp recurrence rate of 41.4% vs 50.7% for those on placebo (not statistically significant) *(217)*. In three small trials of polyp recurrence in familial polyposis patients, two testing 3.0 g ascorbic acid daily *(215,218)* and the other testing 4.0 g ascorbic acid plus 400 mg α-tocopherol daily *(219)* small reductions in polyp formation were suggested. However, more recently, Greenberg et al. *(220)* reported the lack of efficacy of administering 400 mg vitamin E, 25 mg β-carotene, and 1000 mg vitamin C in reducing adenoma recurrence over a 4-yr period. This was an excellent study ($n = 751$) that did exactly what it was designed to do: determine the efficacy of the above treatment regimen on polyp recurrence in established polyp formers over a relatively brief period of time. Based on what was known at the time the study was originally conceived, these results would have led to the conclusion that antioxidants would be ineffective in colon cancer prevention. We now know that this is not the case, and that the question is still rather wide open.

One reason that the Greenberg trial may not have yielded hypothesized results is that when originally designed it did not take into account the as yet unpublished findings of

Vogelstein et al. and others *(221)* that multiple slowly accumulated genetic alterations are usually required to produce a colonic neoplasm in the non-FAP (Familial Adenomatous Polyposis) patient. It would be unrealistic to think that every potential protective factor can protect against cancer by inhibiting every step in this "pathway," and antioxidants are no exception. If a patient already has several cell lines with the requisite accumulated genetic changes to commit the cell lines to adenoma formation, there may be no mechanism whereby antioxidants could block the growth of the committed lines. We know that patients with incident adenoma are likely to form recurrent adenoma; thus, it is likely that by the time a person has an incident adenoma, other cell lines are already genetically altered/committed to form adenomas also. We also now know that the natural history of adenoma growth is rather slower in general than originally thought; so slow, in fact, that the recommended interval for colonoscopic follow-up surveillance for polyp recurrence has now been extended to 5 yr. What this all means, then, is that if a protective agent exerts its action prior to full genetic commitment of a cell to adenoma formation, a reduction in polyp recurrence may not be seen until a substantial proportion of the already committed cell lines have "played out," and this may take longer than the 4 yr of follow-up employed in the Greenberg et al. study. Thus, the findings of the Greenberg et al. study may now be predicted on theoretical grounds that do not exclude antioxidants as protective against colon cancer.

Epidemiologic data are available to support this line of reasoning. In a Finnish male cohort study, prediagnostic serum vitamin E levels were associated with a decreased risk of all cancers combined, but the inverse association was limited to those younger than 70 yr of age *(222)*. In an American female cohort study, vitamin E intake was associated with a decreased risk of colon cancer, and the inverse association was limited to those younger than 65 yr of age in a monotonic fashion *(187)*. Most of the association was attributable to supplemental vitamin E intake, a relatively recent population phenomenon. Older members of the cohort were more likely to have accumulated the requisite number of genetic changes to form polyps, and thus cancer, than the younger members. Beginning vitamin E supplements at a young age may maximize the potential for protecting against colon cancer since at that point the progression of genetic changes is at a point at which vitamin E is effective; conversely, beginning vitamin E at an older age, for some persons, may simply be too late for it to do much good. The fact that Greenberg et al. did not find treatment differences by age does not negate this argument since all patients in the trial were already adenoma formers, regardless of age.

Despite these comments, it should be pointed out that adenoma patients are still very appropriate subjects for studying the efficacy of various interventions on endpoints earlier in the carcinogenic process than adenomas. Because a sporadic adenoma patient has had a polyp does not mean that all cell lines have been committed to polyp formation. Earlier endpoints, such as colonic epithelial cell proliferative abnormalities, still exist and can be normalized. Normalization of such early endpoints can still be used as evidence that the tested intervention may be effective for cancer prevention in patients who have not yet formed polyps as well as in polyp patients once they have been treated long enough and all the cell lines already committed to polyp formation have played out.

Another factor that could have been operative in the Greenberg trial is that it only partially addressed the complex, multifaceted antioxidant system and potential antioxidant interactions. Perhaps a more complete set of antioxidant-related substances, i.e., including selenium, and so forth, would have been more effective. Additionally, a higher dose of vitamin E may have been more effective.

Finally, it should be remembered that another, albeit smaller, trial similar to the Greenberg et al. trial found a statistically significant reduction in polyp recurrence *(216)*. Chance always remains an explanation for the results of any study in which inference is required.

9.6. Antioxidants and Cancer: Clinical Trials

There are few clinical trial data pertaining to the efficacy of antioxidants in reducing cancer incidence or mortality of cancer; however, the colon cancer data are limited. There have been two reported clinical trials testing the efficacy of antioxidants in reducing cancer incidence or mortality, one in a Western population (Finland) *(223)*, and one in an Eastern population (China) *(194)*. The Finnish study, a randomized, double-blind, placebo-controlled trial in 29,133 50–69-yr-old male smokers, tested 50 mg α-tocopherol daily and 20 mg β-carotene daily, each alone and in combination, vs placebo over 5–8 yr. The primary endpoint of the trial was lung cancer incidence, but colon cancer incidence was monitored. There was an 18% increase in the incidence of lung cancer in men on β-carotene alone, but no increase in those on α-tocopherol alone or in combination with β-carotene (perhaps again emphasizing their interdependence). There was a nonstatistically significant decrease in the incidence of colon cancer in those on α-tocopherol, but no apparent effect of β-carotene alone. Data on α-tocopherol and β-carotene in combination in relation to colon cancer were not presented. In the Chinese trial, there was a statistically significant reduction in mortality from all cancers combined for those who were on the daily combination of 15 mg β-carotene, 30 mg α-tocopherol, and 50 μg selenium. Data on colon cancer were not reported separately.

9.7. Summary

In summary, the rationale for a causal role of oxidative damage and a protective role of antioxidant micronutrients in carcinogenesis in general, and in colon carcinogenesis in particular, is very strong, buttressed by a massive basic science literature. The existing data from experimental animal studies are strong, but are of uncertain relevance to humans. Although a few consistent patterns appear to be emerging from the observational epidemiologic studies, by and large, the results of these studies have been unclear. These studies are hampered by the homogeneity of dietary constituents within populations, the multitude of dietary factors and their interactions, and the limited accuracy of current dietary measures. It would, therefore, appear that carefully designed, sufficiently long clinical trials will be the best way to evaluate this group of potential protective factors. Clinical trials would address the following gaps of knowledge: whether antioxidants can:

1. Effectively modulate endpoints early in the carcinogenic process (e.g., colorectal epithelial cell proliferation);
2. Reduce colon polyp recurrence after 5 yr of treatment;
3. Reduce of incidence of adenomatous polyps after 5 yr of treatment;
4. Reduce incidence of, or mortality from, colon cancer after five or more years of treatment.

Clinical trials to address gaps 2–4, the adenoma or carcinoma endpoints, would require extremely large sample sizes, prolonged follow-up, or both; consequently, they would be extremely expensive and may not be justified by the current level of evidence.

However, full-scale clinical trials using biomarkers or precursors for colon cancer, such as colorectal epithelial cell proliferation, that can be measured easily and allow the use of small sample sizes and short interventions are indicated to determine whether adenoma or colon cancer trials of sufficient duration and sample size/statistical power should be undertaken.

10. FOLATE

Folate intake as a potential protective factor against colon carcinogenesis has been of recent interest. Global DNA hypomethylation is consistently found in colon neoplasms *(224–226)*. It also appears to be an early event in the multistep process of colon carcinogenesis, occurring in nonneoplastic tissue prior to the development of the neoplasm. Hypomethylation may be initiated by inadequate cellular levels of the methyl donor, S-adenosylmethionine *(227)*, the production of which is dependent on the vitamin, folate, and the amino acid, methionine *(228)*. Diets deficient in folate and methionine may cause DNA hypomethylation *(228)*. In addition, alcohol, a methyl group antagonist, may cause DNA hypomethylation *(228)*. Thus, a high alcohol intake, in combination with a diet low in folate and methionine, may cause even greater DNA hypomethylation. A major source of dietary folate is plant foods, and that of methionine, animal products, including red meat as well as poultry, fish, seafood, and dairy products.

In addition to these biochemical findings providing biological plausibility for the hypothesis that folate and methionine may protect against colon cancer is the finding that methyl-deficient diets have been shown to cause various cancers in animals *(229–233)*. In human analytic observational epidemiologic studies, an inverse association between folate and risk of colon cancer has been reported in two recent case-control studies *(140,234)* and in a male cohort study *(235)*. The authors of the cohort study also found, using the same food frequency questionnaire as in the male cohort study, an inverse association with colon adenoma in two cohorts *(236)*. In the cohort studies the association was strongest in those with high alcohol consumption.

11. A MODEL OF DIET AND NUTRITION IN THE ETIOLOGY AND PRIMARY PREVENTION OF COLON CANCER

Colon carcinogenesis can be thought of as a long-term, multistep process, in which multiple somatic genetic defects are accumulated *(221)*. The possibility exists that various factors can influence the occurrence or even the reversal of each of the steps (*see* Fig. 3). By inference, the possibility exists that, even after several steps have occurred, the entire process can be reversed. It would seem that the likelihood of reversing some steps would be greater than that of others, and that the likelihood of reversing the entire process would be greater when few rather than many steps have occurred. Naturally occurring foods, food processing, and food preparation methods introduce into the diet multiple factors hypothesized to either increase or decrease the risk of colon cancer. Considering the multistep process of colon carcinogenesis, and the multiple biologically plausible and well-supported dietary factors (although none have acquired consensus status for being established as causal), it would seem likely that risk is a balance of genetic susceptibility, levels of several dietary and other risk factors that increase risk, and levels of several dietary and other risk factors that decrease risk. Some dietary components may influence risk at different steps than do other dietary components;

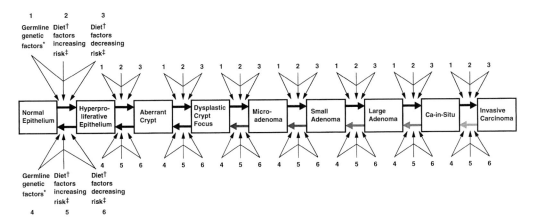

Fig. 3. A model of diet and nutrition in the etiology and primary prevention of colon cancer. *Regarding germ-line genetic factors; a given germ-line genetic factor may play a role at one or more than one step in the multistep process of accumulated somatic genetic changes that lead from normal colon epithelium to invasive colon cancer; one or more than one germ-line genetic factor may be important at any given step, and may be important in pushing the pathway in either direction, although the further one is along the pathway, the less likely it is that the pathway can be pushed back to the preceding step. † Diet = Dietary and other environmental risk factors for colon cancer. ‡ Regarding dietary and other environmental risk factors for colon cancer: the balance of factors that increase vs decrease risk may be important at any step; a given environmental factor may play a role at one or more than one step; one or more environmental factors may be important at any given step; and these factors may be important in pushing the pathway in either direction, although the further one is along the pathway, the less likely it is that the pathway can be pushed back to the preceding step.

some may influence risk at more than one step; some, because of genetic reasons, may influence risk in some individuals and not in other individuals; some may influence risk only in association with other dietary components; and some may interact with other dietary components in other ways.

Thus, a magic bullet approach to prevention, particularly from the public health standpoint, would seem naive and inadequate. A multifactorial approach to prevention would seem most prudent at this time. The diet that would appear ideal, based on current knowledge, for preventing colon cancer would be most like the paleolithic diet (described in ref. *74*), the diet of the earliest evolving/evolved *Homo sapiens*. It is mostly current deviations from this diet that are associated with increased risk for colon cancer: diets high in fat, sucrose, and alcohol, and low in vegetables and fruit and all their associated constituents, including fiber, antioxidants, folate, calcium (wild plant foods were a high source of calcium, thus providing 1500–2000 mg daily compared to the current American average intake of 740 mg), and other nutrients and nonnutrients. The role of meat, apart from fat, is unclear. Meat was clearly a component of the paleolithic diet and is a source of methionine. Wild meat, even red wild meat, is low in fat. The observational epidemiologic literature would suggest increased risk with modern red meat, which is largely high in fat, but no or decreased risk with seafood and skinless white poultry, probably the closest approximations to the wild meat of the paleolithic period. Contributions of current cooking methods remain to be determined.

The diet that protects, then, is likely to be low in fat (and thus in domesticated high-fat red meat), sucrose, and alcohol, and dense in micronutrients (calcium, antioxidants, folate, and others), fiber, and various plant-derived nonnutrient compounds. Because of modern agri-business practices designed to produce vegetables and fruit for transportability and shelf life, for more succulence and less fiber, for more sweetness and less tartness, and so forth, many are concerned that even with a vegetarian diet the modern American eating these commercially grown foods cannot achieve the nutrient and fiber density of the paleolithic diet. The optimum solution would be, as is already occurring in the red meat industry and others, to move to foods that more closely approximate wild foods in being low in fat and dense in micronutrients. An obvious, but unanswered, question is whether nutritional supplements, such as vitamins and minerals, can overcome some of the nutritional deficiencies (relative to the paleolithic diet) in diets based on modern commercial vegetables and fruit, and thus provide some protection against colon cancer, especially in high-risk persons who fail to increase their intake of vegetables and fruit or change other high-risk characteristics of their diets.

12. SUMMARY

Diet and nutrition clearly play a role in the etiology and primary prevention of colon cancer. The most consistent dietary factor associated with colon cancer is vegetable and fruit intake, with a high intake being associated with a decreased risk. Many of the dietary constituents that have been less well studied, but are emerging as at least fairly consistently associated with a decreased risk of colon cancer, are nutritive and nonnutritive substances that are most abundant (or could be most abundant; e.g., calcium) in vegetables and fruit, fiber, calcium, antioxidants, and folate. In addition to many of these relatively well-studied constituents of vegetables and fruit, there is a myriad of other compounds in vegetables and fruit that plausibly may reduce the risk of colon cancer but have not yet received a great deal of study. Many of the dietary constituents of the modern American diet that are most consistently associated with an increased risk of colon cancer are found in abundance in diets low in vegetables and fruit: fat, sucrose, and high-fat red meat cooked at high temperatures.

13. RECOMMENDATIONS

Based on current knowledge, perhaps the most prudent diet would be one modeled after the paleolithic diet: a diet high in vegetables (including grains) and fruit, and low in alcohol and fatty meats and other sources of fat. Evidence from studies of several dietary constituents that are found in most abundance in vegetables and fruit would suggest that changes in agricultural practices to return to more micronutrient-rich vegetable and fruit varieties may be helpful. Until that time, dietary supplementation with such micronutrients as calcium, antioxidants, and folate should receive further study as measures for high-risk individuals unable or unwilling to achieve the ideal diet, realizing that this would not be optimum since current supplements would not be able to address all of the deficiencies of a low vegetable and fruit diet. The current literature provides optimism that colon cancer can be prevented and that diet and nutrition will be key.

REFERENCES

1. Boring CC, Squires TS, Tong T. Cancer statistics. Cancer 1991; 41:19–36.
2. Peto R, Doll R. The Causes of Cancer. Oxford University Press, Oxford; 1981.
3. Schottenfeld D, Winawer SJ. Large intestine. In: Schottenfeld D, Fraumeni JF, eds. Philadelphia; Saunders, 1982; 703–727. Cancer Epidemiology and Prevention.

4. Willett WC, MacMahon B. Diet and cancer—an overview. N Engl J Med 1984; 310:697–703.
5. Potter JD. Reconciling the epidemiology, physiology, and molecular biology of colon cancer. JAMA 1992; 268:1573–1577.
6. Sugarbaker JP, Gundersen LL, Wittes RE. Cancer: principles and practices of oncology. In: Colorectal Cancer 2nd ed. Devita VT, Hellman S, Rosenberry, SF, eds. Philadelphia: Lippincott, 1985; 800–803.
7. Armstrong B, Doll R. Environmental factors and cancer incidence and mortality in different countries, with special reference to dietary practices. Int J Cancer 1975; 15:617–631.
8. Rose DP, Boyar AP, Wynder EL. International comparisons of mortality rates for cancer of the breast, ovary, prostate, and colon, and per capita food consumption. Cancer 1986; 58:2363–2371.
9. Reddy BS. Diet and excretion of bile acids. Cancer Res 1981; 41:3766–3768.
10. Reddy BS, Mangat S, Sheinfil A, Weisburger JH, Wynder EL. Effect of type and amount of dietary fat and 1,2-dimethylhydrazine on biliary bile acids, fecal bile acids, and neutral sterols in rats. Cancer Res 1977; 37:2132–2137.
11. Hill MJ. The role of unsaturated bile acids in the etiology of large bowel cancer. In: Origins of Human Cancer. Hiatt HH, Watson JD, Winsten JA, eds. Cold Spring Harbor, NY: Cold Spring Harbor Laboratory, 1977; 1627–1640.
12. Kandell RL, Bernstein C. Bile salt/acid induction of DNA damage in bacterial and mammalian cells: implications for colon cancer. Nutr Cancer 1991; 16:227–238.
13. Ranken R, Wilson R, Bealmear PM. Increased turnover of intestinal mucosal cell of germfree mice induced by cholic acid. Proc Soc Exp Biol Med 1971; 138:270–242.
14. Chomchai C, Bhadrachari N, Nigro ND. The effect of bile on the induction of experimental intestinal tumors in rats. Dis Colon Rectum 1974; 17:310–312.
15. Narisawa T, Magadia NE, Weisburger JH, Wynder EL. Promoting effect of bile acids on colon carcinogenesis after intrarectal instillation of N-methyl-N´-nitro-N-nitroguanidine in rats. J Natl Cancer Inst 1974; 53:1093–1097.
16. Nigro ND, Singh DV, Campbell RK, Sook M. Effect of dietary beef fat on intestinal tumor formation by azoxymethane in rats. J Natl Cancer Inst 1975; 54:439–442.
17. Reddy BS, Narisawa T, Vukusich C, Weisburger JH, Wynder EL. Effect of quality and quantity of dietary fat and dimethylhydrazine in colon carcinogenesis in rats. Proc Soc Exp Biol Med 1976; 151:237–239.
18. Broitman SA, Vitale JJ, Vavrousek-Jakuba E, Gottlieb LS. Polyunsaturated fat cholesterol and large bowel tumorigenesis. Cancer 1977; 37:2132–2137.
19. Nauss KM, Locniskar M, Newberne PM. Effect of alterations in the quality and quantity of dietary fat on 1,2-dimethylhydrazine-induced colon tumorigenesis in rats. Cancer Res 1983; 43:4083–4090.
20. Hill MJ, Crowther MS, Drasar BE, Hawksworth C, Aries V, Williams REO. Bacteria and aetiology of cancer of large bowel. Lancet 1971; 1:95–100.
21. Reddy BS, Wynder EL. Metabolic epidemiology of colon cancer: fecal bile acids and neutral sterols in colon cancer patients and patients with adenomatous polyps. Cancer 1977; 39:2533–2539.
22. Hill MJ, Drasar BE, Williams REO. Faecal bile-acids and clostridia in patients with cancer of the large bowel. Lancet 1975; 1:535–539.
23. Reddy BS, Mastromarino A, Wynder EL. Further leads on metabolic epidemiology of large bowel cancer. Cancer Res 1975; 35:3403–3406.
24. Mudd DG, McKelvey ST, Norwood W, Elmore DT, Roy AD. Faecal bile acid concentration of patients with carcinoma or increased risk of carcinoma in the large bowel. Gut 1980; 21:587–590.
25. Reddy BS, Watanabe K, Weisberger JH, Wynder EL. Promoting effect of bile acids in colon carcinogenesis in germ-free and conventional F344 rats. Cancer Res 1977; 37:3238–3242.
26. Goldin BR, Swenson L, Dwyer J, Sexton M, Gorbach SL. Effect of diet and Lactobacillus acidophilus supplements on human fecal bacterial enzymes. J Natl Cancer Inst 1980; 64:255–261.
27. Reddy BS, Hanson D, Mangat B, Mathews L, Sbaschnig M, Sharma C, Simi B. Effect of high-fat, high-beef diet and of mode of cooking of beef in the diet on fecal bacterial enzymes and fecal bile acids and neutral sterols. J Nutr 1980; 110:1880–1887.
28. Corpet D, Stamp D, Medline A, Minkin S, Archer M, Bruce WR. Promotion of colonic microadenoma growth in mice and rats fed cooked sugar or cooked casein and fat. Cancer Res 1990; 50:6955–6958.
29. Sugimura T, Sato S. Mutagens-carcinogens in foods. Cancer Res 1983; 43:2415s–2421s.
30. Babbs CF. Free radicals and the etiology of colon cancer. Free Rad Biol Med 1990; 8:191–200.
31. Potter JD, Slattery ML, Bostick RM, Gapstur SM. Colon cancer: a review of the epidemiology. Epidemiol Rev 1993; 15:499–545.
32. Phillips R. Role of life-style and dietary habits in risk of cancer among Seventh-Day Adventists. Cancer Res 1975; 35:3513–3522.

33. Manousos O, Day NE, Trichopoulos D, Gerovassilis G, Tzonou A. Diet and colorectal cancer: a case-control study in Greece. Int J Cancer 1983; 32:1–5.

34. Pickle LW, Greene MH, Ziegler RG, Toledo A, Hoover R, Lynch HT, Fraumeni JF Jr. Colorectal cancer in rural Nebraska. Cancer Res 1984; 44:363–369.

35. Macquart-Moulin G, Riboli E, Cornée J, Charnay B, Berthezene P, Day N. Case-control study on colorectal cancer and diet in Marseilles. Int J Cancer 1986; 38:183–191.

36. LaVecchia C, Negri E, Decarli A, D'Avanzo B, Gallotti L, Gentile A, Franceschi S. A case-control study of diet and colo-rectal cancer in northern Italy. Int J Cancer 1988; 41:492–498.

37. Benito E, Obrador A, Stiggelbout A, Bosch FX, Mulet M, Munoz N, Kaldor J. A population-based case-control study of colorectal cancer in Majorca. I. Dietary factors. Int J Cancer 1990; 45:69–76.

38. Peters RK, Pike MC, Garabrant D, Mack TM. Diet and colon cancer in Los Angeles County, California. Cancer Cause Control 1992; 3:457–473.

39. Willett WC, Stampfer MJ, Colditz GA, Rosner BA, Speizer FE. Relation of meat, fat and fiber intake to the risk of colon cancer in a prospective study among women. New Engl J Med 1990; 323:1664–1672.

40. Hirayama T. A large-scale cohort study on the relationship between diet and selected cancers of digestive organs. In: Gastrointestinal Cancer: Endogenous Factors; Banbury report 7. Bruce WR, Correa P, Lipkin M, Tannenbaum SR, Wilkins TD eds. Cold Spring Harbor, NY: Cold Spring Harbor Laboratory, 1981; 409–426.

41. Phillips RL, Snowdon DA. Dietary relationships with fatal colorectal cancer among Seventh-Day Adventists. J Natl Cancer Inst 1985; 74:307–317.

42. Bostick RM, Potter JD, Steinmetz KA, Kushi LH, Sellers TA, McKenzie DR, Gapstur SM, Folsom AR. Sugar, meat, and fat intake and non-dietary risk factors for colon cancer incidence in Iowa women (United States). Cancer Cause Control 1994; 5:38–52.

43. Stemmermann GN, Nomura AMY, Heilbrun LK. Dietary fat and the risk of colorectal cancer. Cancer Res 1984; 44:4633–4637.

44. Willett WC, Stampfer MJ. Total energy intake: implications for epidemiologic analyses. Am J Epidemiol 1986; 124:17–27.

45. Jain M, Cook GM, Davis FG, Grace MG, Howe GR, Miller AB. A case-control study of diet and colorectal cancer. Int J Cancer 1980a; 26:757–768.

46. Potter JD, McMichael AJ. Diet and cancer of the colon and rectum: a case-control study. J Natl Cancer Inst 1986; 76:557–69.

47. Lyon JL, Mahoney AW, West DW, Gardner JW, Smith KR, Sorenson AW, Standish W. Energy intake: its relationship to colon cancer risk. J Natl Cancer Inst 1987; 78:853–861.

48. Graham S, Marshall J, Haughey B, Mittelman A, Swanson M, Zielezny M, Byers T, Wilkinson G, West D. Dietary epidemiology of cancer of the colon in western New York. Am J Epidemiol 1988; 128: 490–503.

49. Slattery ML, Schumacher MC, Smith KR, West DW, Abd-Elghany N. Physical activity, diet, and risk of colon cancer in Utah. Am J Epidemiol 1988; 128:989–999.

50. Whittemore AS, Wu-Williams AH, Lee M, Shu Z, Gallagher RP, Deng-ao J, Lun Z, Xianghui W, Kun C, Jung D, The CZ, Chengde L, Yao XJ, Paffenbarger Jr. RS, Henderson BE. Diet, physical activity, and colorectal cancer among Chinese in North American and China. J Natl Cancer Inst 1990; 82:915–926.

51. Peltomäki P, Aaltonen LA, Sistonen P, Pylkkänen L, Mecklin JP, Järvinen H, Green JS, Jass JR, Weber JL, Leach FS, Peterson GM, Hamilton SR, de la Chapelle A, Vogelstein B. Genetic mapping of a locus predisposing to human colorectal cancers. Science 1993; 260:810–812.

52. Kadlubar FF, Butler MA, Kaderlik KR, Chou HC, Lang NP. Polymorphisms for aromatic amine metabolism in humans: relevance for human carcinogenesis. Environ Health Persp 1992; 98:69–74.

53. Anti M, Marra G, Armelao F, Percesepe A, Ficarelli R, Ricciutu GM, Valenti A, Rapaccini GL, De Vitis I, D'Agostino G, Brighi S, Vecchio FM. Effect of ω-3 fatty acids on rectal mucosal cell proliferation in subjects at risk for colon cancer. Gastroenterology 1992; 102:883–891.

54. Burkitt D. Related disease—related cause? Lancet 1969; 2:1229–1231.

55. Steinmetz KA, Potter JD. Vegetables, fruit, and cancer. II. Mechanisms. Cancer Cause Control 1991; 2:427–442.

56. Greenwald P, Lanza E. Dietary fiber and colon cancer. In Contemporary Nutrition. Minneapolis, MN: General Mills Nutrition Department, 1986: Vol. 11, No. 1.

57. National Research Council (US), Committee on Diet and Health. Diet and Health: Implications for Reducing Chronic Disease Risk. National Academy Press, United States, 1989.

58. Potter JD. The epidemiology of fiber and colorectal cancer: why don't the epidemiologic data make better sense: In: Dietary Fiber. Kritchevsky D, Bonfield C, Anderson JW, eds. New York: Plenum, 1990; 431–446.

59. Trock B, Lanza E, Greenwald P. Dietary fiber, vegetables, and colon cancer: critical review and meta-analyses of the epidemiologic evidence. J Natl Cancer Inst 1990; 82:650–661.
60. Howe GR, Benito E, Castelleto R, Cornee J, Esteve J, Gallagher RP, Isocovich JM, Deng-ao J, Kaaks R, Kune GA, Kune S, L'Abbe KA, Lee HP, Lee M, Miller AB, Peters RK, Potter JD, Riboli E, Slattery ML, Trichopoulos D, Tuyns A, Tzonou A, Whittemore AS, Wu-Williams AH, Shu Z. Dietary intake of fiber and decreased risk of cancers of the colon and rectum: evidence from the combined analysis of 13 case-control studies. J Natl Cancer Inst 1992; 84:1887–1896.
61. Steinmetz KA, Kushi LH, Bostick RM, Folsom AR, Potter JD. Vegetables, fruit, and colon cancer in the Iowa Women's Health Study. Am J Epidemiol 1994; 139:1–15.
62. Bueding E, Asher S, Dolan P. Anticarcinogenic and other protective effects of dithiolthiones. In: Antimutagenesis and Anticarcinogenesis Mechanisms. Shankel DM, Hartman PE, Kada T, Hollaender A, eds. New York, NY: Plenum, 1986; Vol. 39: 483–489.
63. Wattenberg LW. Chemoprevention of cancer. Cancer Res 1985; 45:1–8.
64. Hocman G. Prevention of cancer: vegetables and plants. Comp Biochem Physiol 1989; 93:201–212.
65. Stich HF, Rosin MP. Naturally occurring phenolics as antimutagenic and anticarcinogenic agents. Adv Exp Med 1984; 177:1–29.
66. Schelp FP, Pongpaew P. Protection against cancer through nutritionally-induced increase of endogenous protease inhibitors—a hypothesis. Int J Epidemiol 1988; 17:287–292.
67. Raicht RF, Cohen BI, Fazzini EP, Sarwal AN, Takahashi M. Protective effect of plant sterols against chemically induced colon tumors in rats. Cancer Res 1980; 40:403–405.
68. Messina M, Barnes S. The role of soy products in reducing risk of cancer. J Natl Cancer Inst 1991; 83:541–546.
69. Messina M, Messina V. Increasing use of soyfoods and their potential role in cancer prevention. J Am Dietetic Assoc 1991; 91:836–840.
70. Aldercreutz H. Western diet and western diseases: some hormonal and biochemical mechanisms and associations. Scand J Clin Lab Invest 1990; 50:3–23.
71. You WC, Blot WJ, Chang YS, Ershow A, Zang ZT, An Q, Henderson BE, Fraumeni JF Jr, Wang TG. Allium vegetables and the reduced risk of stomach cancer. J Natl Cancer Inst 1989; 81:162–164.
72. Potter JD. The epidemiology of diet and cancer: evidence of human maladaptation. In: Nutrition and Cancer Prevention. Investigating the Role of Macronutrients. Moon TE, Micozzi MS, eds. New York: Dekker, 1992; 55–84.
73. Steinmetz KA, Potter JD. Vegetables, fruit, and cancer. I. epidemiology. Cancer Cause Control 1991; 2:325–357.
74. Eaton SB, Shostak M, Konner M. The Paleolithic Prescription. Harper and Row, New York; 1988.
75. Trowell HC. Refined carbohydrate foods and fibre. In: Refined Carbohydrates: Food and Disease. Burkitt DP, Trowell HC, eds. Oxford: Academic, 1975; 23–41.
76. Food and Agricultural Organization. Food Balance Sheets 1975–1977 Average. Rome; FAO, 1980.
77. Stamp D, Zhang X-M, Medline A, Bruce WR, Archer MC. Sucrose enhancement of the early steps of colon carcinogenesis in mice. Carcinogenesis 1993; 14:777–779.
78. Stich HF, Rosin MP, Wu CH, Powrie WD. Clastogenicity of furans found in food. Cancer Lett 1981; 13:89–95.
79. Nishi Y, Miyakawa Y, Kato K. Chromosome aberrations induced by pyrolysates of carbohydrates in Chinese hamster V79 cells. Mutat Res 1989; 227:117–123.
80. Archer MC, Bruce WR, Chan CC, Medline A, Stamp D, Zhang X-M. Promotion of colonic microadenoma in rats by 5-hydroxymethyl-2-furaldehyde in thermolysed sugar. Proc AACR 1992; 33:130.
81. Kruis W, Forstmaier G, Sheurlen C, Stellaard F. Effect of diets low and high in refined sugars on gut transit, bile acid metabolism, and bacterial fermentation. Gut 1991; 32:367–371.
82. Miller AB, Howe GR, Jain M, Craib KJP, Harrison L. Food items and food groups as risk factors in a case-control study of diet and colorectal cancer. Int J Cancer 1983; 32:155–161.
83. Tuyns AJ, Kaaks R, Haelterman M. Colorectal cancer and the consumption of foods: a case-control study in Belgium. Nutr Cancer 1988; 11:189–204.
84. Bristol JB, Emmett PM, Heaton KW, Williamson RCN. Sugar, fat, and the risk of colorectal cancer. Br Med J 1985; 291:1467–1470.
85. Macquart-Moulin G, Riboli E, Cornee J, Kaaks R, Berthezene P. Colorectal polyps and diet: a case-control study in Marseilles. Int J Cancer 1987; 40:179–188.
86. Bidoli E, Franceschi S, Talamini R, Barra S, La Vecchia C. Food consumption and cancer of the colon and rectum in north-eastern Italy. Int J Cancer 1992; 50:223–229.
87. Newmark HL, Wargovich MJ, Bruce WR. Colon cancer and dietary fat, phosphate and calcium: a hypothesis. J Natl Cancer Inst 1984; 72:1323–1325.

88. Bleiberg H, Buyse M, Galand P. Cell kinetic indicators of premalignant stages of colorectal cancer. Cancer 1989; 56:124–129.

89. Paganelli GM, Santucci R, Biasco G, Miglioli M, Barbara L. Effect of sex and age on rectal cell renewal in humans. Cancer Lett 1990; 53:117–121.

90. Paganelli GM, Biasco G, Santucci R, Brandi G, Lalli AA, Miglioli M, Barbara L. Rectal cell proliferation and colorectal cancer risk level in patients with nonfamilial adenomatous polyps of the large bowel. Cancer 1991; 68:2451–2354.

91. Ponz de Leon M, Roncucci L, Di Donato P, Tassi L, Smerieri O, Grazia M, Malagoli AG, De Maria D, Antonioli A, Chahin N, Perini M, Rigo G, Barberini G, Manenti A, Biasco, G, Barbara L. Pattern of epithelial cell proliferation in colorectal mucosa of normal subjects and of patients with adenomatous polyps or cancer of the large bowel. Cancer Res 1988; 48:4121–4126.

92. Lipkin M, Blattner WE, Fraumeni JF, Lynch HT, Deschner E, Winawer S. Tritiated thymidine ($\emptyset_p,\emptyset_h$) labeling distribution as a marker for hereditary predisposition to colon cancer. Cancer Res 1983; 43:1899–1904.

93. Lipkin M, Uehara K, Winawer S, Sanchez A, Bauer C, Phillips R, Lynch HT, Blattner WA, Fraumeni Jr JF. Seventh-Day Adventist vegetarians have quiescent proliferative activity in colonic mucosa. Cancer Lett 1985; 26:139–144.

94. Lipkin M, Enker WE, Eilers GAM. Tritiated-thymidine labeling of rectal epithelial cells in "non-prep" biopsies of individuals at increased risk for colonic neoplasia. Cancer Lett 1987; 37:155–161.

95. Risio M, Lipkin M, Candelaresi G, Bertone A, Coverlizza S, Rossini F. Correlations between rectal mucosa cell poliferation and the clinical and pathological features of nonfamilial neoplasia of the large intestine. Cancer Res 1991; 51:1917–1921.

96. Stadler J, Yeung KS, Furrer R, Marcon N, Himal HS, Bruce WR. Proliferative activity of rectal mucosa and soluble fecal bile acids in patients with normal colons and in patients with colonic polyps or cancer. Cancer Lett 1988; 38:315–320.

97. Terpstra OT, Strautenstein MV, Dees J, Eilers GAM. Abnormal pattern of cell proliferation in the entire mucosa of patients with colon adenoma or cancer. Gastroenterology 1987; 92:704–708.

98. Deschner EE, Lewis DM, Lipkin M. In vitro study of human rectal epithelial cells. 1. Atypical zone of H^3 thymidine incorporation in mucosa of multiple polyposis. J Clin Invest 1963; 42:1922–1928.

99. Biasco G, Lipkin M, Minarini A, Higgins P, Miglioli M, Barbara L. Proliferative and antigenic properties of rectal cells in patients with chronic ulcerative colitis. Cancer Res 1984; 44:5450–5454.

100. Bleiberg H, Mainguet P, Galand P, Chretien J, Dupont-Mairesse N. Cell renewal in the human rectum: in vitro autoradiographic study on active ulcerative colitis. Gastroenterology 1970; 58:851–855.

101. Gerdes H, Gillin JS, Zimbalist E, Urmacher C, Lipkin M, Winawer SJ. Expansion of the epithelial proliferative compartment and frequency of adenomatous polyps in the colon correlate with the strength of family history of colorectal cancer. Cancer Res 1993; 53:279–282.

102. Roncucci L, Ponz de Leon M, Scalmati A, Malgoli G, Pratissoli S, Perini M, Chahin NJ. The influence of age on colonic epithelial cell proliferation. Cancer 1988; 48:235–245.

103. Anti M, Marra G, Armelao F, Percesepe A, Ficarelli R, Ricciuto GM, Valenti A, Rapaccini GL, De Vitis I, D'Agnostino G, Brighi S, Vecchio FM. Rectal epithelial cell proliferation patterns as predictors of adenomatous colorectal polyp recurrence. Gut 1993; 34:525–530.

104. Scalmati A, Roncucci L, Ghidini G, Biasco G, Ponz de Leon M. Epithelial cell kinetics in the remaining colorectal mucosa after surgery for cancer of the large bowel. Cancer Res 1990; 50:7937–7941.

105. Risio M, Coverlizza M, Ferrari A, Candelaresi G, Rossini F. Immunohistochemical study of epithelial cell proliferation in hyperplastic polyps, adenomas, and adenocarcinomas of the large bowel. Gastroenterology 1988; 94:899–906.

106. Newmark HL, Lipkin M. Calcium, vitamin D, and colon cancer. Cancer Res 1992; 52:2067s–2070s.

107. Wargovich MJ, Baer AR. Basic and clinical investigations of dietary calcium in the prevention of colorectal cancer. Prev Med 1989; 18:672–679.

108. Bostick R, Potter JD, Fosdick L, Grambsch P, Lampe J, Wood J, Louis T, Ganz R, Grandits G. Calcium and colorectal epithelial cell proliferation: a preliminary randomized, double-blinded, placebo-controlled clinical trial. J Natl Cancer Inst 1993; 85:132–141.

109. Rozen P. An evaluation of rectal epithelial proliferation measurement as biomarker of risk for colorectal neoplasia and response in intervention studies. Eur J Cancer Prev 1992; 1:215–224.

110. Grambsch PM, Randall BL, Bostick RM, Potter JD, Louis TA. Modeling the labeling index distribution: an application of functional data analysis. J Am Stats Assoc 1995; 90:813–821.

111. Potten CS, Kellett M, Roberts SA, Rew DA, Wilson GD. Measurement of in vivo proliferation in human colorectal mucosa using bromodeoxyuridine. Gut 1992; 33:71–81.

112. Wargovich MJ, Eng VWS, Newmark H. Calcium inhibits the damaging and compensatory proliferative effects of fatty acids on mouse colon epithelium. Cancer Lett 1984; 23:253–258.
113. Bird RP, Schneider R, Stamp D, Bruce WR. Effect of dietary calcium and cholic acid on the proliferative indices of murine colonic epithelium. Carcinogenesis 1986; 7:657–661.
114. Wargovich MJ, Eng WWS, Newmark HL, Bruce WR. Calcium ameliorates the toxic effect of deoxycholic acid on colonic epithelium. Carcinogenesis 1983; 4:1205–1207.
115. Lipkin M, Newmark H. Effect of added dietary calcium on colonic epithelial cell proliferation in subjects at high risk for familial colonic cancer. New Engl J Med 1985; 313:1381–1384.
116. Buset M, Lipkin M, Winawer S, Swaroop S, Friedman E. Inhibition of human colonic epithelial cell proliferation in vivo and in vitro by calcium. Cancer Res 1986; 46:5426–5430.
117. Rozen P, Fireman A, Fine N, Wax Y, Ron E. Oral calcium suppresses increased rectal epithelial proliferation of persons at risk of colorectal cancer. Gut 1989; 30:650–655.
118. Lipkin M, Friedman E, Winawer SJ, Newmark H. Colonic epithelial cell proliferation in responders and non-responders to supplemental dietary calcium. Cancer Res 1989; 49:248–254.
119. Wargovich MJ, Isbell G, Shabot M, Winn R, Lanza F, Hochman L, Larson E, Lynch P, Roubein L, Levin B. Calcium supplementation decreases rectal epithelial cell proliferation in subjects with sporadic adenoma. Gastroenterology 1992; 103:92–97.
120. Gregoire R, Stern HS, Yeung KS, Stadler J, Langley S, Furrer R, Bruce WR. Effect of calcium supplementation on mucosal cell proliferation in high risk patients for colon cancer. Gut 1989; 30:376–382.
121. Bostick RM, Fosdick L, Wood JR, Grambsch P, Grandits G, Lilliemoe JT. Calcium and colorectal epithelial cell proliferation in sporadic adenoma patients. J Natl Cancer Inst 1995; 87:1307–1315.
122. Alder R, McKeown-Eyssen G, Bright-See E. Randomized trial of the effect of calcium supplementation on fecal risk factors for colorectal cancer. Am J Epidemiol 1993; 138:804–814.
123. Lapré JA, De Vries HT, Termont DSML, Kleibeuker JH, De Vries EGE, Van der Meer R. Mechanism of the protective effect of supplemental dietary calcium on cytolytic activity of fecal water. Cancer Res 1993; 53:248–253.
124. Van der Meer R, Welberg JWM, Kuipers F, Kleibeuker JH, Mulder NH, Termont DSML, Vonk RJ, De Vries HT, De Vries EGE. Effects of supplemental dietary calcium on the intestinal association of calcium, phosphate, and bile acids. Gastroenterology 1990; 99:1653–1659.
125. Van der Meer JWM, Kleibeuker JH, Van der Meer R, Kuipers F, Cats A, Van Rijsbergen H, Termont DSML, Boersma-Van Ek W, Vonk FJ, Mulder NH, De Vries EGE. Effects of oral calcium supplementation on intestinal bile acids and cytolytic activity of fecal water in patients with adenomatous polyps of the colon. Euro J Clin Invest 1993; 23:63–68.
126. Yang K, Cohen L, Lipkin M. Lectin soybean agglutinin: measurements in colonic epithelial cells of human subjects following supplemental dietary calcium. Cancer Lett 1991; 56:65–69.
127. Whitfield JF, Boynton AL, MacManus JP, Rixon RH, Sikorska M, Tsang B, Walker PR. The roles of calcium and cyclic AMP in cell proliferation. Ann NY Acad Sci 1980; 339:216–240.
128. Rasmussen CD, Means AR. Calmodulin is involved in regulation of cell proliferation. EMBO J 1987; 6:3961–3968.
129. Arlow FL, Walczak SM, Luk GD, Majumdar APN. Attenuation of azoxymethane-induced colonic mucosal ornithine decarboxylase and tyrosine kinase activity by calcium in rats. Cancer Res 1989; 49:5884–5888.
130. Su L-K, Vogelstein B, Kinzler KW. Association of the APC tumor suppressor protein with catenins. Science 1993; 262:1734–1737.
131. Rubinfeld B, Souza B, Albert I, Müller O, Chamberlain SH, Masiarz FR, Munemitsu S, Polakis P. Association of the APC gene product with β-catenin. Science 1993; 262:1731–1734.
132. Llor X, Jacoby RF, Teng B, Davidson NO, Sitrin MD, Brasitus TA. K-ras mutations in 1, 2-dimethylhydrazine-induced colonic tumors: effects of supplemental dietary calcium and vitamin D deficiency. Cancer Res 1991; 51:4305–4309.
133. Paganelli GM, Biasco G, Brandi G, Santucci R, Gizzi G, Villani V, Cianci M, Miglioli M, Barbara L. Effect of vitamin A, C, and E supplementation on rectal cell proliferation in patients with colorectal adenomas. J Natl Cancer Inst 1992; 84:47–51.
134. Garland C, Barrett-Connor E, Rossof AH, Shekelle RB, Criqui MH, Ogelsby P. Dietary vitamin D and calcium and risk of colorectal cancer: a 19-year prospective study in men. Lancet 1985; 1:307–309.
135. Stemmerman GN, Nomura A, Chyou P-H. The influence of dairy and non-dairy calcium on subsite large-bowel cancer risk. Dis Colon Rectum 1990; 33:190–194.
136. Kune S, Kune GM, Watson F. Case-control study of dietary etiologic factors: the Melbourne colorectal cancer study. Nutr Cancer 1987; 9:21–42.

137. Slattery ML, Sorenson AW, Ford MH. Dietary calcium as a mitigating factor in colon cancer. Am J Epidemiol 1988; 128:504–514.
138. Lee HP, Gourly L, Duffy SW, Esteve J, Day NE. Colorectal cancer and diet in an Asian population—a case-control study among Singapore Chinese. Int J Cancer 1989; 43:1007–1016.
139. Wu AH, Paganini-Hill A, Ross RK, Henderson BE. Alcohol, physical activity and other risk factors for colorectal cancer: a prospective study. Br J Cancer 1987; 55:687–694.
140. Benito E, Stiggelbout A, Bosch FX, Obrador A, Kaldor J, Mulet M, Munoz N. Nutritional factors in colorectal cancer risk: a case-control study in Majorca. Int J Cancer 1991; 49:161–167.
141. Tuyns AJ, Haelterman M, Kaaks R. Colorectal cancer and the intake of nutrients: oligosaccharides are a risk factor, fats are not. A case-control study in Belgium. Nutr Cancer 1987; 10:181–196.
142. Negri E, LaVecchia C, D'Avanzo B, Franceschi S. Calcium, dairy products and colorectal cancer. Nutr Cancer 1990; 13:255–262.
143. Bostick RM, Potter JD, Sellers TA, McKenzie DR, Kushi LH, Folsom AR. Relation of calcium, vitamin D, and dairy food intake to incidence of colon cancer among older women: the Iowa Women's Health Study. Am J Epidemiol 1993; 137:1302–1317.
144. Kampman E, Goldbohm RA, van den Brandt PA, van't Veer P. Fermented dairy products, calcium and colorectal cancer in the Netherlands cohort study. Cancer Res 1994; 54:3186–3190.
145. Haynes RC, Murad F. In: The Pharmacologic Basis of Therapeutics. 7th ed. Gilman AG, Goodman LG, Rall TW, Murad F, eds. New York, NY: MacMillan, 1985.
146. Lointier P, Wargovich MJ, Saez S, Michzel J, Levin B, Wildrick DM, Boman BM. The role of vitamin D_3 in the proliferation of a human colon cancer cell line in vitro. Anticancer Res 1987; 7:817–822.
147. Pence BC, Buddingh F. Inhibition of dietary fat-promoted colon carcinogenesis in rats by supplemental calcium or vitamin D_3. Carcinogenesis 1988; 9:187–190.
148. McSherry CK, Cohen BI, Bokkenheuser VD, Mosbach EH, Winter J, Matoba N, Scholes J. Effects of calcium and bile acid feeding on colon tumors in the rat. Cancer Res 1989; 49:6039–6043.
149. Kawaura A, Takahashi A, Tanida N, Oda M, Sawada K, Sawada Y, Mae Karva S, Shimoyama T. 1 α-Hydroxyvitamin D_3 suppresses colonic tumorigenesis induced by repetitive intrarectal injection of N-methyl-N-nitrosourea in rats. Cancer Lett 1990; 55:149–152.
150. Garland CF, Garland FC, Shaw EK, Comstock GN, Helsing KJ, Gorham ED. Serum 25-hydroxyvitamin D and colon cancer: eight-year prospective study. Lancet 1989; 2:1176–1178.
151. Tajima K, Tominga S. Dietary habits and gastro-intestinal cancers: a comparative case-control study of stomach and large intestinal cancers in Nagoya Japan. Jpn J Cancer Res 1985; 76:705–716.
152. Ursin G, Bjelke E, Heuch I, Vollset SE. Milk consumption and cancer incidence: a Norwegian prospective study. Br J Cancer 1990; 61:454–459.
153. Ames BN. Mutagenesis and carcinogenesis: endogenous and exogenous factors. Env Mol Mut 1989; 14:66–77.
154. Ames BN. Endogenous DNA damage as related to cancer and aging. Mutat Res 1989; 214:41–46.
155. Ames BN. Endogenous oxidative damage, aging, and cancer. Free Rad Res Comms 1989; 7:121–128.
156. Frankel EN. Chemistry of free radical and singlet oxidation of lipids. Prog Lipid Res 1985; 23:197–221.
157. Halliwell B, Aruoma OI. DNA damaged by oxygen-derived species. Its mechanism and measurement in mammalian systems. FEBS Lett 1991; 281:9–19.
158. Ames BN. Dietary carcinogens and anticarcinogens: oxygen radicals and degenerative diseases. Science 1983; 221:1256–1264.
159. Cerutti PA. Pro-oxidant states and tumor promotion. Science 1985; 227:375–380.
160. Cross CE, Halliwell B, Borish ET, Pryor WA, Ames BN, Saul RL, McCord JM, Harman D. Oxygen radicals and human disease. Ann Int Med 1987; 107:526–545.
161. Halliwell B, Gutteridge JMC. Role of free radicals and catalytic metal ions in human disease: an overview. Methods Enzymol 1990; 186:1–85.
162. Machlin LJ, Bendick A. Free radical tissue damage: protective role of antioxidant nutrients. FASEB J 1987; 1:444–445.
163. Frenkel K. Carcinogen-mediated oxidant formation and oxidative DNA damage. Pharm Ther 1992; 53:127–166.
164. Halliwell B, Chirico S. Lipid peroxidation: its mechanism, measurement, and significance. Am J Clin Nutr 1993; 57(Suppl):715s–725s.
165. Djuric Z, Heilbrun LK, Reading BA, Boower A, Valeriote FA, Martino S. Effects of a low-fat diet on levels of oxidative damage to DNA in human peripheral nucleated blood cells. J Natl Cancer Inst 1991; 83:766–769.

166. Dorgan JF, Schatzkin A. Antioxidant micronutrients in cancer prevention. Hematol Oncol Clinics N Am 1991; 5:43–68.

167. Salonen JT, Salonen R, Lappetelainen R, Maenpaa PH, Alfthau G, Paska R. Risk of cancer in relation to serum concentrations of selenium and vitamins A and E: matched case control analysis of prospective data. Br Med J 1985; 290:417–420.

168. Menkes M, Comstock GW, Vuilleamier JP, Helsing VJ, Rider AA, Brookmeyer R. Serum beta carotene, vitamins A and E, selenium, and the risk of lung cancer. New Eng J Med 1986; 315:1250–1254.

169. Horvath PM, Ip C. Synergistic effect of vitamin E and selenium in the chemoprevention of mammary carcinogenesis in rats. Cancer Res 1983; 43:5335–5341.

170. Thompson HJ, Meeker LK, Becci PJ. Effect of combined selenium and retinyl acetate treatment on mammary carcinogenesis. Cancer Res 1981; 41:1413–1416.

171. Bendich A, Machlin LJ, Scandarra O, Burton GW, Wagner DM. The antioxidant role of vitamin C. Adv Free Radical Biol Med 1986; 2:419–444.

172. Bendich A, Diapolito P, Gabriel E, Machlin LJ. Interaction of dietary vitamin C and vitamin E in guinea pig immune response to mitogens. J Nutr 1984; 114:1588–1593.

173. Urbach C, Hickman K, Harris PL. Effect of individual vitamins A, C, E, and carotene administered at high levels and their interactions in the blood. Exp Med Surg 1951; 10:7–20.

174. Combs JF. Protective roles of minerals against free radical tissue damage. Nutr 1987. Bethesda: Am Inst Nutr.

175. Ganther HE, Hafeman DG, Lawrence RW, Serfass RE, Hockstra WG. Selenium and glutathione peroxidase in health and disease. A review. Prascil. In: Trace Elements in Human Health and Disease, Vol. 2. Prasad AS, Oberlea SD, eds. New York: Academic; 1976; 165–235.

176. Kandaswami C, Perkins E, Solonink DS, Drzewieki G, Middleton E. Ascorbic acid-enhanced antiproliferative effect of flavanoids on squamous cell carcinoma in vitro. Anti-Cancer Drugs 1983; 4:91–96.

177. Ip C. Chemoprevention of mammary tumorigenesis by a combined regimen of selenium and vitamin A. Carcinogenesis 1981; 2:915–918.

178. Ip C. Attenuation of the anticarcinogenic action of selenium by vitamin E deficiency. Cancer Lett 1985; 25:325–331.

179. Mergens WJ, Bhagavan HN. α-Tocopherols (vitamin E). In: Nutrition and Cancer Prevention, Investigating the Role of Micronutrients. Moon TE, Micozzis MS, eds. New York: Marcel Dekker, 1990; 305–340.

180. Mirvish SS. Effects of vitamins C and E on N-nitroso compound formation, carcinogenesis, and cancer. Cancer 1986; 58:1842–1850.

181. Okuzumi J, Nishino H, Murakoshi M, Yamane T, Kitao Y, Inagake M, Ohya K, Yoshida M, Takahashi T. Palm carotene inhibits tumor-promoting activity of bile acids and intestinal carcinogenesis. Oncology 1992; 49:492–497.

182. Medina D. Mechanisms of selenium inhibition of tumorigenesis. J Am Coll Toxicol 1986; 5: 21–27.

183. Reddy BS, Rivenson A, Kulkarni N, Upadhyaya P, El-Bayoumy K. Chemoprevention of colon carcinogenesis by the synthetic organoselenium compound 1, 4-phenylenebis(methylene)selencyanate. Cancer Res 1992; 52:5635–5640.

184. Birt DF. Update on the effects of vitamins A, C, and E and selenium on carcinogenesis. Proc Soc Exp Biol Med 1986; 183:311–320.

185. Byers T, Perry G. Dietary carotenes, vitamin C, and vitamin E as protective antioxidants in human cancers. Ann Rev Nutr 1992; 12:139–159.

186. Block G, Patterson B, Subar A. Fruit, vegetables, and cancer prevention: a review of the epidemiologic evidence. Nutr Cancer 1992; 18:1–29.

187. Bostick RM, Potter JD, McKenzie DR, Sellers TA, Kushi LH, Steinmetz KA, Folsom AR. Reduced risk of colon cancer with high intake of vitamin E: the Iowa Women's Health Study. Cancer Res 1993; 53:4230–4237.

188. Longnecker MP, Martin-Moreno J, Knekt P, Nomura AMY, Schober SE, Stähelin HB, Wald NJ, Gey KF, Willett WC. Serum alpha-tocopherol concentration in relation to subsequent colorectal cancer: pooled data from five cohorts. J Natl Cancer Inst 1992; 4: 430–435.

189. Schrauzer GN, White DA, Schneider CJ. Cancer mortality correlation studies-III. Statistical associations with dietary selenium intake. Bioinorganic Chem 1977; 7:23–31.

190. Clark LC. The epidemiology of selenium and cancer. Fed Proc 1985; 44:2584–2589.

191. van den Brandt PA, Goldbohm RA, van `t Veer P, Bode P, Dorant E, Hermus RJJ, Sturmans F. A prospective cohort study on toenail selenium levels and risk of gastrointestinal cancer. J Natl Cancer Inst 1993; 85:224–229.

192. Leonard TK, Mohs ME, Ho EE, Watson RR. Nutrient intakes: cancer causation and prevention. Prog Food Nutr Science 1986; 10:237–277.
193. Nelson RL. Dietary minerals and colon carcinogenesis. Anticancer Res 1987; 7:259–270.
194. Blot WJ, Li J-Y, Taylor PR, Guo W, Daysey S, Wang G-Q, Yang CS, Zheng S-F, Gail M, Li G-Y, Yu Y, Liu B, Tangrea J, Sun Y, Fusheng L, Fraumeni JF, Zhang Y-H, Li B. Nutrition intervention trials in Linxian, China: supplementation with specific vitamin/mineral combinations, cancer incidence, and disease-specific mortality in the general population. J Natl Cancer Inst 1993; 85:1483–1492.
195. Fraga CG, Motchnik PA, Shigenaga MK, Helbock HJ, Jacob RA, Ames BN. Ascorbic acid protects against endogenous oxidative DNA damage in human sperm. Proc Natl Acad Sci USA 1991; 88:11,003–11,006.
196. Simic MG, Bergtold DS. Dietary modulation of DNA damage in humans. Mutat Res 1991; 250:17–24.
197. Garrido A, Garrido F, Guerra R, Valenzuela A. Ingestion of high doses of fish oil increases the susceptibility of cellular membranes to the induction of oxidative stress. Lipids 1989; 24:833–835.
198. Hu ML, Frankel EN, Tappel AL. Effect of dietary menhaden oil and vitamin E on in vivo lipid peroxidation induced by iron. Lipids 1990; 25:194–198.
199. Laganiere S, Yu BP, Fernandes G. Studies on membrane lipid peroxidation in omega-3 fatty acid-fed autoimmune mice: effect of vitamin E supplementation. Adv Exp Med Biol 1992; 262:95–102.
200. Haglund O, Luostarinen R, Wallen R, Wibell L, Saldeen T. The effects of fish oil on triglycerides, cholesterol, fibrinogen and malondialdehyde in humans supplemented with vitamin E. J Nutr 1991; 121:165–169.
201. Meydani M, Natiello F, Goldin B, Free N, Woods M, Skchaeffer E, Blumberg JB, Gorbach SL. Effect of long-term fish oil supplementation on vitamin E status and lipid peroxidation in women. J Nutr 1991; 121:484–491.
202. Shamberger RJ. Increase of peroxidation in carcinogenesis. J Natl Cancer Inst 1972; 48:1491–1497.
203. Gottlieb K, Zarling EJ, Mobarhan S, Bowen P, Sugerman S. β- Carotene decreases markers of lipid peroxidation in healthy volunteers. Nutr Cancer 1993; 19:207–212.
204. Mobarhan S, Bowen P, Andersen B, Evans M, Stacewicz-Sapuntzakis M, Sugerman S, Simms P, Luchesi D, Friedman H. Effects of β-carotene repletion on β-carotene absorption, lipid peroxidation, and neutrophil superoxide formation in young men. Nutr Cancer 1990; 14:195–206.
205. Tolonen M, Sarna S, Halme M, Tuominen SE, Westermarck T, Nordberg UR, Keinonen M, Schrijver J. Anti-oxidant supplementation decreases TBA reactants in serum of elderly. Biol Tr Elem Res 1988; 17:221–228.
206. Dragan I, Ploesteanu E, Cristea E, Mohora M, Dinn V. Studies on selenium in top athletes. Physiologie 1988; 25:187–190.
207. Colette C, Pares-Herbute N, Monnier LH, Cartry E. Platelet function in type I diabetes: effects of supplementation with large doses of vitamin E. Am J Clin Nutr 1988; 47:256–261.
208. Dion PW, Bright-See EB, Smith CC, Bruce WR. Mutat Res 1982; 102:27–37.
209. Lok E, Ratnayake WMN, Scott FW, Mongeau R, Fernie S, Nera EA, Malcolm S, McMathew E, Jee P, Clayson DB. Effect of varying type of fat in a semi-purified AIN-76A diet on cellular proliferation in the mammary gland and intestinal crypts in female Swiss Webster mice. Carcinogenesis 1992; 13:1735–1741.
210. Nayini JR, Sugie S, El-Bayoumy K, Rao V, Rigotty J, Sohn O, Reddy BS. Effect of dietary benzylselenocyanate on azoxymethane-induced colon carcinogenesis in male F344 rats. Nutr Cancer 1991; 15:129–139.
211. Goettler D, Rao AV, Bird RP. The effects of a "low-risk" diet on cell proliferation and enzymatic parameters of preneoplastic rat colon. Nutr Cancer 1987; 10:149–162.
212. Cameron GS, Pence BC. Effects of multiple application of tumor promoters and ultraviolet radiation on epidermal proliferation and antioxidant status. J Invest Dermatol 1992; 99:189–192.
213. Cahill RJ, O'Sullivan KR, Mathias PM, O'Morain B, Beatti S, Hamilton H, O'Morain C. Cell kinetic effects of vitamin E and selenium supplementation in patients with adenomatous polyps. Eur J Cancer Prev 1991; 1:27.
214. Cahill RJ, O'Sullivan KR, Mathias PM, Beattie S, Hamilton H, O'Morain C. Effects of vitamin antioxidant supplementation on cell kinetics of patients with adenomatous polyps. Gut 1993; 34:963–967.
215. Bussey HJR, DeCosse JJ, Deschner EE, Eyes AA, Lesser ML, Morson BC, Ritchie SM, Thomson JPS, Wadsworth J. A randomized trial of ascorbic acid in polyposis coli. Cancer 1982; 50:1434–1439.
216. Roncucci L, DiDonato P, Carati L, Ferrari A, Perini M, Bertoni G, Badogni G, Paris B, Svanoni F, Girola M, Ponz de Leon M. Antioxidant vitamins or lactulose for the prevention of the recurrence of colorectal adenomas. Dis Colon Rectum 1993; 36:227–234.

217. McKeown-Eyssen G, Holloway C, Jazmaji V, Bright-See E, Dion P, Bruce WR. A randomized trial of vitamins C and E in the prevention of recurrence of colorectal polyps. Cancer Res 1988; 48:4701–4705.

218. DeCosse JJ, Adams M, Kuzma JF, LoGerto P, Condon RE. Effect of ascorbic acid on rectal polps patients with familial polyposis. Surgery 1975; 78:608–612.

219. DeCosse JJ, Miller HH, Lesser ML. Effect of wheat fiber and vitamins C and E on rectal polyps in patients with familial adenomatous polyposis. J Natl Cancer Inst 1989; 81:1290–1297.

220. Greenberg ER, Baron JA, Tosteson TD, Freeman DH Jr, Beck GJ, Bond JH, Colacchio TA, Coller JA, Frankl HD, Haile RW, Mandel JS, Nierenberg DW, Rothstein R, Snover DC, Stevens MM, Summers RW, van Stolk RU. A clinical trial of antioxidant vitamins to prevent colorectal adenoma. New Eng J Med 1994; 331:141–147.

221. Vogelstein B, Knizler KW. The multi-step nature of cancer. Trends Genet 1993; 9:138–141.

222. Knekt P, Aromaa A, Maatela J, Aaran RK, Nikkari T, Hakama M, Hakulinen T, Peto R, Saxén E, Teppo L. Serum vitamin E and risk of cancer among Finnish men during a 10-year follow-up. Am J Epidemiol 1988; 127:28–41.

223. Alpha-Tocopherol, Beta Carotene Cancer Prevention Study Group. The effect of vitamin E and beta carotene on the incidence of lung cancer and other cancers in male smokers. New Eng J Med 1994; 330:1029–1035.

224. Feinberg AP, Vogelstein B. Hypomethylation distinguishes genes of some human cancers from their normal counterparts. Nature 1983; 301:89–92.

225. Goelz SE, Vogelstein B, Hamilton SR, Feinberg AP. Hypomethylation of DNA from benign and malignant human colon neoplasms. Science 1985; 228:187–190.

226. Hoffman RM. Altered methionine metabolism, DNA methylation and oncogene expression in carcinogenesis. A review and synthesis. Biochem Biophys Acta 1984; 738:49–87.

227. Cooper AJ. Biochemistry of sulfur-containing amino acids. Ann Rev Biochem 1983; 52:187–222.

228. Finkelstein JD, Cello JP, Kyle WE. Ethanol-induced changes in methionine metabolism in rat liver. Biochem Biophys Res Commun 1974; 61:525–531.

229. Shivapurkar N, Poirer LA. Tissue levels of S-adenosylmethionine and S-adenosylhomocysteine in rats fed methyl-deficient diets for one to five weeks. Carcinogenesis 1983; 4:1052–1057.

230. Wainfan E, Dizik M, Stender MC, Judith K. Rapid appearance of hypomethylated DNA in livers of rats fed cancer-promoting, methyl-deficient diets. Cancer Res 1989; 49:4094–4097.

231. Pascale R, Simile MM, Ruggiu ME, Seddaiu MA, Satta G, Sequenza MJ, Daino L, Vannini MG, Lai P, Feo F. Reversal by 5-azacytidine of the S-adenosyl-L-methionine-induced inhibition of the development of punative preneoplastic foci in rat liver carcinogenesis. Cancer Lett 1991; 56:259–265.

232. Cravo ML, Mason JB, Dayal Y, Hutchinson M, Smith D, Selhub J, Rosenberg I. Folate deficiency enhances the development of colonic neoplasia in dimethylhydrazine-treated rats. Cancer Res 1992; 52:5002–5006.

233. Newberne PM, Rogers AE. Lipotropic factors and carcinogenesis. In: Human Nutrition: Cancer and Nutrition Alfin-Slater RB, Kritchevsky D, eds. New York: Plenum, 1991; 159–185.

234. Freudenheim JL, Graham S, Marshall JR, Haughey BP, Cholewinski S, Wilkinson G. Folate intake and carcinogenesis of the colon and rectum. Int J Epidemiol 1991; 20:368–374.

235. Giovannucci E, Rimm EB, Ascherio A, Stampfer MJ, Colditz GA, Willett WC. Alcohol, low-methionine-low-folate diets, and risk of colon cancer in men. J Natl Cancer Inst 1995; 87:265–273.

236. Giovannucci E, Stampfer MJ, Colditz GA, Rimm EB, Willett NC. Folate methionine, and alcohol intake and risk of colorectal adenoma. J Natl Cancer Inst 1993; 85:875–884.

5 Nutrition and Breast Cancer

Geoffrey R. Howe

1. INTRODUCTION

Breast cancer is the most significant cancer occurring among women in the United States in terms of incidence. In 1995 it has been estimated that there were 182,000 new cases of the disease among women and 46,000 deaths attributable to breast cancer (1). High rates of breast cancer are also seen in Western European and similar populations, including Canada and Australia. Rates of this disease are generally lower in Asian countries, such as Japan and China, but in these latter populations rates have substantially increased over the past several decades (2).

It appears unlikely that the differences between international rates is caused by genetic pools in the various countries with differing susceptibilities. The arguments against such genetic determinants include evidence from migration studies as well as the recent rapid secular changes in rates seen in many previously low-risk countries. As an example of evidence from migrant studies, the patterns seen among migrants from Japan to both Hawaii and the continental United States are of particular interest. Japanese women living in Hawaii have approximately four times the rate of breast cancer compared to women in Japan, although the rates are still lower than among non-Japanese residents of Hawaii (2), strongly suggesting that lifestyle or environmental factors are of critical importance in determining breast cancer risk.

Epidemiologic studies over the past three decades have clearly established the importance of markers of hormonal status as determinants of breast cancer risk. Such markers include age at menarche, age at first full-term birth, number of pregnancies, and age at natural menopause (3). Although such studies are of importance in addressing the issue of the hormonal mechanism of breast cancer induction, the factors so identified do not offer any realistic approach to modification of breast cancer risk for an individual woman. Thus, the recent focus of epidemiologic studies of breast cancer has been on factors that could potentially be subject to individual modification and hence reduction in risk. It is in this context that substantial public and scientific interest has recently focused on various dietary hypotheses, including the possibility that fat intake may be associated with increased risk and that antioxidant vitamins or other dietary factors associated with fruit and/or vegetable intake may be associated with reduction in risk.

In this chapter epidemiologic approaches to addressing dietary hypotheses relating to breast cancer are discussed, followed by a detailed assessment of the epidemiologic evidence relating to such hypotheses. Finally, overall conclusions, including the need for future research, are discussed.

From: *Preventive Nutrition: The Comprehensive Guide for Health Professionals*
Edited by A. Bendich and R. J. Deckelbaum Humana Press Inc., Totowa, NJ

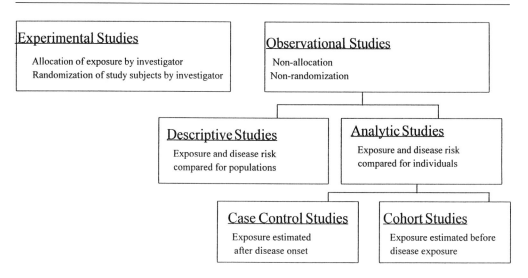

Fig. 1. Types of epidemiologic studies.

2. TYPES OF EPIDEMIOLOGIC EVIDENCE

Several research approaches have been used to study various dietary hypotheses. These include in vitro, animal, and human metabolic studies. These studies provide substantial evidence particularly as to potential mechanisms. In addition, both survey and intervention protocols are critical to provide rationales for changes in dietary habits.

There are several types of epidemiological studies. Some compare breast cancer incidence between or within human populations which are characterized by group or individual dietary patterns.

Figure 1 shows a schematic representation of the types of epidemiologic studies. There is a fundamental distinction between experimental and observational studies. In experimental studies the exposure of interest (e.g., dietary fat intake) of individuals in the study is determined by the experimenter with randomization being the usual mode chosen. To date no large scale experimental study of dietary intervention targeted against breast cancer in women has been completed. However, such an experiment, the Women's Health Initiative, has recently been initiated, and has as one of the interventions being tested the effect of a low fat/high fiber diet (4). Results of the study, however, are not anticipated to be available for a number of years.

Although, theoretically, results of such an experiment could be regarded as being the most definitive form of epidemiologic evidence, there are problems with such studies. First, there is the need to monitor compliance with the dietary intervention being allocated. The most direct method for assessing compliance depends on the self-reporting of diet, which is subject to substantial error in free-living populations (5). Indirect assessment may be based on biological measures, e.g., serum cholesterol, but such measures provide only indirect measures of compliance. A second problem arises because of the potential for "contamination" among the control group, i.e., they may change their diet in the direction of the intervention because of publicity associated with the dietary hypothesis. Again, determining the extent to which this has happened is difficult.

Finally, perhaps the major difficulty with the major intervention studies is the resources that are required. Repetition of such large and expensive trials is, therefore, unlikely, and consequently, the results may be given greater credence than is justifiable. It may also be that the intervention being tested, such as intensive nutritional counseling and guidance, cannot be realistically repeated in the general population.

In observational studies, the investigator takes advantage of what has been called a "natural experiment," comparing the disease rates among individuals who self-select their own diet, i.e., there is no intervention by the investigator. Observational studies may be classified as either descriptive or analytic. In descriptive studies, disease rates and the prevalence of dietary factors are measured at the group or population level, e.g., correlating breast cancer rates with estimated per capita fat intake among various countries. In analytic studies risk and exposure are measured at the individual level.

Although evidence from descriptive studies of breast cancer and diet have received considerable public attention, these are subject to serious biases that severely limit their interpretation. In particular, the quality of the dietary data and the quality of the breast cancer rate data may vary across populations being studied, which could lead to a spurious association. Further, many factors other than diet may vary across the populations being studied, leading to confounding at both the group and the individual level *(6)*. For these reasons, other than one illustrative example (Section 3.), evidence from descriptive studies will not be further considered in the present chapter.

Analytic studies themselves may be subdivided into case-control and cohort studies. In case-control studies dietary estimates are made after the women have developed breast cancer retrospectively, and compared with dietary patterns among a group of women who have not developed breast cancer. In cohort studies, dietary patterns are measured prospectively among a large group of women who are then followed to monitor the subsequent occurrence of breast cancer.

In general, cohort studies are less susceptible to bias than case-control studies and, thus, are the preferred design of analytic study. There are two particular concerns among case-control studies: the possibility of recall bias, in which cases differentially report their diet as compared to controls because of the presence of disease, and selection bias, which will occur if cases and controls have differential participation rates; these rates are related to dietary practices. Contradictory empirical evidence for the existence of such biases in case-control studies of breast cancer and diet has been reported *(7,8)*, but nevertheless, the potential for such biases suggests a cautious interpretation of results of case-control studies of diet and breast cancer.

3. DIETARY FAT INTAKE AND BREAST CANCER RISK

The hypothesis that dietary fat intake, particularly saturated or animal fat, might increase the risk of breast cancer was derived both from animal studies *(9–11)* and ecologic studies *(12)*. Despite the weaknesses in the ecologic studies discussed above, it is of interest to consider the results of such studies in view of the substantial interest they have generated.

There is a strong positive correlation between breast cancer rates in various countries and the corresponding estimated per capita intake of dietary fat. The basic pattern is that low rates of breast cancer are generally seen in Asian and African countries, which traditionally have low-fat diets. Much higher rates of breast cancer are seen in western Eu-

Table 1
Estimated Relative Risks (CI 95%)[a] of Breast Cancer for Women from Regression Analyses
for a 50% Reduction from the US Value in Per Capita Fat Disappearance (12)

Risk factor	Relative risk	
	Age 30–44	Age 55–69
International geographic data		
Total fat	0.53 (0.37–0.78)	0.39 (0.27–0.55)
Saturated fat	0.64 (0.46–0.90)	0.57 (0.42–0.78)
Monounsaturated fat	1.15 (0.76–1.74)	0.99 (0.59–1.67)
Polyunsaturated fat	0.49 (0.26–0.93)	0.45 (0.22–0.93)
International time-trend data		
Total fat	0.40 (0.21–0.76)	0.23 (0.13–0.40)
Animal fat	0.65 (0.35–1.20)	0.57 (0.32–1.00)
Vegetable fat	0.61 (0.30–1.26)	0.39 (0.19–0.80)

[a]Approximate estimates.

ropean, northern American, and similar populations, which have much higher intakes of dietary fat. A recent analysis of the relationship between estimated per capita fat intake and breast cancer incidence was reported based on the relative risk of breast cancer if there was a drop in fat intake by 50% from current US intakes (12). Table 1 shows the relative risks by age for the intakes of total, saturated, mono-, and polyunsaturated fats. The two age groups correspond approximately to breast cancer occurring pre- and post-menopausally. The strong positive relationship between breast cancer rates and total, saturated, and polyunsaturated fat is reflected in the substantially reduced relative risk corresponding to a 50% reduction in intake. However, there is no suggestion of a reduction in relative risk, with a similar reduction in the intake of monounsaturated fat.

Prentice and Sheppard (12) also presented a similar analysis of time-trend data, i.e., correlating changes in breast cancer rates over a 15 yr time period should there be the corresponding estimated changes in the intake of fat for a number of countries. The results (Table 1) correspond closely to those based on the international correlation. There are positive associations with total fat intake and both animal and vegetable fat intakes. The time-trend data were not available in terms of saturated, monounsaturated, and polyunsaturated fats, but animal and saturated fats are highly correlated, as are vegetable and polyunsaturated fats. Thus, ecologic studies support the existence of a positive relationship between fat intake (with the exception of monounsaturated fat) and breast cancer risk.

A second group of ecological studies consists of the migrant studies exemplified by studies of Japanese migrants to Hawaii (13). As well as demonstrating the importance of lifestyle or environmental factors in determining risk of breast cancer, these migrant studies also support the fat hypothesis in the sense that fat intakes are relatively low among women in Japan, are higher among Japanese residents of Hawaii, but are still less than those of non-Japanese women in Hawaii.

The most definitive evidence with respect to the fat hypothesis from epidemiologic studies to date comes from the analytic studies, i.e., the case-control and cohort studies. Many of the earlier studies were based on assessing the intake of a limited number of

Table 2
Relative Risk (CI 95%) of Breast Cancer in Postmenopausal Women, per 45 g/D Saturated Fat Intake Case-Control Studies Included in Formal Combined Analysis *(14)*

Study location	Ref.	Relative risk	CI 95%
Greece	*15,16*	0.39	0.08–1.99
Canada I	*17*	0.90	0.59–1.35
Hawaii (white)	*18*	1.01	0.46–2.20
Canada II	*19*	1.40	1.03–1.92
Israel	*20*	1.45	0.98–2.14
Australia	*21*	1.48	0.90–2.41
Hawaii (Japanese)	*18*	1.58	0.68–3.68
China I	*22*	2.20	0.75–6.48
China II	*23*	2.44	1.25–4.74
Italy II	*24*	3.97	1.89–8.37
Italy I	*25*	4.76	1.15–19.90
Combined	—	1.46	1.24–1.73

high-fat foods among study subjects. The studies are somewhat difficult to interpret, given the lack of complete dietary data. The problem is that in general, intakes of many foods are positively correlated and are also correlated with total energy intake. Therefore, an association between a particular food and risk could arise from a real association between some other food or, indeed, total energy intake itself and risk, i.e., the apparent effect is because of confounding. Meaningful evidence on the fat hypothesis comes mainly from studies with relatively complete assessment of dietary intake that can be used as a basis for estimating the intake of nutrients, such as total and saturated fat, and can also be used to estimate total energy intake.

Results based on a relatively complete diet history have been reported for a number of case-control studies of breast cancer. A combined analysis of 12 of these studies has recently been reported *(14)*. This analysis was based on original data records and thus it was possible to analyze the data in a uniform fashion and directly examine the consistency of findings across studies. All the studies included had estimates of total energy intake available and, hence, it was possible to adjust for any potential effect of energy intake. Overall, there was evidence of a positive association between total fat intake and breast cancer risk. In particular, there was a fairly consistent finding of increased risk associated with saturated fat intake in postmenopausal women. The latter results are shown in Table 2. Of the 11 studies that had estimates for saturated fat intake, eight showed some evidence of a positive effect. Although individual estimates of relative risk varied from study to study, for most of those with positive results, variation was no more than might have occurred by chance. Overall, the relative risk between two individuals who differed in their saturated fat intake by 45 g/d was 1.46 (Confidence Interval [CI] 95%: 1.24–1.73).

A number of other case-control studies of diet and breast cancer have been reported in which complete diet histories were collected, but that were unavailable for the combined analysis discussed above. Table 3 summarizes the results of these studies in a form as compatible as possible with the results shown in Table 2; i.e., focusing on saturated or animal fat intake in postmenopausal women where possible. Again, the prepon-

Table 3
Relative Risk (CI 95%) of Breast Cancer in Women, High- vs Low-Fat Intake,
Other Case-Control Studies

Study location	Ref.	Conditions	Relative risk	95% CI
New York State I	26	Animal fat, all women	0.89	—
New York State II	27	Saturated fat, postmenopausal women	1.04	0.71–1.53
Japan	28	Animal fat, postmenopausal women	1.17	0.62–2.19
Denmark	29	Total fat, all women	1.45	1.17–1.80
Russia	30	Saturated fat, postmenopausal women	1.67	0.24–11.78
France	31	Saturated fat, postmenopausal women	3.3	1.4–7.8
Holland	32	Total fat, all women	3.5	1.6–7.6
Argentina	33	Total fat, postmenopausal women	4.02	2.13–7.58

derance of these studies show positive associations, several of which appear unlikely to be caused by chance.

Thus, overall, the case-control studies of diet and breast cancer with relatively complete dietary assessment do provide evidence in support of the hypothesis that higher than average fat intake, particularly saturated fat, in postmenopausal women increases the risk of breast cancer. However, the potential problems of case-control studies referred to above, namely, the possibility of recall or selection bias, suggests caution in interpreting these findings.

Cohort studies are not subject to recall bias and are potentially less prone to selection bias than the case-control studies. In the past decade the results of a number of cohort studies have appeared in which sufficiently complete dietary data were collected to permit individual estimation of the intakes of both fat and total energy. The results of these studies have been mixed, with some showing no evidence of a positive association, whereas others have suggested a weak positive association. Recently, a combined analysis of the individual records from the eight major dietary cohort studies in women in which at least 200 breast cancer cases have been observed has been published (34). This analysis parallels that previously reported for the case-control studies (14). Table 4 shows a summary of the results of the pooled analysis of the cohort studies; overall, there is no evidence of any meaningful positive association with total fat intake, with the variation across individual studies being no greater than might be expected by chance. Thus, based on the most definitive epidemiologic evidence to date, there is little support for the hypothesis that total fat intake increases breast cancer risk. Similarly, in the combined analysis of the cohort studies, there is essentially no association with the three major fat components, namely, saturated, monounsaturated, or polyunsaturated fat. There was no evidence in the latter analysis that total fat (or any of the fat components) affected breast cancer risk in pre- or post-menopausal women.

Two food items related to fat intake have recently received specific attention. In a cohort study conducted in New York City, Toniolo et al. (51) reported a positive association between red meat intake and breast cancer risk. The other dietary item that has received attention is olive oil, where two case-control studies (52,53) conducted in Mediterranean populations have reported a reduced risk associated with consumption of olive oil. To date no results with respect to these two factors, i.e., red meat or olive oil,

Table 4
Relative Risks of Breast Cancer Highest vs Lowest Quintile of Energy-Adjusted Total Fat
Intake Based on Pooled Analysis of Eight Cohort Studies (34)

Study	Ref.	Relative risk	95% CI
Adventist Health Study	35–38	1.35	0.72–2.51
Canadian Breast Screening Study	39–40	1.07	0.71–1.59
Iowa Women's Health Study	41–43	1.34	1.02–1.76
Netherlands Cohort Study	44–46	0.94	0.64–1.36
New York State Cohort	47	1.19	0.81–1.75
Nurses' Health Study (a)	48	0.89	0.72–1.11
Nurses' Health Study (b)	49	1.00	0.79–1.26
Sweden Mammography Cohort	50	1.04	0.79–1.37
Combined	—	1.04	0.94–1.16

have been reported from the combined analysis of the cohort studies and it would be premature to make any judgment regarding the effects of these food items at this time.

4. ANTIOXIDANT VITAMINS AND FIBER

A number of epidemiologic studies have reported results with respect to breast cancer risk and the intake of vitamins A, C, E, and fiber, or with such foods as fruits, vegetables, and cereal products, which are some of the sources of these dietary factors. Overall, there have been no consistent findings with respect to any of these factors in particular, but generally, there has been some evidence of an inverse association with one or another of these factors or some combination of them.

In terms of fruits and vegetables, a number of epidemiologic studies have suggested inverse associations between consumption of these foods and breast cancer risk (16,53–61). Steinmetz and Potter (54) have suggested a number of potential anticarcinogenic agents in fruits or vegetables, although no specific agent has been established with respect to breast cancer.

There have also been a number of epidemiologic studies in which specific nutrients obtained from fruits, vegetables, or cereal products have been examined. Some studies have suggested inverse relationships between total vitamin A intake and breast cancer risk (14,16,62,63), but others have not (54). Retinol (preformed vitamin A) is involved in the regulation of cell differentiation and has been shown experimentally to reduce carcinogenesis. However, in epidemiologic studies generally no association with retinol intake has been seen (14,56,60,61), but one showed a positive association (31) and two others provided some evidence of an inverse association (16,62). β-Carotene, a precursor of vitamin A, has been postulated to lower cancer risk through its action as an antioxidant. A number of epidemiologic studies of breast cancer have shown inverse relationships with β-carotene (30,61,64,65) although others have shown no such association (31,60,61).

With respect to vitamin C, the combined analysis of 12 case-control studies referred to earlier (14) showed a strong inverse association, as did two other case-control studies (27,30). However, two other case-control studies (26,61) and two cohort studies (62,66) showed little evidence of any association with total vitamin C intake. Two studies also failed to show evidence of any association with supplemental vitamin C intake *(27,62)*.

The possibility that fiber intake might reduce risk of breast cancer has been hypothesized on the basis of the possibility that fiber-rich foods might alter estrogen metabolism. Fiber-rich foods appear to be capable of interfering with the intrahepatic cycling of estrogen either by binding unconjugated estrogens in the gut *(67)* or by reducing deconjugating enzyme activity *(68)*. In addition, phytoestrogens, which can be produced by bacterial action on the precursors in unrefined grains, may reduce the bioavailability of estrogens *(69)*. Several epidemiologic studies have shown inverse relationships with fiber intake *(14,21,27,32)*. However, one major cohort study failed to find evidence of such an association *(49)*.

5. SUMMARY AND CONCLUSIONS

There have been many epidemiologic studies of the relationship between a number of dietary factors and breast cancer risk. The hypothesis that has received the most attention is that total fat or one of the fat components increases risk, particularly in postmenopausal women. Although in general, this hypothesis is supported by ecologic studies and case-control studies, there is now a substantial body of evidence from the methodologically strongest type of observational study, the cohort study, that there is no association between fat intake and breast cancer risk, corroborated in the recent combined analysis *(34)*. Presumably, therefore, the associations seen in the ecologic and case-control studies are most likely to have been because of the inherent limitations of the methodologies. However, the cohort studies also have limitations. These have all been conducted in countries with high fat intakes and high breast cancer rates. Thus, the possibility that very low fat intakes might be associated with reduced risk could not be examined in cohort studies. However, the recent combined analysis was able to pool sufficient women with low fat intakes (< 20% energy from fat) to address this issue, and that analysis provided no evidence that such women were indeed at lower risk *(34)*.

A major limitation of the cohort studies is that these have all focused on diets of women as measured in adulthood. It has been hypothesized that diet could play a role in the provenance of breast cancer at the time of puberty, with lower energy intakes leading to later age at menarche and, hence, reduced risk. However, this hypothesis is yet to be tested in epidemiologic studies, so overall, at this time there is essentially no evidence to support the contention that reduction of total fat intake in adulthood could reduce subsequent breast cancer risk. Recent findings of a positive association with meat intake in a large cohort study *(51)*, and inverse associations with olive oil consumption in two case-control studies *(52,53)*, are interesting findings that, however, need substantially more verification before they can be confirmed.

Although overall there is evidence of an inverse relationship between fruit, vegetable, and/or cereal product consumption and breast cancer risk, many of these associations have been reported from case-control studies, and the experience with respect to the fat hypothesis from the case-control studies suggests considerable caution in interpreting such findings. In addition to the problems of selection and recall bias, a number of these studies have failed to adjust for total energy intake or for the potential confounding effects of other dietary factors. Although isolated results from cohort studies with respect to these dietary factors have been reported, as yet no comprehensive pooled analysis of the cohort data has been published; such results will certainly be of considerable interest when they are reported.

In terms of future research, the continued follow-up of the various dietary cohort studies of women should shed further light on the various dietary hypotheses. The results of the Women's Health Initiative Intervention Study *(4)* will also be of considerable interest, although these are not expected for a number of years. Studies of specific populations, such as women in Mediterranean countries with a high intake of olive oil, could provide insight into some of the specific dietary hypotheses. Long-term studies of the effect of diet before and at the time of menarche would certainly be of interest, but will likely have to depend on biological markers of breast cancer risk to provide results within some reasonable time frame.

5.1. Recommendations

Unfortunately, the balance of the epidemiologic evidence at the present time does not support the possibility that women can meaningfully reduce their breast cancer risk by dietary change. However, given the possibility that increased consumption of fruits, vegetables, and cereal products might possibly be associated with reduced risk, this is certainly consistent with the recommendation to follow the so-called prudent diet *(70)*, which advocates reduced fat intake with corresponding increased consumption of foods rich in antioxidants, fiber, and similar dietary factors.

REFERENCES

1. Cancer Facts and Figures—1995, American Cancer Society, Atlanta; 1995.
2. Parkin DM, Muir CS, Whelan SL, Gao Y-T, Ferlay J, Powell J. Cancer Incidence in Five Continents, Vol VI. Lyon: WHO International Agency for Research on Cancer, 1992.
3. Kelsey JL. Breast Cancer Epidemiology: Summary and Future Direction. Epidemiol Rev 1993; 15:256–263.
4. Prentice R, Calker F, Hurting S, Chopart L, Kleig R, Kushi LH. Aspects of the rational for the Women's Health Trial. J Natl Cancer Inst 1988; 80:802–814.
5. Willett WC. Nutritional Epidemiology. Oxford University Press, 1990.
6. Greenland S, Morganstern H. Ecological bias, confounding, and effect modification (erratum appears in 1991; 20:824). Int J Epidemiol 1989; 18:269–274.
7. Friedenreich CM, Howe GR, Miller AB. The effect of recall bias on the association of calorie-providing nutrients and breast cancer. Epidemiology 1990; 2:424–429.
8. Giovannucci E, Stampfer MJ, Colditz GA, Manson J, Rosner B, Longnecker M, et al. A comparison of prospective and retrospective assessments of diet in the study of breast cancer. Am J Epidemiol 1991; 7:714 (abstract).
9. Tannenbaum A. Genesis and growth of tumors. III. Effects of a high fat diet. Cancer Res 1942; 2:468–475.
10. Carroll KK. Experimental studies of dietary fat and cancer in relation to epidemiological data. Prog Clin Biol Res 1986; 222:231–248.
11. Boissoneault GA, Elson CE, Pariza MW. Net energy effect of dietary fat on chemically induced mammary carcinogenesis in F344 rats. J Natl Cancer Inst 1986; 76:335–338.
12. Prentice RL, Sheppard L. Dietary fat and cancer: consistency of the epidemiologic data, and disease prevention that may follow from a practical reduction in fat consumption. Cancer Causes Control 1990; 1:81–97.
13. Tominga S. Cancer incidence in Japanese in Japan, Hawaii and western United States. Natl Cancer Inst Monogr 1985; 69:83–92.
14. Howe GR, Hirohata T, Hislop TG, Iscovich JM, Yuan JM, Katsouyanni K, et al. Dietary factors and risk of breast cancer: combined analysis of 12 case-control studies. J Natl Cancer Inst 1990; 82:561–569.
15. Katsouyanni K, Trichopoulos D, Boyle P, Xirouchaki E, Trichopoulou A, Lisseos B, et al. Diet and breast cancer: a case-control study in Greece. Int J Cancer 1986; 38:815–820.
16. Katsouyanni K, Willett W, Trichopoulos D, Boyle P, Trichopoulo A, Vasilaros S, et al. Risk of breast cancer among Greek women in relation to nutrient intake. Cancer 1988; 61:181–185.
17. Miller AB, Kelly A, Choi NW. A study of diet and breast cancer. Am J Epidemiol 1978; 107:499–509.
18. Hirohata T, Nomura A, Hankin JH, Kolonel LN, Lee J. An epidemiologic study on the association between diet and breast cancer. J Natl Cancer Inst 1987; 78:595–600.

19. Hislop TG, Coldman AJ, Elwood JM, Brauer G, Kan L. Childhood and recent eating patterns and risk of breast cancer. Cancer Detect Prev 1986; 9:47–58.
20. Lubin F, Wax YK, Modan B. Role of fat, animal protein and dietary fiber in breast cancer etiology: a case-control study. J Natl Cancer Inst 1986; 77:605–612.
21. Rohan TE, McMichael AJ, Baghurst PA. A population-based case-control study of diet and breast cancer in Australia. Am J Epidemiol 1988; 128:478–489.
22. Yu S. Risk factors of breast cancer in Shanghai. Tumor 1984; 4:1–21.
23. Yuan JM, Yu MC, Ross RK, Gao Y-T, Henderson BE. Risk factors for breast cancer in Chinese women in Shanghai. Cancer Res 1988; 48:1949–1953.
24. Toniolo P, Riboli E, Protta F, Charrel M, Cappa APM. Calorie-providing nutrients and risk of breast cancer. J Natl Cancer Inst 1989; 81:278–286.
25. Marubini E, Decarli A, Costa A, Mazzoleni C, Andreoli C, Barbieri A, et al. The relationship of dietary intake and serum levels of retinol and beta-carotene with breast cancer: results of a case-control study. Cancer 1988; 61:173–180.
26. Graham S, Marshall J, Mettin C, Rzepka T, Nemoto T, Byers T. Diet in the epidemiology of breast cancer. Am J Epidemiol 1982; 116:68–75.
27. Graham S, Hellmann R, Marshall J, Rudenheim J, Vena J, Swanson M, et al. Nutritional epidemiology of postmenopausal cancer in western New York. Am J Epidemiol 1991; 134:552–566.
28. Hirohata T, Shigematsu T, Nomura AMY, Nomura Y, Horie A, Hirohata I. Occurrence of breast cancer in relation to diet and reproductive history: a case-control study in Fukuoka, Japan. Natl Cancer Inst Monogr 1985; 69:187–190.
29. Ewertz M, Gill C. Dietary factors and breast cancer risk in Denmark. Int J Cancer 1990; 46:779–784.
30. Zaridze D, Lifanova Y, Maximovitch D, Day NE, Duffy SW. Diet, alcohol consumption and reproductive factors in a case-control study of breast cancer in Moscow. Int J Cancer 1991; 48:493–501.
31. Richardson S, Gerber M, Cenee S. The role of fat, animal protein and some vitamin consumption in breast cancer: a case control study in southern France. Int J Cancer 1991; 48:1–9.
32. Van't Veer P, Kok FJ, Brants HAM, Ockhuizen T, Sturmans F, Hermus RJJ. Dietary fat and the risk of breast cancer. Int J Cancer 1990; 19:12–18.
33. Iscovich J, Howe GR, Kaldor JM. A case-control study of breast cancer in Argentina. Int J Cancer 1990; 44:770–776.
34. Hunter DJ, Spiegelman D, Adami HO, Beeson L, van den Brandt PA, Folsom AR, et al. Cohort studies of fat intake and risk of breast cancer: a pooled analysis. New Eng J Med 1996; 334:356–361.
35. Beeson WL, Mills PK, Phillips RL, Andress M, Fraser GE. Chronic disease among Seventh Day Adventists, a low risk group. Cancer 1989; 64:570–581.
36. Mills PK, Beeson WL, Phillips RL, Fraser GE. Dietary habits and breast cancer incidence among Seventh Day Adventists. Cancer 1989; 64:582–590.
37. Phillips RL, Kuzma JW. Estimating major nutrient intake from self-administered food frequency questionnaires. Am J Epidemiol 1976; 104:354–355 (abstract).
38. Abbey DE, Andress M, Fraser GE, Morgan J, Kuzma J. Validity and reliability of alternative nutrient indices based on a food frequency questionnaire. Am J Epidemiol 1988; 4:934 (abstract).
39. Howe GR, Friedenreich CM, Jain M, Miller AB. A cohort study of fat intake and risk of breast cancer. J Natl Cancer Inst 1991; 83:336–340.
40. Jain MG, Harrison L, Howe GR, et al. Evaluation of a self-administered dietary questionnaire for use in a cohort study. Am J Clin Nutr 1982; 36:931–935.
41. Kushi LH, Sellers TA, Potter JD, et al. Dietary fat and postmenopausal breast cancer. J Natl Cancer Inst 1992; 84:1092–1099.
42. Bostick RM, Potter JD, McKenzie DR, et al. Reduced risk of colon cancer with high intake of vitamin E: the Iowa Women's Health Study. Cancer Res 1993; 53:4230–4237.
43. Munger RG, Folsom AR, Kushi LH, Kaye SA, Sellers TA. Dietary assessment of older Iowa women with a food frequency questionnaire: nutrient intake, reproducibility, and comparison with 24-hour dietary recall interviews. Am J Epidemiol 1992; 136:192–200.
44. van den Brandt PA, Goldbohm RA, van't Veer P, Volovics A, Hermus RJ, Sturman F. A large-scale prospective cohort study on diet and cancer in the Netherlands. J Clin Epidemiol 1990; 43:285–295.
45. van den Brandt PA, van't Veer P, Goldbohm RA, et al. A prospective cohort study on dietary fat and the risk of postmenopausal breast cancer risk. Cancer Res 1993; 53:75–82.
46. Goldbohm RA, van den Brandt Pa, Brants HA, et al. Validation of a dietary questionnaire used in a large-scale prospective cohort study on diet and cancer. Eur J Clin Nutr 1994; 48:253–265.

47. Graham S, Zielezny M, Marshall J, et al. Diet in the epidemiology of postmenopausal breast cancer in the New York State cohort. Am J Epidemiol 1992; 136:1327–1337.

48. Willett WC, Stampfer MJ, Colditz GA, Rosner BA, Speizer FE. Relation of meat, fat and fiber intake to the risk of colon cancer in a prospective study among women. New Engl J Med 1990; 323:1664–1672.

49. Willett WC, Hunter DJ, Stampfer MJ, et al. Dietary fat and fiber in relation to risk of breast cancer: an 8-year follow-up. JAMA 1992; 268:2037–2044.

50. Holmberg L, Ohlander EM, Byers T, et al. Diet and breast cancer risk: results from a population-based, case-control study in Sweden. Arch Intern Med 1994; 154:1805–1811.

51. Toniolo P, Riboli E, Shore RE, Pasternack BS. Consumption of meat, animal products, protein, and fat and risk of breast cancer: a prospective cohort study in New York. Epidemiology 1994; 5:391–397.

52. Martin-Moreno JM, Willett WC, Gorgojo L, et al. Dietary fat, olive oil intake and breast cancer risk. Int J Cancer 1994; 58:774–780.

53. Trichopoulo A, Katsouyanni K, Stuver S, Tzala L, Gnardellis C, Rimm E, Trichopoulos D. Consumption of olive oil and specific food groups in relation to breast cancer risk in Greece. J Natl Cancer Inst 1995; 87:110–116.

54. Steinmetz KA, Potter JD. Vegetables, fruit, and cancer. I. Epidemiology. Cancer Causes Control 1991; 2:325–357.

55. Block G, Patterson B, Subar A. Fruit, vegetables, and cancer prevention: a review of the epidemiological evidence. Nutr Cancer 1992; 18:1–29.

56. Graham S, Hellmann R, Marshall J, et al. Nutritional epidemiology of postmenopausal breast cancer in western New York. Am J Epidemiol 1991; 134:552–566.

57. Baghurst PA, Rohan TE. High-fiber diets and reduced risk of breast cancer. Int J Cancer 1994; 56:173–176.

58. Lanza E, Shankar S, Trock B. In: Macronutrients. Investigating Their Role in Cancer. Miczzi MS, Moon TE, eds. New York: Marcel Dekker, 1992; 293–319.

59. Potischman N, McCulloch CE, Byers T, et al. Breast cancer and dietary and plasma concentrations of carotenoids and vitamin A. Am J Clin Nutr 1990; 52:909–915.

60. La Veechia C, Decarli A, Franceschi S, Gentile A, Negri E, Parazzini F. Dietary factors and the risk of breast cancer. Nutr Cancer 1987; 10:208–214.

61. Ingram DM, Nottage E, Roberts T. The role of diet in the development of breast cancer: a case-control study of patients with breast cancer, benign epithelial hyperplasia, and fibrocystic disease of the breast. Br J Cancer 1991; 64:187–191.

62. Hunter DJ, Stampfer MJ, Colditz GA, et al. A prospective study of consumption of vitamins A, C and E and breast cancer risk. Am J Epidemiol 1991; 134:715 (abstract).

63. Graham S, Marshall J, Mettlin C, Rzepka T, Nemoto T, Byers T. Diet in the epidemiology of breast cancer. Am J Epidemiol 1982; 116:68–75.

64. van't Veer P, Kolb CM, Verhoef P, et al. Dietary fiber, beta carotene and breast cancer: results from a case-control study. Int J Cancer 1990; 45:825–828.

65. Lee HP, Gourley L, Duffy SW, Esteve J, Lee J, Day NE. Dietary effects on breast cancer risk in Singapore. Lancet 1991; 337:1197–1200.

66. Rohan TE, Howe GR, Friedenreich CM, et al. Dietary fiber, vitamins A, C and E, and risk of breast cancer: a cohort study. Cancer Causes Control 1993; 4:29–37.

67. Schultz TD, Howe BJ. In vitro binding of steroid hormones by natural and purified fibers. Nutr Cancer 1986; 8:141–147.

68. Rose DP. Dietary fiber and breast cancer. Nutr Cancer 1990; 13:1–8.

69. Adlecreutz H, Fotsis T, Bannwart C, et al. Determination of urinary lignans and phytoestrogen metabolites, potential antiestrogens and anticarcinogens in urine of women on various habitual diets. J Steroid Biochem 1986; 25:791–797.

70. Diet and Health, Implications for Reducing Chronic Disease Risk. Washington, D.C.: National Academy Press, 1989.

6 Preventive Nutrition and Lung Cancer

George W. Comstock and Kathy J. Helzlsouer

1. INTRODUCTION

In searching for the causes of any cancer, it is natural to think first of substances that come into direct contact with the organs and cells that are involved. For lung cancer, the early suspects were smokes, dusts, and gases, particularly smoke from burning tobacco; dusts containing carcinogens, such as arsenic or asbestos; and radon gas. At present, these and other airborne substances have become accepted carcinogens (1). Tobacco smoke is by far the most important because of the intensity, prevalence, and ubiquity of exposures to this complex mixture of known and suspected toxins and carcinogens.

Not everyone exposed to even high concentrations of these inhalants develops lung cancer, however, and lung cancer occurs among some persons with little or no known exposures. These observations suggest that there are other causes of lung cancer and perhaps substances that prevent or inhibit carcinogenesis. Neither carcinogens nor protective substances have to arrive at the lungs by way of the airways. Anything that is absorbed into the bloodstream has the potential to reach every cell in the body. In this way, dietary components can also affect the tracheo-bronchial tree and the pulmonary parenchyma.

2. CELL TYPES

A potential problem with much of the literature on lung cancer is that this disease is treated as a single entity. Reports usually ignore the possibility that different histologic cell types might indicate different, although related, tumors. One reason for lumping cell types together is the heterogeneity of histologic features even within cell types and the consequent unreliability of cell-type classification (2). Fortunately, the associations of each reported cell type with sex, smoking, most occupational exposures, and nutritional factors appear to differ mainly in degree and not in direction. In any case, very few reports dealing with nutrition specify cell types; hence, cell type will have to be ignored in this chapter.

3. STUDY DESIGNS

3.1. Types

Nutritional studies that relate to the prevention of lung cancer involve many study designs. Those that produce the clearest evidence are experiments on animals in which

From: *Preventive Nutrition: The Comprehensive Guide for Health Professionals*
Edited by A. Bendich and R. J. Deckelbaum Humana Press Inc., Totowa, NJ

virtually all known variables can be controlled. Such studies have led the way to numerous advances in human nutrition. However, appealing as they may be, they can be considered only rough guides to human studies of cancer. Animals often metabolize carcinogens and nutrients differently than humans, it is difficult to mimic most human environments, and no suitable laboratory animal survives long enough to show the effects of long-term exposures.

Similar experimental studies on humans have to be conducted on metabolic wards, are expensive, and rarely involve more than a few subjects. Most important, carcinogens cannot be administered and long-term observations are not feasible. Experimentally, about the most that can be done with adequate numbers of people is to assess the effects of various dietary components on the endogenous production of various harmful oxidation products or their markers, such as breath ethane. However, it is possible to conduct observational studies among free-living general populations to see what outcomes are associated with what people eat.

The simplest observational studies among humans are ecologic in nature. In these studies, population characteristics of various sized geographic units are correlated with the incidence or mortality of lung cancer. Their major advantage lies in the fact that nutritional exposures may differ much more between populations than within them, thereby producing sharper contrasts. On the other hand, data on production, sales, or consumption in geographic units are available for only a few nutrients, and none of these indices can accurately reflect what is actually eaten by individuals in the populations.

Cross-sectional surveys and case-control studies come closer to being able to evaluate differences in dietary intakes of persons with lung cancer and similar persons who have not developed lung cancer. Cross-sectional surveys suffer from the fact that at the time of study, the case group is heavily weighted with survivors. The experience of those who survive may or may not be typical of those who have already died. Cross-sectional studies, in which information about diet and cancer are obtained for the same time period, also suffer from the fact that dietary histories tend to be influenced by current diet, which may be altered considerably by symptoms of the disease or the effects of treatment. Case-control studies of newly diagnosed cases not only can have the same problems, but are beset by the difficulties of obtaining accurate and unbiased histories of dietary habits that existed a long time prior to diagnosis.

Prospective studies, such as cohort or nested case-control studies, are more suitable for investigating the associations between nutrients and lung cancer than cross-sectional or case-control studies. Because dietary histories in these types of studies are obtained before cancer has been diagnosed, they cannot be influenced by the presence of disease.

Such considerations are even more pertinent for investigating associations of serum* components with cancers that cause symptoms or systemic effects that could affect concentrations of nutrients in the serum. In both cross-sectional and case-control studies, serum is drawn after lung cancer is diagnosed, and it is impossible to tell how much of the difference in serum concentrations between cases and noncases is caused by differences that existed long before the cancer was recognized, and how much is because of the effect of a manifest cancer and consequent illness on serum concentrations. As a result, cross-sectional and case-control studies of associations of serum components with lung cancer will not be considered further.

---

*"Serum" will be used to denote either serum or plasma.

In all of these observational studies, it is possible to conclude only that dietary intake is *associated* with lung cancer prevalence, incidence, or mortality. A statistically significant association merely indicates that chance was unlikely to have produced the observation. It tells nothing about the likelihood that some unsuspected flaw in design or some unknown confounder might have been responsible. Only when the result is replicated in different populations and by different study designs is one entitled to believe that the association is true and general. Even so, there is always the possibility that the association with nutrient X came about because it was a "fellow-traveler" with the true but unsuspected causal agent.

Controlled trials produce the most convincing evidence of causation. However, even with this study design, replication in a different population is highly desirable. Rare events, such as statistically significant but false outcomes, can occur. Replication in other populations can reduce such a probability almost to the vanishing point, and also reduce the possibility that the initial finding resulted from some unsuspected interaction of the treatment with a peculiarity of a particular study population. Even so, there are disadvantages to controlled trials. For relatively uncommon outcomes, the study population must be very large. Dosages and methods of administration have to be fixed, and only a few preventive agents or regimens can be tested. Most important, if the event that initiates carcinogenesis occurs long before cancer becomes manifest, or if the initiating event occurs prior to adult life, a controlled preventive trial must continue over a very long period.

In summary, controlled trials are the only study design capable of proving causation. They are limited to investigating only a few preventive agents and regimens, and may require very long periods to study effects on initiation of carcinogenesis. Prospective studies also require long periods of observation and can only determine associations. Case-control and cross-sectional studies are not suitable for most major cancers; cross-sectional studies cannot clearly differentiate whether the tumor affected the diet or vice versa. Ecologic studies are quick and inexpensive, but do not lend themselves to studies of minor nutrients and are rarely more than suggestive. The most reliable information comes from careful consideration of all available evidence.

For all observational studies, consistent failure of a nutrient to be associated with prevention is probably good evidence that it is not a protective agent. In contrast, demonstration that a nutrient is associated with a decrease in cancer, even if consistently observed in a variety of circumstances, does not mean that the observed protection is because of that particular nutrient. It may only be associated with the true protective factor. It behooves us always to think about what might accompany the substances we are studying.

3.2. Smoking and Diet

Because smoking is so strongly implicated in the pathogenesis of lung cancer, many authors have felt compelled to remove the effects of smoking by matching or statistical adjustment. The wisdom of this approach is debatable. Numerous studies have shown that the diets of smokers and nonsmokers differ. The diets of nonsmokers married to spouses that smoke are also likely to be different from nonsmokers married to nonsmokers. Both active and passive smokers (exposed nonsmokers) are usually reported to eat fewer fruits and vegetables than nonsmokers *(3–11)*. Dietary intake is an important determinant of the level of nutrients that reach the cells. If smoking is the cause of a lower intake of fruits and vegetables, then the dietary deficit associated with smoking is a link in the chain of causation with respect to the protective effect of fruits and vegetables (or any specific nutrients they contain) against lung cancer. Under such circumstances, adjustment or matching is usually not appropriate. The adjusted values merely show the effect of a nutrient after the effect of the reduced value as a result of smoking and its associated dietary changes have been removed. If, on the other hand, one considers smoking to be independent of dietary change, then smoking is a confounder and adjustment is entirely appropriate. In any case, the most informative way to report results with respect to smoking is to show the findings both unadjusted and adjusted for smoking, or much better, separately for smokers and nonsmokers. Unfortunately, neither approach is common.

4. NUTRIENTS

4.1. Cholesterol and Fat

Interest in the possible effects of diet on the development of lung cancer appears to have arisen from several sources: trials of cholesterol-lowering diets (12), a general belief in the health promoting effects of fruits and vegetables (13a,b); and possibly an early animal study of vitamin A deficiency (14). One of the first trials of the effects of substituting polyunsaturated for saturated fats in the diet showed an encouraging reduction in mortality from causes related to atherosclerosis, although this finding was not confirmed in similar trials (12). An alarming finding was that an excess of cancer developed during the course of the study among the group fed polyunsaturated fats (15). Case-control studies designed to confirm and elucidate that finding have tended to show, contrary to the finding of the early trial, that persons with the highest intake of cholesterol had an increased risk of lung cancer, even after adjustment for smoking (16–19). In two of the studies, the association was strongest among men and for squamous and small cell cancers (16,17). Cohort studies have yielded divergent results, one in Illinois finding a significant association of lung cancer risk with increased cholesterol intake (20), whereas studies in Hawaii and Finland failed to demonstrate this association (21,22).

The frequency of lung cancer has been reported among participants in two large cohort studies and in five controlled trials of regimens designed to reduce serum cholesterol. Among 160,135 participants in a screening program, 528 cases of lung cancer developed among men and 315 among women two or more years after serum cholesterol was determined (23a). Among men, those in the lowest fifth of the cholesterol distribution had a risk of developing lung cancer 1.92 times that of men in the highest fifth; for women, the relative risk was 2.28.

Among 151 men and 59 women with lung cancer reported in the NHANES I follow-up study, the odds ratio for developing this disease was 1.66 times greater among men in the lowest fourth of the cholesterol distribution than among men with cholesterol levels of 190–216 mg/dL. Among women, the odds ratio was 2.58 compared to those with cholesterol levels of 186–216 mg/dL (23b). However, in neither of the two studies was the dose-response-trend monotonically linear. In two controlled trials, lung cancer death rates were higher in the group under treatment designed to lower cholesterol (24,25), in one there was no difference between the two groups (26), and in two, lung cancer deaths were more frequent among the controls (28,27).

Table 1
Differences in Serum Cholesterol at Baseline Among Lung Cancer Cases
and Comparison Groups

Ref. no. and author	Area	No. of cases	Sex	Difference (case mean–comparison mean)	
				%	p
(36) Cambien	France	27	M	+4.5	.33
(37) Dyer	Illinois	36	M	+1.4	.62
		7	F	−1.4	.84
(38)[a] Kagan	Hawaii	33	M	−9.3	<.01
(39)[b] Keys	United States	29	M	−2.7	.44
	N. Europe	50	M	−1.8	.51
	S. Europe	44	M	−6.6	.04
	Japan	5	M	−4.0	.03
(40) Menkes	Maryland	99	M&F	−1.1	.62
(41)[c] Kok	Netherlands	18	M&F	+0.4	.93
(42) Stähelin	Switzerland	68	M	+1.2	<.01

[a]Includes some prevalent cases
[b]Cancer deaths in first five years of follow-up excluded
[c]Cases in first year of follow-up excluded

Closely related to the cholesterol studies are those that dealt with dietary fat intake. Ecologic studies have shown strong correlations between per capita fat consumption and lung cancer mortality, more marked among men than among women (29,30). Case-control studies have also found that high fat intake was associated with lung cancer (16,31,32). The degree of saturation of the fat was rarely mentioned. One case-control study among nonsmoking women found a much stronger association of saturated fat in the diet with subsequent lung cancer than total fat, cholesterol, oleic acid (monounsaturated), or linoleic acid (polyunsaturated) (32). Confirmation came from a 20-yr follow-up study among Finnish men (33). High intakes of milk, butter, and meat were associated with higher rates of subsequent lung cancer. A protective association with margarine was based on a small number of users and was attributed to a lifestyle consistent with a high degree of health consciousness.

In keeping with the majority of these findings, a review in 1989 concluded that there was an association of high dietary intakes of cholesterol and fat with lung cancer (34). Another commentary listed a number of potential biologic mechanisms by which fat might contribute to a cancer risk (35). Equally appealing as the hypothesis that cholesterol and fat in diets might contribute in some way to carcinogenesis is the possibility that such diets are low in nutrients that might be protective (3,5–10).

Serum cholesterol is closely related to fat and cholesterol in the diet. Summaries of prospective studies of serum cholesterol and lung cancer, representing 10 different populations, are shown in Table 1. Baseline levels of serum cholesterol tend to be slightly but nonsignificantly lower among persons who subsequently developed lung cancer. The study in Hawaii, which showed the greatest difference, was based on lung cancer deaths and probably included a few prevalent cases at the time serum cholesterol was determined *(38)*. If there is an association of serum cholesterol with subsequent lung cancer, it does not appear to be of much importance.

4.2. Alcohol

Relatively little attention has been paid to alcohol intake as a risk factor for lung cancer. Studies in Switzerland, Hong Kong, China, and the United States have agreed that there is an excess risk of lung cancer among moderate to heavy users of alcohol *(43–48)*. In most of them, the findings were adjusted for the effects of smoking and no mention was made of any interactions of smoking and alcohol intake. In the study involving women in Hong Kong who had never smoked, the risk associated with moderate use was close to twice that for nonusers *(44)*.

4.3. Fruits and Vegetables

Numerous investigators have examined the possibility that fruits and vegetables might not only be "good for you" but that they might in some way protect against cancer. A thorough review of this topic was published in 1991 *(13)*. It concluded that "consumption of higher levels of vegetables and fruit is associated consistently, although not universally, with a reduced risk of cancer at most sites." Included in this review were five cohort and eight case-control studies of lung cancer. A weak to moderate association was found between a low intake of vegetables and/or fruit and an increased risk of lung cancer in most of these studies.

In the four years since that review was published, the number of papers on this topic has more than doubled. A small ecologic study of lung cancer in northern and southern Italy, showed that death rates were lower in southern Italy, where the diet was low in saturated and polyunsaturated fats and high in vegetables, even though smoking habits were similar in the two areas *(30)*. Included in this number is a recent comprehensive review of nutritional factors related to lung cancer *(13b)*.

Among the recent studies there is a nested case-control study from Finland *(33)*, two new cohort studies among insurance policy holders in the Lutheran Brotherhood *(47)* and residents in a California retirement community *(49)*, and an updated report of a cohort of women in Iowa *(48)*. These recent results are summarized in Table 2. Evidence from the earlier and later cohort studies strongly favors a decreased risk of lung cancer associated with an increased intake of fruits. For vegetables, the evidence points in the same direction, but not as strongly and consistently.

In addition to the eight case-control studies summarized by Steinmetz and Potter *(13)*, 11 later reports were identified (Table 2). In these studies, evidence regarding the intake of fruits is split between positive and negative associations with lung cancer. However, those favoring a protective association are more numerous and the associations are stronger. Nearly all the case-control studies agree in finding that increased intakes of vegetables are associated with a decreased lung cancer risk.

Few of these studies have looked at interactions between dietary intakes and sex or smoking. When both sexes and all smoking groups have been included in the same study, the cases among women and nonsmokers have usually been too few for mean-

Table 2
Association of Dietary Intakes of Fruits and Vegetables with Lung Cancer in Selected
Studies by Type of Study, Sex, and Smoking History of Participants and by Nature
of Association

Ref. no. and author	Dietary component	Sex	Smoking[a]	Direction[b]	Strength[c]	p-Trend
Cohort and nested case-control						
(33)	Fruits	M	Non	Negative	+++	<.01
Knekt		M	Current	Positive	0	.89
	Vegetables	M	Non	Negative	+	.12
		M	Current	Positive	0	.81
(49)	Fruits	M	All	Negative	0[d]	NC
Shibata		F	All	Negative	+[d]	NC
	Vegetables	M	All	Positive	+[d]	NC
		F	All	Negative	++[d]	NC
(47)	Fruits	M	All	Negative	+[d]	.01
Chow	Vegetables	M	All	Positive	0[d]	.85
	Cruciferous vegetables	M	All	Negative	0[d]	.93
(48)	Fruits	F	All	Negative	++	<.01
Steinmetz	Vegetables	F	All	Negative	+	.07
Case-control						
(50)	Fruits	F	Non	Negative	+++	.02
Kallandidj	Vegetables	F	Non	Positive	0	.86
(45)	Fresh fruits	F	All	Positive	+[d]	<.01
Wu-Williams	Vegetables, low carotene	F	All	Negative	±[d]	.67
	Vegetables, high carotene	F	All	Negative	±[d]	.60
(18)	Fruits	M&F	All	Positive	±[d]	.76
Jain	Vegetables	M&F	All	Negative	+[d]	.01
(51)	Carotene-rich fruits and vegetables	M	All	Negative	++	.14
Harris	Yellow fruits	M	All	Negative	+	.40
	Green vegetables	M	All	Negative	+	.34
(52)	Fruits	M	All	Positive	0[d]	NC
Forman	Vegetables	M	All	Negative	++[d]	NC
(53)	Fruits	F	Never	Negative	+	.04
Candelora	Green-yellow vegetables	F	Never	Negative	+++	<.01
(54)	Fresh fruit	M	All	Negative	0[d]	.31
Swanson	Green vegetables	M	All	Negative	+++[d]	<.01
(55)	Fruits	WM	All	Negative	0[d]	>.05
Dorgan		WF	All	Negative	++[d]	<.01
		BM	All	Positive	++[d]	<.05
		BF	All	Positive	+[d]	>.05
	Vegetables	WM	All	Negative	±[d]	>.05
		WF	All	Negative	++[d]	<.01

(continued)

Table 2 Continued

Ref. no. and author	Dietary component	Characteristics of participants		Association		
		Sex	Smoking[a]	Direction[b]	Strength[c]	p-Trend
		BM	All	Positive	0[d]	>.05
		BF	All	Negative	+[d]	>.05
		All	None[e]	—	0	NS
		All	Ex[f]	Negative	+	NS
		All	Current	Negative	+	NS
(32) Alavanja	Fruits	F	Non	Positive	±	.99
	Vegetables	F	Non	Negative	0	.89
(56) Gao	Fruits	M	Never	Negative	+	.40
		M	Ex	Negative	++	.04
		M	Current	Negative	++	<.01
	Green vegetables	M	Never	Negative	+++	.46
		M	Ex	Negative	+	.47
		M	Current	Negative	++	.04
(57) Mayne	Fruit/fruit juices	M	Non	Negative	+[d]	NS
	Vegetables	M	Non	Negative	++[d]	NS
	Fruit/fruit juices	F	Non	Negative	++[d]	<.10
	Vegetables	F	Non	Negative	++[d]	<.03
	Raw fruits & vegetables	M&F	Never	Negative	+	NS
	Raw fruits & vegetables	M&F	Ex	Negative	++	<.05
(58) Sankaranarayanan	Vegetables	M	All	Negative	+++	.02

NC: Not calculable.

[a]All = nonsmokers and smokers; Never = never smoked; Non = never and former smokers; Ex = former smokers; Current = smoking at time of study.

[b]Positive = level higher in cases; Negative = level higher in noncases.

[c]Strength	Relative risks or odds ratios	% difference in means
0	(0.91–1.09)	± 0–4.9
±	(0.80–0.90) or (1.10–1.25)	± 5–9.9
+	(0.60–0.79) or (1.26–1.67)	± 10–19.9
++	(0.40–0.59) or (1.68–2.50)	± 20–29.9
+++	(<0.40) or (>2.50)	± 30+

[d]Adjusted for smoking.

[e]Never and former light smokers.

[f]Former heavy smokers.

ingful comparisons. When studies are limited to women and nonsmokers, comparisons with men and smokers within the same setting are impossible. As a result, meaningful conclusions cannot be drawn about interactions of diet with sex or smoking at the present time.

Although carrots and cruciferous vegetables are often among the individual food items that are mentioned as being associated with decreased risk, in most instances the broader, more inclusive categories such as "vegetables" or "green and yellow

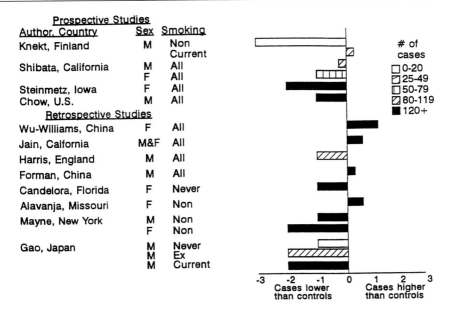

Fig. 1. Strength and direction of associations of dietary intake of fruits with subsequent lung cancer in 12 studies, by sex and smoking status. *See* footnote to Table 2 for strength of association: 1/2 = ±; 1 = +; 2 = ++; 3 = +++.

vegetables" tend to be more strongly associated with decreased risk than individual vegetables.

The associations of fruits and vegetables with lung cancer are shown separately in Figs. 1 and 2. The associations of increased dietary intake of vegetables with subsequent lung cancer are stronger and more consistent than those with an increased intake of fruits.

The findings summarized here and earlier *(13)* show that a diet that includes a high proportion of fruits and vegetables is associated with protection against lung cancer. On balance, their results are more than sufficient to support public health action, such as the recommendations for increasing intake of fruits and vegetables in the dietary guidelines issued by governmental and private health agencies *(59,60)*.

4.4. Retinol

In 1925, it was reported that rats deprived of "fat-soluble A vitamin" showed "replacement of various epithelia by stratified squamous keratinizing epithelium" *(14)*. These changes, generally considered to be precancerous, were noted throughout the respiratory tract, including the bronchi. When butter, a source of retinol, was added to the diet, these changes were prevented. It was 50 years later before a study among humans reported that lung cancer was associated with diets deficient in "vitamin A" as indicated by the consumption of carrots (a source of β-carotene) and milk and eggs (sources of retinol) *(45)*.

Many of the earlier dietary reports referred to "vitamin A" without specifying whether this was retinol, some of the carotenoids (mainly β-carotene), or both. Such studies have been omitted from further consideration. Ten that specifically dealt with di-

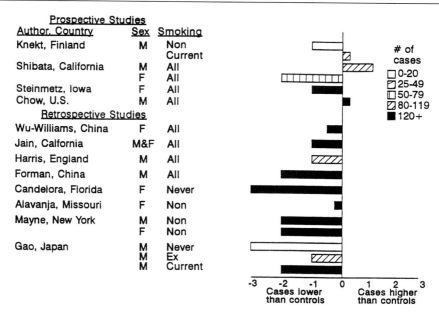

Fig. 2. Strength and direction of associations of dietary intake of vegetables with subsequent lung cancer in 12 studies, by sex and smoking status. *See* footnote to Table 2 for strength of association: 1/2 = ±; 1 = +; 2 = ++; 3 = +++.

etary retinol are summarized in Table 3. Only two showed a strong negative association, indicating possible protection. Most of the others showed weak positive associations *(62,64)*.

As a serum biomarker, retinol has a number of advantages for cancer studies. It is relatively stable when stored in serum at −20°C *(65)*. Serum levels tend to be constant for individuals, falling appreciably only when liver stores are badly depleted, and rising only temporarily after ingestion of large doses. These characteristics make it unsuitable as an index to adequacy of individual body stores. However, because most individuals' serum retinol concentrations are likely to be constant over long periods of time, the serum level to which cells are exposed at the time of blood drawing is likely to represent a long-term exposure. How retinol might act in protecting against cancer is uncertain, but it seems more likely to be involved in repair of oxidative damage than in its prevention.

Ten studies that compared serum retinol concentrations at baseline among persons who subsequently developed lung cancer and persons who did not are summarized in Table 4. There are more negative than positive associations, but few are strong and only one is statistically significant. Only in the Finnish study were findings among smokers and nonsmokers reported. The evidence for a protective association was stronger among nonsmokers than smokers *(72a)*. More decisive is the β-carotene and retinol efficacy trial (CARET), which was limited to smokers, former smokers, and persons exposed to asbestos *(72b)*. Approximately 9000 persons were assigned to a daily regimen of 25,000 IU of retinol and 30 mg of β-carotene; a similar number was assigned to placebo. After 4 yr of follow-up, the incidence of lung cancer was 28% higher among the treated group. It seems un-

Table 3
Association of Dietary Retinol with Lung Cancer in Selected Observational Studies, by Type of Study, Characteristics of Study Participants, and Nature of Association

Ref. no. and author	Type of study	Characteristics of participants				Association		
		Number	Residence	Sex	Smoking[a]	Direction[b]	Strength[c]	p-Trend
(33) Knekt	Cohort	2121	Finland	M	Non	Negative	+	.72
		2417	Finland	M	Current	Positive	+	.08
(47) Chow	Cohort	17,633	United States	M	All	Negative	+	
(62) Pastorino	Case-control	206	Italy	F	All	Negative	+++	.02
(63) LeMarchand	Case-control	827	Hawaii	M	All	Positive	0[d]	.70
		370	Hawaii	F	All	Positive	0[d]	.75
(64) Dartigues	Case-control	318	France	M&F	All	Negative	+++[d]	.17
(50) Kallandidj	Case-control	211	Greece	F	Non	Positive	+	.06
(51) Harris	Case-control	193	England	M	All	Positive	+[d]	.41[e]
(53) Candelora	Case-control	387	Florida	F	Never	Positive	±	.70
(32) Alavanja	Case-control	1450	Missouri	F	Non	Positive	+	.76
(57) Mayne	Case-control	424	New York	M	Non	Negative	0	>.05
		402	New York	F	Non	Positive	0	>.05
		364	New York	M&F	Never	Negative	±	>.05
		462	New York	M&F	Ex	Positive	0	>.05

[a]All = nonsmokers and smokers; Never = never smoked; Non = never and former smokers; Ex = former smokers; Current = smoking at time of study.
[b]Positive = level higher in cases
Negative = level higher in non-cases

[c]Strength	Relative risks or odds ratios	% difference in means
0	(0.91–1.09)	± 0–4.9
±	(0.80–0.90) or (1.10–1.25)	± 5–9.9
+	(0.60–0.79) or (1.26–1.67)	± 10–19.9
++	(0.40–0.59) or (1.68–2.50)	± 20–29.9
+++	(<0.40) or (>2.50)	± 30+

[d]Adjusted for smoking.
[e]p value for difference in means.

Table 4
Serum Retinol and Subsequent Lung Cancer: Differences Between Cases and Comparison
Groups and/or Risk Ratios of Highest to Lowest Category of Serum Retinol Concentrations

Ref. no. and author	Area	No. of cases	Sex and smoking[a]	Difference (Case mean– comparison mean)		Risk ratio		
				%	p	Group	Ratio[b]	p-Trend
(66) Willett	United States H.D.F.P.	17	M&F	−1.4	.50	Fifths	1.1[c]	.98
(67) Nomura	Hawaii	74	M	+7.0	>.50			
(68) Wald	England	656	M	−0.8				
(69) Friedman	California	151	M&F	−0.2	.93	Fifths	0.8[c]	.94
			M	−3.4				
			F	+6.4				
(40) Menkes	Maryland	99	M&F	−1.1	.71	Fifths	0.9	.68
(41) Kok	Netherlands	18	M&F	−2.9	.76			
(70) Connett	United States MRFIT	66	M	−4.4	.25			
(71) Knekt	Finland	144	M	−3.3	<.01	Fifths	0.7	.02
		8	F	−2.8	.08	Fifths	1.5	.08
(42) Stahelin	Switzerland	68	M	+3.4	>.05			
(72) Knekt	Finland	22	M, Non[d]			Thirds	0.2	>.05
		121	M, Current			Thirds	0.7	>.05

[a]If smoking is not specified, data were not stratified by smoking status.

[b]A risk ratio below 1.0 signifies that the group (third, fifth, and so forth) with the highest concentration of serum retinol had less lung cancer develop after baseline than the group with the lowest concentration, i.e., this is a protective association.

[c]Adjusted for smoking.

[d]Non—never smokers and ex-smokers at baseline; Current—smokers at baseline.

likely that retinol protects against lung cancer in humans, although such a possibility exists for nonsmokers. If there is a protective effect of retinol against lung cancer in humans, it is not yet demonstrable, and seems to be no more than weak, if indeed there is any protective effect at all.

4.5. Carotenoids

For many years, β-carotene was considered to be important in human nutrition only because it is a precursor of retinol. That it might play an important role in protection against cancer was brought to wide attention by Peto and Doll (73,74). Study of its potential role was delayed because earlier food composition tables did not distinguish between retinol and β-carotene, and because the carotenoids are not stable when stored at temperatures appreciably warmer than −70° C (65).

Hundreds of carotenoids have been identified, but only six have been found to exist in appreciable concentrations in human serum: α-carotene, β-carotene, cryptoxanthin, lutein, lycopene, and zeaxanthin *(75)*. Table 5 summarizes the associations of lung cancer with dietary carotenoids. Almost all are negative, signifying that higher levels are associated with decreased risk. These negative associations tend to be strongest with α- and β-carotene intake. Only the Finnish study *(33)* examined the association among current smokers, finding essentially none; the protective association was moderately strong among nonsmokers.

Two of the earlier studies of serum carotenoids, those done among participants in the Hypertension Detection and Follow-up Program (HDFP) and the Multiple Risk Factor Intervention Trial (MRFIT), measured total serum carotenoids *(66,70)*. The results were discrepant (Table 6). In the former, the association was positive but nonsignificant; in the latter, the association was negative, moderately strong, and significant. The two populations differed in several ways. The HDFP enrolled both women and men and a considerable proportion of blacks; the MRFIT was limited to men and was heavily weighted with smokers. Unfortunately, neither group stratified their findings on these characteristics, a failing common to many studies of nutritional relationships with lung cancer.

Serum β-carotene has been more extensively studied than total carotenoids (Table 6). Most found strong and significant negative associations. Current smokers in an analysis limited to men also showed a nonsignificant positive association whereas a strong protective association was found among nonsmokers *(72)*.

More definitive answers regarding the potential of β-carotene supplementation to prevent lung cancer are the results of three controlled trials. The first to be reported was the Alpha-Tocopherol Beta-Carotene study, a controlled trial involving more than 29,000 male smokers in Finland *(81a)*. After 5–8 yr of follow-up, the group receiving 20 mg β-carotene/d had a cancer rate 18% higher than those given placebo. As previously noted, the CARET study found that persons receiving 30 mg of β-carotene and 25,000 IU of retinol daily had a lung cancer increase rate 28% higher than the placebo group *(72b)*. The third trial, the Physicians' Health Study, found essentially no differences between the 11,000 men receiving 50 mg of β-carotene every other day for 12 yr and those receiving placebo *(82a)*. There were slight but far from significant reductions in lung cancer among smokers and nonsmokers.

A potential problem with these three trials has been pointed out *(82b)*. If the effect of β-carotene (or other antioxidants) is to protect against the initiation of carcinogenesis, all three trials were much too short in duration. More cogent is the possibility that β-carotene in the observational studies has merely been a "fellow-traveler" with some other substance or substances that are the real causes of the observed protective associations, so that the trial did not test the proper dietary component. None of these explanations accounts for the increased risk of lung cancer among persons who took β-carotene supplements. There is a possibility that a large intake of β-carotene might inhibit the absorption of other protective substances. The evidence on this possibility is still conflicting. Two studies have shown that supplementary β-carotene was associated with a decrease in serum levels of lycopene *(83)* and lutein *(84)*. In contrast, another found that the increase in serum β-carotene following supplementation was accompanied by a rise in the serum concentration of α-carotene and lycopene, and essentially no change in the concentrations of cryptoxanthin or lutein/zeaxanthin *(85)*.

Table 5

Association of Dietary Carotenoids with Lung Cancer in Selected Observational Studies, by Type of Study, Characteristics of Study Participants, and Nature of Association

Ref. no. and author	Type of study	Characteristics of participants				Association		
		Number	Residence	Sex	Smoking[a]	Direction[b]	Strength[c]	p-Trend
Total carotenoids								
(33) Knekt	Cohort	2121	Finland	M	Non	Negative	++	.04
		2417	Finland	M	Current	Negative	0	.91
(47) Chow	Cohort	17,633	United States	M	All	Negative	+	<.01
(53) Candelora	Case-control	387	Florida	F	Never	Negative	+++	.85
(32) Alavanja	Case-control	1450	Missouri	F	Non	Negative	±	>.05
(55) Dorgan	Case-control	1284	New Jersey	WM	All	Negative	±[d]	<.01
		1333	New Jersey	WF	All	Negative	++[d]	>.05
		435	New Jersey	BM	All	Positive	+[d]	>.05
		133	New Jersey	BF	All	Positive	+[d]	>.05
α-Carotene								
(33) Knekt	Cohort	4538	Finland	M	All	Negative	++[d]	.06
(53) Candelora	Case-control	387	Florida	F	Never	Negative	+++	<.01
(76) LeMarchand	Case-control	827	Hawaii	M	All	Negative	++[d]	<.01
		370	Hawaii	F	All	Negative	++[d]	.02
β-Carotene								
(77) Krumhout	Cohort	878	Netherlands	M	All	Negative	+[d]	.19
(33) Knekt	Cohort	4538	Finland	M	All	Negative	+[d]	.13[e]
(78) Shekelle	Cohort	1960	Illinois	M	All	Negative	++[d]	<.01
(49) Shibata	Cohort	24,218 p. yr	California	M	All	Positive	0[d]	
		45,941 p. yr	California	F	All	Negative	+++[d]	
(47) Chow	Cohort	17,633	United States	M	All	Negative	+	.06
(62) Pastorino	Case-control	208	Italy	F	All	Negative	++	
(64) Dartigues	Case-control	318	France	M&F	All	Negative	+++[d]	.34[e]
(50) Kallandidj	Case-control	211	Greece	F	Non	Positive	0	.96
(51) Harris	Case-control	193	England	M	All	Negative	++[d]	.05
(53) Candelora	Case-control	387	Florida	F	Never	Negative	++	.06

Reference	Design	n	Location	Sex	Smoking[a]	Direction[b]	Strength[c]	p
(48) Steinmetz	Nested	2952	Iowa	F	All	Negative	+	.35
(76) LeMarchand	Case-control	827	Hawaii	M	All	Negative	++[d]	<.01
		370	Hawaii	F	All	Negative	+++[d]	<.01
(32) Alavanja	Case-control	1450	Missouri	F	Non	0	0	.83
(57) Mayne	Case-control	424	New York	M	Non	Negative	+	<.05
		402	New York	F	Non	Negative	±	<.05
		364	New York	M&F	Never	Negative	+	>.05
		462	New York	M&F	Ex	Negative	+	>.05
γ-Carotene								
(33) Knekt	Cohort	4538	Finland	M	All	Negative	0	.82[e]
Cryptoxanthin								
(53) Candelora	Case-control	387	Florida	F	Never	Negative	++	.02
(76) LeMarchand	Case-control	827	Hawaii	M	All	Negative	±[d]	.81
		370	Hawaii	F	All	Negative	±[d]	.99
Lutein								
(33) Knekt	Cohort	4538	Finland	M	All	Negative	0	.28[e]
(48) Steinmetz	Nested	2952	Iowa	F	All	Positive	±	.34
(53) Candelora	Case-control	387	Florida	F	Never	Negative	±	.52
(76) LeMarchand	Case-control	827	Hawaii	M	All	Negative	++[d]	.04
		370	Hawaii	F	All	Negative	+++[d]	<.01
Lycopene								
(33) Knekt	Cohort	4538	Finland	M	All	Negative	0	.67[e]
(48) Steinmetz	Nested	2952	Iowa	F	All	Positive	+	.11
(53) Candelora	Case-control	387	Florida	F	Never	Negative	+	.13
(76) LeMarchand	Case-control	827	Hawaii	M	All	Negative	+[d]	.07
		370	Hawaii	F	All	Negative	+[d]	.83

[a]All = nonsmokers and smokers; Never = never smoked; Non = never and former smokers; Ex = former smokers; Current = smoking at time of study.

[b]Positive = level higher in cases; Negative = level higher in non-cases.

[c]Strength	Relative risks or odds ratios	% difference in means
0	(0.91–1.09)	± 0–4.9
±	(0.80–0.90) or (1.10–1.25)	± 5–9.9
+	(0.60–0.79) or (1.26–1.67)	± 10–19.9
++	(0.40–0.59) or (1.68–2.50)	± 20–29.9
+++	(<0.40) or (>2.50)	± 30+

[d]Adjusted for smoking.

[e]p value for difference in means.

123

Table 6
Serum Carotenoids and Subsequent Lung Cancer: Differences Between Cases and Comparison
Groups and Risk Ratio of Highest to Lowest Category of Serum Carotenoid Concentrations

Ref. no. and author	Area	No. of cases	Sex and smoking	Difference (Case mean–comparison mean)		Risk ratio		
				%	p	Group	Ratio	p-Trend
Total carotenoids								
(66) Willett	United States (HDFP)	17	M&F	±[a]	.59			
(70) Connett	United States (MRFIT)	66	M	−12.3	.03	Fifths	0.5[a]	
β-Carotene								
(67) Nomura	Hawaii	74	M	−31.0	<.01	Fifths	0.5[a]	.04
(40) Menkes	Maryland	99	M&F	−13.7	.04	Fifths	0.5[a]	.04
(79) Wald	England	50	M	−22.2	<.01	Fifths	0.4[a]	<.01
(70) Connett	United States (MRFIT)	66	M	−22.4	.07	Fifths	0.4[a]	
(62) Pastorino	Italy	47	F			Thirds	0.2	<.01
(71) Knekt	Finland	144	M	−20.7	<.01	Fifths	0.8	>.05
		8	F	−39.5	.14	Fifths	0.6	>.05
(42) Stahelin	Switzerland	68	M	−47.8	<.01	Eighths	0.6[a]	<.05
(80) Orentreich	California	123	M&F	−15.4	.13	Fifths	0.3[a]	.01
(72) Knekt	Finland	22	M, Non			Thirds	0.4	>.05
		121	M, Current			Thirds	1.2	>.05

[a]Adjusted for smoking.

4.6. Vitamin E

Four tocopherols and four tocotrienols have vitamin E activity, but α-tocopherol is
the major form found in human tissues. Vitamin E is present in human serum at much
greater concentrations than retinol or the carotenoids, being reported in milligrams per
deciliter rather than micrograms per liter. Three studies of the association of vitamin E
intake with lung cancer are summarized in Table 7. Of considerable interest is the strong
associations reported with γ- and δ-tocopherol from the study in Finland, raising questions of whether the usual emphasis on α-tocopherol is justified. Serum concentrations
of vitamin E have been studied more extensively than dietary intakes (Table 8). In this
instance, the results are almost evenly split between negative and positive associations,
with only a few being statistically significant. It is once more noteworthy that current
smokers in Finland showed no evidence of a protective association either with dietary
intake or serum levels of vitamin E (33,72).

Table 7
Associations of Dietary Vitamin E and Specific Tocopherols with Lung Cancer in Selected Studies, by Type of Study, Observations of Participants, and Nature of Association

Ref. no. and author	Type of study	Characteristics of participants				Association		
		Number	Residents	Sex	Smoking[a]	Direction[b]	Strength[c]	p-Trend
(33) Knekt	Cohort (E)[e]	2121	Finland	M	Non	Negative	+++	.12
	(E)	2417	Finland	M	Current	Positive	±	.58
	(α)	4538	Finland	M	All	Negative	0[d]	.71[f]
	(β)	4538	Finland	M	All	0	0[d]	∝.99[f]
	(γ)	4538	Finland	M	All	Negative	+++[d]	.02[f]
	(δ)	4538	Finland	M	All	Negative	+++[d]	<.01[f]
(16) Byers	Case-control (E)	883	New York	M	All	Negative	+[d]	.22
	(E)	469	New York	F	All	Negative	±[d]	.91
(32) Alavanja	Case-control	1450	Missouri	F	Non	Positive	++	.18

[a]All = nonsmokers and smokers; Never = never smoked; Non = never and former smokers; Ex = former smokers; Current = Smoking at time of study.
[b]Positive = level higher in cases; Negative = level higher in non-cases.
[c]

Strength	Relative risks or odds ratios	% difference in means
0	(0.91–1.09)	± 0–4.9
±	(0.80–0.90) or (1.10–1.25)	± 5–9.9
+	(0.60–0.79) or (1.26–1.67)	± 10–19.9
++	(0.40–0.59) or (1.68–2.50)	± 20–29.9
+++	(<0.40) or (>2.50)	± 30+

[d]Adjusted for smoking.
[e]E: Total vitamin E; α, β, γ, δ: Specific tocopherols.
[f]p value for difference in means.

125

Table 8
Serum Vitamin E and Lung Cancer: Differences Between Cases and Comparison Groups
and/or Risk Ratio of Highest to Lowest Category of Serum Vitamin E Concentrations

Ref. no. and author	Area	No. of cases	Sex and smoking	Difference (Case mean– comparison mean) %	p	Risk ratio Group	Ratio	p-Trend
(66) Willett	United States (HDFP)	17	M&F	−7.9	.23			
(67) Nomura	Hawaii	74	M	+7.0	>.50			
(40) Menkes	Maryland	99	M&F	−11.8	<.01	Fifths	0.4[a]	.04
(41) Kok	Netherlands	18	M&F	−9.4	.33	Fifths	0.2[a]	<.05
(86) Knekt	Finland	144	M	−3.6	.25	Fifths	0.7[a]	.71
		8	F	+2.2	.80			
(70) Connett	United States (MRFIT)	66	M	−4.4	.51			
(42) Stahelin	Switzerland	68	M	+1.5	<.01	Eighths	0.68[a]	>.05
(80) Orentreich	California	123	M&F	+4.3		Fifths	1.7[a]	
(72) Knekt	Finland	22	M, Non			Thirds	0.2	<.05
		121	M, Current			Thirds	1.2	>.05

[a]Adjusted for smoking.

Again, the strongest evidence is provided by the Alpha-Tocopherol Beta-Carotene Trial among smokers. In this instance, lung cancer rates were essentially the same among persons taking vitamin E supplements and those taking placebo. Essentially the same criticisms can be raised with respect to the α-tocopherol arm as were mentioned for the β-carotene arm of the trial. In addition, some critics feel that the dose of α-tocopherol was too low to be effective (82b).

Based on currently available evidence, it does not appear that α-tocopherol is likely to have a protective effect against lung cancer. Further studies with the γ and δ forms need to be done.

4.7. Vitamin C

There has been considerable public interest in the possible benefits of taking large doses of vitamin C, largely because of the influence of the Nobel Laureate, Linus Pauling (87). Seven prospective and eight retrospective (case-control) dietary studies are summarized in Table 9. Although most showed a negative, protective association, only five were statistically significant, one being the study among Finnish nonsmokers. Again the finding among Finnish smokers was discrepant.

Because vitamin C degrades rapidly in serum that has not been treated with a preservative, only the study that assayed sera shortly after blood had been drawn has been able to report on serum concentrations of vitamin C (42). In this study, there was virtually no

Table 9
Association of Dietary Vitamin C with Lung Cancer in Selected Studies, by Type of Study, Characteristics of Participants, and Nature of Association

Ref. no. and author	Type of study	Characteristics of participants				Association		
		Number	Residence	Sex	Smoking[a]	Direction[b]	Strength[c]	p-Trend
(88) Kvale	Cohort	10,602	Norway	M	All	Negative	±[d]	.65
(77) Krumhout	Cohort	878	Netherlands	M	All	Negative	+++[d]	<.01
(33) Knekt	Cohort	2121	Finland	M	Non	Negative	+++	<.01
	Cohort	2417	Finland	M	Current	Positive	±	.36
(90) Enstrom	Cohort	4479	United States	M	All	Negative	±	.82
		6869	United States	F	All	Negative	++	.32
(49) Shibata	Cohort	24,218 p yr	California	M	All	Positive	±[d]	
		45,941 p yr	California	F	All	Negative	++[d]	
(47) Chow	Cohort	17,633	United States	M	All	Negative	±	
(48) Steinmetz	Nested	2982	Iowa	F	All	Negative	+	.11
(89) Hinds	Case-control	705	Hawaii	M	All	Negative	+[d]	
		286	Hawaii	F	All	Positive	+[d]	
(31) Byers	Case-control	991	New York	M	All	Negative	0[d]	.52
(16) Byers	Case-control	883	New York	M	All	Negative	±[d]	.70
		469	New York	F	All	Negative	±[d]	.51
(44) Koo	Case-control	137	Hong Kong	F	Never	Negative	++	.02
(63) LeMarchand	Case-control	827	Hawaii	M	All	Negative	++[d]	.01
		370	Hawaii	F	All	Positive	++[d]	.08
(50) Kallandidj	Case-control	211	Greece	F	Non	Negative	+	.08
(53) Candelora	Case-control	387	Florida	F	Never	Negative	++	<.01
(32) Alavanja	Case-control	1450	Missouri	F	Non	Positive	+	.26

[a]All = nonsmokers and smokers; Never = never smoked; Non = never and former smokers; Ex = former smokers; Current = smoking at time of study.
[b]Positive = level higher in cases; Negative = level higher in non-cases.

[c]Strength	Relative risks or odds ratios	% difference in means
0	(0.91–1.09)	± 0–4.9
±	(0.80–0.90) or (1.10–1.25)	± 5–9.9
+	(0.60–0.79) or (1.26–1.67)	± 10–19.9
++	(0.40–0.59) or (1.68–2.50)	± 20–29.9
+++	(<0.40) or (>2.50)	± 30+

[d]Adjusted for smoking.

127

difference in mean serum levels between the 68 men who died from lung cancer and the 2421 survivors after 12–14 yr of follow-up. The available evidence suggests that vitamin C is also associated with protection against lung cancer.

4.8. B Vitamins

Serum levels of vitamins B_1, B_2, and B_6 were assayed in the cohort study in Switzerland (43). There were essentially no differences in the concentrations of these vitamins between cases and noncases in a nested case-control study. On the other hand, there is an indication that a daily regimen of 10 mg of folate plus 500 μg of vitamin B_{12} may reduce the severity of atypical bronchial squamous metaplasia among smokers and thereby reduce the risk of subsequent lung cancer (91). Among 36 smokers with metaplasia on this treatment regimen, 39% showed improvement compared to only 16% among 37 smokers on placebo. If this protective effect of folate is confirmed by observational studies, a more definitive trial would be indicated.

4.9. Selenium

The trace metal selenium was discovered in 1818 by Berzelius, who named it for the moon because of its companionship with tellurium, named for the earth (92). Its importance with relation to cancer comes from the fact that it is a component of the antioxidant enzyme, glutathione peroxidase. Selenium is a convenient marker for this enzyme because it is much easier to assay serum for selenium than for the entire enzyme. The concentration of selenium in soils and crops varies considerably from place to place, making dietary assays difficult when foods are imported from a variety of regions. Only in Finland has such a study been attempted, probably because when the study started, the selenium content of available foods was low, a situation that has changed during the course of the study. In this instance, there was only a slight, nonsignificant negative association among smokers, and essentially no association among nonsmokers (33).

In contrast to the dietary assay situation, 14 prospective studies of selenium as a biomarker for lung cancer risk have been done and are shown in Table 10. These include two in which selenium was measured in toenail clippings rather than in serum (100,102). Selenium is concentrated in hair and nails. Hair is unsuitable because of selenium-containing shampoos, so clippings from the nail of the big toe are used. Depending on their length, these reflect the circulating selenium levels over a period of days or even weeks. As can be seen in Table 10, in almost all instances the associations are negative, consistent with a protective effect of higher levels of selenium. With respect to smoking, the Finnish study found similar protective effects among smokers and nonsmokers. In the Netherlands, the percent difference in toenail selenium concentration between cases and noncases was greater for nonsmokers, less for ex-smokers, and least for smokers, although it must be noted that none of the differences were statistically significant. The situation with respect to selenium may best be summed up by the Scottish verdict, "not proven" in either direction.

4.10. Zinc

Zinc is reported to be one of the factors associated with mobilization of retinol from the liver. In a single cohort study from Japan, a slight and nonsignificant negative association was reported (101).

Table 10
Serum or Toenail Selenium and Lung Cancer: Differences Between Cases and Comparison Groups and/or Risk Ratios of Highest to Lowest Category of Serum Selenium Concentrations

Ref. no. and author	Area	No. of cases	Sex and smoking	Difference (Case mean–comparison mean) %	p	Risk ratio Group	Ratio	p-Trend
(93) Willett	United States (HDFP)	18	M&F	−6.9	.21			
(94) Salonen	Finland	23	M&F	−6.5	.28			
(40) Menkes	Maryland	99	M&F	+2.7	.16	Fifths	1.5[a]	.07
(95) Nomura	Hawaii	71	M	+0.4	>.50	Fifths	0.9[a]	.46
(41) Kok	Netherlands	18	M&F	−4.0	.49			
(96) Coates	Washington	11	M&F			Thirds	0.8	.73
(97) Ringstad	Norway	7	M&F	−8.2	.25			
(98) Knekt	Finland	189	M	−6.8	<.01	Fifths	0.3[a]	<.01
		9	F	−1.0	.93			
(99) Criqui	California	27	M&F	+0.7	.74			
(100)[b] Van den Brandt	Netherlands	285	M	−3.3	.13	Fifths	0.5[a]	.01
		32	F	−6.6	<.01	Fifths	0.4[a]	.10
		6	Never	−10.1	.25			
		122	Ex	−2.6	.16	Fifths	0.5	.24
		189	Current	−1.7	.58	Fifths	0.6	
(72) Knekt	Finland	22	M, Non			Thirds	0.6	>.05
		121	M, Current			Thirds	0.4	<.05
(101) Kabuto	Japan	77	M&F	−4.4	.16	Fourths	0.6	.10
(102)[b] Garland	United States	47	F	−9.6	.03	Thirds	0.5	.19
						Thirds	4.3[a]	.17

[a]Adjusted for smoking.
[b]Toenail selenium was exposure biomarker.

5. CONCLUSIONS

The available evidence is strong that certain factors in fruits and vegetables inhibit the initiation or promotion of lung cancer. If inhibition depends largely on a single substance, it is likely to be something associated with the carotenes or vitamin C and not with vitamin E or selenium. The strong protective associations of γ- and δ-tocopherol in a single study suggests they need further investigation. Of great potential importance, both for indicating mode of action and for public health application, is the possible interaction of smoking and potentially protective substances. Future studies should stratify their results by smoking status and possibly also by sex.

Collaboration with cellular biologists is highly desirable. Knowledge of oxidative reactions within cells that could damage DNA might point to the class of antioxidants most likely to yield protection. How such antioxidants penetrate into cells will also indicate which ones are most likely to affect intracellular reactions.

With respect to dietary recommendations, the findings at present confirm general advice to decrease the ingestion of fat to 30% of caloric intake and to increase the amount of fruits and vegetables in the diet. Specific dietary supplements do not seem indicated at this time. Finally, the available evidence, admittedly scanty, suggests that dietary changes are unlikely to reduce the risk of lung cancer among persons who continue to smoke.

REFERENCES

1. Doll R. Introduction and overview. In: Epidemiology of Lung Cancer. Samet JM, ed. New York: Marcel Dekker, Inc. 1994, 1–14.
2. Churg A. Lung cancer cell type and occupational exposure. In: Epidemiology of Lung Cancer. Samet JM, ed. New York: Marcel Dekker, Inc., 1994, pp. 413–436.
3. Fehily AM, Phillips KM, Yarnell JWG. Diet, smoking, social class, and body mass index in the Caerphilly Heart Disease Study. Am J Clin Nutr 1984; 40:827–833.
4. Sidney S, Caan BJ, Friedman GD. Dietary intake of carotene in nonsmokers with and without passive smoking at home. Am J Epidemiol 1989; 129:1305–1309.
5. Morabia A, Wynder EL. Dietary habits of smokers, people who never smoked, and exsmokers. Am J Clin Nutr 1990; 52:933–937.
6. Subar AF, Harlan LC, Mattson ME. Food and nutrient intake differences between smokers and nonsmokers in the US. Am J Public Health 1990; 80:1323–1329.
7. Cade JE, Margetts BM. Relationships between diet and smoking—Is the diet of smokers different? J Epidemiol Community Health 1991; 45:270–272.
8. La Vecchia C, Negri E, Franceschi S, Parazzini F, Decarli A. Differences in dietary intakes with smoking, alcohol, and education. Nutr Cancer 1992; 17:297–304.
9. Hulsholf KFAN, Wedel M, Löwik MRH, Kok FJ, Kistemaker C, Hermus RJJ, ten Hoor F, Ockhuizen T. Clustering of dietary variables and other lifestyle factors (Dutch Nutritional Surveillance System). J Epidemiol Community Health 1992; 46:417–424.
10. Järvinen R, Knekt P, Seppänen R, Reunanen A, Heliövaara M, Maatela J, Aromaa A. Antioxidant vitamins in the diet: relationships with other personal characteristics in Finland. J Epidemiol Community Health 1994; 48:549–554.
11. Matanoski G, Kanchanaraksa S, Lantry D, Chang Y. Characteristics of nonsmoking women in NHANES I and NHANES II epidemiologic follow-up study with exposure to spouses who smoke. Am J Epidemiol 1995; 142:149–157.
12. McMichael AJ, Jensen OM, Parkin DM, Zaridze DG. Dietary and endogenous cholesterol and human cancer. Epidemiol Rev 1984; 6:192–216.
13a. Steinmetz KA, Potter JD. Vegetables, fruit, and cancer. I. Epidemiology. Cancer Causes Control 1991; 2:325–357.
13b. Ziegler RG, Mayne ST, Swanson CA. Nutrition and cancer. Cancer Causes Control 1966; 7:157–177.
14. Wolbach SB, Howe PR. Tissue changes following deprivation of fat-soluble A vitamin. J Exp Med 1925; 42:753–777.
15. Pearce ML, Dayton S. Incidence of cancer in men on a diet high in polyunsaturated fat. Lancet 1971; 1:464–467.
16. Byers TE, Graham S, Haughey BP, Marshall JR, Swanson MK. Diet and lung cancer risk: findings from the Western New York Study. Am J Epidemiol 1987; 125:351–363.
17. Goodman MT, Kolonel LN, Yoshizawa CN, Hankin JH. The effect of dietary cholesterol and fat on the risk of lung cancer in Hawaii. Am J Epidemiol 1988; 128:1241–1255.
18. Jain M, Burch JD, Howe GR, Risch HA, Miller AB. Dietary factors and risk of lung cancer: results from a case-control study, Toronto, 1981–1985. Int J Cancer 1990; 45:287–293.

19. Stockwell HG, Candelora EC. Re: Dietary cholesterol and incidence of lung cancer: the Western Electric Study (letter). Am J Epidemiol 1992; 136:1167.

20. Shekelle RB, Rossof AH, Stamler J. Dietary cholesterol and incidence of lung cancer: the Western Electric Study. Am J Epidemiol 1991; 134:480–484.

21. Heilbrun LK, Nomura AMY, Stemmerman GN. Dietary cholesterol and lung cancer risk among Japanese men in Hawaii. Am J Clin Nutr 1984; 39:375–379.

22. Knekt P, Seppanen R, Jarvinen R, Virtamo J, Hyvonen L, Pukkala E, Teppo L. Dietary cholesterol, fatty acids, and the risk of lung cancer among men. Nutr Cancer 1991; 16:267–275.

23a. Hiatt RA, Fireman BH. Serum cholesterol and the incidence of cancer in a large cohort. J Chron Dis 1986; 39:861–870.

23b. Steenland, K, Nowlin S. Palu S. Cancer incidence in the National Health and Nutrition Survey I follow-up data: diabetes, cholesterol, pulse, and physical activity. Cancer Epidemiol Biomarkers Prev 1995; 4:807–811.

24. Report of the Committee of Principal Investigators. WHO cooperative trial on primary prevention of ischaemic heart disease with clofibrate to lower serum cholesterol: final mortality follow-up. Lancet 1984; 2:600–604.

25. The Multiple Risk Factor Intervention Trial Research Group. Mortality rates after 10.5 years for participants in the Multiple Risk Factor Intervention Trial. Findings related to a priori hypotheses of the trial. JAMA 1990; 263:1795–1801.

26. Frick MH, Elo O, Haapa K, Heinonen OP, Heinsalmi P, Helo P, et al. Helsinki Heart Study: primary-prevention trial with gemfibrozil in middle-aged men with dyslipidemia. New Engl J Med 1987; 317:1237–1245.

27. Multiple Risk Factor Intervention Trial Research Group. Multiple Risk Factor Intervention Trial. Risk factor changes and mortality results. JAMA 1982; 248:1465–1477.

28. Lipid Research Clinics Program. The Lipid Research Clinics Coronary Primary Prevention Trial results. 1. Reduction incidence of coronary heart disease. JAMA 1984; 251:351–364.

29. Gantt RC, Lincoln JE. Dietary factors and cancer (letter). Int J Epidemiol 1988; 17:231, 232.

30. Taioli E, Nicolosi A, Wynder EL. Possible role of diet as a host factor in the aetiology of tobacco-induced lung cancer: An ecological study in southern and northern Italy. Int J Epidemiol 1991; 20:611–614.

31. Byers T, Vena J, Mettlin C, Swanson M, Graham S. Dietary vitamin A and lung cancer risk: an analysis by histologic subtypes. Am J Epidemiol 1984; 120:769–776.

32. Alavanja MCR, Brown CC, Swanson C, Brownson RC. Saturated fat intake and lung cancer risk among nonsmoking women in Missouri. J Natl Cancer Inst 1993; 85:1906–1916.

33. Knekt P, Järvinen R, Seppänen R, Rissanen A, Aromaa A, Heinonen OP, Albanes D, Heinonen M, Pukkala E, Teppo L. Dietary antioxidants and the risk of lung cancer. Am J Epidemiol 1991; 134:471–479.

34. Freudenheim JL, Graham S. Toward a dietary prevention of cancer. Epidemiol Rev 1989; 11:229–235.

35. Kolonel LN. Lung cancer: another consequence of a high-fat diet? (editorial) J Natl Cancer Inst 1993; 85:1886,1887.

36. Cambien F, Ducimetiere P, Richard J. Total serum cholesterol and cancer mortality in a middle-aged male population. Am J Epidemiol 1980; 112:388–394.

37. Dyer AR, Stamler J, Paul O, Shekelle RB, Schoenberger JA, Berkson DM, Lepper M, Collette P, Shekelle S, Lindberg HA. Serum cholesterol and risk of death from cancer and other causes in three Chicago epidemiological studies. J Chron Dis 1981; 34:249–260.

38. Kagan A, McGee DL, Yano K, Rhoads GG, Nomura A. Serum cholesterol and mortality in a Japanese-American population. The Honolulu Heart Program. Am J Epidemiol 1981; 114:11–20.

39. Keys A, Aravanis C, Blackburn H, Buzina R, Dontas AS, Fidanza F, Karvonen MJ, Menotti A, Nedeljkovic S, Punsar S, Toshima H. Serum cholesterol and cancer mortality in the Seven Countries Study. Am J Epidemiol 1985; 121:870–883.

40. Menkes MS, Comstock GW, Vuilleumier JP, Helsing KJ, Rider AA, Brookmeyer R. Serum beta-carotene, vitamins A and E, selenium, and the risk of lung cancer. New Engl J Med 1986; 315:1250–1254.

41. Kok FJ, van Dujn CM, Hofman A, Vermeeren R, de Brujn AM, Valkenburg HA. Micronutrients and the risk of lung cancer (letter). New Engl J Med 1987; 316:1416.

42. Stähelin HB, Gey KF, Eichholzer M, Lüdin E, Bernasconi F, Thurneysen J, Brubacher G. Plasma antioxidant vitamins and subsequent cancer mortality in the 12-year follow-up of the Prospective Basel Study. Am J Epidemiol 1991; 133:766–775.

43. Stähelin HB, Rösel F, Buess E, Brubacher G. Dietary risk factors for cancer in the Basel Study. Biblthca Nutr Dieta 1986; 37:144–153.

44. Koo LC. Dietary habits and lung cancer risk among Chinese females in Hong Kong who never smoked. Nutr Cancer 1988; 11:155–172.
45. Wu-Williams AH, Dai XD, Blot W, Xu ZY, Sun XW, Xiao HP et al. Lung cancer among women in northeast China. Br J Cancer 1990; 62:982–987.
46. Bandera EV, Freudenheim JL, Graham S, Marshall JR, et al. Alcohol consumption and lung cancer in white males. Cancer Causes Control 1992; 3:361–369.
47. Chow WH, Schuman LM, McLaughlin JK, Bjelke E, Gridley G, Wacholder S, Chien HTC, Blot WJ. A cohort study of tobacco use, diet, occupation, and lung cancer mortality. Cancer Causes Control 1992; 3:247–254.
48. Steinmetz KA, Potter JD, Folsom AR. Vegetables, fruit, and lung cancer in the Iowa Women's Health Study. Cancer Res 1993; 53:536–543.
49. Shibata A, Paganini-Hill A, Ross RK, Henderson BE. Intake of vegetables, fruits, beta-carotene, vitamin C and vitamin supplements and cancer incidence among the elderly: a prospective study. Br J Cancer 1992; 66:673–679.
50. Kalandidi A, Katsouyanni K, Voropoulou N, Bastas G, Saracci R, Trichopoulos D. Passive smoking and diet in the etiology of lung cancer among non-smokers. Cancer Causes Control 1990; 1:15–21.
51. Harris R, Key T, Silcocks P, Bull D, Wald N. A case-control study of dietary carotene in men with lung cancer and in men with other epithelial cancers. Nutr Cancer 1991; 15:63–68.
52. Forman MR, Yao SX, Graubard BI, Qiao YL, McAdams M, Mao BL, Taylor PR. The effect of dietary intake of fruits and vegetables on the odds ratio of lung cancer among Yunnan tin miners. Int J Epidemiol 1992; 21:437–441.
53. Candelora E, Stockwell H, Armstrong A, Pinkham P. Dietary intake and risk of lung cancer in women who never smoked. Nutr Cancer 1992; 17:263–270.
54. Swanson CA, Mao BL, Li JY, Lubin JH, Yao SX, Wang JZ, Cai SK, Hou Y, Luo QS, Blot WJ. Dietary determinants of lung-cancer risk: Results from a case-control study in Yunnan Province, China. Int J Cancer 1992; 50:876–880.
55. Dorgan JF, Ziegler RG, Schoenberg JB, Hartge P, McAdams MJ, Falk RT, Wilcox HB, Shaw GL. Race and sex differences in associations of vegetables, fruits, and carotenoids with lung cancer risk in New Jersey (United States). Cancer Causes Control 1993; 4:273–281.
56. Gao C, Taioma K, Kuroishii T, Hirose K, Inoue M. Protective effects of raw vegetables and fruit against lung cancer among smokers and ex-smokers: a case-control study in the Tokai area of Japan. Jpn J Cancer Res 1993; 84:594–600.
57. Mayne ST, Janerich DT, Greenwald P, Chorost S, Tucci C, Zaman MB, Melamed MR, Kiely M, McKneally MF. Dietary beta carotene and lung cancer risk in U. S. nonsmokers. J Natl Cancer Inst 1994; 86:33–38.
58. Sankaranarayanan R, Varghese C, Duffy SW, Padmakumary G, Day NE, Nair MK. A case-control study of diet and lung cancer in Kerala, South India. Int J Cancer 1994; 58:644–649.
59. Butrum RR, Clifford CK, Lanza E. NCI dietary guidelines: rationale. Am J Clin Nutr 1988; 48:888–895.
60. Willett WC. Diet and health: What should we eat? Science 1994; 264:532–537.
61. Bjelke E. Dietary vitamin A and human lung cancer. Int J Cancer 1975; 15:561–565.
62. Pastorino U, Pisani P, Berrino F, Andreoli C, Barbieri A, Costa A, Mazzoleni C, Gramegna G, Marubini, E. Vitamin A and female lung cancer: a case-control study on plasma and diet. Nutr Cancer 1987; 10:171–179.
63. LeMarchand L, Yoshizawa CN, Kolonel LN, Hankin JH, Goodman MT. Vegetable consumption and lung cancer risk: a population-based case-control study in Hawaii. J Natl Cancer Inst 1989; 81:1158–1164.
64. Dartigues J-F, Dabis F, Gros N, Moise A, Bois G, Salamon R, Dilhuydy J-M, Courty G. Dietary vitamin A, beta carotene and risk of epidermoid lung cancer in south-western France. Europ J Epidemiol 1990; 6:261–265.
65. Comstock GW, Alberg AJ, Helzlsouer KJ. Reported effects of long-term freezer storage on concentrations of retinol, B-carotene, and a-tocopherol in serum or plasma summarized. Clin Chem 1993; 39:1075–1078.
66. Willett WC, Polk BF, Underwood BA, Stampfer MJ, Pressel S, Rosner B, Taylor JO, Schneider K, Hames CG. Relation of serum vitamins A and E and carotenoids to the risk of cancer. New Engl J Med 1984; 310:430–434.
67. Nomura AMY, Stemmermann GN, Heilbrun LK, Salkeld RM, Vuilleumier JP. Serum vitamin levels and the risk of cancer of specific sites in men of Japanese ancestry in Hawaii. Cancer Res 1985; 45:2369–2372.

68. Wald N, Boreham J, Bailey A. Serum retinol and subsequent risk of cancer. Br J Cancer 1986; 54:957–961.
69. Friedman GD, Blaner WS, Goodman DS, Vogelman JH, Brind JL, Hoover R, Fireman BH, Orentreich N. Serum retinol and retinol-binding protein levels do not predict subsequent lung cancer. Am J Epidemiol 1986; 123:781–789.
70. Connett JE, Kuller LH, Kjelsberg MO, Polk BF, Collins G, Rider A, Hulley SB. Relationship between carotenoids and cancer. The Multiple Risk Factor Intervention Trial (MRFIT) Study. Cancer 1989; 64:126–134.
71. Knekt P, Aromaa A, Maatela J, Aaran R-K, Nikkari T, Hakama M, Hakulinen T, Peto R, Teppo L. Serum vitamin A and subsequent risk of cancer: cancer incidence follow-up of the Finnish Mobile Clinic Health Examination Survey. Am J Epidemiol 1990; 132:857–870.
72a. Knekt P. Vitamin E and smoking and the risk of lung cancer. Ann NY Acad Sci 1993; 686;280–287.
72b. Omenn GS, Goodman GE, Thornquist MO, Balmes J, Cullen MR, Glass A, Keogh JP, Meyskens FL Jr, Valanis B, Williams JH Jr, Barnhart S, Hammar S. Effects of a combination of beta carotene and vitamin A on lung cancer and cardiovascular disease. New Engl J Med 1996; 334:1150–1155.
73. Peto R, Doll R, Buckley JD, Sporn MB. Can dietary beta-carotene materially reduce human cancer rates? Nature 1981; 290:201–208.
74. Doll R, Peto R. The Causes of Cancer. Oxford: Oxford University Press, 1981; 1–1312.
75. Bieri JG, Brown ED, Smith Jr JC. Determination of individual carotenoids in human plasma by high performance liquid chromatography. J Liquid Chromatogr 1985; 8:473–484.
76. LeMarchand L, Hankin JH, Kolonel LN, Beecher GR, Wilkens LR, Zhao LP. Intake of specific carotenoids and lung cancer risk. Cancer Epidemiol Biomarkers Prev 1993; 2:183–187.
77. Kromhout D. Essential micronutrients in relation to carcinogenesis. Am J Clin Nutr 1987; 45: 1361–1367.
78. Shekelle RB, Tangney CC, Rossof AH, Stamler J. Serum cholesterol, beta-carotene, and risk of lung cancer. Epidemiol 1992; 3:282–287.
79. Wald NJ, Thompson SG, Densem JW, Boreham J, Bailey A. Serum beta-carotene and subsequent risk of cancer: results from the BUPA study. Br J Cancer 1988; 57:428–433.
80. Orentreich N, Matias JR, Vogelman JH, Salkeld RM, Bhagavan H, Friedman GD. The predictive value of serum B-carotene for subsequent development of lung cancer. Nutr Cancer 1991; 16:167–169.
81. The Alpha-Tocopherol Beta Carotene Cancer Prevention Study Group. The effect of vitamin E and beta carotene on the incidence of lung cancer and other cancers in male smokers. New Engl J Med 1994; 330:1029–1035.
82a. Hennekens CH, Buring JE, Manson JE, Stampfer M, Rosner B, Cook NR, Belanger C, LaMotte F, Gaziano JM, Ridker PM, Willett W, Peto R. Lack of effect of long-term supplementation with beta carotene on the incidence of malignant neoplasms and cardiovascular disease. New Engl J Med 1996; 334:1145–1149.
82b. Blumberg J, Block G. The Alpha-tocopherol, Beta-carotene Cancer Prevention Study in Finland. Nutr Rev 1994; 52:242–245.
83. Gaziano JM, Johnson EJ, Russell RM, Manson JE, Stampfer MJ, Ridker PM, Frei B, Hennekens CH, Krinsky NI. Discrimination in absorption or transport of β-carotene isomers after oral supplementation with either all-trans- or 9-cis-β-carotene. Am J Clin Nutr 1995; 61:1248–1252.
84. Kostic D, White WS, Olson JA. Intestinal absorption, serum clearance, and interactions between lutein and β-carotene when administered to human adults in separate or combined oral doses. Am J Clin Nutr 1995; 62:604–610.
85. Wahlquist ML, Wattanapenpaiboon N, Macrae FA, Lambert JR, MacLennan R, Hsu-Hage B H-H, Australian Polyp Prevention Project Investigators. Changes in serum carotenoids in subjects with colorectal adenomas after 24 months of β-carotene supplementation. Am J Clin Nutr 1994; 60:936–943.
86. Knekt P. Serum alpha-tocopherol and the risk of cancer. Publications of the Social Insurance Institution, Finland, ML:83. Helsinki, Social Insurance Institution; 1988.
87. Cameron E, Pauling L. Ascorbic acid and the glycosaminoglycans: an orthomolecular approach to cancer and other diseases. Oncology 1973; 27:181–192.
88. Kvale G, Bjelke E, Gart JJ. Dietary habits and lung cancer risk. Int J Cancer 1983; 31:397–405.
89. Hinds MW, Kolonel LN, Hankin JH, Lee J. Dietary vitamin A, carotene, vitamin C and risk of lung cancer in Hawaii. Am J Epidemiol 1984; 119:227–237.
90. Enstrom JE, Kanim LE, Klein MA. Vitamin C intake and mortality among a sample of the United States population. Epidemiol 1992; 3:194–202.

91. Heimburger DC, Alexander CB, Birch R, Butterworth Jr CE, Bailey WC, Krumdieck CL. Improvement in bronchial squamous metaplasia in smokers treated with folate and vitamin B_{12}. JAMA 1988; 259:1525–1530.

92. Subcommittee on Nutrition, Committee on Animal Nutrition, Board on Agriculture, National Research Council. Selenium in Nutrition, Revised Edition. Washington: National Academy Press, 1983; 1.

93. Willett WC, Polk BF, Morris JS, Stampfer MJ, Pressel S, Rosner B, Taylor JO, Schneider K, Hames CG. Prediagnostic serum selenium and risk of cancer. Lancet 1983; 2:130–134.

94. Salonen JT, Alfthan G, Huttunen JK, Puska P. Association between serum selenium and the risk of cancer. Am J Epidemiol 1984; 120:342–349.

95. Nomura AMY, Heilbrun LK, Morris JS, Stemmermann GN. Serum selenium and the risk of cancer, by specific sites: a case-control analysis of prospective data. J Natl Cancer Inst 1987; 79:103–108.

96. Coates RJ, Weiss NS, Daling JR, Morris JS, Labbe RF. Serum levels of selenium and retinol and the subsequent risk of cancer. Am J Epidemiol 1988; 128:515–523.

97. Ringstad J, Jacobsen BK, Tretli S, Thomassen Y. Serum selenium concentration associated with risk of cancer. J Clin Path 1988; 41:454–457.

98. Knekt P, Aromaa A, Maatela J, Alfthan G, Aaran R-K, Hakama M, Hakulinen T, Peto R, Teppo L. Serum selenium and subsequent risk of cancer among Finnish men and women. J Natl Cancer Inst 1990; 82:864–868.

99. Criqui MH, Bangdiwala S, Goodman DS, Blaner WS, Morris JS, Kritchevsky S, Lippel K, Mebane I, Tyroler HA. Selenium, retinol, retinol-binding protein, and uric acid associations with cancer mortality in a population-based prospective case-control study. Ann Epidemiol 1991; 1:385–393.

100. van den Brandt PA, Goldbohm RA, van't Veer P, Bode P, Dorant E, Hermus RJJ, Sturmans F. A prospective cohort study on selenium status and the risk of lung cancer. Cancer Res 1993; 53:4860–4865.

101. Kabuto M, Imai H, Yonezawa C, Neriishi K, Akiba S, Kato H, Suzuki T, Land CE, Blot WJ. Prediagnostic serum selenium and zinc levels and subsequent risk of lung and stomach cancer in Japan. Cancer Epidemiol Biomarkers Prev 1994; 3:465–469.

102. Garland M, Morris JS, Stampfer MJ, Colditz GA, Spate VL, Baskett CK, Rosner B, Speizer FE, Willett WC, Hunter DJ. Prospective study of toenail selenium levels and cancer among women. J Natl Cancer Inst 1995; 87:497–505.

7   Nonnutritive Components in Foods as Modifiers of the Cancer Process

John A. Milner

1. INTRODUCTION

Cancer, once thought to be an inevitable consequence of aging, is now thought to be primarily associated with a host of environmental factors, including dietary habits *(1)*. Changes in cancer death rates during relatively short periods of time indicate that environmental factors, rather than a genetic predisposition, are primary determinants of risk. Since evidence exists that environmental factors correlate with approx 90% of all cancer cases, it becomes of paramount importance to identify those factors of greatest importance *(1)*. Within the many possible factors, dietary practice is one that likely deserves special attention *(1,2)*. Dietary habits have been correlated with 60% of cancers in women and more than 40% in men. Geographic correlations of per capita intake of fruits and vegetables are routinely, although not universally, observed to be inversely related to cancer risk *(3–10)*.

In a recent prospective cohort study of 41,837 women aged 55–69 yr an inverse association was observed between lung cancer and the intakes of all vegetables and fruit, all vegetables, and green leafy vegetables. Each of these dietary food sources was associated with an approximate halving of risk *(3)*. Unfortunately, only between 10 and 20% of the US population consumed the recommended five or more daily servings of fruits and vegetables *(5,6)*. Serdula et al. *(6)* assessed the daily fruit and vegetable consumption among 23,699 adults in 16 US states using a random-digit dialing telephone survey. In this study, men were found to consume fewer servings per day (3.3) than women (3.7). The recognized protective relationship existing between fruit and vegetable consumption and cancer risk reinforces the needed to enhance their contribution to the diet among all Americans.

A large number of potentially anticarcinogenic agents are found in fruits and vegetables, including carotenoids, vitamins C and E, selenium, and dietary fiber. However, a host of other compounds existing within these foods, including dithiolthiones, glucosinolates, indoles, isothiocyanates, flavonoids, phenols, sterols, sulfhydryls, and monoterpenes, may also modify the incidence and severity of some types of cancer. These dietary components likely have both complementary and overlapping mechanisms of action, including the induction of detoxification enzymes, inhibition of carcinogen formation including nitrosamines, provision of precursors for antineoplastic compounds, dilution and binding of carcinogens to cellular DNA and proteins in the di-

From: *Preventive Nutrition: The Comprehensive Guide for Health Professionals*
Edited by A. Bendich and R. J. Deckelbaum Humana Press Inc., Totowa, NJ

Table 1
Compounds in Fruits, Vegetables and Spices with Potential
Anticarcinogenic Effects in Humans

Compound	Food source
Allyl compounds	Allium vegetables: garlic and onions
Cinnamic acid	Fruit, coffee beans, soybeans
Flavonoids	Vegetables, fruits, citrus
Indoles	Cruciferous vegetables
Isothiocyanates	Cruciferous vegetables
Terpenes	Citrus, spices

gestive tract, alteration of hormone metabolism, antioxidant effects, and possibly several others. Some of these agents are reviewed in more detail below.

Fruit and vegetable consumption is not the only dietary factor that can influence cancer risk. Ingestion of green and black tea, and herbs and spices has been reported to be inversely associated with cancer risk (11–13). Some of these food items and their associated nonnutritive components are also addressed in subsequent parts of this chapter.

Although dietary correlations with cancer risk are insufficient to establish a causal relationship, they are useful in the generation of a testable hypothesis. Several essential and nonessential nutrients may actually be involved in the observed correlation between dietary habits and cancer risk. Although several macronutrients have been given special attention in recent years, a clear and dominant nutrient has not been forthcoming. The increasing recognition that nonessential nutrients can significantly modify experimentally induced cancer is continuing to foster greater interest in functional foods by scientists and consumers (see Chapter 4).

Clearly, variability in detecting an association between dietary practices and cancer risk is logical since such a relationship must depend on a host of environmental and genetic factors. The complexity of this issue becomes evident when one considers the multitude of interactions that can occur between essential and nonessential food components. Likewise, since all metabolic and phenotypic characteristics are linked by heredity, it is almost inconceivable that a simple solution will alter susceptibility equally in all individuals. Clearly, a greater understanding of the interrelationships among diet, environment, and genetics is needed. Acquiring this information should assist in tailoring dietary recommendations that can help minimize cancer risk in specific target populations.

To date more than 500 compounds have been identified as potential modifiers of experimentally induced cancer. Some of these dietary nonessential compounds that possess potential protective effects against human cancers are broadly presented in Table 1.

This chapter is limited to those nonessential nutrients where ample information is available to establish an effect on the process of carcinogenesis and generally to those dietary constituents where possible mechanisms can be explored. It must be emphasized that purified constituents are not consumed and that single nutrients must be considered as part of a complete, complex diet.

2. ALLYL COMPOUNDS

Recent studies have provided evidence that plants of the genus *Allium* may reduce human cancer risk *(14–16)*. Interestingly, these plants, which include garlic, onions, leek, and chive, have been used in various parts of the world for their antimicrobial activity, ability to repel insects, and their characteristic aroma and flavor. Recently evidence has begun to emerge that these foods may not only reduce hypercholesterolemia *(17)*, but may also reduce the risk of some types of cancer.

2.1. Garlic

Epidemiological evidence continues to accumulate that reveals an inverse relationship between garlic intake and human cancer mortality *(14,18,19)*. Residents in Cangshan County, Shandong Province, China who habitually consume garlic (20 g) have a 10 times lower gastric cancer mortality and lower nitrite concentration in the gastric juices than those who consume less garlic (2 g) *(18)*. Although these are massive intakes, a protection by lower intakes, and those more typical of intakes in the United States, is suggested in the study of Steinmetz et al. *(14)*, indicating significantly lower colon cancer risks. In their study *(14)* mean garlic consumption was 0.7 servings/wk in noncancerous subjects. Precise consumption measurements for garlic and related foods are not readily available. Additional attention needs to be given to monitoring the actual consumption of these foods.

Garlic has long been recognized for its ability to control microbial growth. Garlic extracts have broad-spectrum antimicrobial activity against bacteria and fungi *(20,21)*. This antimicrobial property may partially account for garlic's ability to suppress bacteria and fungi-mediated synthesis of nitrite and nitrosamines. Garlic also has the ability to suppress the spontaneous formation of nitrosamines *(22)*. Since most nitrosamines are recognized for their carcinogenic potential, this alone may have significant human health implications.

Mei et al. *(22)* found that providing 5 g fresh crushed garlic to human subjects resulted in a marked depression in nitrosation reactions as indicated by decreased urinary *N*-nitrosoproline content following consumption of nitrate and proline supplements. Thus, the observed lower incidence of gastric cancer in populations consuming larger quantities of garlic may relate to a reduced capacity to form nitrosamines. Since a positive relationship is known to exist between the sulfhydryl content of foods and their ability to bind nitrite *(23)*, other *Allium* plants may have similar inhibitory effects against nitrosamine and possibly tumor formation.

Recent studies from our laboratory have shown that dietary garlic effectively inhibits the occurrence of DNA adducts in liver resulting from the in vivo formation of nitrosamines *(24)*. In addition, garlic inhibited adduct formation in rats treated with preformed nitrosamines. This reduction in adducts suggest that garlic is also effective in altering the bioactivation of these potentially carcinogenic compounds. Finally, garlic has also been observed to be effective in reducing adducts caused by treatment with methylnitrosurea (MNU), a direct acting carcinogen *(25)*. Together, these data suggest that garlic may also provide protection against cancer by modifying DNA repair. Thus, garlic's ability to inhibit nitrosamine-induced tumors in animals, and possibly human beings, probably results not only from a reduction in carcinogen formation, but a depression in the metabolic activation/detoxification of these carcinogens.

Table 2
Important Sulfur Compounds Found in Garlic

3,5-Diethyl-1,2,4-trithiolane	Diallyl sulfide
Allyl 1-propenyl disulfide	Diallyl trisulfide
Allyl 1-propenyl trisulfide	Methyl allyl trisulfide
Allyl alcohol	Methyl allyl disulfide
Diallyl disulfide	S-allyl cysteine

Although several compounds within garlic may account for the observed anticarcinogenic properties, evidence is accumulating that suggest that one or more allyl sulfur compounds are likely involved. An extensive overview of the chemistry of organosulfur compounds in both intact and crushed garlic has been summarized *(26)*. Table 2 lists some of the major sulfur compounds found in garlic.

Both water-soluble and lipid-soluble allyl sulfur compounds offer protection against chemically induced tumors in experimental animals. The protection provided by garlic and related compounds occurs during both the initiation and promotion phases of carcinogenesis *(27)*. Diallyl sulfide, an oil-soluble flavor component of garlic, completely inhibited *N*-nitrosomethylbenzylamine-induced esophageal tumors *(28)* and reduced the incidence of colon cancer in mice treated with dimethylhydrazine *(29)*. Topical application of garlic oil substantially reduces skin cancers in dimethylbenz(a)anthracene (DMBA)-treated mice *(30)*. Diallyl disulfide, allyl mercaptan, and allyl methyl disulfide have been reported to reduce the risk of forestomach cancers in mice treated with diethylnitrosamine *(31)*. Water-soluble allyl compounds in garlic, such as S-allyl cysteine, do inhibit the metabolism of the mammary carcinogen 7, 12 DMBA *(32)*. Most recently, Liu et al. *(25)* reported that supplying either S-allyl cysteine or diallyl disulfide in the diet of rats markedly reduced the incidence of MNU-induced mammary tumors.

Some garlic compounds are recognized to modify enzymatic activities involved in carcinogen activation and deactivation. Treatment with diallyl sulfide decreases the activity of hepatic cytochrome P450IIE1 *(33)*. Glutathione and glutathione-S-transferases (factors involved in phase II detoxification) increase following the feeding of processed garlic powder to the rat *(34, 35)*. Oral treatment with allyl methyl trisulfide also enhanced glutathione-S-transferase activity in the forestomach, small bowel mucosa, liver, and lung of mice *(35)*. Induction of detoxification enzymes and an increase in glutathione by garlic are consistent with an increased removal of carcinogenic compounds and possibly accounts for the ability of processed garlic and its associated components to depress adduct formation in target tissue and to reduce the incidence of experimentally induced cancer *(27,29,32)*.

Garlic preparations likely vary in the amount of specific organosulfur compounds. Thus, not all garlic can be assumed to be equally effective inhibitors of chemically induced tumors in experimental animals or possibly in humans. The quantity of a water-soluble sulfur compound, S-allyl cysteine, present in various garlic preparations has been shown to correlate with the ability of these preparations to inhibit the in vivo formation of DNA adducts resulting from DMBA treatment *(32)*. Additional attention needs to be given to the impact of processing on the content of individual organosulfur compounds present in garlic and related foods, and their subsequent ability to inhibit the cancer process. Nevertheless, studies from our laboratory have shown that crushed and dehydrated garlic, commercially processed high sulfur garlic, and commercially processed deodorized garlic are all effective in reducing the binding of DMBA metabolites to mammary cell DNA and, therefore, presumably in reducing the incidence of mammary tumors resulting from treatment with this carcinogen (32). Clearly, our studies demonstrate that odor is not a necessary prerequisite for the ability of garlic preparations to inhibit chemically induced tumors.

Specific compounds within garlic may also inhibit the growth of neoplasms (36–38). Choy et al. (36) found that garlic feeding suppressed the growth of Ehrlich ascites tumor cells inoculated into mice. Recent studies by Sundaram and Milner (37) have shown that tumor cells in culture are sensitive to the oil-soluble allyl sulfur compound, diallyl disulfide, but not to the water-soluble allyl sulfur compound, S-allyl cysteine. Several human tumor cell lines are sensitive to diallyl disulfide, both in vitro and in vivo (38,39). Although the mechanism by which diallyl disulfide inhibits tumor proliferation remains unknown, marked changes in calcium homeostasis suggest that changes in intercellular thiols may be a mechanism (38).

Various components of the diet may influence the protection provided by garlic against the cancer process. Ip et al. (40) and Amagase and Milner (41) have shown that dietary selenium in the diet or as a component of garlic can enhance the protection provided by garlic. Amagase and Milner (41) have also shown that the quantity and type of lipid consumed by rats can also influence the ability of garlic to depress adducts resulting from treatment with the carcinogen DMBA.

Overall, several laboratory investigations demonstrate that garlic and/or its components inhibit all phases of the cancer process. Furthermore, these studies reveal that the benefits of garlic are not limited to a specific species, to a particular tissue, or to a specific carcinogen. Finally, odor is not a prerequisite for the protection provided by garlic against the initiation of carcinogenesis. The effective intake of sulfur compounds in humans needed to minimize cancer risk remains to be determined.

2.2. Onions

Much less information exists about the potential anticancer properties of onions. However, an inverse relationship between the consumption of onions and leeks with lung carcinoma has been reported. Dorant et al. (42) found in 484 lung carcinoma patients and 3123 members of a randomly sampled subcohort that a lower lung carcinoma risk was observed in the highest onion intake [rate ratio=0.65, confidence interval (CI) 95%: 0.45–0.95] compared to the lowest consumption. Steinmetz and Potter (14) also found in a case-control study in Australia that a greater intake of onions and legumes was associated with a decreased risk of colon cancer. This study involved 220 individuals with a histologically confirmed colon adenocarcinoma compared to 438 age- and gender-matched controls and revealed in women a protein-adjusted odds ratio of 0.48 (CI 95%: 0.22–1.03) and 0.53 (CI 95% 0.26–1.07) for onions and legumes, respectively. For males, greater intakes of onions, green leafy vegetables, legumes, carrots, and cabbage were all associated with a reduction in cancer risk.

Onions are also recognized to contain a variety of sulfur compounds, as indicated in Table 3. Some of these compounds have been examined for their ability to modify various stages of the cancer process, as indicated below.

Table 3
Important Sulfur Compounds Found in Onions

1-Propenyl propyl disulfide	Methyl 1-propenyl trisulfide
1-Propenyl propyl trisulfide	Methyl propyl disulfide
1-Propenyl methyl disulfide	Methyl propyl trisulfide
Dimethyl trisulfide	Dipropyl trisulfide
Dipropyl disulfide	
Dipropyl tetrasulfide	

Belman *(30)* reported that onion oil inhibited skin tumor yield and incidence following phorbol-myristate-acetate promotion in a dose-dependent manner over the range of 10–10,000 µg when applied three times per week. Interestingly, onion oil was more effective than the oil of garlic in the inhibition of these tumors. However, the intake of onions may not always provide protection against cancer. Takada et al. *(43)* have found that some sulfur compounds (isothiocyanic acid isobutyl ester, dipropyl trisulfide, and allyl mercaptan) promoted liver cell proliferation, suggesting that under some circumstances the consumption of onions, and possibly garlic, may increase cancer risk. It remains to be determined how important these findings are in humans, especially since Matsuda et al. *(44)* reported methyl propyl disulfide and propylene sulfide depressed hepatocarcinogenesis in the rat. Supplying both compounds resulted in a dose-dependent inhibition of glutathione S-transferase placental form (GST-P)-positive foci in the liver. Again, such an inhibition is generally associated with a reduction in cancer risk.

Extracts and essential oils of onions and garlic are recognized to have other physiological effects, including inhibiting platelet aggregation *(45,46)*. The inhibition of human platelet aggregation induced by ADP, epinephrine, collagen, thrombin, and arachidonate possibly relates to perturbations in the plasma membrane.

Although the health benefits of onion consumption have not been extensively examined, available evidence does suggest there is little reason to reduce its use as part of a healthy diet. Nevertheless, it remains to be determined the minimum quantity of onion and related sulfur compounds needed to reduce cancer risk and what factors might modify the efficacy.

3. GLUCOSINOLATES AND ISOTHIOCYANATES IN VEGETABLES

Glucosinolates, naturally occurring constituents of cruciferous vegetables, actually refers to more than 100 sulfur-containing glycosides that yield thiocyanate, nitrile, and isothiocyanate derivatives on hydrolysis. Cruciferous vegetables are particularly noteworthy for their high content of isothiocyanates. Several of these vegetables, including cabbage, Brussels sprouts, and broccoli, found in the genus *Brassica*, generally are viewed as potentially cancer-preventative foods *(47)*.

Organic isothiocyanates have been reported to block the production of tumors in rodents induced by such diverse carcinogens as polycyclic aromatic hydrocarbons, azo dyes, ethionine, N-2-fluorenylacetamide, and nitrosamines. Several thiocyanates or isothiocyanates appear to be effective inhibitors of carcinogen metabolism as reflected by a reduction in carcinogen binding to DNA in the target tissue *(48)*. Phenethyl isothiocyanate is present in rather high concentrations in cabbage, Brussels sprouts, cauliflower, kale, and turnips. Overall, α-naphthyl-, β-naphthyl-, phenyl-, benzyl-, phenethyl-, and other arylalkyl isothiocyanates can inhibit tumor development in liver, lung, mammary gland, forestomach, and esophagus *(48–50)*. Thus, widely diverse isothiocyanates may have importance in the human diet in inhibiting tumors occurring at a variety of sites.

The anticarcinogenic effects of isothiocyanates appear to be mediated by suppression of carcinogen bioactivation by cytochrome P450 and induction of Phase 2 enzymes, such as glutathione transferases and NAD(P)H:quinone reductase *(48)*. Isothiocyanates may also modify the proliferation of neoplasms. Early studies revealed isothiocyanic esters inhibited the growth of Ehrlich ascites carcinoma cells inoculated into mice *(51)*.

3.1. Indoles

Several indole compounds are produced in cabbage, broccoli, Brussels sprouts, and other members of the genus *Brassica* during the hydrolysis of indolyl-methyl glucosinolate *(47)*. Indole-3-acetonitrile, indole-3-carbinol, and 3,3′-diindolylmethane have been recognized as naturally occurring inducers of phase I enzymes, including aryl hydrocarbon hydroxylase *(52)*.

Several indoles have been examined for their ability to alter experimentally induced carcinogenesis. Although indole-3-carbinol has been more frequently examined for its anticarcinogenic properties, studies with brassinin [3-(*S*-methyldithiocarbamoyl) aminomethyl indole], a phytoalexin first identified as a constituent of cabbage, has been found to offer protection *(53)*. Unfortunately, many studies have used large dietary indole concentrations (1–3%). However, consumption of these large quantities of indoles has not always resulted in a consistent effect on tumorigenesis *(43)*. The protection provided by indole-3-carbinol is likely dependent on the species and tissue examined. Evidence does exist that it is effective in inhibiting both the initiation and promotion phases of some chemically induced cancers *(54)*. In several studies, indoles have been found to delay the onset of tumors and result in the occurrence of benign rather than malignant neoplasms *(55)*.

Indole-3-carbinol has been reported to inhibit 7,12 dimethylbenz(a)anthracene-induced mammary tumors, reduce the metabolism of *N*-nitrosodimethylamine as indicated by a reduction in DNA binding, and enhance pathways for carcinogen removal as indicated by an increase in glutathione S-transferase activity *(55)*. Marked increases in activities of cytochrome P450-dependent mono-oxygenases and in a variety of Phase II drug-metabolizing enzymes have been observed following indole consumption in both rodents and humans *(54)*. The ability of indole-3-carbinol to inhibit virally induced tumors comes from studies showing that it inhibits the spontaneous occurrence of endometrial adenocarcinoma in female Donryu rats *(56)*.

Indole-3-carbinol can also alter the rate of growth of transformed cells. It is known to inhibit the growth of the estrogen-responsive human mammary cell line MCF-7, but has little effect on the estrogen-nonresponsive cell line MDA-MB-231 *(57)*. Indole-3-carbinol was found to enhance C-2 hydroxylation of estrogen and induce cytochrome P4501A1 in MCF-7, but not in MDA-MB-231 cells. Thus, the antiproliferative effects of indole-3-carbinol may involve selective induction of estradiol metabolism and/or the related cytochrome P450 system that limited estrogen-sensitivity. Studies by Jellinck *(58)* revealed oral administration of indole-3-carbinol almost doubled the ability of female rat livers to convert estradiol to catechol estrogens. Michnovicz and Bradlow *(59)*

Table 4
Examples of Classes of Flavonoids Found in the Food Supply

Class	Food sources
Flavones	
Tangeretin	Citrus
Nobiletin	Citrus
Flavonols	
Quercetin	Fruits, vegetables, cereal grains
Kaempferol	Fruits, vegetables
Catechins	Tea
Flavanones	
Naringenin	Grapefruit
Isoflavones	
Genistein	Soybeans
Daidzein	Soybeans

investigated the effects in humans of short-term oral exposure to indole-3-carbinol (6–7 mg/kg/d over 7 d). They found urinary excretion of 2-hydroxyestrone relative to that of estriol was significantly increased by indole-3-carbinol, suggesting the induction of 2-hydroxylation. Overall, the potential benefits of indole-3-carbinol against cancer may relate to its ability to alter endogenous estrogen metabolism toward increased catechol estrogen production.

3.2. Flavonoids

The flavonoids are a group of organic molecules ubiquitously distributed in vascular plants. Approximately 2000 individual members of flavonoids have been described. Typical dietary intakes of flavonoids average 1 g daily. As typical phenolic compounds, they can act as potent antioxidants and metal chelators. Overall, several of these flavonoids appear to be effective antipromoters. In addition, some appear to be effective in inhibiting the metabolism of some carcinogens.

Flavonoids are generally classified on the basis of substitutions occurring on one or more of the rings. These classes include flavones, flavonols, flavanones, and isoflavones. Table 4 lists some compounds within each class that have been examined for their anticarcinogenic properties.

3.2.1. FLAVONES

Tangeretin and nobiletin are two polymethoxylated flavonoids in citrus foods that have been examined for their anticarcinogenic properties. These unhydroxylated compounds have been shown to modify cytochrome P450 enzymes. However, depending on the compound examined and the specific enzyme examined the influence is sometimes stimulatory but in other cases inhibitory *(60)*. The mechanisms by which flavones modify P450 is extremely complex and deserves further investigation.

Kandaswami et al. *(61)* have found that both nobiletin and tangeretin were effective in inhibiting the growth of neoplastic cells in culture. Both markedly inhibited the proliferation of a squamous cell carcinoma (HTB 43) and a gliosarcoma (9L) cell line when added to the medium at 2–8 µg/ml. However, a human lung fibroblast-like cell line (CCL 135) was relatively insensitive to these flavonoids. In addition to their antiproliferative effects, both nobiletin and tangeretin have been found to inhibit the invasiveness of MO4 cells into embryonic chick fragments in vitro *(62)*.

3.2.2. FLAVONOLS

3.2.2.1. QUERCETIN AND KAEMPFEROL

Although two of the most common flavonols, quercetin and kaempferol, do exhibit some mutagenicity in the Ames assay, they also appear to be effective modifiers of cancer risk. Quercetin is recognized as a potent inhibitor of P450 reactions *(63)*. In studies by Verma et al. *(64)* up to 5% quercetin was fed without apparent ill consequences to the rat. However, this quantity of quercetin was found to significantly reduce the incidence of both DMBA- and MNU-induced mammary tumors *(64)*. Furthermore, quercetin is known to inhibit the promotion phase of DMBA- and MNU-induced skin tumors *(65)*. Since quercetin is extensively metabolized by intestinal bacteria the quantity reaching tissues is likely limited and, therefore, may explain its relatively low toxicity.

The anticarcinogenic properties of these flavonols are not limited to their ability to modify carcinogen bioactivation. Nakayama et al. *(66)* found these compounds were very effective in reducing oxygen-induced toxicity. Quercetin, kaempferol, catechin, and taxifolin were all found to suppress the cytotoxicity of active oxygen species (O_2^- and H_2O_2) in Chinese hamster V79 cells.

Some of these compounds may also modify the proliferation of existing neoplasms. Ranelletti et al. *(67)* found that the addition of quercetin (10 n*M* and 10 µ*M*) to several colon cancer cell lines resulted in a dose-dependent, reversible inhibition of cell proliferation. Cell-cycle analysis revealed that the growth-inhibitory effect was because of a blocking action in the G0/G1 phase. Alterations in hormonal binding may partially account for the observed effects of quercetin *(67)*. All tumor cells may not be equally sensitive to quercetin since Kandaswami et al. *(61)* were unable to detect an effect of this compound on the growth of human squamous cell carcinomas.

3.2.2.2. GREEN AND BLACK TEA FLAVONOLS

Tea, grown in about 30 countries, is consumed in greatly varying quantities worldwide *(68)*. It is the most widely consumed beverage, apart from water, with a per capita worldwide consumption of approx 0.12 L/yr. Tea is manufactured in three basic forms: unoxidized or green tea, oxidized or black tea, and partially oxidized or oolong tea. Only about 20% of the tea produced is green, and <2% is oolong. Green tea is consumed primarily in China, Japan, and a few countries in North Africa and the Middle East.

Fresh tea leaf is unusually rich in polyphenols known as catechins that may constitute up to 30% of the dry leaf weight. Other polyphenols include flavonols and their glycosides, and depsides, such as chlorogenic acid, coumarylquinic acid, and one unique to tea, theogallin (3-galloylquinic acid). Various quinones are produced by oxidation and condense to form a series of compounds, including bisflavanols, theaflavins, epitheaflavic acids, and thearubigens, which give rise to the characteristic taste and color properties of black tea *(69)*. Green tea composition is very similar to that of the fresh leaf except for a few enzymatically catalyzed changes that occur following harvesting.

Thearubigens constitute the largest mass of the extractable matter in black tea. Oolong tea is intermediate in composition between green and black teas.

Although inconsistencies exist, green tea consumption has frequently been associated with a reduction in cancer *(69,70)*. Gao et al. *(71)* found in a Shanghai population-based, case-control study of esophageal cancer that green tea consumption was associated with protection.

Many investigators have shown that in a variety of animal tumor bioassay systems the administration of green tea, specifically the polyphenolic fraction isolated from green tea leaves, affords protection against chemically induced cancers *(72,73)*. Green tea has also been reported to inhibit chemically induced tumors of the large intestine, forestomach, liver, lung, and mammary tissue *(74–80)*.

Several of the tea preparations have been reported to inhibit the formation of nitrosamines. Since the vast majority of these compounds are known carcinogens in animal models, these studies may have particular significance in humans. Wu et al. *(81)* demonstrated that the amounts of *N*-nitrosomorpholine formed in vitro depended on the molecular structure of tea catechin derivatives and their molar ratios to nitrite. Not only can tea preparations decrease the formation of nitrosamines, but they can also reduce the bioactivation of these compounds to carcinogenic agents. Both green tea and black tea have been reported to block nitrosamine-induced tumorigenesis *(82)*.

One of the main polyphenolic constituents in green tea, (-)-epigallocatechin gallate (EGCG), has been found to be an antitumor promoter in *N*-ethyl-*N'*-nitro-*N*-nitrosoguanidine-induced duodenal tumors and 4-(methyl-*N*-nitrosamino)-1-(3-pyridyl) 1-butanone (NNK)-induced lung cancer *(83,84)*. In the mouse skin tumor bioassay systems, topical application of green tea polyphenols results in protection against 3-methylcholanthrene-induced skin tumorigenicity, 7,12-dimethylbenz(a)anthracene (DMBA)-induced skin tumor initiation, 12-*O*-tetradecanoylphorbol-13-acetate (TPA) and other tumor promoter-caused tumor promotion in DMBA-initiated skin, and benzoyl peroxide- and 4-nitroquinoline N-oxide-caused enhanced malignant progression of nonmalignant lesions. Huang et al. *(85)* found the individual polyphenolic compounds in green tea indicated that topical application of (-)-epigallocatechin gallate, (-)-epigallocatechin, and (-)-epicatechin gallate inhibited TPA-induced inflammation in mouse epidermis.

Green tea extract has also been shown to cause partial regression of established skin papillomas in mice *(72)*. The inhibitory effect of EGCG on spontaneous hepatoma in mice was shown by Nishida et al. *(74)*. Komori et al. *(76)* found EGCG and green tea extracts inhibited the growth of lung and mammary cancer cell lines with similar potencies. Part of the antiproliferative effects of green tea may relate to its ability to modify estrogen binding to membrane receptors *(76)*.

Similarly, chronic oral feeding of green tea polyphenols or water extract of green tea has also been shown to result in protection against ultraviolet B radiation-induced skin tumorigenicity *(82)*. Administration of black tea was comparable to green tea as an inhibitor of UVB-induced skin carcinogenesis in DMBA-initiated SKH-1 mice *(82)*. Oral administration of decaffeinated black tea or green teas also significantly inhibited UVB-induced skin carcinogenesis in these mice.

Collectively, considerable information provides support for a chemopreventive effect of green tea against each stage of carcinogenesis. The mechanism by which green tea affords these diversified effects appear to be multifold, with an alteration in both

Phase I and II enzymes *(86–88)*. Shi et al. *(74)* found (-)-epigallocatechin-3-gallate inhibited the catalytic activities of several P450 enzymes and was more potent against P450 1A and 2B1 than 2E1. Katiyar et al. *(89)* provided evidence that green tea inhibits both stage I and stage II of skin tumor promotion and that the inhibition of tumor promotion depends on the duration of tea treatment.

3.2.3. FLAVANONES IN GRAPEFRUIT

Naringin is the most abundant flavonoid in grapefruit. It has been shown to inhibit the activation of aflatoxin B_1 *(90)*. Part of the protection provided by naringin likely relates to its ability to induce Phase II enzymes, including those associated with both glutathione and glucuronide conjugation *(91)*.

3.2.4. ISOFLAVONES IN SOYBEANS

Recent studies suggest a possible cancer-protective role of some flavonoids in soybeans. Soybeans, compared to several other foods, supply relatively large amounts of four different types of compounds that may have anticarcinogenic properties: glycosides, phytosterols, protease inhibitors, and phytic acid. Soybeans are known to contain about 2% glycosides, which are composed of soyasaponins and isoflavonoids. Plant isoflavonoid glycosides are generally converted by intestinal bacteria to hormone-like compounds with weak estrogenic and antioxidative activity. Much of the attention of soybean isoflavonoids has been directed at daidzein, equol, and genistein. Wei et al. *(92)* has provided evidence that the antioxidant properties of isoflavones are structurally related and the hydroxy group at position 4′ is crucial.

Although many isoflavones are weak estrogens, they can function both as estrogen agonists and antagonists depending on the hormonal milieu and the target tissue and species being examined *(93)*. Evidence now points to the ability of these compounds to not only influence sex hormone metabolism and associated biological activity but also influence intracellular enzymes, protein synthesis, growth factors, malignant cell proliferation, differentiation, and angiogenesis *(94)*.

Considerable evidence points to the ability of isoflavonoids to inhibit the promotion phase of carcinogenesis. Genistein has attracted considerable attention because of its ability to inhibit several enzymes, including protein tyrosine kinases and those involved in signal transduction *(7)*. Recently, genistein was reported to significantly inhibit TPA-induced proto-oncogene expression *(c-fos)* in mouse skin in a dose-dependent manner *(92)*. Furthermore, in a two-stage skin carcinogenesis study, low levels of genistein (1 and 5 µmol) significantly prolonged tumor latency and decreased tumor multiplicity *(92)*.

Lamartiniere et al. *(95)* has provided rather convincing evidence that neonatal genistein exposure has long lasting effects of the ability to withstand carcinogen exposure. Mammary tumor incidence and multiplicity in rats treated on d 2, 4, and 6 postpartum with genistein and subsequently exposed to DMBA on d 50 of age, were substantially reduced compared to untreated controls *(95)*. Part of this protection may relate to the ability of genistein to reduce the number of terminal end buds and increase the number of lobular structures within mammary tissue.

Vasculature has an important role in several steps of the cancer metastatic process, including the site of metastasis since vessels capture cancerous cells and provide the entry route into secondary organs and through angiogenesis since vascular endothelial cells supply nutrients for tumor growth. The linings of all blood vessels are covered with endothelial cells, which play an active role in both processes. Several studies suggest the consumption of plant foods can prevent or retard angiogenesis or neovascularization. Fotsis et al. *(96)* found that genistein was a potent inhibitor of endothelial cell proliferation and in vitro angiogenesis.

4. OTHER PHENOLIC ACID: ELLAGIC ACID

Ellagic acid is a naturally occurring plant phenol that is related to the coumarins, a subclass of lactones found in a variety of fruits and vegetables. It occurs in particularly high concentrations in grapes and nuts. Several studies indicate ellagic acid's potential effectiveness as a chemopreventive agent *(97,98)*. Although the mechanism by which ellagic acid inhibits the cancer process remains unclear, it appears to inhibit both the activation and detoxification of potentially carcinogenic agents. Its ability to alter epoxide hydrolase and increase glutathione S-transferase activity *(98)* may explain its ability to inhibit DNA adducts caused by carcinogenic nitrosamines and benz(a)pyrene *(99)*.

Other phenolic compounds found in fruits and vegetables also may alter the cancer process. Hydroxycinnamic acids also possess potential chemopreventive properties, as indicated by Shugart and Kao *(97)*. However, caffeic acid and related compounds are only minimally effective inhibitors of experimentally induced tumors.

5. TERPENES

D-limonene is probably the terpene most extensively examined for its ability to inhibit experimentally induced carcinogenesis. This compound, found as a natural constituent of citrus oils, also occurs in oils from mint, caraway, thyme, cardamom, and coriander. Currently, d-limonene is widely used as a flavor and fragrance and is listed as generally recognized as safe (GRAS) in food by the Food and Drug Administration.

Limonene has been shown to inhibit skin carcinomas induced by benzo(a)pyrene *(100)*. Feeding of this terpene has also been reported to depress the incidence of mammary tumors in rats treated with DMBA and lung tumors induced by 4-(methylnitrosamino)-1-(3-pyridyl)-1-butanone (NNK) *(101,102)*.

Induction of phase I and phase II enzymes account for the chemotherapeutic effects of limonene against the initiation phase of chemically induced tumors in rodents *(101,103,104)*. Chemopreventive activity during the promotion/progression may be due to depressed posttranslational isoprenylation of growth-controlling small G proteins, such as p21*ras*. Ruch and Sigler *(105)* have provided evidence that the ability of limonene to inhibit some types of tumors may relate to a depression in genes other than *ras*.

An inhibition of 3-hydroxy-3-methyl-glutaryl-coenzyme A (HMG-CoA) reductase activity is known to deplete intermediates required for the posttranslational modification of proteins, a process giving the proteins lipophilic anchors that bind to membranes. Consequently, nuclear lamins and *ras* oncoproteins remain in nascent states and cells do not proliferate. Thus, the ability of D-limonene to suppress tumor proliferation may also relate to its ability to suppress hepatic HMG-CoA reductase activity *(106)*.

Interestingly, limonene has been reported to cause a complete regression of mammary carcinomas *(107,108)*. Some of the terpenes, although possibly not limonene, may induce apoptosis *(109)*. The multiple anticarcinogenic effects of limonene influencing all phases of the cancer process suggest that related monoterpenes may also be efficacious in the chemoprevention and chemotherapy of malignancies.

D-Limonene has been found to cause kidney tumors when given at high doses to male rats and is associated with the development of hyaline droplet nephropathy *(110)*. The mechanism of D-limonene leading to these tumors does not appear to be possible in humans. Thus, D-limonene likely does not pose any carcinogenic or nephrotoxic risk to humans.

Another monoterpene, D-carvone, is a major constituent of caraway seed oil. Both D-carvone and caraway seed oil have been shown to inhibit the activation of dimethyl-nitrosamine and decrease the induction of forestomach tumors *(31)*.

6. SUMMARY AND CONCLUSIONS

Data obtained from epidemiological, clinical, and laboratory investigations provide rather convincing evidence that dietary habits can significantly modify cancer risk. Interestingly, a rather large number of chemical compounds found in foods appear to offer protection against the cancer process. Some of the non-essential nutrients modify the carcinogenic process at specific sites, including carcinogen formation and metabolism, initiation, promotion, and tumor progression; cellular and host defenses, cellular differentiation, and tumor growth.

Unquestionably, dietary habits are not the sole determinant of cancer, but represent a significant point for which intervention is possible. Adjustment of dietary practices to conform to generalized dietary goals may not be necessary, or even appropriate, for all segments of the population.

7. RECOMMENDATIONS

Sophisticated techniques and procedures are desperately needed to adequately assess the potential merit of nutritional intervention for each individual in relationship to his/her cancer risk. A thorough appreciation or understanding of how dietary components contribute to or modify the cancer process will require the continuation of carefully controlled and probing investigations. Hopefully, future research will lead to the recognition of the critical sites where nutrition intervention would be appropriate and allow for sound and realistic recommendations for dietary practices. Until this information is available it remains prudent to eat a variety of foods and avoid excesses. Surely the benefits of fruits, vegetables, and spices must relate to one or more constituents and their interactions with other components of the diet. Although experimental evidence strongly supports nonessential nutrients as modifiers of the cancer process it remains to be determined if humans will benefit from the intake of one or more of these nutrients as supplements. Although individual supplements of nonessential nutrients may well be as effective in modifying cancer risk, their safety must be thoroughly examined, not only for toxicity but their dependence on other components of the diet.

REFERENCES

1. Raunio H, Husgafvel-Pursiainen K, Anttila S, Hietanen E, Hirvonen A, Pelkonen O. Diagnosis of polymorphisms in carcinogen-activating and inactivating enzymes and cancer susceptibility—a review. Gene 1995; 159:113–21.

2. Wynder EL, Gori GB. Contribution of the environment to cancer incidence: an epidemiologic exercise. J Natl Cancer Inst 1977; 58:825–832.

3. Steinmetz KA, Potter JD, Folsom AR. Vegetables, fruit, and lung cancer in the Iowa Women's Health Study. Cancer Res 1993; 53:536–543.

4. Steinmetz KA. Kushi LH, Bostick RM, Folsom AR, Potter JD. Vegetables, fruit, and colon cancer in the Iowa Women's Health Study. Am J Epidemiol 1994; 139:1–15.

5. Block G. Dietary guidelines and the results of food consumption surveys. Amer J Clin Nutr 1991; 53:356S, 357S.

6. Serdula MK, Coates RJ, Byers T, Simoes E, Mokdad AH, Subar AF. Fruit and vegetable intake among adults in 16 states: results of a brief telephone survey. Am J Public Hlth 1995; 85:236–239.

7. Yu MW, Hsieh HH, Pan WH, Yang CS, Chen CJ. Vegetable consumption, serum retinol level, and risk of hepatocellular carcinoma. Cancer Res 1995; 55:1301–1305.

8. Landa MC, Frago N, Tres A. Diet and the risk of breast cancer in Spain. Eur J Cancer Prev 1994; 3:313–320.

9. Stavric B. Role of chemopreventers in human diet. Clin Biochem 1994; 27:319–332.

10. Kennedy AR. The evidence for soybean products as cancer preventive agents. J Nutr 1995; 125:733S–743S.

11. Yang CS, Wang ZY. Tea and cancer. J Natl Cancer Inst 1993; 85:1038–1049.

12. Jin ZC, Qian J. Inhibitory effects of fifteen kinds of Chinese herbal drugs, vegetables and chemicals on SOS response. Chin J Prev Med 1994; 28:147–150.

13. Singletary KW, Nelshoppen J. Inhibition of 7,12-dimethylbenz[a]anthracene (DMBA)-induced mammary tumorigenesis and *in vivo* formation of mammary DMBA-DNA adducts by rosemary extract. Cancer Lett 1991; 60:169–175.

14. Steinmetz KA, Potter JD. Food-group consumption and colon cancer in the Adelaide Case-Control Study. I. Vegetables and fruit. Food-group consumption and colon cancer in the Adelaide Case-Control. Int J Cancer 1993; 53:711–719.

15. Milner JA. Reducing the risk of cancer. In: Functional Foods. New York: Van Nostrand Reinhold, NY, 1994; 39–70.

16. Dorant E, van den Brandt PA, Goldbohm RA, Hermus RJ, Sturmans F. Garlic and its significance for the prevention of cancer in humans: a critical view. Br J Cancer 1933; 67:424–429.

17. Jain AK, Vargas R, Gotzkowsky S, McMahon FG. Can garlic reduce levels of serum lipids? A controlled clinical study. Am J Med 1993; 94:632–635.

18. Mei X, Wang ML, Xu HX, et al. Garlic and gastric cancer I: the influence of garlic on the level of nitrate and nitrite in gastric juice. Acta Nutrimenta Sinica 1982; 4:53–56.

19. You WC, Blot WJ, Chang, YS, et al. Allium vegetables and reduced risk of stomach cancer. J Natl Cancer Inst 1989;81:162–164.

20. Mei X, Wang ML, Han N. Garlic and gastric cancer II—The inhibitory effect of garlic on the growth of nitrate reducing bacteria and on the production of nitrite. Acta Nutrimenta Sinica 1985;7:173–176.

21. Adetumbi MA, Lau BH. Allium sativum (garlic)—a natural antibiotic. Med Hypotheses 1983; 12:227–237.

22. Mei X, Lin X, Liu J, et al. The blocking effect of garlic on the formation of N-nitrosoproline in humans. Acta Nutrimenta Sinica 1989; 11:141–145.

23. Shenoy NR, Choughuley AS. Inhibitory effect of diet related sulphydryl compounds on the formation of carcinogenic nitrosamines. Cancer Lett 1992; 65:227–232.

24. Lin XY, Liu JZ, Milner JA. Dietary garlic suppresses DNA adducts caused by N-nitroso compounds. Carcinogenesis 1994; 15:349–352.

25. Liu JZ, Schaffer EM, Pegg AE, Milner JA. Dietary garlic inhibits mammary carcinogenesis induced by N-methylnitrosourea. FASEB J1995; 9:A991.

26. Block E. The organosulfur chemistry of the genus *Allium*—implications for the organic chemistry of sulfur. Angewandte Chemie Inter Ed Eng 1992; 31:1135–1178.

27. Liu JZ, Lin RI, Milner JA. Inhibition of 7,12-dimethylbenz(a)- anthracene induced mammary tumors and DNA adducts by garlic powder. Carcinogenesis 1992; 13:1847–1851.

28. Wargovich MJ, Woods C, Eng VWS, Stephens LC, Gray KN. Chemoprevention of nitrosomethylbenzylamine-induced esophageal cancer in rats by the thioether, diallyl sulfide. Cancer Res 1988; 48:l6872–6875.

29. Sumiyoshi H, Wargovich MJ. Chemoprevention of 1,2-dimethylhydrazine-induced colon cancer in mice by natural occurring organosulfur compounds. Cancer Res 1990; 50:5084–5087.

30. Belman S. Onion and garlic oils inhibit tumor promotion. Carcinogenesis 1983; 4: 1063–1067.

31. Wattenberg LW, Sparnins VL, Barany G. Inhibition of N-nitrosodiethylamine carcinogenesis in mice by naturally occurring organosulfur compounds and monoterpenes. Cancer Res 1989; 49:2689–2692.

32. Amagase H, Milner JA. Impact of various sources of garlic and their constituents on 7,12-dimethylbenz(a)-anthracene binding to mammary cell DNA. Carcinogenesis 1993; 14:1627–1631.

33. Brady JF, Wang MH, Hong JY, et al. Modulation of rat hepatic microsomal monooxygenase enzymes and cytotoxicity by diallyl sulfide. Toxic Appl Pharmacol 1991; 108:342–354.

34. Liu JZ, Lin XY, Milner JA. Dietary garlic powder increases glutathione content and glutathione S-transferase activity in rat liver and mammary tissues. FASEB J 1992; 6(4):A1493.

35. Sparnins VL, Barany G, Wattenberg LW. Effects of organosulfur compounds from garlic and onions on benzo(a)pyrene-induced neoplasia and glutathione S-transferase activity in the mouse. Carcinogenesis 1988; 9:131–134.

36. Choy YM, Kwok TT, Fung KP, Lee CY. Effect of garlic, Chinese medicinal drugs and amino acids on growth of Erlich ascites tumor cells in mice. Amer J Chinese Med 1983; 11:69–73.

37. Sundaram SG, Milner JA. Impact of organosulfur compounds in garlic on canine mammary tumor cells in culture. Cancer Lett 1994; 74:85–90.

38. Sundaram SG, Milner JA. Diallyl disulfide inhibits the proliferation of human colon tumor cells in culture. Biochem Biophys Acta, 1996; 1315:15–20.

39. Sundaram SG, Milner JA. Diallyl disulfide suppresses the growth of human colon tumor cell xenographs in athymic nude mice. J Nutr 1996; 126:1355–1361.

40. Ip C, Lisk DJ, Stoewsand GS. Mammary cancer prevention by regular garlic and selenium-enriched garlic. Nutr Cancer 1992; 7:279–286.

41. Amagase H, Schaffer E, Milner JA. Dietary components modify the ability of garlic to suppress 7,12 dimethylbenz(a)anthracene-induced mammary DNA adducts. J Nutr 1996; 126:817–824.

42. Dorant E, van den Brandt PA, Goldbohm RA. A prospective cohort study on Allium vegetable consumption, garlic supplement use, and the risk of lung carcinoma in The Netherlands. Cancer Res 1994; 54:6148–6153.

43. Takada N, Kitano M, Chen T, Yano Y, Otani S, Fukushima S. Enhancing effects of organosulfur compounds from garlic and onions on hepatocarcinogenesis in rats: association with increased cell proliferation and elevated ornithine decarboxylase activity. Jpn J Cancer Res 1994; 85:1067–1072.

44. Matsuda T, Takada N, Yano Y, Wanibuchi H, Otani S, Fukushima S. Dose-dependent inhibition of glutathione S-transferase placental form-positive hepatocellular foci induction in the rat by methyl propyl disulfide and propylene sulfide from garlic and onions. Cancer Lett 1994; 86:229–234.

45. Apitz-Castro R, Cabrera S, Cruz MR, Ledezma E, Jain MK. Effects of garlic extract and of three pure components isolated from it on human platelet aggregation, arachidonate metabolism, release reaction and platelet ultrastructure. Thromb Res 1983; 32:155–169.

46. Srivastava KC, Tyagi OD. Effects of a garlic-derived principle (ajoene) on aggregation and arachidonic acid metabolism in human blood platelets. Prost Leuk Essen Fatty Acids 1993; 49:587–595.

47. Beecher CW. Cancer preventive properties of varieties of Brassica oleracea: a review. Amer J Clin Nutr 1994; 59:1166S–1170S.

48. Zhang Y, Talalay P. Anticarcinogenic activities of organic isothiocyanates: chemistry and mechanisms. Cancer Research 1994; 54:1976s–1981s.

49. Wattenberg LW. Inhibition of neoplasia by minor dietary constituents. Cancer Res 1983; 43:2448s–2453s.

50. Sugie S, Okumura A, Tanaka T, Mori H. Inhibitory effects of benzyl isothiocyanate and benzyl thiocyanate on diethylnitrosamine-induced hepatocarcinogenesis in rats. Jpn J Cancer Res 1993; 84:865–870.

51. Daehnfeldt JL. Cytostatic activity and metabolic effects of aromatic isothiocyanic acid esters. Biochem Pharm 1968; 17:511–518.

52. Loub WD, Wattenberg LW, Davis DW. Aryl hydrocarbon hydroxylase induction in rat tissues by naturally occurring indoles of cruciferous plants. J Natl Cancer Inst 1975; 54:985–988.

53. Mehta RG, Liu J, Constantinou A, et al. Cancer chemopreventive activity of brassinin, a phytoalexin from cabbage. Carcinogenesis 1995; 16:399–404.

54. Bjeldanes LF, Kim JY, Grose KR, Bartholomew JC, Bradfield CA. Aromatic hydrocarbon responsiveness-receptor agonists generated from indole-3-carbinol in vitro and in vivo: comparisons with 2,3,7,8-tetrachlorodibenzo-p-dioxin. Proc Natl Acad Sci 1991; 88:9543–9547.

55. Shertzer HG. Indole-3-carbinol protects against covalent binding of benzo[a]pyrene and N-nitrosodimethylamine metabolites to mouse liver macromolecules. Chem-Biol Interactions 1984; 48:81–90.

56. Kojima T, Tanaka T, Mori H. Chemoprevention of spontaneous endometrial cancer in female Donryu rats by dietary indole-3-carbinol. Cancer Res 1994; 54:1446–1449.

57. Tiwari RK, Guo L, Bradlow HL, Telang NT, Osborne MP. Selective responsiveness of human breast cancer cells to indole-3-carbinol, a chemopreventive agent. J Natl Cancer Inst 1994; 86:126–131.

58. Jellinck PH, Michnovicz JJ, Bradlow HL. Influence of indole-3-carbinol on the hepatic microsomal formation of catechol estrogens. Steroids 1991; 56:446–450.

59. Michnovicz JJ, Bradlow HL. Altered estrogen metabolism and excretion in humans following consumption of indole-3-carbinol. Nutr Cancer 1991; 16:59–66.

60. Li Y, Wang E, Patten CJ, Chen L, Yang CS. Effects of flavonoids on cytochrome P450-dependent acetaminophen metabolism in rats and human liver microsomes. Drug Metab Disp 1994; 22:566–571.

61. Kandaswami C, Perkins E, Drzewiecki G, Soloniuk DS, Middleton Jr E. Differential inhibition of proliferation of human squamous cell carcinoma, gliosarcoma and embryonic fibroblast-like lung cells in culture by plant flavonoids. Anti-Cancer Drugs 1992; 3:525–530.

62. Bracke M, Vyncke B, Opdenakker G, Foidart JM, De Pestel G, Mareel M. Effect of catechins and citrus flavonoids on invasion in vitro. Clin Exper Metastasis 1991; 9:13–25.

63. Das M, Mukhtar H, Bik DP, Bickers DR. Inhibition of epidermal xenobiotic metabolism in SENCAR mice by naturally occurring plant phenols. Cancer Res 1987; 47:760–766.

64. Verma AK, Johnson JA, Gould MN, Tanner MA. Inhibition of 7,12-dimethylbenz(a)anthracene- and N-nitrosomethylurea-induced rat mammary cancer by dietary flavonol quercetin. Cancer Res 1988; 48:5754–5758.

65. Mukhtar H, Das M, Khan WA, Wang ZY, Bik DP, Bickers DR. Exceptional activity of tannic acid among naturally occurring plant phenols in protecting against 7,12-dimethylbenz(a)anthracene-, benzo(a)pyrene, 3-methylcholanthrene-, and N-methyl-N-nitrosourea-induced skin tumorigenesis in mice. Cancer Res 1988; 48:2361–2365.

66. Nakayama T, Yamada M, Osawa T, Kawakishi S. Suppression of active oxygen-induced cytotoxicity by flavonoids. Biochem Pharm 1993; 45:265–267.

67. Ranelletti FO, Ricci R, Larocca LM, et al. Growth-inhibitory effect of quercetin and presence of type-II estrogen-binding sites in human colon-cancer cell lines and primary colorectal tumors. Int J Cancer 1992; 50:486–492.

68. Graham HN. Green tea composition, consumption, and polyphenol chemistry. Prev Med 1992; 21:334–350.

69. Yang CS, Wang ZY, Hong JY. Inhibition of tumorigenesis by chemicals from garlic and tea. Adv Exp Med Biol 1994; 354:113–122.

70. La Vecchia C, Negri E, Franceschi S, D'Avanzo B, Boyle P. Tea consumption and cancer risk. Nutr Cancer 1992; 17:27–31.

71. Gao YT, McLaughlin JK, Blot WJ, Ji BT, Dai Q, Fraumeni Jr JF. Reduced risk of esophageal cancer associated with green tea consumption. J Natl Cancer Inst 1994; 86:855–858.

72. Mukhtar H, Katiyar SK, Agarwal R. Green tea and skin—anticarcinogenic effects. J Invest Derm 1994; 102:3–7.

73. Narisawa T, Fukaura Y. A very low dose of green tea polyphenols in drinking water prevents N-methyl-N-nitrosourea-induced colon carcinogenesis in F344 rats. Jpn J Cancer Res 1993; 84:1007–1009.

74. Nishida H, Omori M, Fukutomi Y, et al. Inhibitory effects of (-)-epigallocatechin gallate on spontaneous hepatoma in C3H/HeNCrj mice and human hepatoma-derived PLC/PRF/5 cells. Jpn J Cancer Res 1994; 85:221–225.

75. Katiyar SK, Agarwal R, Zaim MT, Mukhtar H. Protection against N-nitrosodiethylamine and benzo[a]pyrene-induced forestomach and lung tumorigenesis in A/J mice by green tea. Carcinogenesis 1993; 14:849–855.

76. Komori A, Yatsunami J, Okabe S, et al. Anticarcinogenic activity of green tea polyphenols. Jpn J Clin Oncol 1993; 23:186–190.

77. Yin P, Zhao J, Cheng S, Zhu Q, Liu Z, Zhengguo L. Experimental studies of the inhibitory effects of green tea catechin on mice large intestinal cancers induced by 1,2-dimethylhydrazine. Cancer Lett 1994; 79:33–38.

78. Shi ST, Wang ZY, Smith TJ, et al. Effects of green tea and black tea on 4-(methylnitrosamino)-1-(3-pyridyl)-1-butanone bioactivation, DNA methylation, and lung tumorigenesis in A/J mice. Cancer Res 1994; 54:4641–4647.

79. Hirose M, Hoshiya T, Akagi K, Futakuchi M, Ito N. Inhibition of mammary gland carcinogenesis by green tea catechins and other naturally occurring antioxidants in female Sprague-Dawley rats pretreated with 7,12-dimethylbenz[alpha]anthracene. Cancer Lett 1994; 83:149–156.

80. Xu Y, Ho CT, Amin SG, Han C, Chung FL. Inhibition of tobacco-specific nitrosamine-induced lung tumorigenesis in A/J mice by green tea and its major polyphenol as antioxidants. Cancer Res 1992; 52:3875–3879.

81. Wu YN, Wang HZ, Li JS, Han C. The inhibitory effect of Chinese tea and its polyphenols on in vitro and in vivo N-nitrosation. Biomed Environ Sci 1993; 6:237–258.

82. Wang ZY, Huang MT, Lou YR, et al. Inhibitory effects of black tea, green tea, decaffeinated black tea, and decaffeinated green tea on ultraviolet B light-induced skin carcinogenesis in 7,12-dimethylbenz[a]anthracene-initiated SKH-1 mice. Cancer Res 1994; 54:3428–3435.

83. Wang ZY, Hong JY, Huang MT, Reuhl KR, Conney AH, Yang CS. Inhibition of N-nitrosodiethylamine- and 4-(methylnitrosamino)-1-(3-pyridyl)-1-butanone-induced tumorigenesis in A/J mice by green tea and black tea. Cancer Res 1992; 52:1943–1947.

84. Fujita Y, Yamane T, Tanaka M, et al. Inhibitory effect of (-)-epigallocatechin gallate on carcinogenesis with N-ethyl-N'-nitro-N-nitrosoguanidine in mouse duodenum. Jpn J Cancer Res 1989; 80:503–505.

85. Huang MT, Ho CT, Wang ZY, et al. Inhibitory effect of topical application of a green tea polyphenol fraction on tumor initiation and promotion in mouse skin. Carcinogenesis 1992; 13:947–954.

86. Bu-Abbas A, Clifford MN, Ioannides C, Walker R. Stimulation of rat hepatic UDP-glucuronosyl transferase activity following treatment with green tea. Food Chem Toxicol 1995; 33:27–30.

87. Sohn OS, Surace A, Fiala ES, et al. Effects of green and black tea on hepatic xenobiotic metabolizing systems in the male F344 rat. Xenobiotica 1994; 24:119–127.

88. Khan SG, Katiyar SK, Agarwal R, Mukhtar H. Enhancement of antioxidant and phase II enzymes by oral feeding of green tea polyphenols in drinking water to SKH-1 hairless mice: possible role in cancer chemoprevention. Cancer Res 1992; 52:4050–4052.

89. Katiyar SK, Agarwal R, Mukhtar H. Inhibition of both stage I and stage II skin tumor promotion in SENCAR mice by a polyphenolic fraction isolated from green tea: inhibition depends on the duration of polyphenol treatment. Carcinogenesis 1993; 14:2641–2643.

90. Guengerich FP, Kim DH. In vitro inhibition of dihydropyridine oxidation and aflatoxin B1 activation in human liver microsomes by naringenin and other flavonoids. Carcinogenesis 1990; 11:2275–2279.

91. Trela BA, Carlson GP. Effect of flavanone on mixed-function oxidase and conjugation reactions in rats. Xenobiotica 1987; 17:11–16.

92. Wei H, Bowen R, Cai Q, Barnes S, Wang Y. Antioxidant and antipromotional effects of the soybean isoflavone genistein. Proc Soc Exp Biol Med 1995; 208:124–130.

93. Molteni A, Brizio-Molteni L, Persky V. In vitro hormonal effects of soybean isoflavones. J Nutr 1995; 125:751S–756S.

94. Herman C, Adlercreutz T, Goldin BR, et al. Soybean phytoestrogen intake and cancer risk. J Nutr 1995; 125:757S-770S.

95. Lamartiniere CA, Moore J, Holland M, Barnes S. Neonatal genistein chemoprevents mammary cancer. Proc Soc Exp Biol Med 1995; 208:120–123.

96. Fotsis T, Pepper M, Adlercreutz H, et al. Genistein, a dietary-derived inhibitor of in vitro angiogenesis. Proc Natl Acad Sci USA 1993; 90:2690–2694.

97. Shugart L, Kao J. Effect of ellagic and caffeic acids on covalent binding of benzo(a)pyrene to epidermal DNA of mouse skin in organ culture. Int J Biochem 1984; 16:571–573.

98. Chang RL, Huang M-T, Wood AW, et al. Effect of ellagic acid and hydroxylated flavonoids on the tumorigenicity of benzo(a)pyrene on mouse skin and in the newborn mouse. Carcinogenesis 1985; 6:1127–1133.

99. Mandal S, Stoner GD. Inhibition of N-nitrosobenzylmethylamine-induced esophageal tumorigenesis in rats by ellagic acid. Carcinogenesis 1990; 11:55–61.

100. Wattenberg LW. Inhibition of carcinogenesis by minor dietary constituents. Cancer Res 1992; 52:2085s-2091s.

101. Elegbede JA, Maltzman TH, Elson CE, Gould MN. Effects of anticarcinogenic monoterpenes on phase II hepatic drug metabolizing enzymes. Carcinogenesis 1993; 14:1221–1223.

102. Wattenberg LW, Coccia JB. Inhibition of 4-(methylnitrosamino)-1-(3-pyridyl)-1-butanone carcinogenesis in mice by D-limonene and citrus fruit oils. Carcinogenesis 1991; 12:115–117.

103. Crowell PL, Gould MN. Chemoprevention and therapy of cancer by d-limonene. Crit Rev Oncogen 1994; 5:1–22.

104. Larsen MC, Brake PB, Parmar D, Jefcoate CR. The induction of five rat hepatic P450 cytochromes by phenobarbital and similarly acting compounds is regulated by a sexually dimorphic, dietary-dependent endocrine factor that is highly strain specific. Arch Biochem Biophys 1994; 315:24–34.

105. Ruch RJ, Sigler K. Growth inhibition of rat liver epithelial tumor cells by monoterpenes does not involve Ras plasma membrane association. Carcinogenesis 1994; 15:787–789.

106. Elson CE, Yu SG. The chemoprevention of cancer by mevalonate-derived constituents of fruits and vegetables. J Nutr 1994; 124:607–614.
107. Elegbede JA, Elson CE, Tanner MA, Qureshi A, Gould MN. Regression of rat primary mammary tumors following d-limonene. J Natl Cancer Inst 1986; 76:323–325.
108. Haag JD, Lindstrom MJ, Gould MN. Limonene-induced regression of mammary carcinomas. Cancer Res 1992; 52:4021–4026.
109. Mills JJ, Chari RS, Boyer IJ, Gould MN, Jirtle RL. Induction of apoptosis in liver tumors by the monoterpene perillyl alcohol. Cancer Res 1995; 55:979–983.
110. Hard GC, Whysner J. Risk assessment of d-limonene: an example of male rat-specific renal tumorigens. Crit Rev Toxicol 1994; 24:231–254.

8 Dietary Fat and Coronary Heart Disease

K. C. Hayes

1. INTRODUCTION

Numerous experimental and epidemiological studies have revealed the relationship between an elevated blood cholesterol value and development of atherosclerosis (1,2). Since the early days when the association was based on gross pathology, a plethora of investigations, including those from cell biology (3), have carefully documented the pathogenesis of the atherosclerotic process, linking thrombogeneis, the inflammatory response, and an elevated LDL/HDL ratio with atherogenesis and coronary heart disease (CHD). More recently, the possible oxidation of the LDL particle within the damaged arterial intima has developed into a promising avenue of atherogenesis research with implications for modulation by diet (3,4).

Nonetheless, the ongoing discussion of how dietary saturated (SFAs), monounsaturated (MUFAs), or polyunsaturated fatty acids (PUFAs) modulate the concentration of plasma cholesterol continues to be among the most confusing aspects of atherogenesis, not just for consumers, but also for investigators researching the subject. Confusion persists because a metamorphosis is in progress from a simple, earlier literature that focused on total plasma cholesterol as affected by individual fats or classes of fats (SFAs, MUFAs, PUFAs) to a newer approach that attempts to coordinate modulation of specific lipoproteins by dietary fatty acids present in the combination of fats being consumed. During this process a number of new observations are forcing reconsideration of previous concepts.

Among the earliest observations indicating that dietary fat was related to elevated blood lipids was the report by Kinsell (5), who noted that PUFAs lowered plasma cholesterol (TC) even as SFAs elevated plasma lipids. Shortly thereafter, Bronte-Stewart (6) noted that simply adding extra PUFAs to the diet (without decreasing SATs) could dramatically lower an elevated TC. Based on these and related observations, an increase in consumption of PUFAs and decrease in SATs has become the standard dogma of nutritionists and clinicians attempting to improve the plasma lipid profile and decrease the risk of CHD. Although this dietary directive, in conjunction with various other intervention procedures, has reduced CHD mortality in the United States by 40% in the past 25 yr, the detail of the dietary fat recommendation continues to be debated in terms of which unsaturated fatty acids (UNSATs) or SFAs are more acceptable.

Because a high intake of polyunsaturates increases the potential for in vivo lipid peroxidation and the need for vitamin E antioxidant protection, it has been suggested that

From: *Preventive Nutrition: The Comprehensive Guide for Health Professionals*
Edited by A. Bendich and R. J. Deckelbaum Humana Press Inc., Totowa, NJ

the LDL particle might be more prone to peroxidative damage during high PUFA intake, thereby reducing the efficacy of PUFAs as an antiatherogenic fat. Rather, it has been recommended that a high-MUFA oil should be substituted for the hi-PUFA oil, based on the assumption (arguably incorrect) that MUFAs lower TC and LDL-C as effectively as hi-PUFAs without rendering the MUFA-rich LDL as susceptible to oxidative stress *(4)*. Although in vitro estimates of LDL oxidizability favor the latter recommendation, certain in vivo evidence questions whether LDL circulating during a high-PUFA diet is normally more prone to peroxidative damage than LDL circulating during high-MUFA intake *(7)* or whether LDL in atheroma are actually limited in antioxidant protection *(8)*. Furthermore, in vivo data concerning CHD risk clearly suggests that risk is inversely related to the plasma 18:2/18:1 cholesteryl ester ratio, which is directly related to 18:2 intake and inversely related to 18:1 consumption *(9)*. In other words, the greater the 18:2-CE pool, the less atherosclerosis is observed in both human and animal studies *(10,11)*. Reducing 18:2 intake below a critical level also increases the 18:1-CE pool, and expanding 18:1-CE at the expense of 18:2-CE is associated with more cholesterol deposition in the arterial intima, not less. Thus, the simple suggestion to "replace PUFAs with MUFAs while reducing SFAs" is not necessarily the best advice, considering that a high-polyunsaturated fat intake (7–10% total energy[en]) induces the greatest decrease in circulating LDL and is associated with the least cholesterol deposition in arterial lesions. Also, a balance between SFAs and PUFAs ironically may produce the most favorable LDL/HDL ratio *(12)*.

The literature on dietary fat and CHD has been substantially detailed and collated by expert committees *(1,2)* wherein the epidemiological, experimental, and clinical data are convincingly marshalled to make the point that our plasma lipids are best kept below180 mg/dL TC with LDL-C <125 mg/dL for good cardiovascular health. However, a moderate TC value is not a fool proof guarantee against CHD because platelet aggregation and thrombogeneis are probably more important than elevated lipids in the develoment of CHD. Generally speaking, both excessive thrombosis and elevated LDL-C appear to be required for advanced CHD to become clinically manifest *(3)*.

Although most of the evidence incriminating fat with CHD risk has involved the modulation of lipoproteins, fat can also influence blood pressure and platelet aggregation through its effect on prostaglandin and leukotriene metabolism. These physiological events have a major impact on atherogenesis *(3)*. Dietary sodium can also factor into the equation by virtue of its influence on blood volume, and indirectly, blood pressure *(1,2)*. However, the scope of these interrelationships is beyond the focus of this review.

2. IMPORTANCE OF LIPOPROTEIN PROFILE

A compelling set of data currently exists that demonstrates the importance of the plasma lipoprotein profile in risk assessment for CHD *(13,14)*. Furthermore, this profile can be modulated by manipulating the quality of dietary fat (fatty acids) and the amount of dietary cholesterol consumed each day. The risk is clearly associated with LDL. Although the specific objective of raising HDL to lower CHD incidence is not a proven means of therapy, certain interventions that lower CHD risk, such as increased physical activity, cessation of smoking, and alcohol consumption, also raise HDL *(15)*. Furthermore, drugs that have raised HDL during intervention trials tended to reduce CHD incidence *(16,17)*.

Most would agree that an elevated LDL/HDL ratio represents a risk for CHD and that lowering blood lipids, particularly LDL, is beneficial. However, full agreement has not been reached on specific recommendations for lowering lipids by dietary fat manipulation, especially pertaining to individual lipoproteins, or whether once lowered, a significant reduction in CHD will result for patients currently diagnosed with the disease. Furthermore, if CHD mortality is reduced, will overall age-adjusted morbidity and mortality be improved? These questions are especially important to patients who have already suffered a myocardial infarct and are looking to diet for corrective therapy. Significant clinical trials have shown that drug intervention (with inhibitors of cholesterol synthesis) for 5 yr reduced LDL-C by 35% and deaths by 30% without increasing non-CHD deaths *(17,18)*. Whether long-term dietary intervention alone can mediate such a result is open to question, but the preliminary evidence is that drastic lifestyle modifications, including diet, do substantially reduce CHD risk *(19)*.

3. DIETARY CHOLESTEROL IMPACT ON TC

Comprehending the difference between dietary cholesterol and dietary fat as they relate to plasma cholesterol regulation is often conceptually difficult for the average consumer, especially since the relative importance of dietary fat is thought to be greater than that for dietary cholesterol, at least in humans. In fact, a normal intake of dietary cholesterol does elevate TC, especially LDL-C, in certain species, including most humans, but not in others. Those species most responsive to cholesterol intake normally do not consume appreciable dietary cholesterol, e.g., herbivorous animals, like the rabbit, hamster, and certain monkeys, like the rhesus and cynomolgus. Highly carnivorous species, like cats and dogs, and certain omnivorous ones, like rats and mice, tend not to respond to ordinary intakes of dietary cholesterol. The omnivorous human reveals an intermediate sensitivity that tends to vary among individuals.

Reasons for species differences are several and relevant to our understanding of the physiology of cholesterol metabolism. The ability of rats to counterbalance dietary cholesterol intake reflects its proportionally great hepatic cholesterol synthesis relative to whole body synthesis *(20)*. Thus, absorbed cholesterol effectively downregulates whole body synthesis by progressively suppressing hepatic synthesis, in effect balancing the overall body pool without expanding the plasma pool. In species like hamsters (and probably to a certain extent humans), with minimal hepatic cholesterol synthesis, the absorbed cholesterol rapidly suppresses hepatic synthetic capacity and simultaneously depresses LDL receptor (LDL_r) activity to cause a back-up in plasma LDL (and HDL) waiting to clear into the liver *(20)*. In all species dietary cholesterol represents a powerful suppressant of hepatic LDL_r activity as the liver becomes "laden" with this sterol. Overload is most readily documented by accumulation of hepatic cholesteryl esters in susceptible species.

Among humans, the impact of dietary cholesterol varies with different circumstances. Individuals can be hypo- or hyper-responders to cholesterol intake, presumably for genetic reasons not completely understood *(21)*. For example, a protein important for uptake and clearance of triglyceride-rich lipoproteins, apoprotein E exists as three major isoforms E2, E3, and E4. The apoprotein E4 phenotype seems to promote slight enhancement of cholesterol absorption, and such individuals may also have imperfect feedback inhibition of hepatic cholesterol synthesis resulting in general expansion of the whole body cholesterol pool. They are also at higher risk for atherosclerosis *(22)*. Furthermore, effective removal of hepatic cholesterol also depends somewhat on bile acid synthesis and excretion via feces. Humans are much less capable of cholesterol removal than rats because their bile acid synthesis rate is substantially less than that of rats *(23)*. Liver cholesterol storage and overload presumably depend, in part, on the balance between hepatic acyl cholesterol:acyl CoA transferase (ACAT) activity, and the previously mentioned excretion route via bile acids. However, the relative capacity for cholesteryl ester formation in human liver is unclear because little evidence exists that human liver ever experiences appreciable cholesterol storage.

The dietary cholesterol impact in humans also seems to depend on other factors in the diet affecting absorption of both cholesterol and bile acids. Plant sterols, like sitosterol, and certain dietary fibers, like psyllium, can deter cholesterol and bile acid absorption, thereby reducing the cholesterol-raising impact of any cholesterol available in the diet. For example, utilization of sitostanol esters and antibiotics to completely block cholesterol absorption in hypercholesterolemic men decreased TC and LDL-C about 35% *(24)*. Accordingly, in quantitative terms the impact of dietary cholesterol in humans is reflected mainly in LDL-C, and is nonlinear. That is, a 100 mg increment of dietary cholesterol between 0–300 mg/d intake appears to have 2–3 times the impact of 100 mg between 500–800 mg/d, increasing total plasma cholesterol by 4–6 mg/dL per 100 mg in the first instance but only 2–4 mg/dL for the 100 mg increment in the second case *(25)*. The implication is that extremely low cholesterol intake (close to zero) may be desirable when lipoprotein metabolism is clinically stressed, a point supported by actual experience *(19)*.

4. DIETARY FAT AND LIPOPROTEIN METABOLISM

The amount and type of dietary fat have a greater influence on human TC and lipoproteins than cholesterol, but cholesterol intake also influences the response to fatty acids by depressing LDL_r activity. Although it is not certain that fat (fatty acids) routinely alters the rate of bile acid synthesis, high intake of PUFAs (>20%en 18:2) may increase bile acid production *(26)*. On the other hand, certain fatty acids, similar to dietary cholesterol, appear to modify LDL_r activity to exert a major impact on plasma LDL and TC pools *(20,27)*.

4.1. Amount of Fat

The American Heart Association (AHA) and National Cholesterol Education Program (NCEP) have published comparable recommendations *(13)* incorporating the rationale for lowering TC and LDL-C by reducing dietary fat to 30% of total dietary energy or less, saturated fat to 10%en or less, and dietary cholesterol to <200–300 mg/d depending on the initial elevation in LDL-C above 130 mg/dL. Generally, TC will decline 10–15% in response to sustained diet changes, but a decline in excess of 20% is not uncommon in the best cases. Hypercholesterolemic lean individuals are more apt to respond to sustained restrictions in saturated fat and cholesterol intake than hypercholesterolemic obese or normocholesterolemic lean subjects *(28)*. The responsiveness of the lean may reflect their relative lack of 18:2 reserves in adipose tissue. Limitations in the availability of 18:2 may ultimately affect the individual responsiveness of the host (*see* Section 4.3).

It has been suggested that a specific decrease in saturated fatty acids (as a class) must be a major aspect of restricting fat to 30%en if TC is to decline *(29)*, but this does not necessarily apply to 16:0-rich or 18:0-rich fats as much as to 14:0-rich fats, i.e., the primary restriction of milkfat from dairy products *(30,31)*.

It is well established that intervention with a high-carbohydrate, low-fat diet (e.g., 20%en from fat with substantial decreases in saturated fatty acids) can induce a substantial 10–20% reduction in plasma cholesterol, even though plasma triglycerides generally increase, at least temporarily *(26)*. Even this rule may not pertain if subjects have normal lipoprotein metabolism and the same fatty acid profile (the exact saturated:monounsaturated:polyunsturated fatty acid configuration) is maintained between the 40 and 20%en fat exchange *(32)*, i.e., it appears that no change in any lipoprotein parameter is induced by reducing the fat load in normolipemic subjects unless the saturated fatty acid mass *and profile* are altered relative to unsaturates. On the other hand, addition of any fat to a high-carbohydrate diet typically increases HDL-C and plasma cholesterol depending on the amount of carbohydrate replaced. Adding saturated fat usually increases LDL-C, as well, whereas monounsaturates increase LDL-C slightly and polyunsaturates produce a minimal change in this pool *(33)*. Even as a high-carbohydrate diet produces a lower LDL-C, it often increases plasma triglycerides, decreases HDL-C, and decreases LDL size *(26,33,34)*.

This latter triad of changes affecting lipoproteins is thought by some to represent an added risk for CHD *(26,34)*. As a result, a program of limiting fat reduction to about 30% energy has been advocated, while emphasizing a residual fat content that favors monounsaturates over polyunsaturates so that HDL will be less likely to decline and the small dense LDL less likely to form. However, polyunsaturates generally do not depress HDL unless they represent >15–20%en in the diet, and evidence has been presented that the most favorable LDL/HDL ratio (i.e., lowest LDL and highest HDL) is induced by a diet with 30%en as fat containing a combination of 16:0-rich saturated fat (to elevate HDL) and PUFAs (to assure removal of LDL by the liver), each representing 8–10%en *(12)*. Thus, in addition to raising LDL, saturates induce the greatest rise in HDL, followed by monounsaturates, and then polyunsaturates. As inferred from the above summary, monounsaturates appear singularly benign in terms of their impact on lipoprotein metabolism, a conclusion in accordance with the most inclusive analysis (i.e., hundreds of human comparisons) on the subject of dietary fat and plasma lipids *(35)*.

Despite the concern (mentioned above) associated with lowering an elevated plasma cholesterol by feeding a high-carbohydrate (high-CO) diet, it is clear from epidemiologic evidence that populations that normally consume high-CHO, low-fat diets (<25%en as fat) are also afflicted with much less diet-related chronic disease, especially CHD, than populations that consume high-fat diets (>30%en as fat) *(1,2)*. The point is that both long-term diet and other environmental circumstances influence those considerations involving the therapeutic manipulation of diet for altering CHD risk. Thus, a relatively lean, physically active population with a history of moderate food consumption (e.g., most developing nations) exemplifies different metabolic characteristics, including lipoproteins, than an overweight, sedentary population consuming excessive calories based on high fat and sugar. The response to a high-carbohydrate diet by the two populations differs, but the evidence suggests that it is probably advantageous for both groups to either maintain or return to a lifestyle that ultimately includes a low-fat, high-carbohydrate diet based on complex carbohydrates (including fiber) represented by cereal grains, vegetables, and fruit *(36)*. To re-establish a "normal" metabolic profile in an overweight population may require severe, sustained reduction in fat intake, e.g.,

10%en as fat advocated by Pritikin or Ornish *(19)*. Such a regimen has been shown to drastically reduce plasma lipids and even causes dissolution of arterial cholesterol deposits and atherosclerotic plaques, clearly indicating that diets extremely high in complex carbohydrate and low in fat can be advantageous even for those at high risk for CHD. But a major consideration is the individual response, i.e., the concept that individuals (or even subpopulations) vary in their lipoprotein response to altered fat (fatty acid) intake.

4.2. Dietary Fat (Fatty Acid) Quality

Although the focus on fat has historically emphasized the key role of saturated fat and certain fatty acids (12:0, 14:0, and 16:0) in raising TC, it now appears evident that the TC response to these fatty acids must be considered in the context of other fatty acids and cholesterol consumed simultaneously in addition to the metabolic status of the subject at the time of dietary intervention. Thus, the concurrent intake of both 18:2 and other saturated fatty acids modifies the impact of any individual saturated fatty acid, which, in turn, reflects the overall metabolism of lipoproteins at the time intervention is initiated.

After dietary fat saturation had been identified as the major factor regulating plasma cholesterol in humans, it was not long before Keys *(37)* and Hegsted *(38)* developed equations that would predict the relative response in TC when switching from one dietary fat profile to another. However, their estimates, although generally applicable to world populations, now appear oversimplified because they fail to distinguish between the impact of specific fatty acids or to discriminate between the considerable variability in host response. Nonetheless, our current understanding of plasma lipid response to dietary fat derives from the Keys-Hegsted studies *(37,38)* and their original regression equations that were used to predict the impact of fat (and in certain cases, fatty acids) on circulating cholesterol in populations eating Western diets. However, those equations (i.e., ΔTC approximately equal to +2Δ SFAs − 1ΔPUFAs + Δ dietary cholesterol) were based on several assumptions that are arguably inappropriate in light of current information.

4.3. Nonlinear Response to Polyunsaturates

Although Keys and Hegsted pointed out the cholesterol-lowering potential of polyunsaturates (primarily 18:2), they assumed this relationship was linear. However, animal model systems where dietary fatty acids and animals can be meticulously controlled, as well as retrospective analysis of the best set of human data, indicate that the decline in plasma cholesterol associated with increasing polyunsaturate consumption is nonlinear *(31,39,40)*, typically reaching a bottom or "threshold" at about 5%en as 18:2 (Fig. 1). Extra 18:2 only produces a minor further decrease in plasma cholesterol. This 18:2 "threshold" presumably exists for humans, and may correspond to maximum upregulation of LDL receptors by 18:2. Once the nonlinear nature of the plasma cholesterol response to 18:2 is appreciated, previous linear responses in human data sets can be reconciled as merely incomplete and representative of a linear portion of the overall curve, and not as contradictory evidence.

Once the 18:2 threshold is achieved, it appears possible to exchange 18:1 or 18:0, and even 16:0, for any extra 18:2 (above threshold) without modulating the plasma lipids appreciably (Fig. 2). This ability to exchange other fatty acids for 18:2 is evident in a

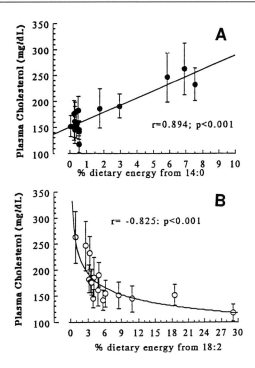

Fig. 1. Correlations between the observed plasma cholesterol response and the percentage of dietary energy from 14:0 reveal a linear relationship (**A**) whereas that with 18:2 is nonlinear (**B**) in monkeys fed cholesterol-free diets (from ref. *31*).

number of human studies *(12,41–45)* and explains much of the confusion and controversy surrounding the ability of certain fatty acids, especially 16:0 and 18:1, to raise or lower plasma cholesterol, respectively, in certain circumstances but not in others. For example, the exclusive intake of a monounsaturated oil (which is not practical) can lower plasma cholesterol effectively because it supplies enough 18:2 to satisfy the 18:2 threshold requirement in the absence of the especially cholesterolemic combination of 12:0+14:0 plus dietary cholesterol found in certain animal fats (*see* ref. *40* for discussion of this point).

Because the plasma cholesterol response to 18:2 is nonlinear, small increments of 18:2 between 1 and 3%en in the diet cause a major decrease in plasma cholesterol, whereas a shift between 15 and 20%en as 18:2 is often without effect (Fig. 1). Whereas LDL receptor activity may be modulated at low intakes of 18:2, the progressive but small decline in LDL-C and plasma cholesterol at higher 18:2 intakes probably reflects decreased VLDL output associated with decreased hepatic triglyceride synthesis.

It is possible that the 18:2 threshold represents the biological requirement for a fixed mass of 18:2 (i.e., mg/kg bd wt/d) as opposed to a %en requirement as originally conceived *(31)*. If so, it would help explain why the percent energy threshold seems to vary somewhat with experimental circumstances in human studies. For example, obese hypercholesterolemic subjects failed to respond to incremental increases in 18:2 from 3–12% energy whereas their lean counterparts did *(28)*. Because the obese tend to eat more food than lean individuals, even at 3% energy the mass of their 18:2 intake (mg/d)

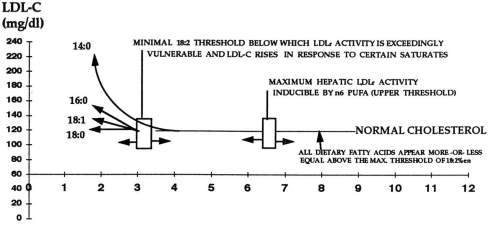

Fig. 2. The scheme depicts the perceived dynamics in humans between the relative importance of 18:2 (as percent dietary energy) and modulation of LDL-C, which in turn is based on the putative antagonism between 18:2 and primarily 14:0. Only 18:2 is thought to exert a positive influence on (i.e., increase) LDL_r activity in humans. By shifting the typical 18:2 intake from low (3%en) to moderate (7%en) the hepatic clearance of LDL-C is increased (lowering LDL-C and plasma cholesterol) to counter the cholesterol-elevating influence of 14:0. Consumption of 16:0 exerts a negative effect (increases LDL-C) only if the 18:2 intake is too low (below threshold), probably because of increased VLDL production, which increases LDL formation *(see text)*. Other factors affecting cholesterol metabolism, such as estrogen and thyroid hormone, presumably affect the 18:2 threshold requirement, accounting for individual and population differences in the threshold.

may be above "threshold" and already maximally effective in terms of LDL_r activity. Or possibly their excess adipose reserves have more than enough 18:2 to act as a "buffer" against any diet shortfall that might otherwise leave them below "threshold."

4.4. Saturated Fatty Acids Are Not Equivalent

The dissimilarity between individual saturated fatty acids regarding their impact on plasma cholesterol was recognized early on by investigators *(26,37,38)* who consistently found that coconut oil and milkfat were more cholesterolemic than other fats. These two dietary fats, along with palm kernel oil, are the richest sources of lauric (12:0) and myristic (14:0) acids, the latter of which was originally identified by Hegsted et al. *(38)* as the most cholesterolemic fatty acid. It has been subsequently shown in monkeys *(31,46)*, humans *(47,48)*, and gerbils *(39)* that 12:0+14:0 (lumped together because they generally occur together, often on the same TG molecule) are, indeed, more cholesterolemic than 16:0 or 18:0. The 14:0-rich triglycerides consumed in their natural form are the only saturated fats that invariably raise TC, and they do so in a linear fash-

Table 1
General Lipoprotein Response (Increase, Neutral, Decrease) to Major Dietary Fatty Acids in Humans (relative to *cis* 18:1)

Fatty acid	Typical %en	VLDL	LDL	HDL	Lp(a)
SFAs					
12:0+14:0	1–4	Incr	Incr	Incr	Decr
16:0	6–12	Incr	Neutr-incr[a]	Incr	Decr
18:0	2–4	Neutr	Neutr[b]	Neutr[b]	Neutr
TRANS (t18:1n9)	2–7	Incr	Incr	Decr	Incr
MUFAs (c18:1n9)	10–18	Neutr	Neutr	Neutr	Neutr
PUFAs (18:2,18:3)	3–8	Decr	Decr	Neutr-decr[c]	Neutr

[a]16:0 response is "conditional" and can increase LDL if present with 14:0 or with dietary cholesterol >300 mg/d or if subject is already severely hypercholestrolemic.

[b]18:0 can decrease LDL and HDL if intake is artificially elevated with modified dietary TG, i.e., unnatural fats.

[c]POLY intake > 20%en typically leads to a decrease in HDL.

ion *(31,39)*. Although both 16:0 and 18:0 can be neutral in the absence of dietary cholesterol, practically speaking in Western diets the main sources of 16:0 and 18:0, i.e., milkfat, beef and chicken fat, and milk chocolate, also contain cholesterol, so that the neutrality of 16:0 can be preempted by its interaction with dietary cholesterol (*see* Section 5.) (Table 1). The 16:0-rich saturates may also raise TC depending on the metabolic status of the host (*see* Section 4.5.). The saturated medium-chain triglycerides (MCTs) composed of 8:0 and 10:0 have been found to be neutral or hypocholesterolemic in limited human studies *(49)*.

When plasma cholesterol rises during saturated fat intake, the major effect is on LDL, although saturated fats containing 12:0, 14:0, and 16:0 are the only fats that consistently raise HDL as well. Stearic acid (18:0) tends not to influence either LDL or HDL at the levels normally consumed (2–5%en), but at atypically high 18:0 intake HDL can be severely depressed along with a major decline in LDL *(48,50)* (Table 1). The peculiar neutrality associated with the consumption of *normal amounts* of stearic acid has been reviewed recently *(51)*.

4.5. Response to 16:0 Is Host Dependent

The plasma cholestrol response to 16:0-rich fats has been problematic because the response seems to vary with experimental conditions and investigative design. Although 16:0 was eventually included with 12:0 and 14:0 by Keys *(37)* and Hegsted *(35)*, the most comprehensive experiments on the subject to date in humans were conducted by Hegsted et al. *(38)*. These unique experiments included 36 diets fed to the same individuals under the *same* environmental circumstances over a span of years. Multiple regression analysis of the data generated under the experimental circumstances employed (middle-aged men with TC of 225 mg/dL on the basal diet), revealed that 14:0 was about four-times more cholesterolemic than 16:0, which was not much more cholesterol-elevating than 18:0 or 18:1. The latter two fatty acids were considered neutral, neither raising nor lowering total cholesterol.

The ability of 16:0 to be truly neutral was initially demonstrated 25 yr ago by Vergroesen *(52)* in a direct comparison with 18:1. He found identical TC values (189,191 mg/dL) in normolipemic Benedictine monks fed liquid formulas containing all their fat (40% energy) as either olive oil or palm oil. The shift between 16:0 and 18:1 intake represented a 15%en exchange between the two fatty acids. A key factor in this comparison was that the 18:2 content of the two oils was essentially identical (at 10% of fatty acids, which represented 4% total energy intake) and dietary cholesterol was restricted to <225 mg/dL. Our investigations in monkeys *(53)* and others in humans *(45,54–56)* elicited the same normocholesterolemic response when these two fatty acids were exchanged by manipulating fats in the diets of subjects with a normal lipoprotein profile.

The "conditional" nature of the host response to 16:0 can be elicited if the circulating lipoproteins are artificially raised *(57)* or when plasma lipoproteins are spontaneously elevated by long-standing metabolic circumstances *(42)*. The later situation is most clearly demonstrated in the data of Mattson and Grundy *(38)*, who essentially fed the Vergroesen liquid formulas of 20 yr earlier *(52)* to elderly men experiencing moderately severe cholesterolemia (average entry cholesterol of 263 mg/dL). In this situation 16:0-rich palm oil lowered the average plasma cholesterol from entry (to 224 mg/dL), but the 16:0-rich fat was decidedly more cholesterolemic than either the 18:1-rich safflower oil (197 mg/dL) or 18:2-rich safflower oil (191 mg/dL). However, as detailed previously *(53,58)*, the sensitivity to 16:0 was highly individualized among the 20 subjects tested. Men with the highest cholesterol values (>240 mg/dL when fed palm oil) were much more responsive to 16:0 than the several men with normal cholesterol values (<200 mg/dL) under the same challenge. In the latter subgroup the response to 16:0, 18:1, and 18:2 was not significantly different, even though 16:0 tended to elicit the highest values and 18:2 the lowest.

The exact determinants of the 16:0-sensitivity are not understood, but it appears to reflect the absolute TC value (LDL-C and probably LDL_r activity as modulated by the 18:2 threshold) (Fig. 2). However, this is not the sole predictor. It probably is affected by BMI, age, sex, insulin responsiveness, thyroid hormone, bile acid synthesis rate, and so forth, i.e., any factor influencing lipoprotein metabolism. The easiest way to increase sensitivity to 16:0 is to impair lipoprotein metabolism by feeding excess dietary cholesterol *(58)*, as detailed elsewhere in cebus monkeys *(57)* and gerbils *(39)*. Dietschy and colleagues *(20)* have also applied this technique of cholesterol-feeding in an attempt to amplify and distinguish the response of the LDL receptor to various dietary fatty acids in their hamster model. When this approach is used, a constant load of 16:0-rich fat (more than other fats) becomes progressively cholesterolemic as the LDL receptors are downregulated by incremental increases in dietary cholesterol *(39,58)*. In a previous report *(31)* the implications of this sensitivity to 16:0 was considered relative to the dietary fat intake and plasma lipids of the world population. Obviously, without knowing exactly all the variables that dictate responsiveness to 16:0, we can only estimate at what point a "stressed" lipoprotein metabolism initiates the 16:0 sensitivity in humans. Perusal of data in the world literature suggests that the cholesterolemic effect of 16:0 is associated with a TC between 200–225 mg/dL for most populations *(31)*, but most likely the response is progressive and related to the "18:2 threshold" and LDL receptor activity. More work is needed to refine these relationships and the implications for cardiovascular health vis-a-vis fatty acid intake.

4.6. Trans *Fatty Acids May Be Worse than Saturates*

Trans fatty acids are mentioned by way of comparison with saturates, primarily because their structure as well as their metabolic impact on cholesterol metabolism are often thought to mimic the dietary saturated fatty acids that they were designed to replace. In fact, recent evidence has revealed that consumption of *trans* fatty acids may be more detrimental than SFAs because of their negative impact on the LDL/HDL ratio and Lp(a) concentration *(59,60)* (*see* Table 1). Consumption of *trans* 18:1, especially the elaidic acid isomer (t18:1n9) in the range of 2–7%en, has been demonstrated to substantially elevate the LDL/HDL ratio because it often depresses HDL-C while raising LDL-C. By contrast, saturated fatty acids that raise LDL-C also raise HDL-C. In addition, most *trans* fat experiments with humans have described a 20–25% increase in Lp(a), the unique lipoprotein in the LDL fraction whose concentration has been identified as an independent risk for CHD.

Epidemiological studies have indicated that the upper range of *trans* fatty acid intake is associated with a substantial increase (+50%) in risk for CHD *(61)*. For example, the Norwegian cohort of the nine-country EURAMIC study described a five-fold increase in CHD risk from the lowest to highest quartiles of *trans* intake, predominately derived from partially hydrogenated fish oil (PHFO) margarine *(62)*. A related clinical study in Norwegian men *(63)* found that 7%en from PHFO elevated the LDL/HDL ratio even more than butter, which had a slightly more negative effect than partially hydrogenated soybean oil (PHSBO). On the other hand, a Malaysian study fed PHSBO and exchanged 5.5%en from t18:1n9 (elaidic acid) for cis18:1n9, 16:0, or 12:0+14:0 in other fat blends and found that elaidic acid increased the LDL/HDL ratio relative to all other fatty acids, including 14:0-rich fat in the form of coconut oil *(64)* (*see* Chapter 13).

5. FATTY ACID AND CHOLESTEROL INTERACTION

The interactive synergy between saturated fat (arguably the 16:0-rich portion) and dietary cholesterol in humans was described a decade ago by Schonfeld et al. *(65)* and again recently by Fielding et al. *(66)*. Similar to the first study, the latter investigators studied four groups of men fed either a modestly polyunsaturated (P/S ratio 0.8) or saturated (P/S ratio 0.3) fat diet with low (200 mg/d) or high (600 mg/d) intakes of dietary cholesterol. Two results were noteworthy. First, at low cholesterol intake (when lipoprotein metabolism would be least compromised) the rise in LDL-C from basal values for all subjects in the presence of saturates was minimal (+3 mg/dL) compared to the polyunsaturates diet (−2 mg/dL), but at the high cholesterol intake the "saturated fat effect" was striking and exaggerated (+25 mg/dL) compared to the polyunsaturates (+16 mg/dL) or compared to the low-cholesterol, saturated fat diet intake (+3 mg/dL). The point is that the saturated fat effect (the major challenge was from relatively neutral 16:0 and 18:0) was only elicited after lipoprotein metabolism was "stressed" by dietary cholesterol. Secondly, the response to dietary fats was surprisingly affected by ethnic background such that Caucasians were significantly more responsive to both saturated fat and cholesterol challenges than non-Caucasians. For example, the LDL-C increase during the high-cholesterol, saturated fat diet was +31 vs +16 mg/dL for the two ethnic groups, respectively. These combined data indicate that the lipoprotein status of the host (affected both by previous and concurrent dietary or longstanding genetic factors) dictates the potential impact of the dietary saturated fat component.

The striking impact of the putative synergy between 16:0 x dietary cholesterol was further elaborated in gerbils by feeding graded intakes of cholesterol in diets rich in 12:0+14:0, 16:0, 18:1, or 18:2 *(39,58)*. Only the 16:0-rich diet elicited a progressive interaction, presumably because 16:0 causes the greatest production of VLDL, which can divert to LDL (or HDL_2 and HDL_3 in gerbils) because the LDL receptors are depressed by cholesterol *(67)*.

6. TRIGLYCERIDE STRUCTURE INFLUENCES FATTY ACID ACTION

Attempts have been made to investigate the cholesterolemic potential of specific saturated fatty acids in humans by enriching the dietary fat with the fatty acid of choice, either by supplementing directly with synthetic triglycerides or by inter-esterifying these specific-fatty acid enriched triglyceride molecules with natural fats. The results may be misleading from a practical point of view because these modified triglycerides appear to render all three trisaturate molecules and their fatty acids (trilaurin, 12:0; trimyristin, 14:0; tripalmitin, 16:0) equally cholesterolemic, i.e., the observed potency of myristic acid as it occurs naturally in triglycerides is reduced whereas the potency of lauric and palmitic acids is raised *(68–70)*. This is especially true if the trimyristin fatty acids are "dispersed" among relatively unsaturated triglycerides by inter-esterification *(31,58)*.

The fact that specific organization of the natural triglyceride probably contributes to the cholesterolemic effect of saturated fat has been hinted at in human studies *(71)*, where randomized butter lowered plasma cholesterol relative to regular butter. This same effect has also been demonstrated extensively in rats *(72)* and most recently in piglets fed from birth for 6 wk on diets with 50%en from fat *(73)*. When a palm oil-rich diet (sn1,3-16:0) in newborn piglets was compared to the same amount of 16:0 from Betapol (sn2-16:0), the plasma cholesterol increased 20% with the Betapol preparation. When a similar study was attempted in adult men and women, no difference in cholesterol was observed *(74)*. However, in the human trial, fat represented only 40% of total energy and the specific fats represented only 70% of total fat intake. Further, the palm oil portion of the fat blend was a solvent-extracted subfraction of crude palm oil, and both fats were prepared as margarine by blending with totally hydrogenated sunflower oil. Thus, the natural fat sources had been modified on the assumption that such modifications would be without effect. More work will be needed in this area before a definitive conclusion can be drawn, but the inference is that age, level of fat in the diet, or relative distribution of other dietary fatty acids situated on the natural triglyceride molecule along with 16:0 may influence the response, all of which makes our understanding of the detailed situation less than definitive.

7. Lp(a) RESPONSE TO FAT CONSUMPTION

An interesting development in the fat-CHD story is the recent report that diets rich in 12:0+14:0 and 16:0, but not 18:0, cause a reduction in the baseline Lp(a) level *(75)*. Only individuals with the highest Lp(a) values were responsive, but these are the persons who appear to be at greatest risk for CHD. Lp(a) is a unique apoprotein found in the LDL fraction of certain individuals that is thought to inhibit fibrinolysis in vivo by virtue of its homology to, and thus competition with, plasminogen. The only other dietary situation known to modulate (in this case, increase) Lp(a) is consumption of *trans*

Table 2
Dietary Fatty Acid Impact on Plasma Cholesterol in Humans: Summary

- 12:0+14:0 > 16:0 ≥ 18:0
- 16:0 ≥ 18:1 ≥ 18:2
- TC decrease with 18:2 appears nonlinear
- 16:0 **x** dietary cholesterol can interact to raise TC
- TC increase with dietary cholesterol appears nonlinear
- Dietary TG structure can influence fatty acid impact on TC
- *Trans* elaidic (t18:1n9) raises LDL, depresses HDL

Table 3
Dietary Recommendations for Cardiovascular Fitness

- Golden rule: maintain body weight (energy balance) at young adult level with BMI of 20–22 kg/Ht m², i.e., "eat less, exercise more."
- Adults keep fat intake <30% of total energy (<33 g/1000 kcal) and SFAs <10%en. Avoid *trans* fatty acid-rich foods and fats
- Derive the major portion of energy from complex carbohydrates in cereal grains, vegetables, and fruits.
- Keep dietary cholesterol <200–300 mg/d or even lower depending on total cholesterol and LDL-cholesterol concentrations.
- Restrict visible fat consumption, especially animal fat sources of saturates and cholesterol (cheese, ice cream, whole milk, fatty meats).
- Assure daily intake of 5%en as 18:2 and 1%en as 18:3 (5 and 1 g/1000 kcal, respectively). Best accomplished with soybean oil- or canola oil-based salad dressing (1 tsp/1000 kcal/d).
- Eat fish at least once per week.
- Consume vitamin E (50 mg) and vitamin C (50 mg) daily as a supplement.

fatty acids, particularly t18:1n9 or elaidic acid, formed during partial hydrogenation of vegetable oils or fish oils *(59,60)*. An underlying theme seems to be that fats (fatty acids) that elevate HDL also depress Lp(a) levels. No relationship has been found between LDL-C and Lp(a), but the correlation between HDL-C and Lp(a), presumably inverse, has never been examined within the data set of a study designed to manipulate lipoproteins by diet. This could be quite revealing, especially since HDL-C, unlike Lp(a), is protective against platelet aggregation and CHD.

8. RECOMMENDATIONS

The evidence concerning diet and chronic disease implies that body weight gain after age 21 should be avoided when possible, especially based on the association among body mass index (BMI), increased serum lipids, and CHD. However, practical reality indicates that this is a difficult assignment in an affluent society where activity levels are reduced and sugar and fat are readily available for consumption.

Having said that, it is also apparent that only approx 50% of the population is genetically prone to experience accelerated CHD risk given the above circumstances of dietary and other environmental insults. Accordingly, one can suggest two approaches, i.e., a general public health recommendation that fits all types or a more specific recommendation for the high-risk subpopulation. In the first instance the recommendation would be to avoid the weight gain readily contributed by dietary fat, in general, with special consideration to dietary fat and cholesterol as outlined in Table 3. The more restricted subpopulation should definitely reduce intake of saturated fat to <10% energy and cholesterol <200 mg/d. In general, the bulk of dietary energy should derive from cereal grains and vegetables with a generous supply of fruit as snack-foods or "treats." In addition, exercise regularly and consume above average amounts of antioxidants such as vitamin E and vitamin C to protect vulnerable lipoprotein lipids (and apolipoproteins) from peroxidation. Also avoid *trans* fatty acids, and consume visible fat only in the form of salad dressing oils. No visible spreads or cheeses should be consumed in the second scenario and milk should be skim or 1% fat only.

REFERENCES

1. Fats and Other Lipids. Diet and Health: Implications for reducing Chronic Disease Risk, National Research Council, Washington, DC, National Academy Press, 1989; 159–258.
2. Coronary Heart Disease. Surgeon's General Report on Nutrition and Health, U.S. Department of Health and Human Services, US Government Printing Office, Washington, DC, 1988; 83–137.
3. Ross R. The pathogenesis of atherosclerosis: a perspective for the 1990s. Nature 1993; 362:801–809.
4. Reaven P, Paarthasarathy S, Grasse BJ, Mille E, Steinberg D, Witztum JL, Effects of oleate-rich and linoleate-rich diets on the susceptibility of low density lipoprotein oxidative modification in mildly hypercholesterolemic subjects. J Clin Invest 1993; 91:668–676.
5. Kinsell LW, Michaels GD, Partridge JW, Boling LA, Balch HE, Cochrane GC. Effect upon serum cholesterol and phospholipids of diets containing large amounts of vegetable fat. J Clin Nutr 1953; 1:231–244.
6. Bronte-Stewart B, Antonis A, Eales L, Brock JF. Effect of feeding different fats on the serum cholesterol level. Lancet 1956; 1:521–527.
7. Turpeinen AM, Alfthan G, Valsta L, Hietanen E, Salonen JT, Schunk H, Nyyssonen K, Mutanen M. Plasma and lipoprotein lipid peroxidation in humans on sunflower and rapeseed oil diets. Lipids 1995; 30:485–492.
8. Suarna, C, Dean, RT, May J, Stocker, R. Human atherosclerotic plaque contains both oxidized lipids and relatively large amounts of α-tocopherol and ascorbate. Arterioscler Thromb Vasc Biol 1995; 15:1616–1624.
9. Siguel EN, Lerman RH. Altered fatty acid metabolism in patients with angiographically documented coronary artery disease. Metabolism 1994; 8:982–993.
10. Kingsbury KJ, Brett C, Stovold R, Chapman A, Anderson J, Morgan DM. Abnormal fatty acid composition and human atherosclerosis. Postgrad Med J 1974; 50:425–440.
11. Rudel LL, Parks JS, Sawyer JK. Compared with dietary monounsaturated and saturated fat, polyunsaturated fat prortects African Green monkeys frm coronary artery atherosclerosis. Arterio Thromb Vasc Biol 1995; 15:2101–2110.
12. Sundram K, Hayes KC, Siru OH. Both dietary 18:2 and 16:0 may be required to improve the serum LDL/HDL cholesterol ratio in normocholesterolemic men. J Nutr Biochem 1995; 6:179–187.
13. Report of the National Cholesterol Education Program (NCEP) Expert Panel on Detection, Evaluation, and Treatment of High Blood Cholesterol in Adults. JAMA 1993; 269:3015–3023.
14. NIH Consensus Panel. Triglyceride, HDL and coronary heart disease. JAMA 1993; 269:505–510.
15. Heiss G, Johnson NJ, Reiland S, Davis CE, Tyroler HA. High-denisty lipoprotein cholesterol levels. The Lipid Research Clinics Program Prevalence Study. Circulation 1980; 62:116s–136s.
16. Gordon DJ, Probstfield JL, Garrison RJ. High-denisty lipoprotein cholesterol and cardiovascular disease. Circulation 1989; 79:8–15.
17. Shepherd J, Cobbe SM, Ford I, Isles CG. Prevention of coronary heart disease with pravastatin in men with hypercholesterolemia 1995. New Engl J Med 1959; 333, 1301–1307.
18. Oliver M, Poole-Wilson P, Shepherd J, Tikkanen MJ. Lower patients' cholesterol now (editorial). Br Med J 1995; 310:1280,1281.
19. Gould KL, Ornish D, Scherwitz L, Brown S, Edens RP, Hess MJ, Mullani N. Changes in myocardial perfusion abnormalities by positron emission tomography after long-term, intense risk factor modificatiom. JAMA 1995; 274,894–901.

20. Dietschy JM, Turley SD, Spady DK. Role of liver in the maintenance of cholesterol and low density lipoprotein homeostasis in different animal species, including humans. J Lipid Res 1993; 34:1637–1659.
21. Katan MB, Beyen AC, de Vries JH, Nobels A. Existence of consistent hypo- and hyper-responders to dietary cholesterol in man. Am J Clin Nutr 1985; 42:190–197.
22. Gylling H, Miettinen TA. Cholesterol absorption and synthesis related to low density lipoprotein metabolism during varying cholesterol intake in men with different apoE phenotypes. J Lipid Res 1992; 33:1361–1371.
23. Botham KM, Bravo E. The role of lipoprotein cholesterol in biliary steroid secretion. Studies with in vivo experimental models. Prog Lipid Res. 1995; 34:71–99.
24. Gylling H, Miettinen TA. The effect of cholesterol absorption inhibition on low density lipoprotein cholesterol level. Atherosclerosis 1995; 117, 305–308.
25. Hopkins PN. Effects of dietary cholesterol on serum cholesterol: a meta-analysis and review. Am J Clin Nutr 1992; 55:1060–1070.
26. Grundy SM, Denke MA. Dietary influence on serum lipids and lipoproteins. J Lipid Res 1990; 31:1149–1172.
27. Nicolosi RJ, Stucchi AF, Kowala MC, Hennessy LK, Hegsted DM, Schaefer EJ. Effect of dietary fat saturation and cholesterol on low density lipoprotein composition and metabolism. In vivo studies of receptor and non-receptor mediated catabolism of LDL in Cebus monkeys. Arteriosclerosis 1990; 10:119–128.
28. Howard BV, Hannah JS, Heiser CC, Jablonski KA, Paidi MC, Alarif L, Robbins DC, Howard WJ. Polyunsaturated fatty acids result in greater cholesterol lowering and less triacylglycerol elevation than do monounsaturated fatty acids in a dose-response comparison in a multiracial study group. Am J Clin Nutr 1995; 62:292–402.
29. Barr SL, Ramakrishnan R, Johnson C, Holleran S, Dell RB, Ginsberg HN. Reducing total dietary fat without reducing saturated fatty acids does not significantly lower plasma cholesterol concentrations in normal males. Am J Clin Nutr 1992; 55:675–681.
30. Hayes KC. Specific dietary fatty acids in predicting plasma cholesterol. Am J Clin Nutr 1993; 57:230,231.
31. Hayes KC, Khosla P. Dietary fatty acid thresholds and cholesterolemia. FASEB J 1992; 6:2600–2607.
32. Nelson GI, Schmidt PC, Kelley DS. Low-fat diets do not lower plasma cholesterol levels in healthy men compared to high-fat diets with similar fatty acid composition at constant caloric intake. Lipids 1995; 30; 969–976.
33. Katan MB, Zock PL, Mensink RP. Dietary oils, serum lipoproteins, and coronary heart disease. Am J Clin Nutr 1995; 61:1368s–1373s.
34. Krauss RM. Dense low density lipoproteins and coronary artery disease. Am J Cardiol 1995; 75:B53–B57.
35. Hegsted DM, Ausman LM, Johnson JA, Dallal GE. Dietary fat and serum lipids: an evaluation of the experimental data. Am J Clin Nutr 1993; 57:875–883.
36. Rimm, EB, Ascherio A, Giovannucci E, Spiegelman D, Stampfer MJ, Willet WC. Vegetable, fruit and cereal fiber intake and risk of coronary heart disease. JAMA 1996; 275:447–451.
37. Keys A, Anderson JT, Grande F. Predication of serum cholesterol response of man to changes in fats in the diet. Lancet 1957; 2:959–966.
38. Hegsted DM, McGandy RB, Meyers ML, Stare FJ. Quantitative effects of dietary fat on serum cholesterol in man. Am J Clin Nutr 1965; 27:281–295.
39. Pronczuk A, Khosla P, Hayes KC. Dietary myristic, palmitic and linoleic acids modulate cholesterolemia in gerbils. FASEB J 1994; 8:1191–1200.
40. Hayes KC, Khosla P, Pronczuk A. A rationale for plasma cholesterol modulation by dietary fatty acids: modulating the human response in animals. J Nutr Biochem 1995; 6:188–194.
41. Baudet MF, Dachet C, Lasserre M, Esteva O, Jacotot B. Modification in the composition and metabolic properties of human LDL and HDL by different fats. J Lipid Res 1984; 25:456–468.
42. Mattson FH, Grundy SM. Comparison of the effects of dietary saturated, monounsaturated, and polyunsaturated fatty acids on plasma lipids and lipoproteins in man. J Lipid Res 1985; 26:194–202.
43. Mensink RP, Katan MB. Effect of a diet enriched with monounsaturated or polyunsaturated fatty acids on levels of low-density and high-density lipoprotein cholesterol in healthy women and men. New Engl J Med 1989; 321:436–441.
44. Berry EM, Eisenberg S, Haratz D, Friedlander Y, Norman Y, Kaufmann NA, Stein Y. Effects of diets rich in monounsaturated fatty acid on plasma lipoproteins—The Jerusalem study: high MUFAs vs. high PUFA. Am J Clin Nutr 1991; 53:899–907.
45. Ghaforunissa, Reddy V, Sesikaran B. Palm olein and groundnut oil have comparable effects on blood lipids and platelet aggregation in healthy Indian subjects. Lipids 1995; 30:1163–1169.

46. Hayes KC, Pronczuk A, Lindsey S, Diersen-Schade D. Dietary saturated fatty acids (12:0,14:0, 16:0) differ in their impact on plasma cholesterol and lipoproteins in nonhuman primates. Am J Clin Nutr 1991; 53:491–498.

47. Sundram K, Hayes KC, Siru OH. Dietary palmitic acid results in a lower serum cholesterol than a lauric-myrsitic acid combination in normolipemic humans. Am J Clin Nutr 1994; 59:841–846.

48. Tholstrup T, Marckmann P, Jespersen J, Sandstrom B. Fat high in stearic acid favorably affects blood lipids and factor VII coagulant activity in comparison with fats high in palmitic acid or high in myristic and lauric acids. Am J Clin Nutr 1994; 59:371–377.

49. Bach AC, Babayan VK. Medium-chain triglycerides: an update. Am J Clin Nutr 1982; 36:950–962.

50. Dougherty RM, Allman MA, Iacono JM. Effects of diets containing high or low amounts of stearic aid on plasma lipoprotein fractions and fecal fatty acid excretion of men. Am J Clin Nutr 1995; 61:1120–1128.

51. Pearson TA. Stearic acid: a unique saturated fatty acid. Am J Clin Nutr 1994; 60:983(s)-1071(s).

52. Vergroesen AJ, Gottenbus JJ. The role of fats in human nutrition: an introduction. In: The Role of Fats in Human Nutrition, 2nd ed. Vergroesen, AJ, Crawford M, eds. New York: Academic, 1975, pp. 1–44.

53. Khosla P, Hayes KC. Comparison between dietary saturated (16:0), monounsaturated (18:1) and polyunsaturated (18:2) fatty acids on plasma lipoprotein metabolism in cebus and rhesus monkeys fed cholesterol-free diets. Am J Clin Nutr 1992; 55:51–62.

54. Ng TKW, Hayes KC, de Witt GF, Jegathesan M, Satgunasingham N, Ong ASH, Tan DTS. Palmitic and oleic acids exert similar effects on serum lipid profile in normocholesterolemic human. J Am Coll Nutr 1992; 11:383–390.

55. Sundram K, Hayes KC, Siru OH. A balance between dietary 18:2 and 16:0 optimizes the serum LDL/HDL cholesterol ratio in normocholesterolemic men. J Nutr Biochem 1995; 6:179–187.

56. Choudry N, Tan L, Truswell AS. Comparison of palmolein and olive oil: effects on plasma lipids and vitamin E in young adults. Am J Clin Nutr 1965; 61:1043–1051.

57. Khosla P, Hayes KC. Dietary palmitic acid raises LDL cholesterol relative to oleic acid only at a high intake of cholesterol. Biochim Biophys Acta 1993; 1210:13–22.

58. Hayes KC. Saturated fats and blood lipids: new slant on an old story. Can J Cardiol 1995; 11:39G–46G.

59. Katan MB, Zock PL, Mensink RP. Trans fatty acids and their effects on lipoproteins in humans. Ann Rev Nutr 1995; 5:473–493.

60. Khosla P, Hayes KC. Dietary trans- monounsaturated fatty acids negatively impact plasma lipids in humans: critical review of the evidence. J Am Coll Nutr 1996; 15:325–339.

61. Willett WC, Ascherio A. Trans fatty acids: Are the effects only marginal? Am J Public Health 1994; 84:722–724.

62. Aro A, Kardinaal AFM, Salminen I, Kark JD, Riemersma RA, Delgado-Rodriguez M, Gomez-Aracena J, Huttunen JK, Kohlmeier L, Martin BC, Martin-Moreno JM, Mazaev VP, Ringstad J, Thamm M, van't Veer P, and Kok FJ. Adipose tissue isomeric trans fatty aids and risk of myocardial infarction in nine countries: the Euramic Study. Lancet, 1995; 345:273–278.

63. Almendingen K, Jordal O, Kierulf P, Sandstad B, Petersen JI. Effects of partially hydrogenated fish oil, partially hydrogenated soybean oil, and butter on serum lipoproteins and Lp(a) in men. J Lipid Res 1995; 36:1370–1384.

64. Sundram K, Anisah I, Hayes KC, Jeyamalara R, Pathmanathan R, Trans-18:1 raises cholesterol more than cis-mono or saturated fats in humans. FASEB J 1995; 9:A440.

65. Schonfeld G, Patsch W, Rudel LL, Nelson C, Epstein M, Olson E. Effects of dietary cholesterol and fatty acids on plasma lipoproteins. J Clin Invest 1982; 9:1072–1080.

66. Fielding CJ, Havel RJ, Todd KM, Yeo KE, Schloetter MC, Weinberg V, Frost PH. Effects of dietary cholesterol and fat saturation on plasma lipoprotein in an ethnically diverse population of healthy young men. J Clin Invest 1995; 95:611–618.

67. Khosla P, Hayes KC. Dietary fat saturation in rhesus monkeys affects LDL concentrations by modulating the independent production of LDL apolipoprotein B. Biochem Biophys Acta 1991; 1083:46–56.

68. McGandy RB, Hegsted DM, Meyers ML. Use of semisynthetic fats in determining the effects of specific fatty acids on serum lipids in man. Am J Clin Nutr 1970; 23:1288–1298.

69. Zock PL, De Vries JHM, Katan MB. Impact of myristic acid versus palmitic acid on serum lipid and lipoprotein levels in healthy women and men. Arterioscler Thromb 1994; 14:567–575.

70. Tholstrup T, Marckman P, Jespersen J, Vessby B, Jart A, Sandstrom B. Effect on blood lipids, coagulation and fibrinolysis of a fat high in myrisitc acid and a fat high in palmitic acid. Am J Clin Nutr 1994; 60:919–925.

71. Christophe A, Matthys F, Geers R, Verdonk G. Nutritional studies with randomized butter. Cholesterolemic effects of butter-oil and randomized butter-oil in man. Arch Internat Physiol Biochim 1978; 86:414,415.
72. Mukherjee S, Sengrupa S. Serum cholesterol lowering effects of butterfats nteresterified with edible oils with or without polyunsaturated acids. Proc 13th World Cong. Intl Soc Fat Res 1976; 23–39.
73. Innis SM, Quinlan P, Diersen-Schade D. Saturated fatty acid chain length and positional distribution in infant formulas: effects on growth and plasma lipids and ketones in piglets. Am J Clin Nutr 1993; 57:382–90.
74. Zock PL, De Vries JHM, de Fauro NJ, Katan MB. Positional distribution of fatty acids in dietary triglycerides: effects on fasting blood lipoprotein concentrations in humans. Am J Clin Nutr 1995; 61:48–55.
75. Tholstrup T, Marckmann P, Vessby B, Sandstrom B. Effect of fats high in individual saturated fatty acids on plasma lipoprotein (a) levels in young healthy men. J Lipid Res 1995; 36:1447–1452.

9 Antioxidant Vitamins and Cardiovascular Disease

Julie E. Buring and J. Michael Gaziano

1. INTRODUCTION

The hypothesis that antioxidant vitamins may reduce risks of cardiovascular disease has been the subject of considerable research attention in recent years. Basic research studies have provided evidence of possible mechanisms for an effect of antioxidants on atherosclerosis, and several observational epidemiologic studies have suggested that risk of coronary heart disease (CHD) may be 20–40% lower among those with high dietary intake or serum levels of antioxidant vitamins. CHD remains the leading cause of death in the United States, as well as most developed countries, accounting for approximately one of every four deaths. For this reason, even the modest reductions in CHD risk suggested by studies to date, if real, could yield substantial public health benefits. At present, however, available data remain inadequate to draw firm conclusions regarding the possible role of antioxidant vitamins in the prevention of cardiovascular disease. This chapter reviews the evidence on antioxidants and cardiovascular disease, discusses its strengths and limitations, and summarizes the trials now ongoing.

2. POSTULATED MECHANISM

Although elevated levels of low-density lipoprotein (LDL) cholesterol have been clearly established as a risk factor for CHD, the precise mechanisms for such an effect are only now being elucidated. An accumulating body of research supports the hypothesis that oxidative damage to LDL cholesterol greatly enhances its atherogenicity *(1)*. In basic research, oxidized LDL has been shown to accelerate several steps in atherosclerosis, including endothelial damage, monocyte/macrophage recruitment, increased uptake of LDL by foam cells, alteration in vascular tone, induction of growth factors, as well as formation of autoantibodies to oxidized LDL *(2)*. These basic research findings have raised the possibility that agents with antioxidant properties—including the dietary antioxidants β-carotene, vitamin E, and vitamin C—might play a role in reducing risks of cardiovascular disease

3. ANIMAL STUDIES

Evidence from several animal studies supports the hypothesis that antioxidants can delay the progression of atherosclerosis. Three such studies have demonstrated decreased formation of atheromatous lesions in animals fed vitamin E compared to con-

From: *Preventive Nutrition: The Comprehensive Guide for Health Professionals*
Edited by A. Bendich and R. J. Deckelbaum Humana Press Inc., Totowa, NJ

trols. One study utilized restricted anovulatory hens, who are prone to hyperlipidemia and subsequent aortic intimal thickening. When fed 1000 mg of vitamin E per kilogram of feed, such hens had reduced levels of plasma peroxides and less aortic intimal thickening compared to controls (3). In a study among hypercholesterolemic mongrel rabbits, those fed 10 mg of vitamin E per kilogram body weight per day experienced a reduction in aortic atherosclerotic lesions compared to controls (4). Finally, in a study of monkeys fed an atherogenic diet, a reduction in carotid ultrasound stenosis was reported among those receiving 108 IU of vitamin E per day compared to controls (5). This reduction was observed among monkeys who received vitamin E prophylactically beginning at the start of the trial and among those administered vitamin E therapeutically after atherosclerosis was established. With respect to vitamin C, dietary deficiency in this vitamin has been reported to promote atherosclerotic lesion formation in guinea pigs (6), and later studies in deficient guinea pigs suggested that administration of vitamin C can lead to regression of early atherosclerotic lesions (7).

Several studies have tested probucol, a cholesterol-lowering agent that also has strong antioxidant properties. One experiment, in Watanabe heritable hyperlipidemic rabbits, controlled for the cholesterol-lowering actions of probucol by giving the cholesterol-lowering drug lovastatin to one of two control groups (8). The probucol group experienced a lower rate of fatty streak formation than the lovastatin-treated group, suggesting that probucol's benefit may, in part, derive from its antioxidant effects. In regard to β-carotene, few animal studies have tested its effects on atherosclerosis development.

4. DESCRIPTIVE STUDIES

Descriptive epidemiologic studies, which assess exposure and disease levels among population groups, also provide some support for the antioxidant vitamin-cardiovascular disease hypothesis, although the findings are not entirely consistent. Two studies in Great Britain found significant inverse relationships between consumption of fresh fruits and vegetables and atherosclerotic disease rates (9,10). Studies in Europe have reported inverse associations between plasma vitamin E levels standardized to plasma cholesterol levels and cardiovascular disease mortality rates (11,12). The findings for selenium and vitamin A were less consistent. In a cross-sectional survey among Finnish men, no association was found between plasma levels of vitamin C or E and prevalent ischemic heart disease (13). Finally, in another plasma study in Europe, a trend for lower heart disease mortality with higher vitamin E levels was seen, but no consistent findings were observed for plasma vitamins A and C (14). Thus, the findings from some, but not all, descriptive studies are suggestive of a correlation between dietary intake or plasma levels of antioxidant vitamins and cardiovascular disease rates.

5. ANALYTIC OBSERVATIONAL STUDIES

The antioxidant vitamin-cardiovascular disease hypothesis has recently been explored in several analytic observational studies, including the Nurses' Health Study, the Massachusetts Elderly Cohort Study, the Health Professionals Follow-up Study, the First National Health and Nutrition Examination Survey (NHANES I), and the Iowa Women's Health Study. It has also been evaluated in three prospective blood-based investigations. Because these studies collect exposure and disease information from individuals and follow them for subsequent development of disease, to the extent that they also collect data on potential confounding variables they can provide a more reliable assessment than descriptive studies of the possible role of antioxidant vitamins in cardiovascular disease prevention.

5.1. Dietary Intake Studies

The largest analytic observational study to evaluate antioxidant vitamins and cardiovascular disease is the Nurses' Health Study, a prospective cohort of 121,700 US female nurses, aged 30–55 at entry, established in 1976. In dietary intake studies, subjects are typically divided into quartiles or quintiles based on their intake of the variable being assessed, and subsequent rate of disease occurrence in the highest intake category is then compared to that in the lowest. The Nurses' Health Study used dietary intake data provided on a semiquantitative food frequency questionnaire to estimate the actual intake of antioxidant vitamins. The analyses were based on 552 incident cases of CHD (nonfatal myocardial infarction [MI] + fatal CHD) occurring over an 8-yr period. For β-carotene, the relative risk for those in the highest β-carotene intake quintile compared with the lowest was 0.78, a 22% reduction in risk, with a significant p value for trend of 0.02 *(15)*. For vitamin E, the relative risk was 0.66, with a p-trend <0.001. However, when vitamin E intake was examined separately from diet and supplements, the observed association was almost entirely a result of use of supplements. For vitamin C, the relative risk was 0.80, but there was no clear trend across intake quintiles, with a p of 0.15 *(16)*. All these estimates were adjusted for age, smoking, and a number of other cardiovascular disease risk factors.

A similar study was conducted among 51,529 US male health professionals, aged 40–75 at baseline in 1986. In the Health Professionals Follow-up Study, after adjusting for age, smoking, and other cardiovascular risk factors, the relative risk of CHD (non-fatal MI + fatal CHD) for those in the highest β-carotene intake quintile was 0.71 (p-trend = 0.03) *(17)*. For vitamin E, the relative risk was 0.60 (p-trend = 0.01). Although the relation was strongest for vitamin E supplement users, an association of borderline significance was still apparent for dietary vitamin E intake alone. Vitamin C intake appeared unrelated to risk of CHD.

A smaller cohort study among 1299 elderly Massachusetts residents evaluated the association between dietary β-carotene intake and subsequent cardiovascular disease mortality. In this study, after an average follow-up of 4.75 yr, those in the highest β-carotene intake quartile had a relative risk of cardiovascular death of 0.57 compared with those in the lowest intake category (p-trend = 0.016) *(18)*. For fatal MI the corresponding relative risk was 0.32, with a p value for trend of 0.02.

The NHANES I evaluated vitamin C intake among 11,348 US adults, aged 25–74, whose mortality experience was followed for a median of 10 yr and compared to that expected based on rates among US whites *(19)*. Among those with the highest vitamin C intake from diet and supplements, the standardized mortality ratio for cardiovascular death was 0.66 (95% confidence interval [CI] 0.53–0.83). The inverse relation of vitamin C from diet alone was of borderline statistical significance, so the overall association appeared to be explained by supplement use. One limitation of this report is that the study did not take into account use of other supplements, which, in other studies, was highly correlated with use of vitamin C.

Finally, the Iowa Women's Health Study evaluated the association between antioxidant vitamin intake and CHD mortality among 34,486 postmenopausal women with no history of cardiovascular disease. Based on approx 7 yr of follow-up, there was an inverse relation of dietary vitamin E intake with CHD mortality among the subgroup of women who did not report any use of vitamin supplements, with those in the highest quintile of dietary vitamin E intake experiencing a relative risk of 0.38 in relation to those in the lowest intake quintile (*p*-trend = 0.004) *(20)*. Vitamin E supplement use, however, was not associated with a lower risk of CHD death, a finding in contrast to the Nurses' Health Study and Health Professionals Follow-up Study, both of which found the most pronounced inverse association among supplement users. Intake of vitamin A, carotenoids, and vitamin C in the Iowa study did not appear to be associated with risk of CHD death.

5.2. Blood-Based Studies

Three blood-based studies have been conducted as nested case-control studies within larger prospective cohort investigations. A Finnish study found no significant association between serum vitamins A and E in frozen samples and subsequent coronary heart disease mortality *(21)*. Another study also reported no association between baseline levels of serum vitamins A and E and subsequent cardiovascular mortality *(22)*. Both of these studies, however, stored samples at −20°C, a temperature at which antioxidant vitamin levels may not remain stable over time. A third study reported a significant inverse association between serum β-carotene in frozen samples and subsequent risk of myocardial infarction *(23)*.

5.3. Limitations of Analytic Observational Studies

Although the data from these analytic observational studies, both prospective dietary intake and blood-based, are compatible with possible cardiovascular benefits of antioxidant vitamins, observational studies are unable to control for potential effects of unknown or unmeasured confounding variables that may explain all or part of any observed associations. It may be, for example, that greater dietary intake of antioxidant vitamins, measured by a diet assessment questionnaire or blood levels, is only a marker for some other dietary practices that are truly protective. It is certainly plausible that intake of antioxidant-rich foods is indeed protective, but that the benefits may result not from their antioxidant properties, but other components these foods have in common. It is also possible that intake of antioxidant vitamins from food or supplements is correlated with other unmeasured or unknown nondietary lifestyle behaviors. Thus, when searching for small to moderate-sized effects—as is the case with antioxidant vitamins and cardiovascular disease—the amount of uncontrolled confounding in all observational studies is likely to be as large as the most plausible alternative hypothesis *(24)*.

Because of these limitations inherent in all observational studies, only randomized trials of sufficient sample size, dose and duration of treatment and follow-up can address conclusively whether antioxidant vitamins actually decrease cardiovascular disease risk. Such a conclusion was reached in 1991 by a consensus conference convened by the National Heart, Lung, and Blood Institute, which supported the need for randomized clinical trials of β-carotene, vitamin E, and/or vitamin C in primary and secondary prevention of cardiovascular disease *(25)*.

6. RANDOMIZED TRIALS

To date, no large-scale randomized trials have been completed that were designed specifically to test antioxidant vitamins in the primary prevention of cardiovascular disease. However, four completed trials that were designed to test antioxidant vitamins in cancer prevention also assessed the relationship of antioxidant vitamin supplementation to cardiovascular disease outcomes.

The Chinese Cancer Prevention Study evaluated antioxidant and other micronutrient supplements among 29,584 residents of four communities in Linxian, a rural county in north-central China. This region suffers from one of the world's highest rates of esophageal and gastric cancer, and dietary intake of several micronutrients is very low. Nine different agents were tested in the trial (retinol, zinc, riboflavin, niacin, vitamin C, molybdenum, β-carotene, vitamin E, and selenium), with participants assigned at random to one of eight different vitamin/mineral supplement combinations. Subjects receiving the combined daily treatment of β-carotene (15 mg), vitamin E (30 mg), and selenium (50 μg) experienced a 10% decrease in cerebrovascular mortality compared with those not receiving this treatment (relative risk = 0.90; 95% CI, 0.76–1.07) *(26)*. Since CHD is rare in this population, it could not be evaluated. In the primary analyses concerning cancer, those assigned to combine treatment with β-carotene, vitamin E, and selenium experienced a 13% decrease in total cancer mortality (relative risk = 0.87; 95% CI, 0.75–1.00) and a significant 21% decrease in gastric cancer deaths (relative risk = 0.79; 95% CI, 0.64–0.99). For total mortality, there was a 9% decrease among those assigned to this regimen (relative risk = 0.91; 95% CI, 0.84–0.99). Because the agents in this trial were evaluated in combined regimens, it was not possible to distinguish the separate effects of any one supplement. Moreover, it is possible that supplementation with these agents may have different effects in poorly nourished individuals than among those with adequate dietary intake of micronutrients.

The Alpha-Tocopherol, Beta Carotene (ATBC) Cancer Prevention Study evaluated vitamin E (50 mg daily) and β-carotene (20 mg daily) in a 2×2 factorial design among 29,133 male smokers in Finland, aged 50–69. After 6 yr of treatment, there was no apparent benefit of either agent on cardiovascular outcomes. Those assigned to β-carotene, in fact, experienced an 8% increase in total mortality, primarily because there were more deaths from lung cancer and ischemic heart disease *(27)*. For vitamin E, there was an increase in deaths caused by cerebral hemorrhage. Regarding lung cancer, the primary trial endpoint, there was no benefit of either agent, and unexpectedly, a significant 18% increase in the β-carotene group. For vitamin E, a potential issue in the interpretation of the ATBC trial results was the low dose, which, at 50 mg/d, is considerably lower than the levels mainly associated with reducing cardiovascular disease risk in observational studies discussed above. Nevertheless, the ATBC findings were in clear contrast to the accumulating body of observational evidence, which indicated possible benefits of both vitamin E and β-carotene. The results suggested that some of the apparent benefits seen in observational studies may have been overestimates, or even that these agents may have harmful effects not previously observed or even postulated *(28)*.

The Beta-Carotene and Retinol Efficacy Trial (CARET) randomized 18,314 men and women at high risk for lung cancer because of cigarette smoking history or occupational asbestos exposure to daily treatment with a combined supplement containing β-carotene (30 mg) and vitamin A (25,000 IU retinyl palmitate) or placebo. The trial was terminated early, after approx 4 yr of treatment, based primarily on interim data analyses suggesting it was unlikely any material benefits would emerge with continuation to its scheduled termination, but also because of emerging data compatible with the ATBC trial findings. Specifically, there was a nonsignificant 26% increase in cardiovascular disease mortality among those assigned the supplement combination (relative risk = 1.26; 95% CI, 0.99–1.61, $p = 0.06$) (29). There was a statistically significant 28% increased risk of lung cancer in the treated group (relative risk = 1.28; 95% CI, 1.04–1.57, $p = 0.02$) and a significant 17% increase in total mortality (relative risk = 1.17; 95% CI, 1.03–1.33, $p = 0.02$). It is important to note, however, that the prespecified stopping boundary for early termination of the trial ($p = 0.007$) was not reached for any of these endpoints, and the finding for cardiovascular disease mortality did not even reach conventional statistical significance at the $p = 0.05$ level. In addition, as with the Chinese Cancer Prevention Study, independent effects of the study interventions could not be established because the study agents were given as a combined regimen.

The Physicians' Health Study (PHS) randomized 22,071 US male physicians to alternate day β-carotene (50 mg), aspirin (325 mg), both active treatments, or both placebos. The aspirin component was terminated early, in 1988, because of the emergence of a statistically significant 44% reduction in risk of a first myocardial infarction among participants assigned to aspirin (30). Regarding β-carotene, after approx 12 yr of treatment and follow-up, which is twice the length of any other trial, there was no significant evidence of any effect of β-carotene supplementation—either beneficial or harmful—on risk of individual cardiovascular disease outcomes or on a combined endpoint consisting of nonfatal myocardial infarction, nonfatal stroke, and total cardiovascular death (31). The relative risks in the β-carotene group were 0.96 for total myocardial infarction (95% CI, 0.84–1.09), 0.96 for total stroke (95% CI, 0.83–1.11), 1.09 for total cardiovascular death (95% CI, 0.93–1.27), and 1.0 for the composite endpoint (95% CI, 0.91–1.08). There was also no significant effect of β-carotene on total cancer incidence (relative risk = 0.98, 95% CI, 0.91–1.06). Among the 11% of participants who were smokers at baseline, there was no significant benefit or harm, although small absolute effects could not be ruled out in this subgroup. Because the PHS has lasted far longer than any other trial of β-carotene, its findings of no significant benefit or harm in this general population are particularly reliable, and exclude the possibility of even small overall benefits or harm with a high degree of assurance. Regarding randomized trial data in secondary prevention or among high-risk patients, for β-carotene, a subgroup analysis of the PHS restricted to the 333 physicians who entered the trial with chronic stable angina or a prior coronary revascularization procedure indicated a possible reduction in vascular disease events among those allocated to β-carotene (32).

For vitamin E, three trials with small samples have reported benefits among patients with claudication (33–35). A fourth trial among patients with angina found no effect of vitamin E, but its 6-mo treatment period may have been inadequate to observe an effect (36). The largest completed trial of antioxidants in secondary prevention is the Cambridge Heart Antioxidant Study (CHAOS), which randomized 2002 men and women with angiographically proven atherosclerosis to vitamin E (400 or 800 IU daily) or placebo for a median treatment duration of 1.4 yr (37). There was a significant benefit associated with vitamin E on the primary trial endpoint of nonfatal myocardial infarction plus cardiovascular death (relative risk = 0.53; 95% CI, 0.34–0.83). This benefit, however, was caused entirely by a significant 77% reduction in nonfatal myocardial infarction (relative risk = 0.23; 95% CI, 0.11–0.47). There was, in fact, a nonsignificant increased risk of cardiovascular death in the vitamin E group (relative risk = 1.18; 95% CI, 0.62–2.27).

7. CONCLUSION

Regarding β-carotene, the totality of evidence now available from large-scale randomized trials indicates that supplementation with this antioxidant appears to confer no material benefit among well-nourished populations in the primary prevention of cardiovascular disease. It remains possible, however, that β-carotene supplementation is beneficial among subgroups at high-risk because of prior CHD or those with low blood levels of antioxidants. Whether there is a true hazard of β-carotene supplementation among current cigarette smokers, as raised by the ATBC and CARET trials, will be evaluated by a collaborative overview of the post-publication results of continued follow-up in all completed trials of β-carotene. If the apparent excess risk observed in those trials is in fact real, it should persist with longer follow-up. Conversely, if, as is still possible, there is eventually some benefit from β-carotene supplementation, then this too may emerge with longer follow-up. A common protocol for a collaborative analysis of the post-publication results of all the β-carotene trials is therefore being devised, with the first analyses planned for sometime around the year 2000. This will provide the most reliable evidence on whether the long-term effects are favorable, unfavorable, or null.

For vitamin E, the ATBC trial showed no evidence of benefit on ischemic heart disease, but the CHAOS study among patients with documented atherosclerosis suggested benefits on subsequent nonfatal myocardial infarction. With respect to vitamin C, there are no completed trials of this agent alone.

Several large-scale trials are now ongoing that will provide reliable answers concerning antioxidant vitamins in the prevention and treatment of cardiovascular disease. In primary prevention, the PHS will continue randomized treatment with β-carotene in order to provide more reliable evidence on this agent. Utilizing a factorial design, the trial will also add vitamin E (600 IU on alternate days), vitamin C (500 mg daily), and a multivitamin in order to also evaluate the effects of these agents on cardiovascular disease as well as cancer. The Women's Health Study is assessing the benefits and risks of vitamin E supplementation (600 IU on alternate days) as well as low-dose aspirin (100 mg on alternate days) among 39,876 apparently healthy US female health professionals, aged 45 and older *(38)*.

With respect to trials in secondary prevention or among high-risk populations, the Women's Antioxidant Cardiovascular Study will evaluate β-carotene (50 mg on alternate days), vitamin E (600 IU on alternate days), and vitamin C (500 mg daily) among approx 8000 US female health professionals, aged 45 and older, who are at high risk because of a prior cardiovascular disease event or the presence of three or more significant coronary risk factors *(39)*. The Heart Outcomes Prevention Evaluation (HOPE) Study is testing vitamin E (400 IU daily) and an angiotensin converting enzyme (ACE) inhibiting drug among 9000 high-risk patients in Canada *(40)*, whereas the Heart Protection Study is testing a daily cocktail of vitamin C (250 mg), vitamin E (600 mg), and β-carotene (20 mg) as well as the cholesterol-lowering drug simvastatin among 20,000 high-risk patients in the United Kingdom *(41)*. Finally, in Italy, the GISSI Prevention Trial is evaluating vitamin E (300 mg daily) and fish oil supplements among 11,000 patients with a recent myocardial infarction *(41)*.

In summary, currently available data raise the possibility that antioxidant vitamins may decrease risks of cardiovascular disease. For β-carotene, however, large-scale randomized trials have not supported a benefit of this supplement among a general, well-nourished population. For other antioxidants, such as vitamin E, as well as for β-carotene among high-risk subjects, additional data are needed from large-scale randomized trials of sufficient sample size, dose, and duration of treatment and follow-up. Several such trials are now ongoing, and their results will contribute reliable data to a totality of evidence on antioxidant vitamins that will permit appropriate clinical recommendations for individual patients as well as rational public health policy for the population as a whole.

RECOMMENDATIONS

With regard to current recommendations concerning vitamin supplement use, there is insufficient evidence for a public health recommendation to use antioxidant vitamins to prevent cardiovascular disease. In contrast, with respect to dietary intake recommendations, increased intake of antioxidant-rich fruits and vegetables would appear to be part of an overall sound dietary program, because such foods provide a range of nutritional benefits beyond any potential effects of antioxidants, and their increased intake may even yield indirect benefits simply by substituting for consumption of high-fat foods. Finally, even if currently ongoing studies demonstrate a net benefit of antioxidant vitamins on cardiovascular disease risk, the use of vitamin supplements—or even increased intake of such agents through dietary change—should always be an adjunct, not alternative, to other measures with demonstrated efficacy in reducing risks of cardiovascular disease. Such known risk modifiers include smoking cessation, control of high blood pressure and elevated cholesterol, avoidance of obesity, and increased physical activity.

REFERENCES

1. Steinberg D, Parthasarathy S, Carew TE, Khoo JC, Witztum JL. Beyond cholesterol: modifications of low-density lipoprotein that increase its atherogenicity. New Engl J Med 1989; 320:915–924.
2. Gaziano JM, Manson JE, Buring JE, Hennekens CH. Dietary antioxidants and cardiovascular disease. NY Acad Sci 1992; 669:249–259.
3. Smith TL, Kummerow FA. Effect of dietary vitamin E on plasma lipids and atherogenesis in restricted anovulatory chickens. Atherosclerosis 1989; 75:105–109.
4. Wojcicki J, Rozewicka L, Barcew-Wiszniewska B, Samochowiec L, Juzwiak S, Kadlubowska D, Tustanowski S, Juzyszyn Z. Effect of selenium and vitamin E on the development of experimental atherosclerosis in rabbits. Atherosclerosis 1991; 87:9–19.
5. Verlangieri AJ, Bush M. Prevention and regression of atherosclerosis by alpha-tocopherol. J Am Coll Nutr 1992; 11:131–138.
6. Willis GC. An experimental study of the intimal ground substance in atherosclerosis. Can Med Assoc J 1953; 69:17–22.
7. Willis GC. The reversibility of atherosclerosis. Can Med Assoc J 1957; 77:106–109.
8. Carew T, Schwenke D, Steinberg D. Antiatherogenic effect of probucol unrelated to its hypercholesterolemic effect: evidence that antioxidants *in vivo* can selectively inhibit low density lipoprotein degrada-

tion in macrophage-rich fatty streaks and slow the progression of atherosclerosis in the Watanabe heritable hypercholesterolemic rabbits. Proc Natl Acad Sci USA 1987; 84:7725–7729.

9. Acheson RM, Williams DRR. Does consumption of fruit and vegetables protect against stroke? Lancet 1983; 1:1191–1193.
10. Armstrong BK, Mann JL, Adelstein AM, Eskin F. Commodity consumption and ischemic heart disease mortality, with special reference to dietary practices. J Chronic Dis 1975; 36:673–677.
11. Gey KF, Brubacher GB, Stahelin HB. Plasma levels of antioxidant vitamins in relation to ischemic heart disease and cancer. Am J Clin Nutr 1987; 45:1368–1377.
12. Gey KF, Puska P. Plasma vitamins E and A inversely correlated to mortality from ischemic heart disease in cross-cultural epidemiology. Ann NY Acad Sci 1989; 570:268–282.
13. Salonen JT, Solonen R, Seppanen K, Kantola M, Parviainen M, Alfthan G, Maenpaa PH, Taskinen E, Rauramaa R. Relationship of serum selenium and antioxidants to plasma lipoproteins, platelet aggregability and prevalent ischemic heart disease in eastern Finnish men. Atherosclerosis 1988; 70:155–160.
14. Riemersma RA, Oliver M, Elton RA, Alfthan G, Vartiainen E, Salo M, Rubba P, Mancici M, Georgi H, Vuilleumier J-P, Gey KF. Plasma antioxidants and coronary heart disease: vitamins C and E, and selenium. Eur J Clin Nutr 1990; 44:143–150.
15. Stampfer MJ, Hennekens CH, Manson JE, Colditz GA, Rosner B, Willett WC. Vitamin E consumption and the risk of coronary disease in women. New Engl J Med 1993; 328:1444–1449.
16. Manson JE, Stampfer MJ, Willett WC, Colditz GA, Rosner B, Speizer FE, Hennekens CH. A prospective study of vitamin C and incidence of coronary heart disease in women. Circulation 1992; 85:865 (abstract).
17. Rimm EB, Stampfer MJ, Ascherio A, Giovannucci E, Colditz GA, Willett WC. Vitamin E consumption and the risk of coronary heart disease in men. New Engl J Med 1993; 328:1450–1456.
18. Gaziano JM, Branch LG, Manson JE, Colditz GA, Willett WC, Buring JE, Hennekens CH. A prospective study of beta-carotene in fruits and vegetables and decreased cardiovascular mortality in the elderly. Ann Epidemiol 1995; 5:255–260.
19. Enstrom JE, Kanim LE, Klein MA. Vitamin C intake and mortality among a sample of the United States population. Epidemiol 1992; 3:194–202.
20. Kushi LH, Folsom AR, Prineas RJ, Mink PJ, Wu Y, Bostick RM, Dietary antioxidant vitamins and death from coronary heart disease in women, New Engl J Med 1996; 334:1156–1162.
21. Salonen JT, Salonen R, Penttila I, Herranen J, Jauhiainen M, Kantola M, Lappetelainen R, Maenpaa P, Alfthan G, Puska P. Serum fatty acids, apolipoproteins, selenium and vitamin antioxidants and risk of death from coronary artery disease. Am J Cardiol 1985; 56:226–231.
22. Kok FJ, de Bruijn AM, Vermeeren R, Hofman A, VanLaar A, deBruin M, Hermus RJT, Valkenberg HA. Serum selenium, vitamin antioxidants and cardiovascular mortality: a 9 year follow-up study in the Netherlands. Am J Clin Nutr 1987; 45:462–468.
23. Street DA, Comstock GW, Salkeld RM, Schuep W, Klag M. A population based case-control study of serum antioxidants and myocardial infarction. Am J Epidemiol 1991; 134:719, 720.
24. Hennekens CH, Buring JE. Epidemiology in Medicine. Boston: Little, Brown and Company, 1987.
25. Steinberg D and workshop participants. Antioxidants in the prevention of human atherosclerosis: summary proceedings of a National Heart, Lung, and Blood Institute Workshop: September 5–6, 1991; Bethesda, MD. Circulation 1992; 85:2337–2347.
26. Blot WJ, Li J-Y, Taylor PR, Guo W, Dawsey S, Wang GQ, Yang CS, Zheng SF, Gail M, Li GY, Yu Y, Liu BQ, Tangrea J, Sun YH, Liu F, Fraumeni JF, Zhang YH, Li B. Nutrition intervention trials in Linxian, China: supplementation with specific vitamin/mineral combinations, cancer incidence, and disease-specific mortality in the general population. J Natl Cancer Inst 1993; 85:1483–1492.
27. Alpha-Tocopherol, Beta Carotene Cancer Prevention Study Group. The effect of vitamin E and beta carotene on the incidence of lung cancer and other cancers in male smokers. New Engl J Med 1994; 330:1029–1035.
28. Hennekens CH, Buring JE, Peto R. Antioxidant vitamins—benefits not yet proved. New Engl J Med 1994; 330:1080, 1081.
29. Omenn GS, Goodman GE, Thornquist MD, Balmes J, Cullen MR, Glass A, Keough JP, Meyskens FL Jr., Valanis B, Williams JH Jr., Barnhart S, Hammar S. Effects of a combination of beta carotene and vitamin A on lung cancer and cardiovascular disease. New Engl J Med 1996; 334:1150–1155.
30. Steering Committee of the Physicians' Health Study Research Group. Final report on the aspirin component of the ongoing Physicians' Health Study. New Engl J Med 1989; 321:129–135.
31. Hennekens CH, Buring JE, Manson, JE, Stampfer MJ, Rosner B, Cook NR, Belanger C, LaMotte F, Gaziano JM, Ridker PM, Willett W, Peto R. Lack of effect of long-term supplementation with beta-carotene

on the incidence of malignant neoplasms and cardiovascular disease. New Engl J Med 1996; 334: 1145–1149.

32. Gaziano JM, Manson JE, Ridker PM, Buring JE, Hennekens CH. Beta carotene therapy for chronic stable angina (abstract). Circulation 1990; 82(4, Suppl III):III–202.

33. Livingston PD, Jones C. Treatment of intermittent claudication with vitamin E. Lancet 1958; 2:602–604.

34. Williams HTG, Fenna D, MacBeth RA. Alpha-tocopherol in the treatment of intermittent claudication. Surg Gynecol Obstet 1971; 132:662–666.

35. Haeger K. Long-time treatment of intermittent claudication with vitamin E. Am J Clin Nutr 1974; 427:1179–1181.

36. Gillilan RE, Mandell B, Warbassee JR. Quantitative evaluation of vitamin E in the treatment of angina pectoris. Am Heart J 1988; 93:444–449.

37. Stephens NG, Parsons A, Schofield PM, Kelly F, Cheeseman K, Mitchinson MJ, Brown MJ. Randomised controlled trial of vitamin E in patients with coronary disease: Cambridge Heart Antioxidant Study (CHAOS). Lancet 1996; 347:781–786.

38. Buring JE, Hennekens CH, for the Women's Health Study Research Group. The Women's Health Study: summary of the study design. J Myocardial Ischemia 1992; 4:27–29.

39. Manson JE, Gaziano JM, Spelsberg A, Ridker PM, Buring JE, Willett WC, Hennekens CH. A secondary prevention trial of antioxidant vitamins and cardiovascular disease in women: rationale, design and methods. Ann Epidemiol 1985; 5:261–265.

40. The HOPE Study Investigators. The HOPE (Heart Outcomes Prevention Evaluation) Study. The design of a large, simple randomized trial of an angiotensin-converting enzyme inhibitor (ramipril) and vitamin E in patients at high risk of cardiovascular events. Can J Cardiol 1996; 12:127–137.

41. Jha P, Flather M, Lonn E, Farkouh M, Yusuf S. The antioxidant vitamins and cardiovascular disease. A critical review of epidemiologic and clinical trial data. Ann Intern Med 1995; 123:860–872.

10 Iron and Heart Disease

A Review of The Epidemiologic Data

Christopher T. Sempos, Richard F. Gillum, and Anne Condon Looker

1. INTRODUCTION

In 1981 Jerome Sullivan *(1)* proposed a new theory to explain the differences in coronary heart disease (CHD) incidence and mortality between men and women. He noticed that as men and women age the gaps between them in heart disease incidence and in body iron stores both decrease *(2,3)*. Lower stores of iron levels in women are mostly a result of menstrual blood loss and with menopause the differences in iron stores decrease. As a result, he theorized that body iron stores are directly or positively related to CHD risk, i.e., the higher your body iron stores the greater your CHD risk. Until the publication of results from Finland by Salonen et al. *(4)* showing a positive relationship between serum ferritin levels, a measure of body iron stores, and the risk of heart attack in men the hypothesis was largely ignored. Since then, however, there has been an almost explosive interest in the relationship of body iron stores to the risk of heart disease.

Apart from Dr. Sullivan's theory, interest in the relationship between iron and heart disease has been building slowly over the years stemming from several separate lines of research. Many of the early epidemiologic studies looking at heart disease found a correlation between hemoglobin or hematocrit and risk of heart disease *(5–8)*. However, others did not *(9–12)*. At the same time, cancer research was showing a link between fruit and vegetable intake and risk of cancer *(13,14)*. This line of research lead, in part, to the development of the antioxidant theory of disease prevention *(15)*. At the same time several researchers have reported that risk of cancer may be associated with higher levels of body iron stores *(16–23)*. The result is that research on the effects of antioxidant nutrients on heart disease risk *(24–25)* as well as research on the importance of LDL oxidation in the development of atherosclerosis *(26,27)*, iron in myocardial reperfusion injury *(28,29)*, and the publication of Salonen et al. have merged antioxidant research with research on iron's possible role in promoting tissue-damaging oxidation.

The purpose of this chapter is to examine the recent epidemiologic data that are directly related to Dr. Sullivan's hypothesis. Important related topics, e.g., the relationship of antioxidant nutrients, oral contraceptives, estrogen replacement therapy, and menopause to CHD risk, and iron and myocardial reperfusion injury are not discussed (*see* Chapter 9).

From: *Preventive Nutrition: The Comprehensive Guide for Health Professionals*
Edited by A. Bendich and R. J. Deckelbaum Humana Press Inc., Totowa, NJ

Table 1
Geometric[a] Mean Serum Ferritin by Serum Transferrin Saturation Level[b]

Transferrin saturation, %[c]	Men		Women	
	N	Ferritin, (µg/L)	N	Ferritin, (µg/L)
<16%	98	74	107	38
16–19%	99	94	128	54
20–29%	334	94	403	62
30–44%	269	111	195	70
45–59%	39	105	20	89
≥60%	5	231	9	285

[a]Within in each transferrin saturation group the serum ferritin data was transformed using natural logarithms. The antilog of the mean of the log transformed distribution is the geometric mean value shown in the table.
[b]US men and women ages 45–74 yr of age.
[c]Calculated as the ratio of serum iron (µmol/L) divided by total iron binding capacity (µmol/L).
Source: CDC/NCHS: Unpublished data from the second National Health and Nutrition Examination Survey, conducted in 1976–1980.

2. SERUM MEASURES OF BODY IRON STORES

Serum ferritin is currently the best measure of body iron stores that is feasible to use in epidemiologic studies (30). It is a fairly sensitive indicator of changes in body iron stores as you move along the stages of iron status from deficient, to replete, to iron overload in healthy individuals, e.g., not suffering from an infection, inflammation, or cancer. Less direct and sensitive measures of body iron stores are serum iron, total iron binding capacity (TIBC), and transferrin saturation (TS), which is calculated as the ratio of serum iron to total iron binding capacity. TS is the best measure of circulating iron available to tissues and is considered to be a better measure of stores than serum iron or TIBC. Other common iron status measures are even less directly related to body iron stores, e.g., hemoglobin, hematocrit, and erythrocyte protoporphyrin. Hemoglobin and hematocrit are measures of the oxygen-carrying capacity of blood and viscosity.

As body iron stores increase, so do serum ferritin levels (31,32). As a result, serum ferritin can be useful in detecting iron deficiency and overload. A serum ferritin level of < 15 µg/L "has been used as an indicator of iron deficiency" in both men and women (33). Separate upper limits have been suggested for adult men (400 µg/L), menstruating women (200 µg/L), and postmenopausal women (300 µg/L) (33).

TS and serum iron levels also tend to increase as stores increase over the normal range, whereas TIBC levels tend to decrease as stores increase. The opposite trends occur as body iron stores decrease. At very high levels of body iron stores, as in homozygous hemochromatosis (TS >60%), or at depleted levels (TS < 16%), i.e., iron deficiency, TS is considered to be good measure of body iron stores. Within the normal range of TS, i.e., 20–60%, it is not clear how well TS reflects body iron stores. Data from the second national Health and Nutrition Examination Survey (Table 1) show that there does appear to be a positive correlation, albeit low, between the two measurements with the result that with increasing level of TS, mean levels of serum ferritin tend to rise as well, especially in women. The correlation between log-transformed serum ferritin and TS for men and women 45–74 yr of age was $r=0.22$ overall, $r=0.14$ for men, and $r=0.25$ for women.

Serum iron status measures are also affected by inflammation and chronic infection. Serum ferritin levels tend to increase in response to inflammation *(33)*, whereas TS, TIBC, and serum iron levels decrease *(34)*. For example, in response to a heart attack, ferritin levels are initially raised whereas TS, TIBC, and serum iron levels decrease *(35,36)*. In the study by van der Schouw et al. *(37)* serum ferritin levels returned to control levels 6 wk after the heart attack whereas TS and serum iron levels continued to be depressed.

3. BODY IRON STORES AND RISK OF HEART DISEASE: THE EPIDEMIOLOGIC DATA

3.1. Prospective Studies Based on Serum Ferritin

Prospective or cohort studies are ones in which both disease status and risk factors are measured at baseline or time zero. However, under this design, depending on the objectives of the study, participants with CHD at baseline may be eliminated from further analyses. The persons remaining would then be those who are at risk of developing CHD, i.e., for whom it can be reasonably established that the risk factor status preceded the development of clinical signs or symptoms of, in this case, CHD. Those people are then followed over time to see who develops or dies from CHD. A researcher then performs analyses designed to look at what baseline measures affect the risk of developing CHD based on specific hypotheses. It is because the time sequence of risk-factor exposure precedes disease development that prospective studies are considered to be the strongest observational study design *(38)*. Using various measures of body iron stores, a number of researchers have attempted to assess the hypothesis that CHD risk increases with body iron stores.

As stated earlier, the theory was largely ignored until the publication by Salonen et al. *(4)* of results from the Finnish Kuopio Ischemic Heart Disease Risk Factor Study (KIHD). The study consisted of 1931 randomly selected men who were 42, 48, 54, or 60 yr of age and who were free of clinical symptoms of CHD at baseline. During an average of 3 yr of followup, 46 men had either a definite or possible heart attack as defined by ECG or enzyme criteria. Five additional men who were admitted to the hospital for prolonged chest pain did not meet the criteria. The authors reported that the results were not changed substantively by including those men, and the published results were based on 51 heart attacks.

Salonen et al. reported finding a statistically significant linear association between serum ferritin level and the risk of heart attack ($z=2.64$, $p < 0.01$) after adjusting for possible confounding. Thus, as serum ferritin levels increased so did the risk of heart attack. The more surprising finding was, however, that men with a serum ferritin ≥ 200 µg/L had a greater than twofold higher risk of heart attack compared to those with lower serum ferritin values. The difference was statistically significant (relative risk=2.2, CI 95%: 1.2–4.0, $p < 0.01$). Again the results were adjusted for possible confounding in a multivariate model. Additionally, they reported finding that compared to men with serum ferritin levels <200 µg/L, men with a serum ferritin of 200–399 µg/L had a nearly identical risk of heart attack, as did men with serum ferritin levels ≥ 400 µg/L *(4)*.

The study by Salonen et al. *(4)*, although based on a small number of heart attacks, was a well conducted study. (In a letter to the editor, they presented data to indicate that the relationship was still significant after an average of 5 yr of followup and 83 heart attacks *[39]*.) They have been criticized, however, for not having adequately adjusted for inflammation *(40)* and because there was a negative correlation between age and serum ferritin *(41)*. However, neither criticism appears to be entirely justified *(42,43)*. The authors reported that they found no correlation between serum ferritin and plasma fibrinogen (an acute phase protein) in the whole sample or with C-reactive protein in a subsample *(4,42,43)*. Moreover, the authors adjusted for blood leukocyte count in their analyses *(4)*. More importantly, the association between serum ferritin and heart attack was not attenuated when the analysis was repeated after removing heart attacks that occurred within the first 6 mo following blood collection. As was stated earlier, serum ferritin levels go up after a heart attack but return to baseline levels within 6 mo after the heart attack *(37)*.

Only three other prospective studies have looked at the association between serum ferritin and CHD *(44–46)*. None of the three found an association. The largest of these, regrettably, has been published only as an abstract *(44)*. Using a nested case-control design, 238 men participating in the US Physicians Study *(44)* had a heart attack during the period after the 1982 baseline. Stored serum for those men and for 238 controls matched for age and smoking status were analyzed for serum ferritin concentrations. After adjustment for other CHD risk factors, men with serum ferritin levels ≥ 200 µg/L were not found to have a higher risk of heart attack (RR=1.1, CI 95%: 0.7–1.6).

In the study by Magnusson et al. *(45)* 2036 Icelandic men and women ages 25–74 yr were followed for an average of 8.5 yr. During that time 81 participants (63 men and 18 women) had a heart attack. The data analysis strategy they used was different than the one used by Salonen et al., so the results are not directly comparable. In their multivariate models, Magnusson included both serum ferritin, in the normal units or log transformed, and serum TIBC as continuous variables. The interesting finding was that TIBC was shown to have a significant negative association with risk of heart attack (RR=0.95, CI 95%: 0.92–0.98). That is, those with higher TIBC levels had a lower risk of heart attack. Neither serum ferritin (RR=0.999, CI 95%: 0.997–1.001) nor log ferritin (RR=0.781, CI 95%: 0.540–1.129) were significantly associated with risk of heart attack. The authors acknowledge that the results from their study should be interpreted cautiously. However, they interpreted those results as indicating that, in their study, body iron stores as measured by serum ferritin were not associated with risk of heart attack. They further acknowledge that ferritin is a much better index of body iron stores than is TIBC, but TIBC is also know to have antioxidant properties *(47)*. Given the recent results concerning the oxidative modification of LDL cholesterol and the reported protective effects of antioxidant nutrients, Magnusson et al. postulated that "if iron increases the risk of coronary artery disease by oxidizing LDL, as has been postulated, a critical step in its pathogenetic pathway would be the accumulation of free iron in the subendothelial space. The serum iron binding capacity might be a more reliable indicator of this accumulation of free iron in the vessel wall than the total iron stores." *(45, p.107)*. Additionally, they felt that their results "support the concept that iron being an important transition metal might contribute to atherogenesis along with other classic risk factors, although arguing against the recent hypothesis that iron stores *per se* increase risk." *(45, p.107)*.

The fourth study, by Frey and Krider *(46)*, is based on 298 men with serum ferritin measurements seen over a 10-yr period in a West Virginia medical practice. Over a followup period of 1–10 yr (mean 5.16 yr) 32 men had a heart attack. The authors reported finding no difference in mean serum ferritin levels between patients who had or did not have a heart attack, nor was there any association between risk of heart attack and having a serum ferritin level above 200 µg/L. Unfortunately, none of the results appeared to have been adjusted for age or for other CHD risk factors.

3.2. Prospective Studies Based on TS

There have been five papers published looking at the relationship between body iron stores as measured by TS and CHD risk *(12,48–51)* and one where serum iron *(52)* was used. Only the study by Morrison et al. *(52)* reported finding a significant positive association. In that study 9920 men and women 35–79 yr of age were followed for approx 16 yr. During that time 141 men and 83 women died of an acute myocardial infarction (MI) or heart attack. Persons with a serum iron level ≥ 175 µg/L compared to those with a value < 120 µg/L were found to have a significantly higher risk of dying of an acute MI (men: RR=2.18, CI 95%: 1.01–4.74; women: RR=5.53, CI 95%: 1.69–18.12). Unfortunately, for those with a serum iron in the highest category, there were only seven deaths among the men and three among the women. Although the results are consistent with those from Finland, the small numbers of events in the highest category tend to make their results less certain.

The papers by Sempos et al. *(48)* and Liao et al. *(12)* were both based on the same data from NHANES I Epidemiologic Followup Study. Liao et al. *(12)* looked at the relationship of TS, TIBC, serum iron, hemoglobin, and hematocrit and risk of MI. None of the iron status measures were found to be significantly related to the risk of heart attack. Although focusing on TS, Sempos et al. *(48)* found similar results. No relationship was found among the various iron status measures and risk of CHD, MI, death from CHD or MI, or all causes of mortality. Reunanen et al. *(49)*, Baer et al. *(50)*, and van Asperen et al. *(51)* also reported finding no association between TS and risk of CHD using TS as a measure of body iron stores.

The above papers that found no association between iron status and CHD have been criticized for using TS as a measure of body iron stores *(39)* and for using the lowest levels of TS as the comparison group. The relationship between ferritin and TS has been described previously. Because persons with very low TS levels (<16%) as well as those with very high levels (> 60%) are probably sick individuals, persons with the lowest TS levels may not be the most appropriate comparison group.

Table 2 shows the relationship between TS and risk of CHD where TS has been divided into six categories (<16%, 16–19%, 20–29%, 30–44%, 45–59% and ≥ 60%). The analyses were conducted by the authors using data, which are available on public use data tapes, from the NHANES I Epidemiologic Followup Study. For those analyses the TS category of 20–29% was used as the reference category. A TS <16% is used to indicate iron deficiency and a TS of 16–29% is at the low end of the normal range. Based on Sullivan's theory, persons with TS levels of 16–19% should have a lower risk of CHD than those with higher values. However, based on the results in Table 2, that was not the case for either men or women. In fact, persons with TS levels at or above 30% appeared to be possibly at lower risk of CHD than those with a TS of 20–29%. When TS is divided into wider categories that are a better reflection of differences in body iron stores,

Table 2
Multivariate[a] Adjusted Risk of Coronary Heart Disease (CHD)[b]
by Transferrin Saturation Level

	Transferrin saturation level, %					
	<16	*16–19*	*20–29[d]*	*30–44*	*45–59*	*≥60*
Men						
CHD cases, *n*	32	42	211	228	32	9
Sample size, *N*	92	118	613	637	128	30
RR	1.09	1.09	1.00	1.00	0.75	0.76
95% CI	0.75–1.59	0.78–1.53	—	0.84–1.22	0.51–1.09	0.39–1.49
Women						
CHD cases, *n*	36	59	207	136	20	4
Sample size, *N*	147	215	860	617	95	21
RR	1.28	1.18	1.00	0.84	0.97	0.86
95% CI	0.90–1.83	0.88–1.57	—	0.68–1.04	0.61–1.54	0.32–2.33

[a]Adjusted for age, education, cigarette smoking, reported history of diabetes, systolic blood pressure, and serum cholesterol and albumin
[b]Persons with baseline history of heart disease were excluded
[c]White men and women 45–74 yr of age at baseline.
[d]Reference group for calculating relative risk (RR).
Source: CDC/NCHS; Unpublished data from the NHANES 1 Epidemiologic Followup Study (NHEFS). Baseline data collected in 1971–1974 with followup through 1987.

and when the comparison group is one with "healthy" TS values, no evidence was found to support the hypothesis that body iron stores are positively related to CHD risk. Women with very low TS (<16%) values also appear to be at a higher risk of CHD.

3.3. Prospective Studies: TS and All Causes of Mortality

Because it is possible that one factor, although associated with lower risk of death from one cause, may be associated with a higher risk of death from other causes, it is important to examine the relationship of body iron stores to risk of death from all causes. Table 3 shows the relationship between TS and all causes of mortality. Men with a TS <16% had a higher risk of death than those with a TS of 20–29% and although nonsignificant, there was some indication that men with a TS of 16–19% may also be at a higher risk of death. There was, however, no indication that a TS at or above 30% was associated with a greater risk of death. (The analyses shown in Table 3 were also conducted by the authors using data from the NHANES I Epidemiologic Followup Study.)

The relationship was somewhat similar in women, but there was a U-shaped relationship between TS and risk of death. TS levels <16% or ≥60% were associated with a higher risk of death. The fact that TS levels in men ≥60% were not associated with increased risk of death may be a result of the small numbers of deaths in that category. In a letter to the editor, Takkunin et al. *(53)* reported finding a negative association between TS and risk of death in men and women. Their findings may be related to using the lowest quartile of TS as the comparison group.

Table 3
Multivariate[a] Adjusted Risk of Death from All Causes by Transferrin Saturation Level[b]

	Transferrin saturation level, %					
	<16	16–19	20–29[c]	30–44	45–59	≥60
Men						
CHD cases, n	66	82	349	378	75	20
Sample size, N	114	156	749	772	163	35
RR	1.46	1.21	1.00	0.95	1.01	1.01
95% CI	1.12–1.90	0.95–1.54		0.82–1.10	0.78–1.30	0.64–1.59
Women						
CHD cases, n	66	90	337	180	30	11
Sample size, N	179	248	981	705	109	23
RR	1.24	1.00	1.00	0.70	0.81	1.33
95% CI	0.95–1.62	0.79–1.26		0.58–0.84	0.56–1.18	0.73–2.43

[a]Adjusted for age, education, cigarette smoking, reported history of diabetes, systolic blood pressure, and serum cholesterol and albumin.
[b]White men and women 45–74 yr of age at baseline.
[c]Reference group for calculating relative risk (RR).
Source: CDC/NCHS; Unpublished data from the NHANES I Epidemiologic Followup Study (NHEFS). Baseline data collected in 1971–1974 with followup through 1987.

3.4. Prospective Studies: Dietary Iron and CHD Risk

Salonen et al. *(4)* also reported that dietary iron intake was positively associated with the risk of having a heart attack. Other researchers have not been able to corroborate this finding *(12,45,48,49,54)*. Table 4 shows the results of analyses conducted by the authors looking at the relationship between dietary iron and risk of CHD or heart attack using data from the NHANES I Epidemiologic Followup Study. In this case the lowest iron intake group was used as the reference group. As with all studies other than Salonen et al. *(4)*, there was no clear relationship of iron intake to risk of CHD or heart attack.

One paper reported finding an association between heme iron intake and risk of heart attack, but not with total iron intake *(54)*. Although very interesting, these results have not been verified as yet by any other study. In any event, it is not clear what a relationship between dietary iron and CHD would mean in the context of a discussion of the association between body iron stores and CHD risk. Dietary intake methods do not adequately capture long-term dietary patterns, nor do they reflect the influence of growth and development or the effect of menopausal status on body iron stores, all of which are important factors in determining body iron stores. Additionally, an association between dietary iron and CHD risk may be a marker for a high fat, high cholesterol diet or something totally unrelated to body iron stores.

3.5. Case-Control or Cross-Sectional Studies

There have been five studies *(55–59)* that have used a case-control or cross-sectional study design. All of the studies have used serum ferritin as the measure of body iron stores. In only one *(58)* of the five was a significant positive association be-

Table 4

Multivariate[a] Adjusted Risk of Coronary Heart Disease or Myocardial Infarction by Dietary Iron Intake Level[b,c]

Sex and dietary iron (mg/d)	Coronary heart disease		Myocardial infarction	
	Relative risk	95% CI	Relative risk	95% CI
Men				
<8.7[d]	1.00	—	1.00	—
8.7–10.8	0.92	0.70–1.19	1.04	0.69–1.55
10.9–13.2	0.76	0.57–1.01	0.98	0.65–1.49
13.3–17.0	1.08	0.83–1.41	1.17	0.79–1.75
≥17.1	0.76	0.57–1.01	0.93	0.61–1.42
Women				
<6.1	1.00	—	1.00	—
6.1–7.7	0.77	0.57–1.02	0.78	0.49–1.24
7.8–9.6	0.72	0.53–0.97	0.65	0.39–1.08
9.7–12.4	0.60	0.43–0.83	0.65	0.39–1.09
≥12.5	0.75	0.56–1.02	0.84	0.53–1.35

[a]Adjusted for age, education, cigarette smoking, reported history of diabetes, systolic blood pressure, and serum cholesterol and albumin

[b]Intake based on a single 24-h recall

[c]White men and women 45–74 yr of age at baseline.

[d]Reference group for calculating Relative Risk (RR)

Source: CDC/NCHS; Unpublished data from the NHANES I Epidemiologic Followup Study (NHEFS). Baseline data collected in 1971–1974 with followup through 1987.

tween serum ferritin and coronary artery disease found. The other four (55–57,59) found no association.

There are many variations of a case-control study, but classically in this type of study persons with the disease of interest are located, a suitable group of controls is found, and the exposure of interest, in this case serum ferritin, is measured. Cross-sectional studies share many similarities with case-control studies. In cross-sectional studies a sample, usually random, of individuals would have blood drawn to measure serum ferritin and a clinical assessment to determine CHD status. In both case-control and cross-sectional studies, cases of CHD are compared to noncases (controls) to see if they were more or less likely to have higher levels of serum ferritin.

Case-control and cross-sectional studies are not generally considered to be as rigorous as prospective studies (38). The problem with both types of studies is that both disease status, e.g., heart disease, and exposure, e.g., serum ferritin, are measured at the same time. For example, the disease itself may alter body iron stores, i.e., serum ferritin levels. Additionally, people who already know that they have the disease or who know they are sick before they are examined may change their behavior, thus altering their levels of body iron stores. As a result it is difficult to establish if the exposure lead to the disease or vice versa.

As stated before, serum ferritin levels are increased in response to inflammation, infection, cancer, and heart attack. As a result, CHD should increase serum ferritin levels, so that more often than not a false positive association would be found between ferritin and CHD. The fact that four out of five studies in this category found no association is then a somewhat stronger argument against the hypothesis. On the other hand, including persons with CHD in these studies who have changed their diets to lower their serum cholesterol levels would tend to produce false negative results since a reduction in the intake of meat and animal products may also, over time, reduce their levels of body iron stores and, as a result, their serum ferritin levels. However, one way to evaluate this possibility is to assess the association between serum total and low density lipoprotein (LDL) cholesterol and CHD concurrently with the serum ferritin and CHD assessments. In three of the studies that found no association between serum ferritin and CHD *(56,57,59)*, and in the one study that found a positive association *(58)*, LDL cholesterol was positively associated with having CHD, suggesting that it is less likely that changes in behavior have produced false negative results.

3.6. Autopsy Data and Ecological Data

The use of data from autopsy and ecological studies provide relatively weaker evidence than either prospective or case-control studies *(38)*. However, data from autopsy and ecological studies can be very useful in suggesting lines of research or in making an overall assessment of the accuracy and applicability of a particular theory.

Miller and Hutchins *(60)* reviewed over 47,000 consecutive autopsies performed at Johns Hopkins University from May 1889 through October 1992. In that review they identified 41 cases of inherited iron-overload disease, hereditary hemochromatosis (n=33), or hemosiderosis. For each case two controls were then selected. Controls were defined as the previous or next autopsied patient matched for age within one decade, sex, and race. The authors found that coronary artery disease (CAD) was significantly less common among iron-overload cases than among controls. They concluded that "the low prevalence of CAD in subjects with hemochromatosis and multiorgan hemosiderosis does not support the hypothesis that iron overload states enhance coronary atherogenicity." *(60,* p.233*)*.

Lauffer *(61)* looked at the association between nonheme liver (hepatic) iron content and mortality from coronary heart disease for 11 different countries. Liver iron and serum cholesterol levels were found from various published sources. In univariate analyses Lauffer found a higher correlation between hepatic iron (r=0.55) and CHD death than with serum cholesterol (r=0.30). The highest correlation with CHD death was found by multiplying hepatic iron by serum cholesterol (r=0.74). The author interpreted these results as supporting the hypothesis that the body iron stores are positively related to risk of CHD. In addition, he stated that hepatic iron is a useful index in "describing the differences in CAD due to both diet (and/or culture) and sex." *(61,* p.96*)*.

There appear to be a number of problems with this study *(61)*. First, the hepatic iron data come from multiple sources and it is not certain how comparable the measurements are from one study to the next. Second, it is not certain if those measurements are representative of a population. Third, in the correlation analyses the data points for men and women are grouped together even though it is obvious that the correlations are very different for men compared to women. Finally, given the large amount of ecological data showing a strong correlation between serum cholesterol and CHD mortality *(62,63)*, the low correlation cited by Lauffer raises further concerns about the quality of the data used for that report.

4. SUMMARY

In 1981 Jerome Sullivan *(1)* proposed that body iron stores are directly or positively related to CHD risk, i.e., the higher your body iron stores the greater your CHD risk. Until the publication of results from Finland by Salonen et al. *(4)* showing a positive relationship between serum ferritin levels and risk of heart attack in men, the hypothesis was largely ignored. The vast majority of the epidemiologic results published since that study have failed to support the original hypothesis. However, it must also be stated that there have been too few prospective studies that have looked at the relationship between serum ferritin and CHD risk to reach any firm conclusions. Additionally, none of the studies that have been published in more than abstract form replicates the study by Salonen et al. *(4)*. Furthermore, because serum ferritin levels and diagnosis of clinically apparent CHD are made at the same time in case-control and cross-sectional studies, those findings are seen as less conclusive than prospective data.

To better understand the role of body iron stores may play in CHD risk it may be necessary to take into account antioxidant status, e.g., vitamin E status. It has been proposed that iron may be related to CHD by promoting the production of tissue-damaging free radicals *(15,26,29)*. Antioxidant systems, including vitamin E, beta-carotene, and vitamin C, are all involved in reducing free radical activity and damage. Thus, any relationship between iron and CHD that may exist may be more a result of a relative deficiency of antioxidants and not necessarily high body iron levels. Clearly a more integrated research approach is needed for looking at this problem before it can be resolved.

5. RECOMMENDATIONS

The Finnish results and experimental data looking at myocardial reperfusion injury have lead some *(32,64)* to suggest that depletion of body iron stores to a level just short of anemia may be useful in preventing CHD. At the present time we do not agree with that suggestion.

There have not been enough studies done in this area, especially prospective ones, to reach any firm conclusions concerning the relationship of body iron stores and the risk of CHD. However, at this time there is also no consistent and conclusive evidence to support Sullivan's hypothesis. If anything, most of the evidence fails to support the hypothesis. As a result we feel that it is too soon for physicians to give specific advice on this issue to their patients.

REFERENCES

1. Sullivan JL. Iron and the sex difference in heart disease risk. Lancet 1981; 1:1293, 1294.
2. Sullivan JL. The iron paradigm of ischemic heart disease. Am Heart J 1989; 117:1177–1188.
3. Sullivan JL. The sex difference in ischemic heart disease. Perspect Biol Med 1983; 26:657–671.
4. Salonen JT, Nyyssönen K, Korpela H, Tuomilehto J, Seppänen R, Salonen R. High stored iron levels are associated with excess risk of myocardial infarction in eastern Finnish men. Circulation 1992; 86:803–811.
5. Böttiger L-E, Carlson LA. Risk factors for ischemic vascular death for men in the Stockholm Prospective Study. Atherosclerosis 1980; 36:398–408.
6. Paul O, Lepper MH, Phelan WH, et al. A longitudinal study of coronary heart disease. Circulation 1963; 28:20–31.
7. Truett J, Cornfield J, Kannel W. A multivariate analysis of risk of coronary heart disease in Framingham. J Chronic Dis 1967; 20:511–524.

8. Carter C, McGee D, Reed D, Yano K, Stemmermann G. Hematocrit and the risk of coronary heart disease: the Honolulu Heart Program. Ann Heart J 1983; 105:674–679.

9. Cullen KJ, Stenhouse NS, Wearne KL. Raised haemoglobin and risk of cardiovascular disease. Lancet 1981; 2:1288, 1289.

10. Sorlie PD, Garcia-Palmieri MR, Costas R Jr, Havlik RJ. Hematocrit and risk of coronary heart disease: the Puerto Rico Heart Health Program. Am Heart J 1981; 101:456–461.

11. Mayer GA. Hematocrit and coronary heart disease. Can Med Assoc J 1965; 180:63–65.

12. Liao Y, Cooper RS, McGee DL. Iron status and coronary heart disease: negative findings from the NHANES I Epidemiologic Follow-up Study. Am J Epidemiol 1994; 139:704–712.

13. Graham S. Results of case-control studies of diet and cancer in Buffalo, New York. Cancer Res 1983; 2409s–2413s.

14. Ziegler R. Vegetables, fruits and carotenoids and the risk of cancer. Am J Clin Nutr 1991; 53:251s–259s.

15. Diplock AT. Antioxidant nutrients and disease prevention: an overview. Am J Clin Nutr 1991; 53:189s–193s.

16. Stevens RG, Jones DY, Micozzi MS, Taylor PR. Body iron stores and the risk of cancer. New Engl J Med 1988; 319:1047–1052.

17. Stevens RG, Beasley RP, Blumberg BS. Iron-binding proteins and risk of cancer in Taiwan. J Natl Cancer Inst 1986; 76:605–610.

18. Selby JV, Friedman GD. Epidemiologic evidence of an association between body iron stores and risk of cancer. Int J Cancer 1988; 41:677–682.

19. Merk K, Mattsson B, Mattsson A, Holm G, Gullbring B, Björkholm M. The incidence of cancer among blood donors. Int J Epidemiol 1990; 19:505–509.

20. Korn EL, Graubard BI. Epidemiologic studies utilizing surveys: accounting for the sampling design. Am J Public Health 1991; 81:1166–1173.

21. Stevens RG, Graubard BI, Micozzi MS, Nershi K, Blumberg BS. Moderate elevation of body iron level and increased risk of cancer occurrence and death. Int J Cancer 1994; 56:364–369.

22. Knekt P, Reunanen A, Takkunen H, Aromaa A, Heliövaara M, Hakulinen T. Body iron stores and risk of cancer. Int J Cancer 1994; 56:379–382.

23. Nelson RL, Davis FG, Sutter E, Sobin LH, Kikendall JW, Bowen P. Body iron stores and risk of colonic neoplasia. J Natl Cancer Inst 1994; 86:455–460.

24. Jha P, Flather M, Lonn E, Farkouh M, Yusuf S. The antioxidant nutrients and cardiovascular disease. A critical review of epidemiologic and clinical trial data. Ann Intern Med 1995; 123:860–872.

25. Chalmers TC. Antioxidants and cardiovascular disease: why do we still not have the answers. Ann Intern Med 1995; 123:887.

26. Steinberg D, Parthasarathy S, Carew TE, Khoo JC, Witztum JL. Beyond cholesterol. Modifications of low-density lipoprotein that increase its atherogenicity. New Engl J Med 1989; 320:915–924.

27. Esterbauerer H, Gebicki J, Phul H, Jurgens G. The role of lipid peroxidation and antioxidants in oxidative modification of LDL. J Free Rad Biol Med 1992; 13:341–390.

28. Smith C, Mitchinson MJ, Auroma OI, Halliwell B. Stimulation of lipid peroxidation and hydroxyl-radical generation by the contents of human atherosclerotic lesions. Biochem J 1992; 286:901–905.

29. McCord JM. Is iron sufficiency a risk factor for ischemic heart disease. Circulation 1991; 83:1112–1114.

30. Expert Scientific Working Group. Summary of a report on assessment of the iron nutritional status of the United States population. Am J Clin Nutr 1985; 42:1318–1330.

31. Bothwell T, Charlton R, Cook J, Finch C. Iron Metabolism in Man. Oxford, England: Blackwell Scientific, 1979.

32. Herbert V. Everyone should be tested for iron disorders. J Am Diet Assoc 1992; 92:1502–1509.

33. Custer EM, Finch CA, Sobel RE, Zettner A. Populations norms for serum ferritin. J Lab Clin Med 1995; 126:88–94.

34. Yip R, Dallman PR. The roles of inflammation and iron deficiency as causes of anemia. Am J Clin Nutr 1988; 48:1295–1300.

35. Birgegård G, Hällgren R, Venge P, Wide L. Serum ferritin during inflammation. A study on myocardial infarction. Acta Med Scan 1979; 206:361–366.

36. Griffiths JD, Campbell LJ, Woodruff IW, Cruickshank D, Mathews YB, Hunt D, Campbell DG, Cowling DC. Acute changes in iron metabolism following myocardial infarction. Am J Clin Pathol 1985; 84:649–654.

37. van der Schouw YT, van der Veek PMWC, Kok FJ, Koster JF, Schouten EG, Hofman A. Free Radical Biol Med 1990; 8:47–53.

38. Lilienfeld AM, Lilienfeld DE. *Foundations of Epidemiology.* 2nd Ed. New York: Oxford University Press, 1980.

39. Salonen JT, Nyyssönen K, Salonen R. Body iron stores and the risk of coronary heart disease. (Letter). New Engl J Med 1994; 331:1159.

40. Weiss G, Fuchs D, Wachter H. High stored iron levels and the risk of myocardial infarction. (Letter). Circulation 1993; 87:1425.

41. MacDonald HB. High stored iron levels are associated with excess risk of myocardial infarction in Eastern Finnish Men. (Letter). Circulation 1993; 87:2063.

42. Salonen JT, Nyyssönen K, Korpela H, Salonen R, Tuomilehto J, Seppänen R. High storediron levels and the risk of myocardial infarction. (Reply) Circulation 1993; 87:1425,1426.

43. Salonen JT, Nyyssönen K, Korpela H, Salonen R, Tuomilehto J, Seppänen R. High stored iron levels are associated with excess risk of myocardial infarction in Eastern Finnish Men. (Reply). Circulation 1993; 87:2063,2064.

44. Stampfer MJ, Grodstein F, Rosenberg I, Willett W, Hennekens C. A prospective study of plasma ferritin and risk of myocardial infarction in US physicians. Circulation 1993;87:688 (abstract).

45. Magnusson MK, Sigfusson N, Sigvaldason H, Johannesson GM, Magnusson S, Thorgeirsson G. Low iron-binding capacity as a risk factor for myocardial infarction. Circulation 1994; 89:102–108.

46. Frey GH, Krider DW. Serum ferritin and myocardial infarct. WV Med J 1994; 90:13–15.

47. Dormandy TL. Free-radical oxidation and antioxidants. Lancet 1978; 1:647–650.

48. Sempos CT, Looker AC, Gillum RF, Makuc DM. Body iron stores and the risk of coronary heart disease. New Engl J Med 1994; 330:1119–1124.

49. Reunanen A, Takkunen H, Knekt P, Sappänen R, Aromaa A. Body iron stores, dietary iron intake and coronary heart disease mortality. J Intern Med 1995; 238:223–230.

50. Baer DM, Tekawa IS, Hurley LB. Iron stores are not associated with acute myocardial infarction. Circulation 1994; 89:2915–2918.

51. van Asperen IA, Feskensens EJM, Bowels CH, Kromhout D. Body iron stores and mortality due to cancer and ischemic heart disease: a 17-year follow-up study of elderly men and women. Int J Epidemiol 1995; 24:665–670.

52. Morrison HI, Semenciw RM, Mao Y, Wigle DT. Serum iron and fatal acute myocardial infarction. Epidemiology 1994; 5:243–246.

53. Takkunen H, Reunanen A, Knekt P, Aromaa A. Body iron stores and the risk of cancer (Letter). New Engl J Med 1989; 320:1013,1014.

54. Ascherio A, Willett WC, Rimm EB, Giovannucci EL, Stampfer MJ. Dietary iron and risk of coronary heart disease among men. Circulation 1994; 89:969–974.

55. Aronow WS. Serum ferritin is not a risk factor for coronary artery disease in men and women aged ≥ 62 years. Am J Cardiol 1993; 72:347–348.

56. Solymoss BC, Marcil M, Gilfix BM, Gelinas F, Poitras AM, Campeau L. The place of ferritin among risk factors associated with coronary artery disease. Coronary Artery Dis 1994; 5:231–235.

57. Rauramaa R, Väisänen S, Mercuri M, Rankinen T, Penttila I, Bond MG. Association of risk factors and body iron status to carotid atherosclerosis in middle-aged Eastern Finnish men. Eur. Heart J 1994; 15:1020–1027.

58. Kiechl S, Aichner F, Gerstenbrand F, Egger G, Mair A, Rungger G, Spögler F, Jarosch E, Oberhollenzer F, Willeit J. Body iron stores and presence of carotid atherosclerosis. Results from the Bruneck Study. Arteriosclerosis Thromb 1994; 14:1625–1630.

59. Moore M, Folsom AR, Barnes RW, Eckfeldt JH. No association between serum ferritin and asymptomatic carotid atherosclerosis. The Atherosclerosis Risk in Communities (ARIC) Study. Am J Epidemiol 1995; 141:719–723.

60. Miller M, Hutchins GM. Hemochromatosis, multiorgan hemosiderosis, and coronary heart disease. JAMA 1994; 272:231–233.

61. Lauffer RB. Iron stores and the international variation in mortality from coronary artery disease. Med Hypotheses 1990; 35:96–102.

62. Keys A. Coronary heart disease in seven countries. Circulation 1970; 41:1–245.

63. McGill HC, Jr. (ed.). Geographic Pathology of Atherosclerosis. Baltimore, MD; Williams & Wilkins, 1968

64. Sullivan JL. Stored iron and ischemic heart disease. Empirical support for the new paradigm. Circulation 1992; 86: 1036,1037.

11

Homocysteine, Folic Acid, and Cardiovascular Disease Risk

Shirley A. A. Beresford and Carol J. Boushey

1. INTRODUCTION

Homocysteine, an amino acid by-product of methionine metabolism, has been attracting a lot of interest recently in connection with a number of different disease endpoints. Principal among these is cardiovascular disease. Historically, the finding of thrombotic complications in the rare hereditary disease of homocystinuria led to the hypothesis that the carriers for this condition might have an increased frequency of vascular disease. Many studies were, therefore, done to relate elevated homocyst(e)ine blood levels—whether genetic in origin or not—to vascular disease. The majority of these investigations showed an association of hyperhomocyst(e)inemia with coronary artery disease, cerebrovascular disease, and peripheral vascular disease. Some of the interest in homocysteine comes about because of the interconnection between its metabolic pathway and that of folic acid.

In this chapter we review the metabolism of homocysteine, its regulation, and measurement. Next we review the studies, including intervention studies, that provide information on the relationship between folate intake on homocysteine levels. This is followed by a summary of those studies of the association between blood folate levels and homocysteine levels and of the additional roles of pyridoxine and cobalamin in reducing elevated homocysteine. The formal meta-analyses of the association between homocysteine and coronary heart disease (CHD), cerebrovascular disease, and peripheral vascular disease follow. Finally, we review the evidence linking plasma folate and cardiovascular disease and discuss the likely impact of population strategies to change folic acid intake on risk of CHD.

2. HOMOCYSTEINE

2.1. What Is Homocysteine?

When protein is digested, methionine, an essential amino acid, is released. This is true for all forms of protein, whether from meat, fish, or plant protein. During the conversion of methionine to cysteine, the amino acid, homocysteine is formed (Fig. 1). In healthy individuals, methionine and homocysteine cycle metabolically, any excess homocysteine is excreted, and new methionine is released after protein ingestion.

Homocysteine can be metabolized via the transsulfuration pathway to form cystathionine or through a remethylation pathway to form methionine (1,2). The conden-

From: *Preventive Nutrition: The Comprehensive Guide for Health Professionals*
Edited by A. Bendich and R. J. Deckelbaum Humana Press Inc., Totowa, NJ

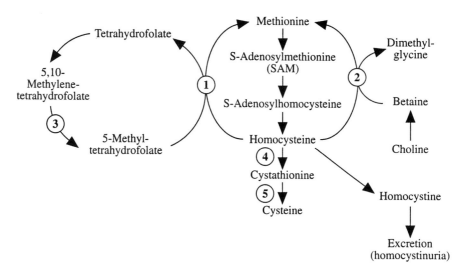

Fig. 1. Homocysteine metabolism in humans. Enzymes [vitamins involved]: 1. N-5-methyltetrahydrofolate: homocysteine methyltransferase (methionine synthase) [folate, vitamin B_{12}], 2. betaine: homocysteine methyltransferase, 3. methylene-tetrahydrofolate reductase (MTHFR) [folate], 4. cystathionine β-synthase [vitamin B_6], 5. γ-cystathionase [vitamin B_6].

sation of homocysteine and serine to form cystathionine is catalyzed by cystathionine β-synthase, an enzyme widely distributed in mammalian tissues. This enzyme requires pyridoxal 5′-phosphate, the biologically active form of vitamin B_6, as a cofactor. Remethylation of homocysteine to methionine is accomplished by two pathways in humans. One pathway is catalyzed by N-5-methyltetrahydrofolate:homocysteine methyltransferase (methionine synthase). This enzyme, widely distributed in animal tissues, requires 5-methyltetrahydrofolate as the methyl donor and cobalamin (vitamin B_{12}) as a cofactor. The enzyme methylenetetrahydrofolate reductase regenerates 5-methyltetrahydrofolate. In the other pathway, betaine acts as the methyl donor and the active enzyme is betaine:homocysteine methyltransferase. This latter reaction is confined to the liver; its quantitative significance in humans is not fully elucidated *(3)*. Thus, the amount of circulating homocysteine is tightly regulated by three B vitamins: folic acid, B_{12}, and B_6.

A hypothesis presented by Selhub and Miller *(4)* postulates that there is a pattern of homocysteine elevation particular to each of these three vitamins based on the central modulating effect of S-adenosylmethionine (S-AdoMet, *see* Fig. 1). In their proposal, S-AdoMet is an activator of cystathionine β-synthase and an allosteric inhibitor of methylenetetrahydrofolate reductase. In folate and vitamin B_{12} deficiency states, the inhibition of the remethylation pathway leads to a depletion of S-AdoMet and, therefore, a relative inhibition of the transsulfuration pathway. In this case, homocysteine would accumulate because of lack of activity in two pathways. In a vitamin B_6 deficiency state, the decrease of S-AdoMet would not occur, metabolism of homocysteine would proceed via the remethylation pathway, and the S-AdoMet generated would promote what residual enzyme activity exists for transsulfuration. However, after a large methionine load, the usual low level of S-AdoMet would temporarily increase beyond the capacity of the B_6-deficient pathway and transient elevated homocysteine levels would occur. The confirmation of this hypothesis and other aspects of homocysteine metabolism have important consequences for clinical application.

Homocysteine exists in plasma in several forms. In normal subjects, about 70–85% of the amino acid homocysteine is protein-bound via disulfide linkages, primarily to albumin *(5,6)*. When plasma is deproteinized with acid, the homocysteine moieties in the acid-soluble portion are referred to as "free-homocysteine" or nonprotein-bound homocysteine. "Free" homocysteine can exist as the disulfide homocystine, where two homocysteine molecules are linked together; or a mixed disulfide (MDS), with homocysteine bound to cysteine. Homocysteine MDS accounts for most of the free homocysteine in plasma. In addition, Araki and Sako *(7)* identified small amounts of reduced homocysteine in blood.

These various moieties of homocysteine are often represented as homocyst(e)ine. The amount of total plasma/serum homocysteine is the sum of the free plus protein-bound homocysteine *(8)* and is referred to as total homocyst(e)ine or total homocysteine *(9)*. Throughout this chapter we have abbreviated this as tHcy. On handling and storage, only trace amounts of free-homocysteine can be detected because most homocysteine becomes protein-bound. Thus, bound homocysteine would be considered tHcy in stored samples. Various methods for measuring tHcy correlate well ($r = 0.95$ and $r = 0.98$) with each other *(10,11)*.

To maximize the differences of tHcy levels between normals and heterozygotes for cystathionine β-synthase deficiency (such as parents of homozygotes with homocystinuria), tHcy levels are frequently measured following a methionine load. The amount of methionine administered for a postmethionine-load (PML) test can be as high as 100 mg/kg of bodyweight, i.e., about four times the dietary intake of a normal Western diet *(12,13)*. Even though distinctions between normal and impaired tHcy levels in heterozygotes have been made with the PML method *(14)*, the sensitivity and specificity of the PML test are not high enough to detect all persons heterozygous for cystathionine β-synthase deficiency *(14,15)*.

2.2. Abnormalities of Homocysteine Regulation

The balance of methionine and homocysteine in the body can be disturbed because of inadequate intake of the three B-vitamins or because of genetic defects leading to low or absent enzyme activity rates in the relevant metabolic pathways. That there is indeed a strong genetic influence on homocysteine levels is supported by twin studies *(16,17)*, whereas familial studies point to a role of shared environment also *(18,19)*. An interruption of the transsulfuration or remethylation pathways of homocysteine (Fig. 1) produces hyperhomocyst(e)inemia. Severe hyperhomocyst(e)inemia (>100 μmol/L) is most often the result of homozygous cystathione β-synthase deficiency and leads to a condition called homocystinuria, characterized by an over-accumulation of tHcy, as evidenced by urinary excretion of homocystine. The frequency of this genetic disorder in the US population has been estimated as 1 in 291,000 *(20)*, with 0.5% of the population being carriers or heterozygotes for cystathione β-synthase deficiency. These carriers have a metabolic defect and slightly elevated homocyst(e)ine levels. Several other autosomal recessive inborn errors of metabolism can cause homocystinuria. These are once again very rare, and include five different vitamin B12 metabolic defects (CbC, D, E, F, G) *(21)*. A homozygous deficiency of the enzyme, methylenetetrahydrofolate reductase (MTHFR), presents with neurological symptoms, but is extremely rare and occurs in

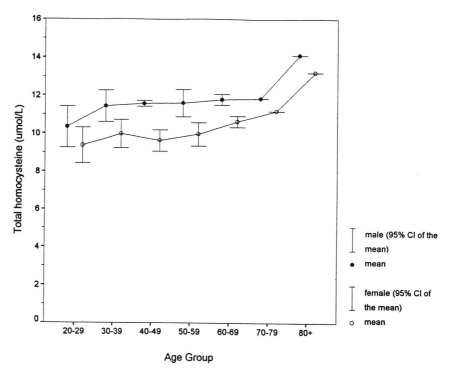

Fig. 2. Mean levels of plasma homocyst(e)ine in males and females (combined from published sources). Figure based on combining mean levels of total homocyst(e)ine from Andersson et al. *(10)*, Berg et al. *(16)*, Brattstrom et al. *(27)*, Brattstrom et al. *(14)*, Selhub et al. *(28)*, and Ueland et al. *(8)*. The age groups 70–79 and 80+ do not include confidence intervals (Selhub *[28]* was the sole source of information for these age groups).

the general population at a rate of about one-tenth that of cystathionine β-synthase deficiency *(22)*.

Of great potential importance here is that a high frequency polymorphism of MTHFR has been identified *(23)*. It is a thermolabile variant that occurs in neurologically normal subjects, and is inherited as an autosomal recessive trait at a frequency of 5%. This implies that 35% of the general population is heterozygous for this trait. The gene for this enzyme has been cloned *(24)*, leading to the identification of the basic molecular defect of the thermolabile variant of MTHFR. The hyperhomocyst(e)inemia of subjects with the MTHFR enzyme variant in the homozygous state has been found to be correctable with oral folic acid supplements *(25,26)*, suggesting that this metabolic block can be overcome with pharmacological doses of folic acid.

2.3. The Measurement of Homocysteine

The concentration of tHcy in plasma among healthy, disease-free individuals ranges between 5 and 15 μmol/L *(8)*. Figure 2 shows mean levels of tHcy for male and female adults by age group based on six reports *(5,8,10,16,27,28)*. The 95% confidence intervals (CI) are shown for five 10-yr age groups from 20–29 to 60–69. Confidence interval information was not available for the 70–79 and 80+ age groups *(28)*. Gartler et al. *(29)*

showed that cystathionine β-synthase activity in healthy subjects decreased with age so that persons above 70 yr and particularly the very old had very low enzyme activity. The finding of higher tHcy levels in the older population generally fits these findings.

Plasma tHcy was dependent on age, gender, and in women, possibly related to menopausal status *(10)*. In general, men have higher tHcy concentrations than women *(16,30)*; the cut-off values for hyperhomocyst(e)inemia reported by Wu et al. *(31)* and Malinow et al. *(32)* support a lower range for females. Large differences between pre- and postmenopausal women when measuring homocysteine-cysteine mixed disulfide *(5,33)* were not found when measuring tHcy.

3. FOLATE AND HOMOCYSTEINE

3.1. The Influence of Folate Intake on Plasma Homocysteine

As described previously *(34)*, the English-language literature was searched for human studies of homocysteine and folic acid using MEDLINE (1988 through November 1995). Beyond the twelve studies summarized previously *(5,27,28,35–43)*, an additional three intervention studies *(44–46)* have been identified in which the effect of folic acid alone could be evaluated, and two other intervention studies that included folic acid in one of their regimens *(47,48)*. More information from the metabolic study by O'Keefe and colleagues *(49)*, previously published only as an abstract *(43)*, is also included. Only data on subjects with normal concentrations of folate, vitamin B_{12}, and vitamin B_6 were included in this analysis. All 14 intervention studies and two metabolic studies that included folic acid in their intervention regimen are summarized in Table 1 *(5,27,35–42,44–49)*. Results are grouped according to the form of homocyst(e)ine measured.

The increases in folic acid intakes in these studies ranged from 74 *(36)* to 10,000 μg/d *(27,41,45,46)*. The majority of studies enrolled persons with elevated homocyst(e)ine and used combinations of pyridoxine, cobalamin, and folic acid at different doses to effect a reduction on homocyst(e)ine, as shown in Table 1. It is apparent that the reduction in tHcy associated with a given dose of folic acid is dependent on the degree of elevation of tHcy before treatment *(45,48)*. When studies provided data on fasting tHcy and folate or folic acid intake and were not restricted to persons with elevated homocyst(e)ine *(28,35,36,49)*, their results were used to construct Fig. 3.

In the study of Brattstrom and colleagues *(35)*, subjects were randomized to receive 5000 μg of folic acid, 1 mg cobalamin, or 40 mg pyridoxine. Only subjects receiving folic acid experienced a significant decrease in plasma tHcy levels. The posttreatment value for tHcy concentration is included in Fig. 3.

Ubbink et al. *(39,42)* showed that 1000 μg of folic acid in combination with cobalamin and pyridoxine significantly lowered fasting tHcy in healthy men with hyperhomocyst(e)inemia (>16.3 μmol/L). In another study of hyperhomocyst(e)inemic men *(41)*, they showed that 650 μg of folic acid alone resulted in a similar reduction to that achieved when folic acid, cobalamin, and pyridoxine were combined. Patients with homocystinuria *(37)* and others with occlusive arterial disease *(27)* experienced significant drops in tHcy levels only after folic acid was added to a regimen of pyridoxine. In identical twins with premature coronary artery disease, Wilcken et al. *(37)* (data not shown in Table 1) reported that 2 wk of treatment with folic acid restored tHcy concentrations (before and after a methionine load) to levels considered normal.

Table 1
Summary of Intervention Studies that Include Folic Acid: Effects on Homocysteine Levels[a]

						Homocyst(e)ine levels	
First author	No. of subjects[b]	Age, yr	Status of subjects	No. of wk	Daily intervention	Before treatment, μmol/L	After treatment, μmol/L
Subjects with elevated homocysteine						*PML Hcy-Hcy and Hcy-cys*	
Dudman (38)	22	16–60	Vascular disease	2	100 mg B₆, 5 mg folic acid, or Both	28.5 / 31.1 / 30.4	.77[c] / .69[c] / .49[c]
Franken (40)	9 m / 55 f-pre / 8 f-post	16–55	Vascular disease	6	250 mg B₆	30.5 / 28.5 / 43.7	17.7[d] / 17.0[d] / 31.1[d]
						PML total Hcy	
Franken (44)	30	<55	Arterial occlusive disease or thromboembolism	6	50 mg B₆, 250 mg B₆, or 250 mg B₆ + 5 mg folic acid	59.6 / 69.7 / 66.3	46.9 / 51.5 / 33.7
van den Berg (47)	72 / 29 m / 35 f-pre / 8 f-post	<50	Arteriosclerotic arterial occlusive disease	6–12	250 mg B₆ + 5 mg folic acid	71 / 69 / 64 / 109	37 / 37 / 33 / 49
						Fasting Hcy-Hcy	
Wilcken (37)	11	NG[‡]	Homocystinuria not responsive to pyridoxine	36	100 mg B₆ + 6 g betaine + 5 mg folic acid	57	8***
						Fasting total Hcy	
Brattstrom (27)	20	24–59	Occlusive arterial disease	2	240 mg B₆ or 240 mg B₆ + 10 mg folic acid	23.3 / 25.6	25.6 / 10.9***

198

Study	n	Age	Population	wk	Treatment	Before	After
Ubbink (39)	30 m	19–71	Hcy > 16.3 µmol/L	6	Placebo or 12.2 mg B6 + 0.4 mg B12 + 1 mg folic acid	24.0 28.6	22.1 11.5***
Ubbink (42)	20 m	18–65	Hcy > 16.3 µmol/L	6	12.2 mg B6 + 0.05 mg B12 + 1 mg folic acid	30.9	14.0*
Ubbink (41)	91 m	20–73	Hcy >16.3 µmol/L	6	Placebo, 10 mg B6, 0.4 mg B12, 0.65 mg folic acid, or combination of 3 vitamins above	30.6 29.1 30.5 28.8 27.1	30.7 27.8 26.0* 16.8****,e 13.6****,e
Franken (44)	30	<55	Arterial occlusive disease or thromboembolism	6	50 mg B6, 250 mg B6, or 250 mg B6 + 5 mg folic +	15.1 17.1 19.9	16.3 14.8 9.4
van den Berg (47)	72 29 m 35 f-pre 8 f-post	<50	Arteriosclerotic arterial occlusive disease	6–12	250 mg B6 + 5 mg folic acid	19 23 15 20	9 10 8 10
Nilsson (46)	4	Mean 76.7	Psychogeriatric department, elevated tHcy	1	10 mg folic acid or 1 mg B12 (im) then 10 mg folic acid	29.8 29.8	14.8 19.4
Landgren (45)	53	28–81	Acute M.I within last 24– 36 hours	6	No folic acid, 2.5 mg folic acid, or 10 mg folic acid	19.4 14.5 17.2 15.4	8.9 15.1 12.5 11.3
Healthy subjects							*Fasting Hcy-cys*
Brattstrom (5)	15	34–63	Healthy	4	5 mg folic acid	3.5	2.4**

(continued)

199

Table 1 (continued)[a]

First author	No. of subjects[b]	Age, yr	Status of subjects	No. of wk	Daily intervention	Before treatment, µmol/L	After treatment, µmol/L
						Homocyst(e)ine levels	
						Fasting total Hcy	
Brattstrom (35)	42	43–56	Free of vascular disease	2	1 mg B$_{12}$, 5 mg folic acid, or 40 mg B$_6$	10.7 19.9 12.0	11.5 9.5** 11.4
Jaccob (36)	10	33–46	Healthy volunteers (periods w/o methionine)	15 1/2	Depletion of 415 µg folate Repletion with 74 µg folate or Supplement with 341 µg folate	8.9 12.8	12.8 13.3
Ubbink (48)	19 m	Mean 20	Hcy < 16.3 µmol/L, not taking vitamin supplements	6	10 mg B$_6$ + 0.4 mg B$_{12}$ + 1.0 mg folic acid	13.3 10.0	8.9 7.3
O'Keefe (49)	17 f	21–27	Nonpregnant, healthy	10	170 µg folic acid, 270 µg folic acid, or 370 µg folic acid in addition to 30 µg dietary folate	NA NA NA	12.6 8.40 7.72

*, **, *** $p < 0.05$, $p < 0.01$, $p < 0.001$ compared with pretreatment values.
‡NG: not given; NA: not available.
[a]Hcy = homocyst(e)ine, Hcy-Hcy = homocystine, Hcy-cys = homocysteine-cysteine, PML = post-methionine load, pre = premenopausal, post = postmenopausal, m = males, f = females.
[b]Unless indicated, subjects include males and females.
[c]After treatment results expressed as a ratio. The 4- and 8-hr PML hcy levels were averaged and the ratio between the mean value after treatment is compared with the mean value before treatment.
[d]After pyridoxine treatment 56% of subjects had normalized PML levels. After further treatment with continued pyridoxine, 5 mg folic acid and/or 6 g betaine, 95% of remaining cases normalized.
[e]Compared with results achieved with placebo supplement, $p < 0.01$ for folic acid and $p < 0.001$ for combination.

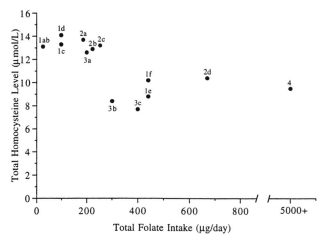

Fig. 3. Mean intakes of folate or folic acid and plasma levels of homocyst(e)ine. Data points based on groups from: Jacob et al. *(36)* (la–lf), mean levels of homocyst(e)ine (tHcy) at three levels of dietary folate; Selhub et al. *(28)* (2a–2d), main levels of tHcy from lowest deciles and highest decile of folate intake; O'Keefe et al. *(49)* (3a–3c), mean levels of tHcy at three levels of dietary folate; Brattstrom et al. *(35)* (4), mean tHcy level after added supplements of 5000 μg folic acid, pretreatment folate intake unknown. Results from Ubbink et al. *(41)* are not included here since the mean level of tHcy is artificially high as subjects were limited to individuals that rescreened as positive for hyperhomocyst(e)inemia.

In a folate depletion and repletion study *(36)* of ten healthy men, dietary folate was controlled to three levels of intake: very low, 25 μg/d; low, 99 μg/d; and desirable, 440 μg/d for two periods with different methionine intakes. Whether methionine was low or high made little difference to tHcy levels. However, the different levels of folate intake were associated with markedly different tHcy levels (Fig. 3). That is, low folate was associated with higher homocysteine levels.

O'Keefe and colleagues *(49)* studied 18 healthy nonpregnant women, with normal blood chemistry profiles, and randomized them into three groups in a metabolic study. Each group consumed 30 μg/d dietary folate with supplemental folic acid, bringing the daily folate dose to 200, 300, or 400 μg/d. After 70 d, levels of tHcy in the group consuming 200 μg/d of folate were statistically significantly higher ($p < 0.05$) than levels in the groups consuming 300 or 400 μg/d of folate (Fig. 3).

Selhub and others *(28)* examined data from 1160 Framingham subjects and found that intake of dietary folate estimated from a food-frequency questionnaire correlated well with plasma folate concentrations ($r = 0.63$). Total homocyst(e)ine values were negatively associated (Fig. 3). THcy levels for the estimated intakes of dietary folate were similar to results obtained in the two metabolic ward studies *(36,49)*. In another observational study, Stampfer et al. *(50)* found a correlation coefficient of –0.27 ($p < 0.001$) between plasma tHcy levels and folate intake among disease-free control men.

Figure 3 appears to show that the association between mean dietary folate and mean tHcy levels may not be linear, but may reach a plateau beyond which plasma tHcy levels remain stable. This existence of a plateau is supported by the result of Ubbink and colleagues *(39)* in which subjects, after 6 wk of treatment with 1000 μg folic acid, 0.4

mg cobalamin, and 12.2 mg pyridoxine, had no additional lowering of tHcy when twice these amounts were given.

3.2. Homocysteine and Blood Folate

Seven studies *(8,10,28,51–54)* of tHcy and folate found that tHcy levels markedly increased as plasma/serum folate levels decreased. Folate levels were determined from blood *(10)*, plasma *(28,52)*, or serum *(8,51)* samples and quantified by radioassay *(51,54)* or microbiological assay *(28,52)*. Five additional studies *(13,30,55–57)* provide support for a strong inverse association between total Hcy levels and plasma/serum folate levels.

Kang et al. *(51)* measured serum protein-bound homocysteine in 239 stored samples representing extreme depletion or sufficiency of folate or vitamin B_{12} among 1826 subjects seen in a 1 yr period at a major metropolitan medical center. The mean age of included subjects was 63.7 yr (range 16–97 yr) in this study, with 56% being female. Among subjects with subnormal serum folate (<4.5 nmol/L), 84% had homocysteine values that exceeded 2 standard deviations (SD) above the mean for a normal group. A level of serum folate concentration above which homocysteine levels did not change significantly appeared to be 9.1 nmol/L*. Since carefully conducted assessment of dietary folate intake reflects biochemically measured folate status *(58)*, these findings are consistent with an inverse association between tHcy levels and dietary folate over the low portion of the range of folate intake, with a flattening out of the relationship at the high end, as was shown in Fig. 3.

3.3. Pyridoxine and Vitamin B_{12}

Cobalamin alone is effective in lowering tHcy levels in cases with overt cobalamin (vitamin B_{12}) deficiency *(27,59–61)*. In 20 subjects with vascular disease with elevated tHcy values *(27)*, treatment with pyridoxine alone improved the result of the methionine loading test, whereas the inclusion of folic acid resulted in a marked decrease in basal tHcy levels, especially in subjects with hyperhomocyst(e)inemia. From this and other studies *(14)*, it appears that pyridoxine may be effective in reducing elevated tHcy following a methionine load test, but not in reducing the elevated fasting tHcy. Dudman et al. *(38)* found treatment with either pyridoxine or folic acid similarly effective to those from combined treatment for subjects with vascular disease as assessed with a post-methionine load test. Folic acid, on the other hand, seems to be the key factor in reducing fasting hyperhomocyst(e)inemia.

4. HOMOCYSTEINE AND CARDIOVASCULAR DISEASE

4.1. Homocysteine and Coronary Heart Disease

As described elsewhere *(34)*, the English-language medical literature was searched to find descriptive, observational, and experimental human studies concerning various kinds of vascular diseases and their relationship to tHcy levels, and/or folate levels, or folate intake. The search has been extended in this chapter to include both the period 1988 to June 1994 and the period June 1994 to November 1995. To the 17 studies iden-

---

*Criteria used to evaluate plasma folate levels in the absence of vitamin B_{12} deficiency in populations. High risk: <6.7 nmol/L, moderate risk: 6.7–11.1 nmol/L, low risk: >11.1 nmol/L *(58)*.

tified in the earlier review *(34)*, three more studies of homocysteine and CHD have been added. These 20 studies are summarized in Table 2. Study designs varied from prospective through cross-sectional to case-control studies in which controls were selected from a source population different from that of the cases. These source populations of controls ranged from volunteers to hospital patients. Other studies recruited controls from screening programs or population-based registries. Some studies included cases of both fatal and nonfatal myocardial infarction, whereas others included only nonfatal cases, sometimes defined by degree of angiographically confirmed occlusion of a coronary vessel. Seven studies measured PML levels of homocyst(e)ine as homocysteine-cysteine *(62,63)*, homocystine *(63)*, homocysteine-cysteine plus homocystine *(12,13,38,64)*, or not specified *(65)*. Of the 15 studies that used fasting levels of homocyst(e)ine, 12 measured tHcy *(31,50,56,66–74)*, one measured homocysteine-cysteine plus homocystine *(64)*, one measured homocysteine-cysteine and homocystine *(63)* and one measured protein-bound homocysteine *(75)*.

Study quality among studies used in the calculations were evaluated based on factors adapted from Friedenreich *(76)*. The areas evaluated were

1. Type of study design;
2. Representativeness of study sample;
3. Inclusion of potential confounders;
4. Homogeneity of case definition;
5. Quality of homocysteine measurement; and
6. For cases and controls, comparability of exclusion criteria.

Common study weaknesses included selection of controls from a different population from that of cases, subjects not representative of the general population, lack of homogeneity of case definition, and lack of information regarding storage-status of biological specimens. The quality scores clustered together such that studies with similar design had similar scores. Therefore, classification by study design also represents ranking by study quality.

Nested case-control studies were those whose controls were sampled from the cohort from which the cases arose; blood samples were obtained (and frozen) before the disease occurred. Population-based case-control studies were retrospective studies in which cases and controls were drawn from the same defined general population. These two study types were classified as "high quality." Cross-sectional studies used no sampling by outcome status and may have included convenience samples. "Other" case-control studies included hospital-based investigations and those whose controls were from a different population than the cases.

Malinow et al. *(32)* introduced the term hyperhomocyst(e)inemia to identify above normal concentrations of plasma/serum tHcy, which they defined as >16 µmol/L *(9)*. At present there is no consensus on the exact level for defining elevated tHcy. The definitions commonly employed are values exceeding the 90th or 95th percentile among a group of healthy subjects or values exceeding the mean of normal controls by more than 2 SD. The cut-off values used by investigators for classification of elevated tHcy levels in their respective studies, therefore, vary according to the distribution among their control subjects.

Based on consideration of all studies, we selected tHcy concentrations of >15 µmol/L as representative of hyperhomocyst(e)inemia in the general population. After

Table 2
Studies of Homocyst(e)ine and Coronary Artery Disease[a]

First author	No. of cases/controls[c]	Age, yr	Component	Homocyst(e)ine levels[b] Mean		Percent elevated	
				Cases	Controls	Cases	Controls
Post-methionine load							
Cross-sectional							
Wilcken (62)	25/22 m	< 50	4h, Hcy-cys	NG	NG	28	5*
Murphy-Chutorian (63)	99/39 m	21–65	6h, Hcy-Hcy	0.7	0.6	16	2*
Wilcken (64)	20/20 m	<50	4h, Hcy-Hcy + Hcy-cys	13.7	12.9	NG	NG
Other case-control							
Clarke (13)	60/27	<55	Peak, Hcy-Hcy + Hcy-cys	18.7[d]	13.4[d]	30	0
Dudman (38)	14/36 f	<52	4h and 8h, Hcy-Hcy + Hcy-cys	NG	NG	19	0
	48/20 m			NG	NG	29	0
	62/56			NG	NG	21	0
Graham, Daly[e] (65,77)	380/810	<55	Hcy	36.1	31.7	NG	NG
Boers (33)	25/40	<50	Peak, Hcy-Hcy + Hcy-cys	NG	NG	0	0
Fasting or basal							
Prospective, nested case-control							
Stampfer (50)	271/271 m	40–84	Total basal	11.1	10.5*	11	5
Alfthan (71)	92/141 m	40–64		9.8	9.8	9[f]	6[f]
	99/128 f		Total basal	9.4	9.3	9[f]	5[f]
Arnesen (72)	122/478	12–61	Total basal	12.7	11.3**	NG	NG

204

Study	Cases/controls	Age	Hcy measure	Control	Cases	Control %	Cases %
Population case-control							
Israelsson (66)	21/36 m	48–58	Total fasting	16.4	13.5*	24	6
Pancharuniti (69)	101/108 m	30–50	Total fasting	13.5[d]	11.9****,[d]	NG	NG
Wu (31)	170/168	≤55 m, ≤65 f	Total fasting	13.4	10.1***	18	4***
Cross-sectional							
Kang (75)	241/202	<69	Protein-bound fasting	5.5	4.3***	10	4
Malinow (67)	64/92 m	65/60	Total fasting	13.1	11.3*	19	5*
	35/167 f	70/62		12.9	10.2*	9	5
	99/259			NG	NG	15	5
Other case-control							
Genest (68)	170/255 m	<60	Total fasting	13.7	10.9***	28	10
Ubbink (56)	163/195 m	555	Total fasting	16.2	13.4	38	17
von Eckardstein (70)	199/156 m	36–65	Total basal	8.9[d]	7.8****,[d]	NG	NG
Dalery (73)	123/380 m	<60	Total fasting	11.7	9.7***	18.1	10
	27/204 f			12.0	7.6**	44.4	10
Robinson (74)	201/185 m	62 ± 11	Total fasting	13.9	11.2**	45	20
	103/46 f			15.3[g]	10.1**	56	20

*, **, *** $p < 0.05$, $p < 0.01$, $p < 0.001$ difference between cases and controls.

[a]Studies are represented in the table only. Two studies reported results for both postmethionine load and fasting values (63,64).

[b]Hcy = homocyst(e)ine, Hcy-Hcy = homocystine, Hcy-cys = homocysteine-cysteine. Elevated Hcy levels are usually determined as above the 95th percentile for the control group or above 2 SD of the control mean. NG = not given.

[c]Unless marked subjects are males and females. m = males, f = females.

[d]Geometric mean level of serum/plasma Hcy.

[e]Exact components of Hcy not given.

[f]Percent with elevated Hcy levels is for myocardial infarction and stroke based on 134 male cases and 131 female cases.

[g]Mean includes the value of a folate-deficient patient, namely 250 μmol/L tHcy.

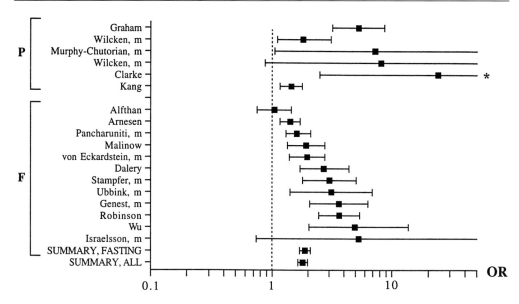

Fig. 4. Elevated homocysteine and CHD risk: odds ratios with 95% CI on a log scale. An odds ratio > 1.0 indicates that elevated homocyst(e)ine (Hcy) levels increase the risk for vascular disease. Unless indicated, odds ratios are for males (m) and females (f). Asterisks (*) indicate that the upper bound of the risk estimate was infinity. The *Summary All* includes all studies (except Graham et al. *[65]* since separate risk estimates for coronary artery disease, cerebrovascular disease, and peripheral vascular disease were not provided) and the *Summary Fasting* includes only studies that measured fasting levels of total homocysteine (tHcy). P: postmethionine load or protein-bound fasting homocysteine. F: fasting or basal total homocysteine.

examining tHcy distributions among controls, we considered a tHcy level of 10 μmol/L as being a "healthy" level, therefore, a 5 μmol/L reduction from 15 to 10 was noted as beneficial.

Of the seven studies that measured homocysteine post methionine load, three were cross-sectional and four were case-control studies whose subjects were not selected on a population basis. Their characteristics are summarized in Table 2. There was one study *(75)* that measured fasting protein-bound homocysteine. The remaining 12 studies all measured tHcy, eight from fasting samples and four from nonfasting samples. The three prospective studies measured basal levels, which are easier to obtain in large cohort investigations. All of the studies measuring tHcy provided mean levels for cases and controls (Table 2).

A significant difference (*P* < 0.05) between mean homocysteine levels of cases and controls was reported in 1 of the 17 studies that reported such data. Six of the 20 studies in Table 2 provided an estimate of the simple effect of homocyst(e)ine levels on coronary artery disease risk (not adjusted for other risk factors) as an odds ratio or relative risk estimate *(13,31,50,63,65,69,77)*. Twelve other studies provided enough data to allow us to calculate odds ratios *(56,62,64,66–68,70–75)*. The odds ratios and confidence intervals of these 18 studies are shown in Fig. 4. Of the two studies providing insufficient data, one showed support *(38)* and one lack of support *(12)* for homocyst(e)ine as a risk factor.

Fig. 4 also shows the pooled or summary odds ratio, calculated by us, for CHD in persons with elevated homocyst(e)ine levels as defined by the investigators in each

Concept of Population Distribution Shift

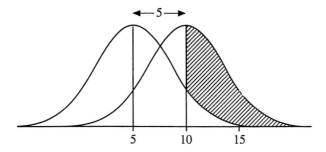

Fig. 5. Concept of population distribution shift. The concept of reducing homocyst(e)ine (Hcy) levels in the population by 5 μmol/L or shifting the population distribution. The potential benefit for reduction in Hcy levels is only assumed for those individuals in the shaded area. Only reductions to 10 μmol/L are considered beneficial for those individuals with Hcy values between 11 and 14 μmol/L. For individuals with Hcy values ≥15 μmol/L, benefit is assumed for the full 5 μmol/L reduction.

study. The summary estimate is 1.8 (CI 95%: 1.6,2.0). An analysis restricted to the 12 studies that measured fasting levels of tHcy *(31,50,56,66–74)* resulted in a similar summary odds ratio of 1.9 (CI 95%:1.7,2.1).

4.2. Potential Risk Reduction in the Population

Although early studies examined the risk of cardiovascular disease associated with elevated homocysteine, many recent studies have found evidence of a graded relationship between homocysteine and risk of cardiovascular disease *(72,74,78–80)*. Indeed, several studies *(69,81,82)* of carotid and coronary arteries indicate that the extent of quantitatively defined arterial narrowing is consistent with a graded response to increasing tHcy levels. Pooling information from studies that used disparate definitions of elevated homocysteine, as described in the previous section, leads to grouping of quite disparate estimates of risk. On the other hand, each of these studies can contribute estimates of the linear association between tHcy and CHD risk. As described in the earlier paper *(34)*, we were able to translate differences in mean values between cases and controls to estimate odds ratios per μmol/L change in tHcy using the linear discriminant function method *(83)*. Although this method is approximate, the assumption of a Gaussian distribution for tHcy leads to conservative estimates *(34)*. We calculated odds ratio estimates for a difference of 5 μmol/L in fasting tHcy concentration, from each study that measured fasting levels of tHcy in cases and controls, combined them using the general variance-based confidence interval method, and calculated summary estimates of the effect of tHcy on vascular disease risk assuming a fixed effects model, and using the methods of Greenland *(83)* and Pettiti *(84)*. The resultant odds ratios estimate the effect of moving the whole population distribution of homocysteine levels down by 5 μmol/L. This shift is shown schematically in Fig. 5. Individuals at each point of the Gaussian curve on the right have tHcy lowered by 5 μmol/L and are represented by a corresponding point of the Gaussian curve on the left.

Therefore, assuming a linear relationship between tHcy levels and risk of coronary artery disease, we calculated a summary odds ratio based on a 5 μmol/L increment in tHcy concentration for 12 studies *(31,50,56,66–74)* that measured fasting levels of tHcy in cases and controls. These are arranged in Fig. 6 in ascending order of odds ratio

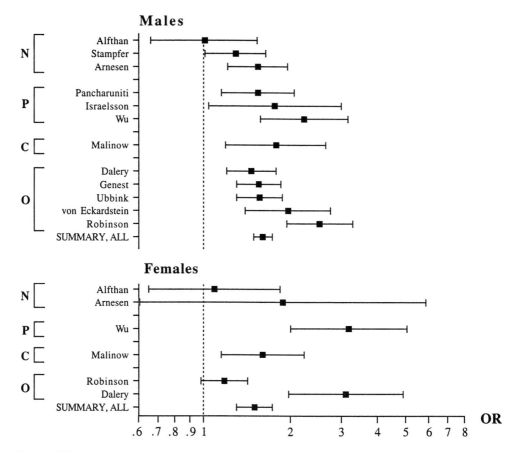

Fig. 6. CHD risk per 5 μmol/L change in homocyst(e)ine: odds ratios with 95% CI on a log scale. An odds ratio > 1.0 indicates that elevated homocyst(e)ine (Hcy) levels increase the risk for vascular disease. For each study, the odds ratio estimate was calculated from the mean levels of total Hcy in cases and controls by the linear discriminant function method. Unless indicated, odds ratios are for males and females. The *Summary All* included all studies in each figure. N: nested case-control studies within prospective studies; P: population-based case-control studies; C: cross-sectional studies; O: other case-control studies.

within study type, for males and females separately. For one study *(74)*, we excluded one very large outlying value of homocysteine from the mean value for female cases, since its inclusion greatly inflated both the mean and variance estimates for that study. The combined odds ratio for a 5 μmol/L increment in tHcy is 1.6 (CI 95%:1.5,1.7) for males and 1.5 (CI 95%: 1.3,1.7) for females. These results were similar when the summary included only the high quality studies. Effectively, there is between a 50 and 60% increase in the odds of CHD in those with higher homocysteine levels (5 μmol/L higher).

4.3. Homocysteine and Cerebrovascular Disease

To the 11 studies of homocysteine and risk of stroke summarized before *(12,13,27,38,57,65,71,77,85–88)*, one recent prospective study was added to the calculations *(80)*. This study, in middle-aged men from 18 different towns around England, Scotland, and Wales, detected a significant risk of stroke associated with homocysteine, in contrast with the other two published nested case-control studies. Characteristics of all 12 studies are summarized in Table 3. Four studies of presymptomatic carotid arteriosclerosis, not included in Table 3, provide additional support for tHcy as a risk factor in cerebrovascular disease. Evidence of carotid atherosclerosis using ultrasound methods was noted in heterozygotes for cystathionine-β-synthase deficiency *(89,90)*. Two larger cross-sectional studies also showed an association of hyperhomocyst(e)inemia with objective evidence of carotid-artery stenosis *(81,82)*.

Ten studies provided odds ratios or provided sufficient data to calculate odds ratios of the effect of elevated homocyst(e)ine on cerebrovascular disease risk *(13,27,57,65, 71,77,80,85–88)*. Odds ratios and 95% confidence intervals are presented in Fig. 7. Two additional studies (12,38), with insufficient data for estimating an odds ratio, also provided support for homocyst(e)ine as a risk factor. The summary estimate of the odds ratio of cerebrovascular disease and elevated homocyst(e)ine concentration is 2.0 (CI 95%: 1.7,2.4) (Fig. 7). When restricted to seven studies that measured fasting or basal levels of tHcy *(27,57,71,80,86–88)*, a combined odds ratio of 1.9 (CI 95%: 1.6,2.3) is obtained.

Since, once again, the definitions of the level of tHcy considered elevated were inconsistent, we calculated a summary odds ratio based on a change of 5 µmol/L in tHcy levels using the seven studies that measured fasting levels of tHcy. The combined odds ratio is 1.8 (CI 95%: 1.6,2.0) and included data from both males and females (Fig. 8). The combined odds ratio of the high quality studies *(57,71,80,88)* is slightly lower: 1.5 (CI 95%: 1.3,1.8).

4.4. Homocysteine and Peripheral Vascular Disease

A recent population-based case-control study by Mansoor and colleagues *(91)* has been added to our previous review of nine studies of homocysteine and peripheral vascular disease *(12,13,27,32,38,65,77,92–94)*, and described in Table 4. Three of the studies in Table 4 included cases of vascular disease other than peripheral vascular disease. The tHcy measurements reported by Malinow et al. *(32)* and Taylor et al. *(92)* include cases of cerebrovascular disease. The odds ratio in the Graham *(65)* and Daly *(77)* study included all vascular diseases.

Two studies estimated the effect of homocyst(e)ine on peripheral vascular disease risk *(13,65,77)*, whereas four provided data to calculate such risks *(27,91,93,94)* (Fig. 9). The summary odds ratio included the four studies that measured fasting levels of tHcy *(27,91,93,94)*. The combined odds ratio is 2.0 (CI 95%: 1.5,2.6). The two studies with insufficient data for estimating an odds ratio also supported homocyst(e)ine as a risk factor *(12,38)*.

5. FOLATE AND CARDIOVASCULAR DISEASE

5.1. Plasma Folate and Risk of Cardiovascular Disease

Many studies of cardiovascular disease and tHcy levels also measured folate, vitamin B_6 and vitamin B_{12} as summarized in Table 5. Mean levels of plasma/serum folate among cases were reported significantly lower than among controls in two studies *(69,94)*. On the other hand, the mean folate concentration between cases and controls

Table 3
Studies on Homocyst(e)ine and Cerebrovascular Disease[a]

First author	No. of cases/controls[c]	Age, yr	Component	Homocyst(e)ine levels[b] Mean		Percent elevated	
				Cases	Controls	Cases	Controls
Post-methionine load							
Other case-control							
Brattstrom (85)	19/17	34–63	4h Hcy-cys	16.0*	11.9*	NG	NG
Boers (12)	25/40	<50	Peak Hcy-Hcy + Hcy-cys	NG	NG	28	0
Clarke (13)	38/27	<55	Peak Hcy-Hcy + Hcy-cys	18.7[d]	13.4*,[d]	42	0
Dudman (38)	27/20 m	<61	Peak Hcy-Hcy + Hcy-cys	NG	NG	15	0
	24/36 f		4h and 8h Hcy-Hcy + Hcy-cys	NG	NG	23	0
	51/56			NG	NG	23	0
Graham, Daly[e] (65,77)	214/810	<55	Hcy	40.5	31.7	NG	NG
Fasting or basal							
Prospective, nested case-control							
Alfthan (71)	42/141 m	40–60	Basal total	10.4	9.8	9[f]	6[f]
	32/128 f			10.1	9.3	9[f]	5[f]
Verhoef (88)	109/427 m	60	Basal total	11.1	10.6	26	20
Perry (80)	107/118 m	40–59	Basal total	13.7[d]	11.9**,[d]	NG	NG
Population case-control							
Brattstrom (14)	54/34 m	38–72	Fasting total	17.4	12.7***	NG	NG
	16/32 f	38–72		14.4	11.1***	NG	NG
	70/66	38–72		16.8	11.9***	31	6
Hospital case-control							
Araki (86)	90/45	39–79	Fasting total	13.1	8.6*	NG	NG
Other case-control							
Brattstrom (27)	18/46	24–63	Fasting total	13.2	11.0*	17	4
Coull (87)	41/31	67/61	Fasting total	15.8	10.7***	NG	NG

[a]See key to Table 2.

210

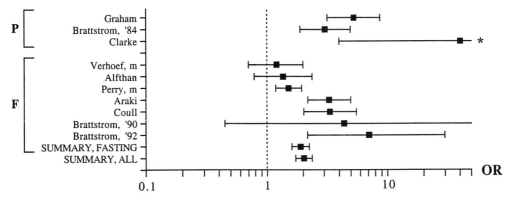

Fig. 7. Elevated homocysteine and cerebrovascular disease risk: odds ratios with 95% CI on a log scale. An odds ratio > 1.0 indicates that elevated homocyst(e)ine (Hcy) levels increase the risk for vascular disease. Unless indicated, odds ratios are for males (m) and females (f). Asterisks (*) indicate that the upper bound of the risk estimate was infinity. The *Summary All* includes all studies (except Graham et al. *[65]* since separate risk estimates for coronary artery disease, cerebrovascular disease, and peripheral vascular disease were not provided) and the *Summary Fasting* includes only studies that measured fasting levels of total Hcy. P: post methionine load homocysteine; F: fasting or basal total homocysteine.

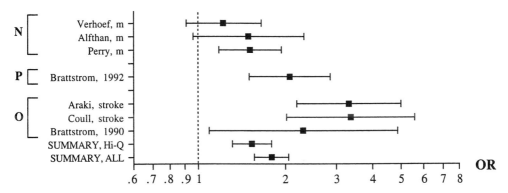

Fig. 8. Cerebrovascular disease risk per 5 μmol/L change in homocyst(e)ine: odds ratios with 95% CI on a log scale. An odds ratio > 1.0 indicates that elevated homocyst(e)ine (Hcy) levels increase the risk for vascular disease. For each study, the odds ratio estiamte was calculated from the mean levels of total Hcy in cases and controls by the linear discriminant function method. Unless indicated, odds ratios are for males (m) and females (f). The *Summary All* included all studies and the *Summary High Quality (Hi-Q)* included only those studies classified as high quality. N: nested case-control studies within prospective studies; P: population-based case-control studies; O: other case-control studies.

were not significantly different in four studies *(27,85,93,95)*. However, in one of these studies *(93)*, elevation of plasma tHcy in subjects with intermittent claudication (a manifestation of peripheral vascular disease) was mainly confined to subjects with serum folate levels of ≤11.0 nmol/L. The univariate odds ratio for coronary artery disease of the highest quartile of plasma folate (9.3 nmol/L) compared to the lowest (<3.5 nmol/L) was 0.4 (CI 95%: 0.3,0.9) in men *(69)*. The National Health and Nutrition Examination

Table 4
Studies on Homocyst(e)ine and Peripheral Vascular Disease[a]

| First author | No. of cases/controls[c] | Age, yr | Component | Homocyst(e)ine levels[b] | | | |
| | | | | Mean | | Percent elevated | |
				Cases	Controls	Cases	Controls
Post-methionine load							
Population case-control							
Mansoor (91)	82/65	36–62	4^h Hcy	39.8	28.1**	NG	NG
Other case-control							
Boers (12)	25/40	<50	Peak Hcy-Hcy + Hcy-cys	NG	NG	28	0
Clarke (13)	25/27	<55	Peak Hcy-Hcy + Hcy-cys	15.8[d]	13.4*[d]	28	0
Dudman (38)	9/20 m	<61	4^h and 8^h Hcy-Hcy + Hcy-cys	NG	NG	22	0
	9/36 f			NG	NG	11	0
	18/56			NG	NG	16	0
Graham, Daly[e,h] (65,77)	154/810	<55	Hcy	39.9	31.7	NG	NG
Fasting							
Population case-control							
Molgaard (93)	78/98 m	45–69	Fasting total	16.7	13.8***	23	5
Bergmark (94)	58/58	<50	Fasting total	NG	NG	28	5
Mansoor (91)	82/65	36–62	Fasting total	15.7	11.7***	NG	NG
Other case-control							
Malinow[h] (32)	26/18 m	70/>60	Fasting total	15.4	10.7*	NG	NG
	21/11 f			17.0	9.0*	NG	NG
	47/29			16.2	10.1*	47	0***
Brattstrom (27)	37/46	24–63	Fasting total	18.7	11.0***	32	4
Taylor[h] (92)	214/29	65/>60	Fasting total	14.4	10.1*	NG	NG

See key to Table 2.
[h]Cases included instances of vascular disease other than peripheral vascular disease
Study by Mansoor evaluated both fasting and postmethionine load tHcy

212

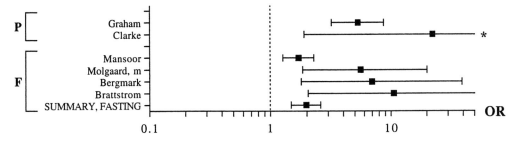

Fig. 9. Elevated homocysteine and peripheral vascular disease risk: odds ratios with 95% CI on a log scale. An odds ratio > 1.0 indicates that elevated homocyst(e)ine (Hcy) levels increase the risk for vascular disease. Unless indicated, odds ratios are for males (m) and females (f). Asterisks (*) indicate that the upper bound of the risk estimate was infinity. The *Summary Fasting* includes only studies that measured fasting levels of total Hcy. P: post methionine load homocysteine; F: fasting or basal total homocysteine.

and Survey (NHANES) Epidemiologic Follow-up Study (95) reported an elevated risk for stroke in men and women, but only the risk for black subjects with folate levels <9.2 nmol/L was significantly elevated (odds ratio 3.6; CI 95%: 1.02–12.71).

When subjects in studies of vascular disease were divided according to levels of tHcy, individuals with reduced tHcy levels had significantly higher levels of blood folate *(56,57)* and red cell folate *(13)* (Table 5). Finally, plasma, red cell, and serum folate levels were significantly and negatively correlated (–0.25 to –0.57) with tHcy levels *(27,31,57,69,93)* among cases with vascular disease. Studies examining the correlation between levels of tHcy and folate among controls were less consistent; three studies *(27,57,93)* reported insignificant results among controls, whereas the correlation among controls (–0.48, $p = 0.0001$) from a community-based case-control study *(69)* was higher than among cases (–0.40, $p = 0.0001$).

6. CONCLUSIONS

6.1. Evidence of a Causal Relationship Between Homocysteine and CHD

The evidence linking homocysteine levels with risk of cardiovascular disease is very strong and consistent, particularly with risk of CHD. Both prospective and case-control studies suggest a positive association. There is also evidence for CHD that hyperhomocyst(e)inemia is a major risk factor independent of some other known major risk factors, such as total-cholesterol *(50,63,66,68,69,75)*, low density lipoprotein (LDL)- or high density lipoprotein (HDL)-cholesterol *(31,50,68,69)*, body mass index *(50,69)*, age *(69)*, and high blood pressure *(50,68,69,75)*. Although the magnitude of the association is not large, it could be estimated with good precision. The summary risk estimate for coronary artery disease for an increase of 5 μmol/L of homocysteine was 1.6 for males and 1.5 for females. This level of risk is similar to other well-established risk factors for CHD.

There is some evidence that elevated tHcy levels precede the occurrence of coronary artery disease. There is no evidence that coronary artery disease or related diagnostic

Table 5

Concentration of Vitamins by Homocyst(e)ine Levels and/or Vascular Disease Status, listed by Folate Measurement

| | | | | Mean (± SD) concentration of vitamins | | | | | |
| | | | | B6, nmol/L | | B12, pmol/L | | Folate, nmol/L | |
First author	No. of cases/No. of controls[a]	Age range	Homocyst(e)ine condition/other conditions[b]	Cases	Controls	Cases	Controls	Cases	Controls
Ubbink[c] (56)	129/195 males	see Table 1	Fasting: > 16.3 µmol/L ≤ 16.3 µmol/L	Plasma: 30.1 ± 21.6 29.8 ± 17.7	—[d]	Plasma: 286.2 ± 291.1 310.6 ± 143.5	—	Blood: 377.0 ± 142.7 533.4 ± 170.4***,e	—
Brattstrom (57)	142/66	38–90	Fasting: > 18.3 µmol/L ≤ 183 µmol/L	Plasma: 21.9 ± 12.3 31.9 ± 16.2**,e	15.3 ± 3.5 25.8 ± 13.6	Serum: 282 ± 159 270 ± 115	175 ± 81.9 254 ± 89.9	Blood: 288 ± 101 364 ± 142***,e	211 ± 60.7 302 ± 78.9
Brattstrom (27)	37[f]–46 18[f]–(46) 17[f]–(46)	24–63	Fasting	Plasma: 17.9 ± 8.6 20.5 ± 8.1 13.7 ± 7.0	39.7 ± 24.9*** Same *** Same ***	Serum: 302 ± 142 271 ± 123 289 ± 103	243 ± 106* Same Same	Red cell: 296 ± 106 330 ± 114 297 ± 147	306 ± 81 same same
Clark[g] (13)	111/27	<55	Peak PML: ≥ 24 µmol/L < 24 µmol/L	— —	— —	Serum: 293 ± 121 374 ± 129**,e	—	Red cell: 653 ± 197 1240 ± 362**,e	—
Pancharutunii (69)	101/108 males	30–50	Fasting	—	—	Plasma: 343.2[h]	331.0[h]	Plasma: 10.2[h]	12.5*,h
Brattstrom (85)	19/17	34–63	Fasting	—	—	Serum: 436.4 ± 57.2[i]	356.1 ± 33.3[i]	Serum: 13.3 ± 1.6[i]	11.8 ± 1.3[i]
Molgaard (93)	78/98	45–69	Fasting	—	—	Serum: 230.6 ± 93.8	210.5 ± 81.2	Serum: 11.2 ± 6.8	11.3 ± 6.4
Bergmark (94)	58/58	<50	Fasting: Smokers Non/exsmokers	Not specified: 26.50 34.13*,j	34.83 42.33*,j	Not specified: 470 393	350 364	Serum: 11.15 15.21*,j	12.78 13.33
Giles (95)	98/1908	25–74		—	—	—	—	Serum: 17.3	18.7

*p < 0.05, **p < 0.01, ***p < 0.001 difference between cases and controls, unless otherwise noted.

[a]Unless otherwise indicated, numbers refer to males and females combined. Numbers in parenthesis indicate controls were used for more than one analysis.

[b]Conditions include postmethionine load test (PML), fasting, or basal levels of homocyst(e)ine, as well as other factors, e.g., smokers and nonsmokers.

[c]Study included 163 coronary artery disease (CAD) cases, however vitamin status assessed for 129 CAD subjects with one, two, or three occluded vessel(s).

[d]— = data not available.

[e]Difference between individuals above and below homocyst(e)ine cut-off levels.

[f]Brattstrom (27) study: n = 37 subjects with intermittent claudication, n = 18 subjects with transient ischemic attacks or stroke, n = 17 subjects with cerebral thrombosis with verified cerebral infection.

[g]Study included 123 vascular disease cases, however vitamin status was assessed for 111.

[h]Geometric mean.

[i]± SEM

[j]Difference between smokers and non/exsmokers within case or control status.

214

manipulations influence tHcy concentrations. In the positive prospective studies *(50,72,80)* high tHcy levels clearly antedated the manifestations of either coronary artery disease or stroke.

6.2. Possible Biological Mechanisms

There are biologically plausible mechanisms by which tHcy might alter risk of developing vascular disease. Atherogenic mechanisms promoted by homocysteine include endothelial cell desquamation, oxidation of LDL, and monocyte adhesion to the vessel wall *(1,22)*. Direct toxicity of homocysteine to the endothelium has been reported in laboratory studies *(96–98)*. Harker et al. showed endothelial desquamation in vivo in baboons infused with homocystine *(99)* or homocysteine *(100)* at the high levels typical of patients with homocystinuria. Tsai and coworkers *(101)* have shown that homocysteine increases DNA synthesis in vascular smooth muscle cells consistent with early arteriosclerotic lesions and induces these cells to proliferate while impeding the regeneration of endothelial cells. Homocysteine may predispose to arteriosclerosis by promoting oxidation of LDL *(102)* or by decreasing thrombomodulin cell-surface expression and inhibiting protein C activation, thus probably contributing to development of thrombosis *(103)*.

In summary, the association between hyperhomocyst(e)inemia and CHD is of the same order as that of other major risk factors for heart disease. We concluded that the association is likely to be causal. Thus, one can calculate an estimate of the population attributable-risk percent (PAR%).

6.3. Reducing Risk Associated with Elevated Homocysteine

The body of work linking hyperhomocyst(e)inemia to coronary artery disease was used to calculate the PAR%, which is the proportion of excess CHD in the population attributable to hyperhomocyst(e)inemia *(104)*. Demographic and mortality data from CHD were obtained from the *Statistical Abstract of the United States 1993*, 113th edition *(105)*.

When the PAR% is calculated for a population shift in the whole distribution of a risk factor, the proportion of the population exposed to that risk factor is 1.0. We took the conservative approach of assuming that the benefit of reduced tHcy (the distribution shift) accrued only in individuals with total tHcy >10 µmol/L, so that no more than 40% of the population was assumed to be exposed to the elevated tHcy in all calculations. This concept is illustrated in the shaded area of Fig. 5. The cutoff of 10 µmol/L was chosen since it is the median value of tHcy in adult males, estimated from population-based studies *(68,69)*. The proportion of the population with tHcy in 1 µmol/L intervals between 10 and 15 µmol/L was estimated for males *(68,69)* and females (16,31,55) using data from population-based studies. The potential benefits of a distribution shift of 5 µmol/L were calculated as the sum of five separately computed PAR% values for reducing tHcy, described in more detail elsewhere *(34)*. Summing these incremental PAR% values, the estimated proportion of potentially preventable deaths from coronary artery disease as a result of a decrease in tHcy in males aged 45+ in the United States is between 11 and 16%, which is between 38,000 and 55,500 deaths per year. The corresponding values for females are between 5 and 10%, the equivalent of between 17,500 and 35,500 deaths per year.

6.4. *Folic Acid and Homocysteine Reduction*

Although there are no studies that directly relate daily intake of folic acid with the postulated reduced risk of coronary artery disease, there are data linking folic acid intake with reduced plasma tHcy levels and other data linking elevated tHcy levels with CHD risk. We inferred that increased folic acid intake would reduce levels of tHcy and that a change in tHcy levels would be reflected in decreased coronary artery disease. We extended the concept of population attributable risk percent to estimate the potential extent of preventable mortality from CHD with defined changes in folate intake in the population. To estimate the corresponding odds ratio for any given change in folic acid intake, we assumed a perfect translation to a change in tHcy. Because the changes in folic acid intake of interest are in the range 50–400 µg/d, we used only information from studies changing folate intake in that range. These were two metabolic studies *(36,49)*, which each provided three data points for estimating the regression line of change in tHcy on change in folate. The estimated slope was 0.0092 with intercept 1.05. Next, we used the linear relationship between tHcy levels and CHD (with slope 0.094 for males and 0.081 for females). We then calculated the contribution to the population-attributable risk percent from changes in elevated tHcy, again assuming that reductions of tHcy below 10 µmol/L would have no further benefit. Three intervention strategies: dietary advice to increase folate, folic acid supplementation in the form of tablets, and food fortification by adding folic acid to grains were considered.

6.4.1. DIETARY CHANGES TO INCREASE FOLATE INTAKE

If the population would change dietary intake of folate by eating two or three more servings daily of fruits and vegetables, dietary folate ingestion would be expected to increase by about 100 µg/d. If the bioavailability of dietary folate is about half that of (unconjugated) folic acid *(106)*, a daily increase of about 50 µg folic acid could be expected. Such an increase of folic acid would be associated with an average decrease in tHcy of about 2 µmol/L. No dietary intervention program can be assumed to be 100% effective; therefore, we calculated expected results for 20, 40, and 80% effectiveness of such a program. We restricted the effect to members of the population not currently taking folic acid supplements. We assumed that all persons with tHcy levels ≥15 µmol/L were not taking supplements *(55)*, that 66% of males and 52% of females with tHcy levels of 10–15 µmol/L were not taking supplements *(107)*. These two considerations modify the calculation of the proportion exposed, which also takes into account the percentage of the population with tHcy levels in the relevant range (above 10 µmol/L). The percentage of male deaths from CHD preventable as a result of this dietary intervention program would be between 0.9 and 5.3%. For females these levels would be between 0.4 and 3.2%. The impact of this intervention strategy as measured by the number of deaths potentially prevented per year is shown in Table 6, always assuming that increased folate intake would affect CHD mortality through reducing tHcy.

6.4.2. FOLIC ACID SUPPLEMENTS

If a person not currently taking supplements with folic acid started taking them, about 400 µg/d folic acid (the level in most supplements) would be added to that individual's daily intake. With such an increase, the average decrease in tHcy levels in a member of the general population would be about 5 µmol/L. We used the same assumptions concerning benefit only to nonsupplement users described above, and calculated the expected effects with programs achieving different success rates. If programs of folic acid supplementation intervention were to successfully reach 10, 25, or 50% of the target population, the proportion of potentially preventable deaths among adult males from CHD would be between 0.9 and 6.6%. For females, these values would be between 0.3 and 3.2% (Table 6).

6.4.3. FOOD FORTIFICATION

Fortification is the addition of a nutrient(s) to foods to prevent or correct a nutrient deficiency, to balance the total nutrient profile of a food, or to restore nutrients lost in processing. Currently, in addition to thiamin, niacin, riboflavin, and iron added to refined grains to enrich them, iodine is added to salt and vitamins A and D are added to dairy products. Proposals *(108,109)* to fortify flours and cereal products with folic acid at 140 μg/100 g or 350 μg/100 g have been discussed by the Food and Drug Administration (FDA) as a public health measure to reduce the incidence of neural tube defects. In calculating the PAR%, we assumed that there would be no change in supplementation habits, that nonsupplement users would accrue no additional benefit, and that 10% of the population would continue to eat only non-fortified grain products. Using food consumption data for males and females (51+ yr) *(109)*, a representative increase in folic acid intake under each fortification scheme would be 170 and 350 μg/day, respectively, for males and 160 and 250 μg/day, respectively, for females. We interpolated these changes in median values from data provided for the 25th and 95th percentiles of the estimated distributions of intake before and after fortification. The corresponding average decrease in tHcy levels would be about 2.6 and 4.3 μmol/L, respectively, for males and slightly lower for females. The proportion of deaths from CHD potentially preventable among males, estimated conservatively, would be between 5.9 and 8.4%, and between 7.1 and 10.2%, respectively, and among females, between 1.7 and 3.6%, and between 2.2 and 4.8%, respectively (Table 6). The values given are the 95% confidence limits of the estimated population-attributable risk percents according to each fortification scheme.

6.5. Limitations

In meta-analysis, results are combined from studies that may differ in methodology and include noncomparable populations. Publication bias, i.e., not publishing small negative studies, is possible. Although negative studies that were published were included in the summary risk ratios, there may have been other negative studies performed whose lack of inclusion may have inflated the summary risk ratios.

There are no studies that directly relate dietary folate to occurrence of vascular disease. The relationship between homocysteine and CHD risk is very strong, but there have been no randomized controlled trials. Although many investigations demonstrate that folic acid reduces tHcy levels, the nature of that relationship is estimated from only a small number of studies. Although various combinations of folic acid, vitamin B_{12}, and vitamin B_6 were often administered, folic acid appeared to be the effective agent since it reduced tHcy levels even when given alone. However, because the interactions of folic acid, vitamin B_{12}, and vitamin B_6 are not fully known, further studies of all three of the vitamins would be useful.

Whether nutritional inadequacy of folic acid alone will raise tHcy levels or whether this response is limited to individuals predisposed genetically to develop hyperhomo-

Table 6
Potential Impact on Prevention of Deaths from Coronary Heart Disease for Males and Females Aged 45+ Based on Three Intervention Strategies

Intervention strategy	Increase in folic acid (μg/d)[a]	Percent of CHD deaths potentially prevented				Annual number of potentially preventable deaths[b]			
		Males		Females		Males		Females	
		Estimate	Range	Estimate	Range	Estimate	Range	Estimate	Range
Nutrition education to increase dietary folate									
20% effective	50	1.1	0.9–1.3	0.6	0.4–0.8	4000	3000–4500	2000	1500–3000
40% effective	50	2.3	1.9–2.7	1.2	0.7–1.6	8000	6500–9500	4500	2500–6000
80% effective	50	4.5	3.8–5.3	2.3	1.5–3.2	15,500	13,000–18,500	8000	5500–11,500
Folic acid supplements									
10% effective	400	1.1	0.9–1.3	0.5	0.3–0.6	4000	3000–4500	1500	1000–2000
25% effective	400	2.8	2.3–3.3	1.1	0.7–1.6	9500	8000–11,500	4000	2500–5500
50% effective	400	5.6	4.6–6.6	2.3	1.4–3.2	19,500	16,000–23,000	8000	5000–11,500
Food fortification of flour and cereal products at:									
140 μg/100 g	m: 170; f: 160	7.1	5.9–8.4	2.6	1.7–3.6	24,500	20,500–29,000	9000	6000–12,500
350 μg/100 g	m: 350; f: 280	8.6	7.1–10.2	3.4	2.2–4.8	30,000	24,500–35,500	12,000	8000–17,000

[a]Bioavailability of dietary folate assumed to be about half that of folic acid (unconjugated).
[b]Mortality data from CHD based on data for males and females 45+ from 1990 in US Bureau of the Census, *Statistical Abstract of the United States: 1993* (113th edition) Washington, DC, 1993.

cyst(e)inemia needs further study. The existence of several different genetic traits (including the common MTHFR polymorphism described in Section 2.2) predisposing to high tHcy levels suggests that genetic variability in response to folic acid intake might be expected. At least until such differences are fully elucidated, a population approach that treats the different genetic and environmental origins of the homocyst(e)ine-folic acid relationship in the same way appears appropriate.

6.6. The Broader Health Context

Are there negative implications of widespread supplementation or fortification with folic acid? It has been known for a long time that folic acid may mask the hematological manifestation of unrecognized pernicious anemia (cobalamin deficiency), allowing its neurological manifestations, which may be severe and include spinal cord damage, to progress (110). However, such effects were mainly observed with high pharmacological doses of folic acid, i.e., 5000 µg or more. It is not clear whether such high doses precipitate or exacerbate the neuropathy of cobalamin deficiency. The effect on the neuropathy of vitamin B_{12} deficiency of lower doses, such as might be expected to occur were grain to be fortified or dietary supplements to be taken on a widespread basis, remains poorly defined (110). Recent studies have estimated among the elderly a 5% prevalence of serum vitamin B_{12} deficiency associated with methylmalonicacidemia (54,61), unrelated to pernicious anemia. This deficiency could be corrected by low doses of cobalamin. If the oral dose of vitamin B_{12} were large enough, even persons with pernicious anemia (estimated to be 1/5000) (111) would derive some benefit, because 1–3% of vitamin B_{12} can be absorbed by simple diffusion (112). In any of the strategies discussed to increase folic acid intake, the highest consumers of folic acid would be those taking vitamin supplements containing 400 µg of folic acid. The current 100% daily values for folic acid, vitamin B_6, and vitamin B_{12} available in supplements are 400 µg, 20 mg, and 6 µg respectively. Were 1 mg (1000 µg) cobalamin to be added to vitamin supplements containing 400 µg folic acid, most vitamin B_{12} deficiencies would be corrected, and concern about the possible masking effects of folic acid would be considerably lessened (110).

What are other implications of such a nutritional policy? There are about 2500 cases of neural tube defects per year in the United States, and about 1500 fetuses with this condition are aborted per year following detection by prenatal diagnosis (113). Women who had children with neural tube defects have slightly elevated tHcy levels. In some women this is because of low folate intake or poor absorption, and in some this is presumably caused by yet undescribed genetic defects or variants predisposing to hyperhomocyst(e)inemia (114). There is excellent evidence from a variety of studies that at least 50% of neural tube defects can be prevented if 400 µg of folic acid is taken daily before and during the first 4 wk of pregnancy (113). Since many women do not realize when they are in the very early stages of pregnancy, folic acid supplementation and dietary counseling are needed before or very early in pregnancy to prevent neural tube defects. Currently, efforts have not been successful in increasing folic acid intake in the population during this critical time (115). It has, therefore, been recommended to add folic acid to the food supply by fortification of grains (109). This recommendation might help to prevent a large number of neural tube defects and, in the light of our meta-analysis, at the same time promises to have the much larger effect in reducing vascular disease in many thousands of men and women (see Chapter 19).

7. RECOMMENDATIONS

On a population basis, fortification of grains with folic acid would be the most logical step to help to prevent a large fraction of neural tube defects. The strength of the evidence suggests that fortification as a public health measure might also be of benefit in the prevention of vascular disease. It appears that the potential benefits far outweigh the available evidence concerning possible risks for neurological impairment with undiagnosed vitamin B_{12} deficiency. Major clinical trials to assess the role of folic acid for vascular disease prevention with careful attention to its possible neurological effects in vitamin B_{12} deficient individuals should be initiated by the National Institutes of Health. Meanwhile, action on a population basis should not wait: A combined strategy to increase both folic acid and vitamin B_{12} intake appears prudent at this stage *(110)*, and would likely improve the potential for lowering the risk of arteriosclerotic vascular disease as well as neural tube defects. We recommend a policy of fortification of grains with folic acid at 350 µg/100 g and the mandatory addition of 1 mg vitamin B_{12} to all vitamin supplements containing 400 µg folic acid.

On an individual basis, we recommend taking a dietary supplement of 400 µg/d folic acid to prevent vascular disease. This recommendation has particular potential benefit for middle aged and older people, both men and women. Such a dose is found in most multivitamins of the one-a-day type.

8. POSTSCRIPT

Since this chapter was written, the FDA has regulated changes in the standards of identity for enriched flour and cereal grain products such that they will contain about 140 µg folic acid/100 g. effective January 1, 1998.

REFERENCES

1. Mudd SH, Levy HL, Skovby F. Disorders of transsulfuration. In: The Metabolic Basis of Inherited Disease, 6th ed. Scriver CR, Beaudet AL, Sly WS, Valle D, eds. New York: McGraw-Hill, 1989; pp.693–734.
2. Ueland PM, Refsum H. Plasma homocysteine, a risk factor for vascular disease: plasma levels in health, disease, and drug therapy. J Lab Clin Med 1989; 114:473–501.
3. Mason JB, Miller JW. The effects of vitamins B_{12}, B_6, and folate on blood homocysteine levels. Ann NY Acad Sci 1992; 669:197–203.
4. Selhub J, Miller JW. The pathogenesis of homocysteinemia: interruption of the coordinate regulation of S-adenosylmethionine of the remethylation and transsulfuration of homocysteine. Am J Clin Nutr 1992; 55:131–138.
5. Brattstrom LE, Hultberg BL, Hardebo JE. Folic acid responsive postmenopausal homocysteinemia. Metabolism 1985; 34:1073–1077.
6. Kang S, Wong PWK, Malinow MR. Hyperhomocyst(e)inemia as a risk factor for occlusive vascular disease. Ann Rev Nutr 1992; 12:279–298.
7. Araki A, Sako Y. Determination of free and total homocysteine in human plasma by high-performance liquid chromatography with fluorescence detection. J Chromatogr 1987; 422:43–52.
8. Ueland PM, Refsum H, Stabler SP, Malinow MR, Andersson A, Allen RH. Total homocysteine in plasma or serum: methods and clinical applications. Clin Chem 1993; 39:1764–1779.
9. Malinow MR. Role of plasma homocyst(e)ine in arterial occlusive diseases. Clin Chem 1994; 40:857,858.
10. Andersson A, Brattstrom L, Israelsson B, Isaksson A, Hamfelt A, Hultberg B. Plasma homocysteine before and after methionine loading with regard to age, gender, and menopausal status. Eur J Clin Invest 1992; 22:79–87.
11. Shipchandler MT, Moore EG. Rapid, fully automated measurement of plasma homocyst(e)ine with the Abbott Imx^r Analyzer. Clin Chem 1995; 41:991–994.

12. Boers GHJ, Smals AGH, Trijbels FJM, Fowler B, Bakkeren JAJM, Schoonderwaldt HC, et al. Heterozygosity for homocystinuria in premature peripheral and cerebral occlusive arterial disease. New Engl J Med 1985; 313:709–715.
13. Clarke R, Daly L, Robinson K, Naughten E, Cahalane S, Fowler B, et al. Hyperhomocysteinemia: an independent risk factor for vascular disease. New Engl J Med 1991; 324:1149–1155.
14. Brattstrom L, Lindgren A. Hyperhomocysteinemia as a risk factor for stroke. Neurol Res 1992; 14:81–84.
15. McGill JJ, Mettler G, Rosenblatt DS, Scriver CR. Detection of heterozygotes for recessive alleles. Homocyst(e)inemia: paradigm of pitfalls in phenotypes. Am J Med Genet 1990; 36:45–52.
16. Berg K, Malinow MR, Kierulf P, Upson B. Population variation and genetics of plasma homocyst(e)ine level. Clin Genet 1992; 41:315–321.
17. Reed T, Malinow MR. Chritian JC, Upson B. Estimates of heritability of plasma homocyst(e)ine levels in aging adult male twins. Clin Genet 1991; 425–428.
18. Genest JJ, McNamara JR, Upson B, Salem DN, Ordovas JM, Schaefer EJ, et al. Prevalence of familial hyperhomocyst(e)inemia in men with premature coronary artery disease. Arteriosclerosis Throb. 1991; 11:1129–1136.
19. Williams RR, Malinow MR, Hunt SC, Upson B, Wu LL, Hopkins PN, et al. Hyperhomocyst(e)inemia in Utah Siblings with early coronary disease. Coronary Artery Dis 1990; 1:681–685.
20. Mudd SH, Levy HL, Skovby F. Disorders of transsulfuration. In: The Metabolic and Molecular Bases of Inherited Disease, 7th ed. Scriver CR, Beaudet AL, Sly WS, Valle D, eds. New York: McGraw Hill, 1995, pp. 1279–1327.
21. Rosenblatt DS, Thomas IT, Watkins D, Cooper BA, Erbe RW. Vitamin B12 responsive homocysteinuria and megaloblastic anemia: heterogeneity in methylcobalamin deficiency. Am J Med Genet 1987; 26:377–383.
22. Rees MM, Rodgers GM. Homocysteinemia: association of a metabolic disorder with vascular disease and thrombosis. Throm Res 1993; 71:337–359.
23. Kang S, Zhou J, Wong PWK, Kowalisyn J, Strokosch G. Intermediate homocysteinemia: a thermolabile variant of methylenetetrahydrofolate reductase. Am J Hum Genet 1988; 43:414–421.
24. Frosst P, Blom HJ, Milos R, Goyette P, Sheppard CA, Matthew RG, et al. A candidate genetic risk factor for vascular disease: a common mutation in methylenetetrahydrofolate reductase. Nat Genet 1995; 10:111–113
25. Kang S, Wong PWK, Susmano A, Sora J, Norusis M, Ruggie N. Thermolabile methylenetetrahydrofolate reductase: an inherited risk factor for coronary artery disease. Am J Hum Genet 1991; 48:536–545.
26. Kang S, Wong PWK, Zhou J, Sora J, Lessick M, Ruggie N, et al. Thermolabile methylenetetrahydrofolate reductase in patients with coronary artery disease. Metabolism 1988; 37:611–63
27. Brattstrom L, Israelsson B, Norrving B, Bergqvist D, Thorne J, Hultberg B, et al. Impaired homocysteine metabolism in early-onset cerebral and peripheral occlusive arterial disease. Atherosclerosis 1990; 81:51–60.
28. Selhub J, Jacques PF, Wilson PWF, Rush D, Rosenberg IH. Vitamin status and intake as primary determinants of homocysteinemia in an elderly population. Jama 1993; 270:2693–2698.
29. Gartler SM, Hornung SK, Motulsky AG. Effect of chronologic age on induction of cystathionine synthase, uroporphyrinogen I synthase, and glucose-6-phosphate dehydrogenase activities in lymphocytes. Proc Natl Acad Sci USA 1981; 78:1919–1919.
30. Jacobsen DW, Gatautis VJ, Green R, Robinson K, Savon SR, Secic M, et al. Rapid HPLC determination of total homocysteine and other thiols in serum and plasma: sex differences and correlation with cobalamin and folate concentrations. Clin Chem 1994; 40: 873–881.
31. Wu LL, Wu J, Hunt SC, James BC, Vincent GM, Williams RR, et al. Plasma homocyst(e)ine as a risk factor for early familial coronary artery disease. Clin Chem 1994; 40:552–561.
32. Malinow MR, Kang S, Taylor LM, Wong PWK, Coull B, Inahara T, et al. Prevalence of hyperhomocyst(e)inemia in patients with peripheral arterial occlusive disease. Circulation 1989; 79:1180–1188
33. Boers GH, Smals AG, Trijbels FJ, Leermarkers AI, Kloppenborg PW. Unique efficiency of methionine metabolism in premenopausal women may protect against vascular disease in the reproductive years. J Clin Invest 1983; 72:1971–1976
34. Boushey CJ, Beresford SAA, Omenn GS, Motulsky AG. A quantitative assessment of plasma homocysteine as a risk factor for vascular disease: probable benefits of increasing folic acid intake. JAMA 1995; 274:1049–1057.
35. Brattstrom LE, Israelsson B, Jeppsson J-O, Hultberg BL. Folic acid: an innocuous means to reduce plasma homocysteine. Scand J Clin Invest 1988; 48:215–221.

36. Jacob RA, Wu M, Henning SM, Swendseid ME. Homocysteine increases as folate decreases in plasma of healthy men during short-term dietary folate and methyl group restriction. J Nutr 1994; 124:1072–1080.
37. Wilcken DEL, Wilcken B, Dudman NPB, Tyrrell PA. Homocystinuria: the effects of betaine in the treatment of patients not responsive to pyridoxine. New Engl J Med 1983; 309:448–453.
38. Dudman NPD, Wilcken DEL, Wang J, Lynch JF, Macey D, Lundberg P. Disordered methionine/homocysteine metabolism in premature vascular disease. Arteriosclerosis Thromb 1993; 13:1253–1260.
39. Ubbink JB, Vermaak WJH, van der Merwe A, Becker PJ. Vitamin B-12. vitamin B-6 and folate nutritional status in men with hyperhomocysteinemia. Am J Clin Nutr 1993; 57:47–53.
40. Franken DG, Boers GHJ, Blom HJ, Trijbels FJM, Kloopenborg PWC. Treatment of mild hyperhomocysteinemia in vascular disease patients. Arteriosclerosis Thromb 1994; 14:465–470.
41. Ubbink JB, Vermaak WJH, van der Merwe A, Becker PJ, Delport R, Potgieter HC. Vitamin requirements for the treatment of hyperhomocysteinemia in humans. J Nutr 1994; 124:1927–1933.
42. Ubbink JB, van der Merwe A, Vermaak WJH, Delport R. Hyperhomocysteinemia and the response to vitamins supplementation. Clin Invest 1993; 71:993–998
43. Davis BA, Hofler SA, Bailey LB, O'Keefe CA, Gregory JF, Cerda JJ. Homocysteine response to dietary folate modification in nonpregnant women. FASEB J 1994; 8:A248.
44. Franken DG, Boers GHJ, Blom HJ, Trijbels JMF. Effect of various regimens of vitamin B6 and folic acid on mild hyperhomocysteinemia in vascular patients. J Inher Metab 1994; 17:159–162.
45. Landgren F, Israelsson B, Lindgren A, Hultberg B, Andersson A, Brattstrom L. Plasma homocysteine in acute myocardial infarction: homocysteine-lowering effect of folic acid. J Int Med 1995;237:381–388.
46. Nilsson K, Gustafson L, Faldt R, Andersson A, Hultberg B. Plasma homocysteine in relation to serum cobalamin and blood folate in a psychogeriatric population. Eur J Clin Invest 1994;24:600–606.
47. van den Berg M, Franken DG, Boers GHJ, Blom HJ, Jakobs C, Stehouwer CDA, et al. Combined vitamin B6 plus folic acid therapy in young patients with arteriosclerosis and hyperhomocysteinemia. J Vasc Surg 1994; 20:933–940.
48. Ubbink JB, Becker PJ, Vermaak WJH, Delport R. Results of B-vitamin supplementation study used in a prediction model to define a reference range for plasma homocysteine. Clin Chem 1995;41:1033–1037.
49. O'Keefe CA, Bailey LB, Thomas EA, Hofler SA, Davis BA, Cerda JJ, et al. Controlled dietary folate affects folate status in nonpregnant women. J Nutr 1995; 125:2717–2725.
50. Stampfer MJ, Malinow MR, Willet WC, Newcomer LM, Upson B, Ullmann D, et al. A prospective study of plasma homocyst(e)ine and risk of myocardial infraction in US Physicians. JAMA 1992; 268:877–881
51. Kang S, Wong PWK, Norusis M. Homocysteinemia due to folate deficiency. Metabolism 1987; 36:458–462
52. Lewis CA, Pancharuniti N, Sauberlich HE. Plasma folate adequacy as determined by homocysteine level. Ann NY Acad Sci 1992; 699:360–362
53. Stabler SP, Marcell PD, Podell ER, Allen RH, Savage DG, Lindenbaum J. Elevation of total homocysteine in the serum of patients with cobalamin or folate deficiency detected by capillary gas chromatography-mass spectrometry. J Clin Invest 1988; 81:466–474.
54. Lindenbaum J, Rosenberg IH, Wilson PWF, Stabler SP, Allen RH. Prevalence of cobalamin deficiency in the Framingham elderly population. Am J Clin Nutr 1994; 60:2–11.
55. Brattstrom L, Lindgren A, Israelsson B, Andersson A, Hultberg B. Homocysteine and cysteine: determinants of plasma levels in middle-aged and elderly subjects. J Intern Med 1994; 236:633–641.
56. Ubbink JB, Vermaak WJH, Bennet JM, Becker PJ, van Staden DA, Bissbort S. The prevalence of homocysteinemia and hypercholesterolemia in angiographically defined coronary heart disease. Klin Wochenschr 1991; 69:527–534.
57. Brattstrom L, Lindgren A, Israelsson B, Malinow MR, Norrving B, Upson B, et al. Hyperhomocysteinaemia in stroke: prevalence, cause, and relationships to type of stroke risk and stroke factors. Eur J Clin Invest 1992; 22:214–221.
58. Sauberlich HE. Evaluation of folate nutrition in population groups. In: Folic Acid Metabolism in Health and Disease. Picciano MF, Stokstad ELR, Gregory JF, eds. New York: Wiley-Liss, 1990, 212–235.
59. Brattstrom L, Israelsson B, Lindgarde F, Hultberg B. Higher total plasma homocysteine in vitamin B_{12} deficiency than in heterozygosity for homocystinuria due to cystathionine β-synthase deficiency. Metabolism 1988; 37:175–178.
60. Lindenbaum J, Healton EB, Savage DG, Brust JCM, Garrett TJ, Podell ER, et al. Neuropsychiatric disorders caused by cobalamin deficiency in the absence of anemia or macrocytosis. New Engl J Med 1988; 318:1720–1728.
61. Allen RH, Stabler SP, Savage DG, Lindenbaum J. Diagnosis of cobalamin deficiency I: usefulness of serum methylmalonic acid and total homocysteine concentrations. Am J Hematol 1990; 34:90–98.

62. Wilcken DEL, Wilcken B. The pathogenesis of coronary artery disease: a possible role for methionine metabolism. J Clin Invest 1976; 57:1079–1082.

63. Murphy-Chutorian DR, Wexman MP, Grieco AJ, Heininger JA, Glassman E, Gaull GE, et al. Methionine intolerance: a possible risk factor for coronary artery disease J Am Coll Cardiol 1985; 6:725–730.

64. Wilcken DEL, Reddy SG, Gupta VJ. Homocysteinemia, ischemic heart disease, and the carrier state for homocystinuria. Metabolism 1983; 32:363–370.

65. Graham I. Interactions between homocysteinaemia and conventional risk factors in vascular disease. Eur Heart J 1994; 15:530(Abstract).

66. Israelsson B, Brattstrom LE, Hultberg BL. Homocysteine and myocardial infraction. Atherosclerosis 1988; 71:227–233.

67. Malinow MR, Sexton G, Averbuch M, Grossman M, Wilson D, Upson B. Homocyst(e)inemia in daily practice: levels in coronary artery disease. Coronary Artery Dis 1990; 1:215–220.

68. Genest JJ, McNamara JR, Salem DN, Wilson PWF, Schaefer EJ, Malinow MR. Plasma homocyst(e)ine levels in men with premature coronary artery disease. J Am Coll Cardiol 1990; 16:1114–1119.

69. Pancharuniti N, Lewis CA, Sauberlich HE, Perkins LL, Go RCP, Alverez JO, et al. Plasma homocyst(e)ine, folate and vitamin B-12 concentrations and risk for early-onset coronary artery disease. Am J Clin Nutr 1994; 59:940–948.

70. von Eckardstein A, Malinow MR, Upson B, Heinrich J, Schulte H, Schonfeld R, et al. Effects of age, lipoproteins, and hemostatic parameters on the role of homocyst(e)inemia as a cardiovascular risk factor in men. Arterioscler Thromb 1994; 14:460–464.

71. Alfthan G, Pekkanen J, Jauhiainen M, Pitkaniemi J, Karvonen M, Tuomilehto J, et al. Relation of serum homocysteine and lipoprotein(a) concentrations to atherosclerotic disease in a prospective Finnish population based study. Atherosclerosis 1994; 106:9–19.

72. Anesen E, Refsum H, Bonaa KH, Ueland PM, Forde OH, Nordrehaung JE. Serum total homocysteine and coronary heart disease. Int J Epid 1995; 24:704–709.

73. Dalery K, Lussier-Cacan S, Selhub J, Davignon J, Latour Y, Genest J, Jr. Homocysteine and coronary heart disease in French Canadian subjects: relation with vitamins B12, B6, pyridoxal phosphate, and folate. Am J Cardiol 1995; 75: 1107–1111.

74. Robinson K, Mayer EL, Miller DP, Green R, van Lente F, Gupta A et al. Hyperhomocysteinemia and low pyridoxal phosphate. Circulation 1995; 92:2825–2830.

75. Kang S, Wong PWK, Cook HY, Norusis M, Messer JV. Protein-bound homocyst(e)ine-A possible risk factor for coronary artery disease. J Clin Invest 1986; 77:1482–1486.

76. Friedenreich CM. Methods for pooled analyses of epidemiologic studies. Epidemiology 1993; 4:295–302.

77. Daly L, Graham I. Hyperhomocysteinaemia: a powerful risk factor of vascular disease. Presented at the Annual Scientific Meeting Working Group/Epidemiology and Prevention of the European Society of Cardiology; April 25, 1994.

78. Stampfer MJ, Malinow MR. Can lowering homocysteine levels reduce cardiovascular risk? New Engl J Med 1995; 332:328–329.

79. den Heijer M, Blom HJ, Gerrits WBJ, Rosendaal FR, Haak HL, Wijermans PW, et al. Is hyperhomocysteinaemia a risk factor for recurrent venous thrombosis? Lancet 1995; 345:882–885.

80. Perry IJ, Refsum H, Morris RW, Ebrahim SB, Ueland PM, Shaper AG. prospective study of serum total homocysteine concentration and risk in middle-aged British men Lancet 1995; 346:1395–1398.

81. Malinow MR, Nieto FJ, Szklo M, Chambless LE, Bond G. Carotid artery intimal-medial wall thickening in plasma homocyst(e)ine in aysmptomatic adults. Circulation 1993; 87:1107–1113.

82. Selhub J, Jacques PF, Bostom AG, D'Agostino RB, Wilson PWF, Belanger AJ, et al. Association between plasma homocysteine concentrations and extracranial carotid-artery stenosis. New Engl J Med 1995; 332:286–291.

83. Greenland S. Quantitative methods in the review of epidemiologic literature. Epidemiol Rev 1987; 9:1–30.

84. Petitti DB, Kelsey JL, Marmot MG, Stolley PD, Vessey MP, eds. Meta-Analysis, Decision-Analysis and Cost-Effectiveness Analysis. New York: Oxford University Press, 1994; 1–246.

85. Brattstrom LE, Harbebo JE, Hultberg BL. Moderate Homocysteinemia: a possible risk factor for arteriosclerotic cerebrovascular disease. Stroke 1984; 15:1012–1016.

86. Araki A, Sako Y, Fukushima Y, Matsumoto M, Asada T, Kita T. Plasma sulfhydryl-containing amino acids in patients with cerebral infarction and in hypertensive subjects. Atherosclerosis 1989; 79:139–146.

87. Coull BM, Malinow MR, Beamer N, Sexton G, Nordt F, de Garmo P. Elevated plasma homocyst(e)ine concentration as a possible independent risk factor for stroke. Stroke 1990; 21:572–576.

88. Verhoef P, Hennekens CH, Malinow MR, Kok FJ, Willett WC, Stampfer MJ. A prospective study of plasma homocyst(e)ine and risk of ischemic stroke. Stroke 1994; 25:1924–1930.

89. Clarke R, Fitzgerald D, O'Brien C, Roche C, Parker RA, Graham I. Hyperhomocysteinaemia: a risk factor for extracranial carotid artery atherosclerosis. Ir J Med Sci 1992; 161:61–65.

90. Rubba P, Faccenda F, Pauciullo P, Carbone L, Mancini M, Strisciuglio P, et al. Early signs of vascular disease homocystinuria: A noninvasive study by ultrasound in eight families with cystathionine-β-synthase deficiency. Metabolism 1990; 39:1191–1195.

91. Mansoor MA, Bergmark C, Svardal AM, Lonning PE. Redox status and protein binding of plasma homocysteine and other aminothiols in patients with early-onset peripheral vascular disease: homocysteine and peripheral vascular disease. Arterioscler Throm Biol 1995; 15:232–240.

92. Taylor LM, DeFrang RD, Harris EJ, Porter JM. The association of elevated plasma homocyst(e)ine with progression of symptomatic peripheral arterial disease. J Vasc Surg 1991; 13:128–136.

93. Molgaard J, Malinow MR, Lassvik C, Holm A-C, Upson B, Olsson AG. Hyperhomocyst(e)inaemia: an independent risk factor for intermittent claudication. J Intern Med 1992; 231:273–279.

94. Bergmark C, Manssor MA, Swedenborg J, de Faire U, Svardal AM, Ueland PM. Hyperhomocysteinemia in patients operated for lower extremity ischeamia below the age of 50—effect of smoking and extent of disease. Eur J Vasc Surg 1993; 7:391–396.

95. Giles WH, Kittner SJ, Anda RF, Croft JB, Casper ML. Serum folate and risk for ischemic stroke. Stroke 1995; 26:1166–1170.

96. Dudman NPB, Hicks C, Wang J, Wilcken DEL. Human arterial endothelial cell detachment in vitro: its promotion by homocysteine and cysteine. Atherosclerosis 1991; 91:77–83.

97. Wall RT, Harlan JM, Harker LA, Striker GE. Homocysteine-induced endothelial cell injury in vitro: a model for the study of vascular injury. Throm Res 1980; 18:113–121.

98. Blann AD. Endothelial cell damage and homocysteine. Atherosclerosis 1994; 94:89–91.

99. Harker LA, Slichter SJ, Scott CR, Ross R. Homocysteinemia. Vascular injury and arterial thrombosis. New Engl J Med 1974; 291:537–543.

100. Harker LA, Ross R, Slichter SJ, Scott CR. Homocystine-induced arteriosclerosis. The role of endothelial cell injury and platelet response in its genesis. J Clin Invest 1976; 58:731–741.

101. Tsai J, Perrella MA, Yoshizumi M, Hsieh C, Haber E, Schlegel R, et al. Promotion of vascular smooth muscle cell growth by homocysteine: a link to atherosclerosis. Proc Natl Acad Sci USA 1994; 91:6369–6373.

102. Heinecke JW, Rosen H, Chait A. Iron and copper promote modification of low density lipoprotein by human arterial smooth muscle cells in culture. J Clin Invest 1984; 74:1890–1894.

103. Lentz SR, Sadler JE. Inhibition of thrombomodulin surface expression and protein C activation by the thrombogenic agent homocysteine. J Clin Invest 1991; 88:1906–1914.

104. Hennekens CH, Buring JE. Epidemiology in Medicine. Boston: Little, Brown and Company, 1987.

105. U.S. Bureau of the Census. Statistical Abstract of the United States: 1993, 113th edition, Washington, DC, 1993.

106. Sauberlich HE, Kretsch MJ, Skala JH, Johnson HL, Taylor PC. Folate requirement and metabolism in nonpregnant women. Am J Clin Nutr 1987; 46:1016–1028.

107. Bender MM, Levy AS, Schucker RE, Yetley EA. Trends in prevalence and magnitude of vitamin and mineral supplement usage and correlation with health status. J Am Diet Assoc 1992; 92:1096–1101.

108. Nightingale SI. From the Food and Drug Administration: proposals for folic acid fortification and labelling of certain foods to reduce the risk of neural tube defects. JAMA 1993; 270:2283.

109. Federal Register. October 14, 1993; 58:53,254–53,297, 55,305–53,317.

110. Savage DG, Lindenbaum J. Folate-cobalamin interactions. In: Folate in Health Disease. Bailey LB, ed. New York: Marcel Dekker, Inc. 1995, 237–285.

111. Schafer LW, Larson DE, Melton LT, Higgins JA, Zinsmeister AR. Risk of development of gastric carcinoma in patients with pernicious anemia: a population-based study in Rochester, Minnesota. Mayo Clin Proc 1985; 60:444–448.

112. Linder MC. Nutrition and metabolism of vitamins. In: Nutritional Biochemistry and Metabolism with Clinical Applications. Linder MC, ed. New York: Elsevier, 1985,69–131.

113. Centers for Disease Control. Recommendations for the use of folic acid to reduce the number of cases of spina bifida and other neural defects. MMWR 1992: 41:1–7.

114. Mills JL, McPartlin JM, Kirke PN, Lee YJ, Conley MR, Weir DG, at el. Homocysteine metabolism in pregnancies complicated by neural-tube defects. Lancet 1995; 345:149–151.

115. Stevenson RE, Dean JH, Allen WP, Kelly M. Prevention program for reducing risk for neural tube defects—South Carolina, 1992–1994. Morbid Mortal Wkly Rpt. 1995; 44:141,142.

12 Omega-3 Fatty Acids from Fish

*Primary and Secondary Prevention
of Cardiovascular Disease*

William E. Connor and Sonja L.Connor

1. INTRODUCTION

Fish and fish oils contain the very long chained and highly polyunsaturated Ω-3* fatty acids, which are derived from phytoplankton, the base of the food chain in the oceans, lakes, and rivers *(1)*. Phytoplankton synthesize the Ω-3 fatty acids, eicosapentaenoic (20:5) (EPA) and docosahexaenoic (22:6) (DHA), which are subsequently incorporated into fish, shellfish, and sea mammals. These fatty acids have profound biological and biochemical effects in the body. Despite a wealth of scientific information (a recent review listed over 120 references about cardiovascular effects alone *[2]*, clinical interest in Ω-3 fatty acids has not been high in the United States despite considerable attention to their use in Europe and Japan. This chapter will focus on the considerable and underappreciated potential benefits of the Ω-3 fatty acids on cardiovascular disease.

In the 1950s it was discovered that polyunsaturated vegetable oils containing the Ω-6 linoleic acid had a pronounced plasma cholesterol lowering effect, yet the mechanism of this action has remained obscure *(1)*. In those early days, it was noted that fish oil, which was also polyunsaturated, had a similar hypocholesterolemic effect. No mention was made of the fact that fish oil contained very long chain Ω-3 fatty acids (C20:5 and C22:6) and that these might act differently than the Ω-6 fatty acid of vegetable oils, linoleic acid (C18:2). These early data about fish oil lay fallow until the pioneering observations of Dyerberg and Bang focused special attention on the Ω-3 fatty acids, EPA (20:5) and DHA (22:6) found in marine oils *(3)*. They observed a lower coronary mortality among the Greenland Eskimos, whose diet was especially rich in marine oils compared to Danish people eating a high saturated fat diet *(4)*. Later it was found that not only were these Ω-3 fatty acids cholesterol lowering, but, in addition, they had a profound plasma triglyceride lowering effect, especially in hypertriglyceridemic patients *(5–7)*. Over a decade of research in humans, animals, profused organs, and tissue cultures has firmly documented the mechanisms of the hypolipidemic actions of these Ω-3 fatty acids from fish and, furthermore, have demonstrated that these fatty acids have many other beneficial effects in cardiovascular disease.

*In this chapter, the terms omega (Ω)-3 and n-3 are used interchangeably as they are in the literature.

From: *Preventive Nutrition: The Comprehensive Guide for Health Professionals*
Edited by A. Bendich and R. J. Deckelbaum Humana Press Inc., Totowa, NJ

This chapter will focus on seven different areas of research that will help to answer the question about the potential benefits of Ω-3 fatty acids from fish oil on primary and secondary prevention of cardiovascular disease. These are listed below and will be discussed in detail subsequently.

PRIMARY PREVENTION:
1. Experimental animal studies to inhibit the growth of atherosclerotic plaques.
2. Lipid and lipoprotein disorders.
3. Diabetes mellitus.
4. Hypertension.

SECONDARY PREVENTION:
5. Antiarrhythmic actions.
6. Thrombosis.
7. Clinical trials and epidemiological observations on coronary disease prevention.

2. EXPERIMENTAL ATHEROSCLEROSIS AND FISH OIL

When menhaden oil (a fish oil product) was incorporated in atherogenic diets fed to rhesus monkeys, aortic plaques and their cholesterol content were much less than in the non- fish-oil fed groups (8). Since the plasma lipid levels were roughly similar in control groups, the inhibition of atherosclerosis may have involved other mechanisms operative in the vessel wall itself. Carotid atherosclerosis was likewise inhibited. Pigs fed an atherogenic diet had much less coronary atherosclerosis when given cod liver oil containing the Ω-3 fatty acids (9). There is good evidence that EPA and DHA from fish oil are even incorporated into advanced human atherosclerotic plaques (10). They are present in complicated plaques as components of cholesterol esters and phospholipids. The incorporation of EPA and DHA from the plasma lipoproteins into the plaques is detectable within a week of fish oil feeding. Perhaps the inhibition of atherosclerosis occurs because EPA and DHA inhibit cellular growth in the arterial wall (11). Atherosclerosis cannot develop even after injury and the influx of low density lipoprotein (LDL) cholesterol and cholesterol ester unless there is also a cellular reaction. Two important cells in atherosclerosis are smooth muscle cells and macrophages. Because of the suppression of cellular growth factors by Ω-3 fatty acids, proliferation of smooth muscle cells was inhibited (12). Likewise, macrophage infiltration into the vessel wall was lessened by Ω-3 fatty acids (8). Even the initial lesion of atherosclerosis—the fatty streak—develops less under the influence of dietary Ω-3 fatty acids (8).

3. EFFECTS ON THE PLASMA LIPIDS AND LIPOPROTEINS

A major effect of dietary Ω-3 fatty acids from fish oil is on the plasma levels of lipids and lipoproteins (6). As will be shown, the science in this area is very clear: Ω-3 fatty acids lower the plasma very low density lipoprotein (VLDL) and triglyceride levels through depression of synthesis of triglyceride in the liver. Ω-3 fatty acids also suppress postprandial lipemia, the chylomicron remnants of which are considered atherogenic. Effects on LDL and high density lipoprotein (HDL) have been variable. HDL either increases or does not change. Like the drug gemfibrozil, Ω-3 fatty acids may cause an increase in LDL because they lower the plasma triglyceride concentration in some hyperlipidemic states, such as familial combined hyperlipidemia, as will be discussed in detail in Section 3.3.

Theoretically, the ideal nutritional program to reduce the plasma lipid and lipoprotein concentrations maximally would be a very low cholesterol and saturated fat diet, which would upregulate the LDL receptor and reduce LDL plasma concentrations, combined with a diet containing fish oil, which would suppress VLDL production and lower plasma triglyceride concentrations.

3.1. Effects of Fish Oil in Normal Subjects

Several recent reviews have documented that Ω-3 fatty acids from fish have a great effect on plasma lipids and lipoproteins, even in normal subjects (1,6). The principal action is on the plasma triglyceride and VLDL concentrations. This hypolipidemic action is well illustrated in a study of 12 healthy adults (six men and six women) who were given three different diets fed in random order for 4 wk each: a saturated control diet, a salmon diet containing considerable amounts of Ω-3 fatty acids, and a vegetable oil diet high in Ω-6 fatty acids (13). Both the salmon diet and the vegetable oil diet decreased the plasma cholesterol similarly, from 188 to 162 mg/dL. Both diets reduced LDL, from 128 to 108 mg/dL. HDL cholesterol levels were not changed by the salmon oil diet. The salmon diet decreased VLDL cholesterol levels and the changes in plasma triglyceride were most striking, from 76 to 50 mg/dL. The polyunsaturated vegetable oils did not lower VLDL and triglyceride levels.

3.2. Studies in Hyperlipidemic Patients

Because of the hypolipidemic effect of n-3 fatty acids in normal subjects, it seemed most reasonable to test their effects in hyperlipidemic patients (7). The two groups of hyperlipidemic patients selected for study were characterized by hypertriglyceridemia, since the depression of the plasma triglyceride and VLDL appeared to be a unique effect of n-3 fatty acids from fish oil.

Twenty hypertriglyceridemic patients volunteered for the study (eight men and 12 women). Ten of the patients presented with increased levels of both VLDL and LDL, consistent with the type II-b phenotype. Their mean plasma lipid levels at time of entry were 337 mg/dL for cholesterol and 355 mg/dL for triglyceride. Clinically, many of these patients had familial combined hyperlipidemia, a disorder characterized by a strong disposition to the development of coronary heart disease (CHD) and by overproduction of lipoproteins, particularly VLDL.

The other 10 patients had apparent type V hyperlipidemia, as characterized by increased chylomicrons and greatly increased VLDL levels in the fasting state. Their mean plasma lipid levels at entry were 514 mg/dL for cholesterol and 2874 mg/dL for triglyceride. Four of the type V patients had concomitant, noninsulin-dependent diabetes mellitus and two had adult-onset, insulin-dependent diabetes mellitus. Their insulin doses and diabetic control remained constant throughout the study despite the salmon oil.

The type V phenotype is characterized by both overproduction of VLDL and impaired clearance of the remnants of chylomicron and VLDL metabolism. Clinically, type V patients have the "chylomicronemia" syndrome, which is characterized by episodes of abdominal pain from enlargement of abdominal viscera (hepatomegaly and splenomegaly) and by episodes of acute pancreatitis. These patients also suffer from eruptive xanthomata, neuropathy, and lipemia retinalis. Although LDL levels are low in type V patients, the presence of the atherogenic remnant particles predisposes them to the development of atherosclerotic complications, including CHD.

Special care was taken to make certain that the patients were in steady-state conditions before entry. Steady-state was defined as a constancy of body weight and diet and an absence of any residual hypolipidemic drug effect. Most of the patients had not been receiving any hypolipidemic drugs just prior to the study. In the patients previously given drugs, these were discontinued and plasma lipid levels were monitored until pre-drug levels were attained.

Two different control diets were used for the two groups of hypertriglyceridemic patients, depending on the phenotype of hyperlipidemia. Type II-b patients received their usual low-cholesterol (100 mg/d), low-fat (20–30% of total calories) diet. Subsequent dietary periods for type II-b patients consisted of a fish oil diet for 4 wk, followed, in some patients, by a 4-wk period of a diet high in a vegetable oil containing a predominance of n-6 fatty acids. Both of these diets were balanced for cholesterol content (approx 250 mg/d) and contained 30% of calories as fat. The diets in all periods were eucaloric, such that the subjects neither gained nor lost weight.

For type V patients, the control diet consisted of a very-low-fat diet (5%), in order to lower plasma triglyceride levels maximally. The next dietary interval contained fish oil at 20 or 30% of total calories. Finally, a polyunsaturated vegetable oil diet was also provided that contained 20–30% of total calories as fat and 200–300 mg of cholesterol/d. Both the fish oil and the vegetable oil diets were initially used cautiously in the type V patients in order to minimize the risk of hepatosplenomegaly, abdominal pain, and acute pancreatitis.

The salmon oil diet provided about 20 g/d of n-3 fatty acids for a 2600-kcal intake, with 30% of total calories as fat. On the other hand, the vegetable oil diet provided about 47 g of the n-6 polyunsaturated fatty acid, linoleic acid. Thus, the fish oil diets actually provided 43–64% fewer total polyunsaturated fatty acids than the vegetable oil diet, gram for gram.

The fish oil diet decreased the plasma LDL-cholesterol levels in the type II-b patients by 26 mg/dL. Of individual lipoprotein cholesterol changes, the decline of VLDL cholesterol was most striking, but LDL and HDL cholesterol also decreased. The plasma triglyceride changes were even greater than the cholesterol changes with the fish oil diet. The plasma triglyceride level decreased from 334 to 118 mg/dL. This occurred largely because of the change in VLDL triglyceride, which was lowered from 216 to 55 mg/dL.

The highly polyunsaturated vegetable oil diet had a much weaker effect on VLDL cholesterol and triglyceride. LDL values were similar; but in contrast, HDL cholesterol was higher after the vegetable oil diet. Plasma apolipoprotein changes reflected the lipoprotein lipid changes. In the type II-b patients, there were significant reductions in apo B and C-III levels in the fish oil period, which paralleled the declines in LDL and VLDL levels.

In the type V patients, effects of the fish oil diet were even more striking (Figs. 1 and 2). With consumption of the very-low-fat control diet, their initial plasma lipid levels declined considerably, but still remained greatly elevated. Many of these patients still had milky-appearing plasma, with chylomicrons present in the fasting state. The first change to occur in these patients after the fish oil diet was the virtual disappearance of fasting chylomicronemia, which had been present in five of the patients. During the fish oil diet, total plasma triglyceride decreased from a control value of 1353 to 281 mg/dL,

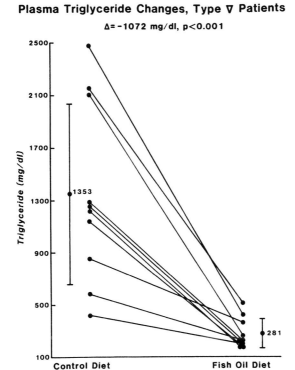

Fig. 1. The changes in plasma triglyceride levels in the 10 type V patients: control diet vs fish oil diet. To convert triglyceride from milligrams per deciliter to millimoles per liter, multiply by 0.0113.

a drop of 79% (Fig. 1). VLDL triglyceride decreased similarly, from 1087 to 167 mg/dL. Plasma cholesterol levels declined into the normal range after the fish diet, from 373 to 207 mg/dL (Fig. 2). Most of this total plasma cholesterol decrease occurred as the result of marked changes in the amount of VLDL cholesterol, which decreased from 270 to 70 mg/dL. Of interest was the 48% concomitant rise of LDL cholesterol, from the low value of 84 to 125 mg/dL. Apolipoprotein levels changed to reflect the altered lipoprotein lipid levels. Apo A-1 levels did not change, whereas apo B, C-III, and E all decreased significantly.

When the n-6-rich vegetable oil replaced the fish oil in the diets of eight type V patients, all patients had increases in plasma triglyceride levels within 3–4 d. After 10–14 d of the vegetable oil feeding, the mean plasma triglyceride values rose 198%, and VLDL triglyceride increased from 171 to 550 mg/dL. Plasma cholesterol also increased, from 195 to 264 mg/dL. LDL-cholesterol levels, on the contrary, were decreased 28% by the vegetable oil diet, another indication that the metabolic abnormality of the type V phenotype was worsening. Because of enhanced hypertriglyceridemia and the risk of development of abdominal pain typical of this type V disorder, the vegetable oil feeding period was discontinued prematurely in all type V patients (7).

3.3. Implications of the Fish Oil Studies in Hypertriglyceridemic Patients

In the 20 hypertriglyceridemic patients, fish oil incorporated in the diet led to an even more profound hypolipidemic effect than had been observed in normal subjects. The

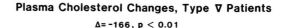

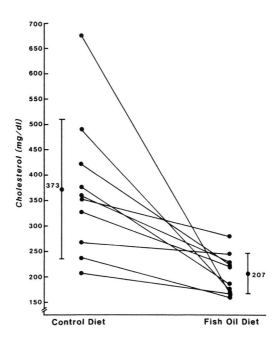

Fig. 2. The changes in plasma cholesterol levels in the 10 type V patients: control diet vs fish oil diet. To convert cholesterol from milligrams per deciliter to millimoles per liter multiply by 0.026.

plasma triglyceride levels decreased in each of the 20 patients, a 79% decrease in the type V patients and a 64% decrease in the type II-b patients; plasma cholesterol levels decreased 45% and 27%, respectively. In the 12 normal subjects previously investigated *(13)*, decreases were less for plasma triglyceride (38%) and much less for plasma cholesterol (14%). Apparently, the greater the hypertriglyceridemia, the greater the reductions brought about by dietary fish oil in plasma lipids, and especially in VLDL.

These results may have considerable therapeutic importance for patients with severe and moderate hypertriglyceridemia. The only dietary treatment to date for severely hypertriglyceridemic type V patients has been the very severe and therapeutically difficult restriction of dietary fat to between 5 and 10% of total calories in an effort to approach normal plasma triglyceride levels. Americans find this possible to do on a short-term basis, but very difficult on a long-term basis because they are accustomed to eating higher quantities of fat; i.e., approx 40% of total calories. Hitherto, all fatty foods have been contraindicated in type V hyperlipidemia. The findings of this study suggest that some fatty, and even high cholesterol, foods (i.e., fish or even shellfish) containing marine n-3 fatty acids are quite appropriate for ingestion and may produce further triglyceride lowering over and above that which results from the very-low-fat diet.

Other studies in familial combined hyperlipidemia and in type IV hyperlipidemia have shown increases in LDL and apo B while plasma VLDL and triglyceride values were declining *(6,14,15)*. Such LDL increases have also occurred in type IV patients given the drug gemfibrozil. Perhaps this is an expected physiological action when hy-

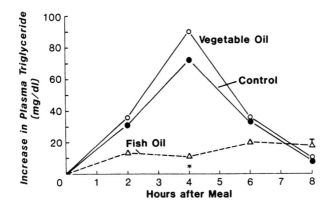

Fig. 3. The increase in plasma triglyceride levels following the ingestion of 50 g of fat. Saturated fat test meal given during the saturated fat diet (closed circles); vegetable oil test meal given during the vegetable oil diet (open circles); salmon oil test meal given during the salmon oil test (triangles). Mean fasting triglyceride levels were 72 ± 19, 76 ± 37, and 46 ± 11 mg/dL before the saturated fat, vegatable oil, and salmon oil, respectively, test meals were administered.

pertriglyceridemia is being corrected. Should the LDL levels become abnormally high after either drugs or fish oil, then further therapy of the LDL specifically is warranted (i.e., bile acid binding resins or lovastatin). Fish oil has also produced plasma cholesterol and triglyceride lowering in type III patients and in familial hypercholesterolemia (16).

3.4. Reduction of Postprandial Lipemia After Fatty Meals

It has been observed that fish oils markedly decreased the usual chylomicronemia that follows fatty meals (17,18). In other words, fat tolerance was greatly improved (see Fig. 3). This improvement could result from diminished absorption, slower synthesis, and slower entry of chylomicrons into the circulation or, alternatively, from a more rapid removal of the chylomicrons that do appear in the circulation. There is no evidence for diminished absorption, and fat balance studies have not shown increased fat excretion in stools after dietary periods enriched with fish oil. Whether reduced chylomicron production or enhanced removal of chylomicrons is responsible has not yet been completely clarified. Fish oil feeding produces smaller VLDL particle size in animals compared to vegetable oil feeding. Smaller VLDL would have, then, an enhanced catabolism. Perhaps, after a background diet of fish oil, chylomicrons are smaller in size and hence, more rapidly catabolized, the result being a much flatter fat tolerance curve (17).

3.5. The Mechanism of the Hypolipidemic Effects of Fish Oil

How Ω-3 fatty acids exert their effects to decrease the levels of plasma triglyceride and cholesterol has been tested in humans in two different sets of experiments: The inhibition by fish oil of the usual hypertriglyceridemia that inevitably results when a high-carbohydrate (CHO) diet is suddenly fed to humans; and the effects of fish oil on apo B, VLDL, and LDL production rates and turnovers.

3.6. *Fish Oil and the Inhibition of Carbohydrate-Induced Hypertriglyceridemia*

The well-known phenomenon of carbohydrate-induced hypertriglyceridemia is a physiologic response. In this model, VLDL triglyceride synthesis is stimulated as the dietary CHO intake abruptly increases. The increased VLDL synthesis leads to hypertiglyceridemia, which may persist for many weeks. If n-3 fatty acids do inhibit VLDL synthesis, then the usual CHO-induced hypertiglyceridemia should not occur when fish oil is incorporated into the high-CHO diet.

Seven mildly hypertriglyceridemic, but otherwise healthy subjects, (ages 22–54 yr) were fed three different experimental diets *(19)*. Each was composed of a liquid formula plus three bran muffins per day to supply fiber. The baseline diet contained 45% of calories from CHO. The high-CHO diets were then divided into control and fish groups; both containing 15, 10, and 75% of calories as fat, protein, and CHO, respectively. In the baseline and high-CHO control diets, a blend of peanut oil and cocoa butter provided the fat, which was replaced by fish oil in the form of a commercially available marine lipid concentrate in the high-CHO fish oil diet. The total amount of fish oil consumed per day was 50 g (in a 3000-kcal diet), equivalent to approx 3.3 tablespoons of oil. This amount provided 8.5 g of EPA and 5.5 g of DHA.

The three experimental diets were fed in three different sequences in the Clinical Research Center (Fig. 3). In the first sequence, the high-CHO control diet preceded the high-CHO fish oil diet (Fig. 4A). In the second sequence, the high-CHO diet was given for 20 d instead of 10 in order to demonstrate that the hypertriglyceridemia did not spontaneously resolve after the first 10 d. It was then followed by the fish oil diet (Fig. 4B). In the third sequence, the fish oil was fed first with the high CHO diet for 25 d and then removed to permit the effects of the high CHO to be manifest for the next 15 d (Fig. 4C). Three subjects were studied with the first sequence and two subjects each were studied with the second and third sequences.

In all seven subjects, the high-CHO control diet increased the plasma triglyceride levels over the baseline diet from 105 to 194 mg/dL *(19)*. The magnitude of the CHO-induced hypertriglyceridemia correlated significantly with each individual's baseline triglyceride levels. The rise in plasma triglyceride levels was complete by d 5 and resulted almost entirely from an increase in the VLDL triglyceride fraction, which more than doubled during the control diet, from 69 to 156 mg/dL (Fig. 4). Although the total plasma cholesterol levels did not change, VLDL cholesterol levels approximately doubled, from 18 to 34 mg/dL; and HDL cholesterol was reduced from 49 to 41 mg/dL.

When the fat of the high-CHO control diet was replaced isocalorically with fish oil, the elevated plasma triglyceride concentration was reduced from 194 to 75 mg/dL, a decrease of 61%. This decrease usually occurred within 3 d (Fig. 4A). Once again, changes in VLDL triglyceride levels were largely responsible for this effect (156 to 34 mg/dL) (Fig. 5). Total cholesterol levels decreased insignificantly during the high-CHO fish oil diet—from 172 to 153 mg/dL—primarily because of the drop in VLDL cholesterol levels (34 to 12 mg/dL) *(19)*.

The hypertriglyceridemia persisted even when the period of CHO induction was prolonged from 10 to 20 d and did not significantly decrease until fish oil was incorporated into the diet (Fig. 4B). When the high-CHO fish oil diet followed the baseline diet, the plasma triglyceride level did not rise, but the level increased when the high-CHO control diet was fed subsequently (Fig. 4C). The high-CHO control diet decreased the lev-

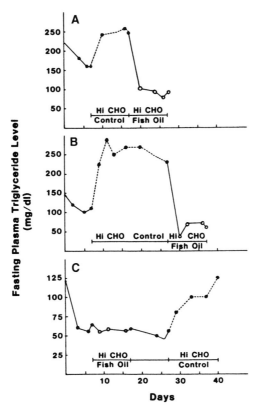

Fig. 4. The effects of the baseline (0 0) diet and the control (0—0) and fish oil (0 0) diets on plasma triglyceride levels in three subjects. We see the reversal of carbohydrate-induced hypertriglyceridemia by dietary fish oil (**A**), the persistence of the hypertriglyceridemia (throughout 20 d) and the subsequent reversal by fish oil (**B**), and the prevention of carbohydrate-induced hypertriglyceridemia by fish oil (**C**).

els of apo B and increased apo C-III concentrations; apo A-1 and E levels did not change. The high-CHO fish oil diet decreased apo A-1 and apo C-III levels; apo B and E concentrations did not change.

The incorporation of corn oil in place of fish oil into the high-CHO regimen failed to prevent the induced hypertriglyceridemia. For the three subjects who participated in this study, the average triglyceride levels were as follows: baseline, 93 ± 23 mg/dL; high-CHO control, 196 ± 58 mg/dL; high-CHO corn oil, 215 ± 90 mg/dL; and high-CHO fish oil, 86 ± 10 mg/dL.

Dietary fish oil not only prevented but also rapidly reversed the dietary, CHO-induced elevations in plasma triglyceride and VLDL levels, whereas the n-6 fatty acid rich corn oil had no effect at all. Since the primary difference between corn oil and the commercial fish oil preparation is the type of polyunsaturated fatty acids present (corn oil, 57% 18:2 n-6; linoleic acid; the commercially available fish oil preparation, 32% n-3 fatty acids), the difference in effect was because of the n-3 fatty acids in the fish oil. This finding implied a probable inhibitory effect of n-3 fatty acids on hepatic VLDL production *(19)* (*see* Chapter 8).

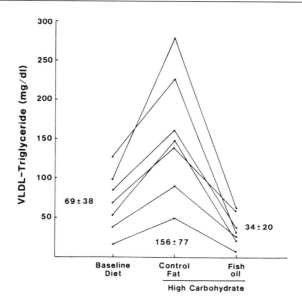

Fig. 5. The effects of the high carbohydrate control and fish oil diets on the plasma VLDL triglyceride levels in the seven subjects.

3.7. Fish Oil and the Synthesis and Turnover of Apo B, VLDL, and LDL

The hypothesis that n-3 fatty acids probably reduced VLDL levels by inhibiting VLDL synthesis was supported by studies designed to elucidate further mechanisms of the hypotriglyceridemic effect of n-3 fatty acids. Dietary fish oil affected either the synthesis or the removal of VLDL. The rates of flux and turnover of VLDL triglyceride were measured after injection of ³H-glycerol into people studied under two dietary protocols, one containing fish oil and the other containing fats typical of the American diet *(20)*. This technique permitted the calculation of both synthetic and removal rates of VLDL.

Ten male subjects were selected on the basis of having a wide range of fasting plasma triglyceride concentrations, from 34 to 4180 mg/dL, so that the hypothesis about the mechanism of action of dietary fish oils could be tested in subjects with greatly different pool sizes of plasma triglyceride. Liquid formula diets containing 15–20% fat, 65–75% CHO, and 10–15% protein were fed during both the control and the fish oil dietary periods. The two diets differed only in the type of fat they contained. In the control diet, a blend of cocoa butter and peanut oil (1:2) was incorporated into the formulas. The fish oil diet containing the commercial preparation was taken in three divided doses daily and was not mixed into the formulas. The principal difference between the two diets was the higher content of linoleic acid (18:2 n-6) in the control diet and the presence of n-3 fatty acids in the fish oil diet. The former diet contained virtually no n-3 fatty acids, whereas the latter provided about 17 g/d of these highly polyunsaturated fatty acids.

The experimental diets were consumed for a period of 3–5 wk before the actual VLDL turnover procedure was conducted. This time was needed for the plasma triglyceride levels to stabilize, particularly in the subjects whose triglyceride levels were above normal. Seven subjects consumed the control diet first, followed by the fish oil diet; in the remaining three, the order was reversed. The order in which the diets were administered did not affect the results.

The isocaloric substitution of fish oil for the control vegetable fat produced the expected significant reductions in the total and lipoprotein lipid levels in all 10 subjects. Total cholesterol levels for all 10 subjects fell from 195 to 144 mg/dL, a reduction of 22%. Decreases in VLDL levels accounted for most of the drop in plasma cholesterol (83 to 21 mg/dL). LDL cholesterol levels did not change significantly, whereas HDL cholesterol concentrations fell from 31 to 24 mg/dL. All of these changes were evident in both the normal and the hypertriglyceridemic groups.

After the administration of ^{3}H-glycerol and its incorporation into the triglyceride of VLDL, the decay curves were analyzed by computer-models so that VLDL synthesis and turnover could be calculated. The incorporation of n-3 fatty acids into the diet caused a 72% decrease in the VLDL triglyceride pool size (11.4 to 3.2 g; $p < .025$). The decreased pool size was associated with a 45% reduction in the VLDL triglyceride synthetic rate (23 to 12.6 mg/h/IW; $p < .005$) and a 45% decrease in the residence time of VLDL triglyceride in the plasma (5.8 to 3.2 h; $p < 0.005$). The reciprocal of the residence time is the fractional catabolic rate (FCR), which was increased by 65% (0.23 to 0.38 h^{-1}, $p < .005$). There was a significant rise in the cholesterol/triglyceride ratio in VLDL during the fish oil interval (0.18–25; $p < .05$). Finally, the ratio of the fast to the slow synthetic pathways did not change with fish oil feeding. The same trends were seen in both normal and hypertriglyceridemic patients. Similar results have also been found by a slightly different dietary plan and with the labeling of VLDL apo B with ^{125}I (21). There was a striking reduction of VLDL synthesis and enhanced turnover.

Direct evidence that the hepatic synthesis of triglyceride and VLDL is suppressed by n-3 fatty acids from fish oil has been seen in three in vitro studies of the perfused rat liver and in studies of liver cells from rats and rabbits in primary culture (22–24). In all of these studies triglyceride synthesis was reduced. In one, enhanced ketone body production resulted; in the others there was a diversion of n-3 fatty acids from triglyceride synthesis into phospholipid synthesis (24). When the net results of the human and animal studies are taken together, the evidence is very strong that suppression of VLDL and triglyceride synthesis is a primary mechanism for the hypolipidemic effects of n-3 fatty acids, coupled with an increased fractional catabolic rate of VLDL.

3.8. Fish Oil and LDL Turnover

Labeled LDL turnover studies have been carried out in normal subjects given fish oil. It was demonstrated that there was a decreased synthesis of LDL and a tendency for an increased fractional catabolic rate (25). Spady and colleagues have shown enhancement of LDL receptor activity after the administration of fish oil in the rat (26). This latter result fits in very well with the increased fractional catabolic rate observed in the normal human subjects. It seems very clear that the Ω-3 fatty acids from fish oil have major effects on all of the major lipoproteins with the exception of HDL.

3.9. Summary and Conclusions: Fish Oil Effects on Plasma Lipids and Lipoproteins

The Ω-3 fatty acids from fish oil and fish have been shown to have a remarkable effect on the synthesis and clearance of triglyceride-rich lipoproteins, especially VLDL and chylomicrons. Even LDL synthesis and clearance have been affected. Because of these significant effects on lipoprotein synthesis and clearance, beneficial effects of fish oil have been demonstrated in a variety of hyperlipidemic states, especially those with such conditions as hypertriglyceridemia and chylomicronemia. Therapeutic implications for fish oil are especially positive in type V, type IV, and type III hyperlipidemia. Recent data indicate a similar effectiveness in hypertriglyceridemic diabetic patients without affecting glucose homeostasis (27).

Difficulty in interpreting the effects of fish oil in various hyperlipidemic patients has occurred because of vastly different experimental conditions (6). In some studies, fish oil was simply added as a supplement to the usual diet in doses of 8–16 g/d. In the control period a placebo oil, such as olive oil or safflower oil, was not always utilized. In other studies, there was the customary diet plus the use of an appropriate placebo oil. Furthermore, various kinds of fish oils have been utilized, some containing a considerable amount of cholesterol and saturated fat. Newer fish oils have fewer saturated fatty acids, higher concentrations of n-3 fatty acids, and a lower cholesterol content.

Some conclusions have emerged from the wide variety of studies, most of which have not been controlled for caloric and body weight stability. Fish oil is most effective when administered at 6–30% of the total calories and when the diet is well controlled. In these studies, LDL lowering has usually occurred as has profound VLDL and triglyceride lowering in normal subjects and in a wide variety of hyperlipidemic states. In our experience, this lowering of plasma cholesterol levels has occurred in patients with types V, II-a, II-b, III, and IV hyperlipidemia, with the most dramatic results occurring in the type V patients who do not tolerate any other kind of dietary fat (6,7,28). In the literature and in our experience, HDL levels have not been greatly affected by fish oil. Clearly, the use of fish oil in hyperlipidemia must be individualized regarding both use and dosage. Lower doses of fish oil (8–15 g/d) particularly lower the plasma triglyceride levels (6).

Why the plasma LDL and apo B have at times increased after fish oil administration when at the same time the plasma VLDL and triglyceride have decreased is a most challenging question and may relate to fundamental aspects of VLDL-LDL metabolism. Normally, LDL is derived from two sources: conversion from VLDL and direct synthesis from the liver. The catabolism of VLDL is likewise in two directions through intermediate density lipoprotein (IDL). This lipoprotein may be removed by the apo E receptor in the liver or converted to LDL. The animal experiments of Huff and Telford suggest why, in some instances, fish oil might increase LDL (29). Turnover studies in the miniature pig revealed that fish oil feeding increased the proportion of VLDL being converted to LDL. Apparently, the n-3 fatty acids of fish oil produce a smaller VLDL particle, which is more likely to be converted to LDL. In this pig study, LDL concentrations, however, did not increase because the direct synthesis of LDL was reduced more by fish oil than the increase in LDL from VLDL. These pig studies await confirmation in humans. They do explain why LDL may increase in some humans fed fish oil: More VLDL is converted to LDL and direct LDL synthesis does not decrease, thus adding up to more LDL. LDL turnover studies have shown decreased production of LDL in normal humans given large amounts of salmon oil vs vegetable oil (25). In this study, the plasma LDL decreased after n-3 fatty acids.

4. FISH OIL IN DIABETIC PATIENTS

In diabetic patients there is enhanced risk for vascular disease, so the use of fish oil might be particularly desirable if glucose control is not disturbed. The literature is controversial with regard to the effects of Ω-3 fatty acids in diabetic patients (30,31).

In type I, insulin-dependent diabetics there is universal agreement that glucose control is not hampered with fish oil supplementation and that the beneficial effects on the plasma lipids and lipoproteins have been demonstrated. In type II, adult-onset diabetic patients, the results have been somewhat conflicting, possibly because such patients are very susceptible to the caloric load imposed. In most studies, the plasma triglyceride and VLDL concentrations have declined, but some studies have shown the deterioration in glucose homeostasis. This literature has recently been reviewed by Heine and colleagues *(30)*. Most of the studies have been short term and, in some, caloric control has been somewhat distorted by the administration of calorie-dense fish oil without there being a suitable placebo. The addition of fish oil to the usual diet would be hypercaloric, thereby disturbing glucose control. When there is attention to the caloric content of the supplement, then there are beneficial effects on the plasma triglyceride and VLDL without disturbing glucose homeostasis, as illustrated in the following experiment.

These problems and objections were considered in an experimental design of a study in 16 adult-onset diabetics who were randomized to a double-blind, placebo-controlled crossover study *(27)*. The subjects of the study were overweight and most were receiving hypoglycemic agents. There was a 3-month stabilization baseline period in which they were given a eucaloric, lower fat (30% of the calories from fat), high complex carbohydrate diet with 55% of calories from carbohydrate. This was followed by two 6-mo intervention periods in which the subjects continued on the same diet and received a supplement of 15 g/d of either olive oil or fish oil. The fish oil contained 6 g/d of Ω-3 fatty acids. The endpoints of the study were plasma lipid and lipoprotein concentrations and glucose homeostasis. The plasma triglyceride concentrations were much lower with the fish oil preparation vs olive oil (260 vs 449 mg/dL). VLDL cholesterol was lower as was VLDL triglyceride. The total plasma cholesterol was unchanged. There was a significant increase in LDL cholesterol, as has been mentioned previously, when hypertriglyceridemic individuals are given fish oil, from 117 to 145 mg/dL. HDL cholesterol did not change.

However, the effects of fish oil on glucose homeostasis revealed no difference from the 6 mo period of olive oil administration. Body weights were unchanged. Fasting glucose levels were 172 and 178 mg/dL, olive oil vs fish oil. Another measure of diabetic control, hemoglobin A-1 C, revealed no difference, nor did the 24-h urinary glucose excretion, the plasma C-peptide, or the 24-h urinary C-peptide.

In view of the extremely high mortality from CHD in adult-onset diabetic patients, this hypolipidemic action of fish oil was of interest because diabetic control did not deteriorate and there were significantly beneficial plasma lipid-lipoprotein effects. The other actions of the Ω-3 fatty acids from fish oil in inhibiting the development of atherosclerosis, in preventing thromboxane A_2 formation, in increasing endothelial-derived relaxing factor, and in inhibiting platelet-derived growth factor would all be additional reasons for postulating a therapeutic benefit from the use of fish oil in diabetic patients.

5. HYPERTENSION

Omega-3 fatty acids in 11 studies have been uniformly associated with a mild uniform decrease in systolic blood pressure and at times a decrease in diastolic blood pressure, particularly in the upright position *(2)*. This has especially occurred in mild hypertensives *(2,32,33)*. The suggested mechanism has been an attenuation in the responses of forearm vascular resistance and blood flow to angiotensin; i.e., less vascular reactivity. Since the decreases in both systolic and diastolic pressures are not great even in the best studies (4.6 and 3.0 mm Hg) *(33)*, fish oil cannot be regarded as a single treatment modality for hypertension. However, when used for other purposes, the mild blood pressure lowering effect of Ω-3 fatty acids would certainly provide an added benefit.

6. ANTI-ARRHYTHMIC ACTIONS

Sudden death from ventricular arrhythmias is a much dreaded complication in patients with CHD. Several experimental studies have addressed this problem with the use of n-3 fatty acids from fish oil. McLennan et al. used coronary artery ligation in the rat to produce an in vivo model of ventricular fibrillation and myocardial infarction *(34)*. They found that the number of ventricular ectopic beats and duration of tachycardia or fibrillation was increased when the rats were fed sheep kidney fat (a saturated fat) when compared to rats fed tuna fish oil, a rich source of n-3 fatty acids. The rats fed tuna fish oil had a significantly reduced incidence and severity of arrhythmias. In another animal study, ventricular fibrillation was prevented by fish oil during both the occlusion of the coronary artery and during reperfusion *(35)*.

In other experiments, Hallaq et al. *(36)* have used isolated neonatal cardiac myocytes (from hearts of 1-d-old rats) as a model for the study of cardiac arrhythmogenic factors that are modified by n-3 fatty acids. They incubated isolated myocytes (for 3–5 d) in a culture medium enriched with arachidonic acid (AA) or EPA (20:5 n-3). The AA-enriched myocytes developed a toxic cytosolic calcium concentration on exposure to ouabain, whereas EPA-enriched myocytes preserved physiologic calcium levels. An increase of EPA in the membrane phospholipids was demonstrated with a small reduction in arachidonic acid in myocytes fed EPA. A second study by the same researchers further indicated the mechanism of action of the fish oil fatty acids in preventing the arrhythmias of these isolated myocytes *(37)*. It was found that n-3 fatty acids prevented a calcium-depleted state in the myocytes caused by the L-type calcium channel blocker nifedipine. The protective effects of the n-3 fatty acids appeared to result from their modulatory effects on nifedipine-sensitive L-type calcium channels. These studies indicated a definite beneficial effect of dietary n-3 fatty acids on the heart—the prevention of cardiac arrhythmias in animals.

More recently, fatty fish consumption was associated with prevention of cardiac arrest from ventricular fibrillation (VF) in coronary patients. VF is the cause of death in most patients with CHD and it accounts for the 20–30% of people whose first indication of coronary disease is cardiac arrest. A recently published study from the University of Washington compared the effects of eating fish with the incidence of cardiac arrest *(38)*. There was a 50% reduction in the risk of cardiac arrest in people who consumed at least one fatty fish meal per week. A typical fatty fish would be salmon. Other fatty fish include sardines, mackerel, and Chilean sea bass. Even those who consumed a less fatty fish, such as tuna, had benefit because all fish and shellfish contain the beneficial Ω-3 fatty acids.

This protection against cardiac arrest occurred from the Ω-3 fatty acids (EPA and DHA) in the fat of the fish. The effects of eating fish were reflected biochemically in the fatty acids of the red blood cells. If the red blood cells had a relatively low level of the Ω-3 fatty acids, 3.3% of total fatty acids, there was a much greater risk of cardiac arrest than in those individuals whose red blood cell Ω-3 fatty acids were 5% or more of the total fatty acids. In other words, there was a 70% reduction in the risk of cardiac arrest in those people with the higher red-blood-cell Ω-3 fatty acid content *(38)*.

This information is particularly valuable because it fits in nicely with the study conducted several years ago by Burr et al. in Wales, in which men who were advised to eat fatty fish or to consume some fish oil capsules had a 29% reduction in total deaths, and, in particular, in deaths from CHD *(39)*. Thus, the evidence becomes stronger and stronger that even some fish (or Ω-3 fatty acid consumption) on a consistent basis (at least one serving a week) may prevent many deaths from CHD.

7. THROMBOSIS

Omega-3 fatty acids have invariably had an antithrombotic effect, particularly a diminution in thromboxane A_2, which produces platelet aggregation and vasoconstriction *(1,40)*. Platelet reactivity and adhesion were, therefore, considerably reduced after fish oil ingestion *(41)*. There have been reductions also of PAI-1, fibrinogen, TPA, and increases in platelet survival and bleeding time *(2)*. Enhanced fibrinolysis has also been observed *(2)*. Perhaps even more significant was a study in baboons showing that Ω-3 fatty acids eliminated both vascular thrombus formation and vascular lesions after vascular injury *(42)*. The baboons treated with fish oil showed decreases in thrombus formation at sites of surgical carotid endarterectomy. The function of the endothelium, important in both thrombosis and atherosclerosis, is affected by Ω-3 fatty acids *(40)*. The production of prostacyclin is enhanced and endothelial-derived relaxation factor (EDRF), or nitric oxide, which is depressed in atherosclerotic disease, was greatly increased by the Ω-3 fatty acids of fish oil *(43–45)*.

8. POPULATION STUDIES AND CLINICAL TRIALS

The epidemiological data and clinical trials of Ω-3 fatty acids and coronary disease are rather extensive and go back to the initial observations of Dyerberg and Bang, who found a much lower rate of CHD in the Greenland Eskimos compared with Danes *(4)*. They deduced by means of extensive studies that it was the Ω-3 fatty acid content of the Eskimo diet that inhibited the atherosclerotic disease despite the fact that the Eskimo diet was a high cholesterol, high fat diet *(3)*. The dietary fat, instead of being pathogenic, was protective since it was derived from the seas (fish, seal, and so forth) and contained the Ω-3 fatty acids. The pathology of atherosclerosis in Alaskan natives was at the same time much less than atherosclerosis found in Caucasians living in Alaska *(46)*.

A number of studies correlating fish consumption (providing Ω-3 fatty acids) and the mortality from CHD have been carried out *(2)*. In Dutch men the mortality from CHD was more than 50% lower among those who consumed at least 30 g of fish per day than among those who did not eat fish *(47)*. In the MRFIT trial n-3 fatty acid consumption correlated inversely with all-cause mortality and coronary mortality *(48)*. Even in the Harvard Health Professionals Follow-up Study of 51,529 men, the consumption of one to two servings of fish per week was associated with a lower incidence of CHD *(49)*.

This information is buttressed by a randomized controlled clinical trial in 2333 men who had recovered from myocardial infarction and who were then asked to increase their intake of fatty fish or fish oil *(39)*. There was a 29% reduction in the 2-y all-cause mortality in subjects advised to eat fatty fish and there was also a reduction in deaths from ischemic heart disease, but no reduction in nonfatal myocardial infarction. This was the first intervention trial in which all-cause mortality was reduced in a coronary intervention program. One likely reason for the reduction in coronary mortality was the decrease in cardiac arrest as documented recently by another study *(38)*. Men who ate fatty fish at least once a week had a 50% reduction in cardiac arrest, which probably resulted from the anti-arrhythmic action of the Ω-3 fatty acids discussed earlier.

9. RECOMMENDATIONS

The intake of Ω-3 fatty acids from fish should definitely be increased to prevent CHD. This could be best in the form of two to three fish meals per week in the context of a low-fat diet. Fish, of course, could be substituted for meat in the diet. At the same time, the diet should be reduced in fat content to 20% of the total calories with a high-CHO, high-fiber intake. The intake of cholesterol should be limited to 100 mg/d.

Table 1 provides the fat content and Ω-3 fatty acid content for a wide variety of fish and shellfish *(50)*. All fish and shellfish contain the Ω-3 fatty acids even when the fat content is rather low, as it is in shellfish. The lower the fat content, the higher the percentage of Ω-3 fatty acids that are present in a given fish or shellfish. The goal of this recommendation is to produce an increased content of the Ω-3 fatty acids, EPA and DHA, in the blood and tissues of the body. This will occur if there is consistent consumption of fish and shellfish of 100–300 g/wk.

Should it be desired to ascertain what the chronic intake of fish and shellfish has been in the past, there are excellent markers to document this point. The markers would be the measurement of the Ω-3 fatty acids in the plasma, which would reflect a more immediate intake, their measurement in red blood cells, which, because of the greater half-life of these cells, would reflect the intake over a longer period of time, and finally biopsies of the adipose tissue, whose fatty acids would reflect the intake over many months and years *(51)*.

For the intensive treatment of various forms of hyperlipidemia as well as the production of an antithrombotic state, fish oils would need to be utilized in addition to the consumption of fish. The dose of fish oil might well be 6–15 g/d, titrated according to the endpoint desired.

For people who are unable to consume fish or shellfish, the use of fish oil would again be advisable. For primary prevention, 2–3 g/d would be desirable. Higher doses, as noted above, should be used for secondary prevention and the attainment of discrete endpoints of plasma lipid and lipoprotein levels and platelet function.

In conclusion, the Ω-3 fatty acids from fish and fish oil greatly inhibit the atherosclerotic process and coronary thrombosis by many actions and should be considered as an important therapeutic modality in patients with CHD and to prevent coronary disease in highly susceptible people.

Table 1
Fat and Ω-3 Fatty Acid Content of Fish and Fish Oils

Fish (100 g, edible portion, raw)	Fat (g)	Ω-3 fatty acids (g)[a]
Anchovy, European	4.8	1.4
Bass, striped	2.3	0.8
Bluefish	6.5	1.2
Carp	5.6	0.3
Catfish, Channel	4.3	0.3
Cod, Atlantic	0.7	0.3
Cod, Pacific	0.6	0.2
Flounder, unspecified	1.0	0.2
Haddock	0.7	0.2
Halibut, Pacific	2.3	0.4
Herring, Atlantic	9.0	1.6
Herring, Pacific	13.9	1.7
Mackerel, Atlantic	13.9	2.5
Mullet, unspecified	4.4	1.1
Ocean perch	1.6	0.2
Pike, Walleye	1.2	0.3
Pompano, Florida	9.5	0.6
Sablefish	15.3	1.4
Salmon, Atlantic	5.4	1.2
Salmon, Chinook	10.4	1.4
Salmon, Pink	3.4	1.0
Salmon, Sockeye	8.6	1.2
Sardines, in sardine oil[b]	15.5	3.3
Shark	1.9	0.5
Snapper, red	1.2	0.2
Sole	1.2	0.1
Sturgeon	3.3	0.3
Swordfish	2.1	0.2
Trout, brook	2.7	0.4
Trout, lake	9.7	1.6
Trout, rainbow	3.4	0.5
Tuna	2.5	0.5
Crustaceans		
Crab, Alaska King	0.8	0.3
Crab, Dungeness	1.0	0.3
Crayfish, unspecified	1.4	0.1
Lobster, Northern	0.9	0.2
Shrimp, unspecified	1.1	0.3
Mollusks		
Abalone, New Zealand	1.0	Trace
Clam, hardshell	0.6	Trace
Clam, littleneck	0.8	Trace
Mussel, blue	2.2	0.5
Octopus, common	1.0	0.2
Oyster, pacific	2.3	0.6
Scallop, unspecified	0.8	0.2
Squid, unspecified	1.0	0.3

[a]EPA plus DHA.
[b]Analysis by the Atherosclerosis Research Laboratory, Portland, OR

REFERENCES

1. Goodnight SHE Jr., Harris WS, Connor WE, Illingworth DR. Polyunsaturated fatty acids, hyperlipidemia and thrombosis. Arteriosclerosis 1982; 2:87–113.
2. Connor WE. N-3 fatty acid and heart disease. In: Nutrition and Disease Update: Heart Disease. Kritchevsky D, Carroll KK, eds. Champaign, IL: American Oil Chemists' Society Press, 1994; 7–42.
3. Bang HO, Dyerberg J, Hyorne N. The composition of food consumed by Greenlandic Eskimos. Acta Med Scand 1973; 200:69–73.
4. Bang HO, Dyerberg J. Lipid metabolism and ischemic heart disease in Greenland Eskimos. In: Advanced Nutrition Research, vol 3. Draper HH, ed. New York: Plenum 1980; pp.1–32.
5. Connor WE. Hypolipidemic effects of dietary omega-3 fatty acids in normal and hyperlipidemic humans: effectiveness and mechanisms. In: Health Effects of Polyunsaturated Fatty Acids in Seafoods. Chapt. 10. Simopoulos AP, ed. Academic, Portland, OR 1986; pp.173–210.
6. Harris WS. Fish oils and plasma lipid and lipoprotein metabolism in humans: A critical review. J Lip Res 1989; 30:785–807.
7. Phillipson BE, Rothrock DW, Connor WE, Harris WS, Illingworth DR. The reduction of plasma lipids, lipoproteins and apoproteins in hypertriglyceridemic patients by dietary fish oil. New Engl J Med 1985; 312:1210.
8. Davis HR, Bridenstine RT, Vesselinovitch D, Wissler RW. Fish oil inhibits development of atherosclerosis in Rhesus monkeys. Arteriosclerosis 1987; 7:441–449.
9. Weiner BH, Ockene IS, Levine PH, Cuénoud HF, Fisher M, Johnson BF, Daoud AS, Jarmolych J, Hosmer, D, Johnson MH, Natale A, Vaudreuil C, Hoogasian JJ. Inhibition of atherosclerosis by cod-liver oil in a hyperlipidemic swine model. New Engl J Med 1986; 315:841–846.
10. Rapp JH, Connor WE, Lin DS, Porter JM. Dietary eicosapentaenoic acid (EPA) and docosahexaenoic acid (DHA) from fish oil: their incorporation into advanced human athero-sclerotic plaques. Arteriosclerosis Thromb 1991; 11:903–911.
11. Fox PL, DeCorleto PE. Fish oils inhibit endothelial cell production of platelet-derived growth factor-like protein. Science 1988; 241:453–456.
12. Kaminski WE, Jendraschak E, Kiefl R, Von Schacky C. Dietary (ω-3 fatty acids lower levels of platelet-derived growth factor mRNA in human mononuclear cells. Blood 1993; 81:1871–1879.
13. Harris WS, Connor WE, McMurry MP. The comparative reduction of the plasma lipids and lipoproteins by dietary polyunsaturated fats: salmon oil versus vegetable oils. Metabolism 1983; 32:179.
14. Friday KE, Failor RA, Childs MT, Bierman EL. Effects of n-3 and n-6 fatty acid-enriched diets on plasma lipoproteins in heterozygous familial hypercholesterolemia. Arteriosclerosis Thromb 1991; 11:47–54.
15. Failor RA, Childs MT, Bierman EL. The effects of omega-3 and omega-6 fatty acid-enriched diets on plasma lipoproteins and apoproteins in familial combined hyperlipidemia. Metabolism 1988; 37:1021–1028.
16. Illingworth DR, Schmidt E. The influence of dietary n-3 fatty acids on plasma, lipids and lipoproteins. Ann NY Acad Sci 1993; 676:60–69.
17. Harris WS, Connor WE, Alam N, Illingworth DR. The reduction of postprandial triglyceride in humans by dietary n-3 fatty acids. J Lipid Res 1988; 29:1451–1460.
18. Weintraub MS, Zechner R, Brown A, Eisenberg S, Breslow JL. Dietary polyunsaturated fats of the ω-6 and ω-3 series reduce postprandial lipoprotein levels: chronic and acute effects of fat saturation on postprandial lipoprotein metabolism. J Clin Invest 1988; 82:1884–1893.
19. Harris WS, Connor WE, Inkeles SB, Illingworth DR. Dietary omega-3 fatty acids prevent carbohydrate-induced hypertriglyceridemia. Metabolism 1984; 33:1016–1019.
20. Harris WS, Connor WE, Illingworth DR, Rothrock DW, Foster DM. Effect of fish oil on VLDL triglyceride kinetics in man. J Lipid Res 1990; 31:1549–1558.
21. Nestel PJ, Connor WE, Reardon MR, Connor S, Wong S, Boston R. Suppression by diets rich in fish oil of very low density lipoprotein production in men. J Clin Invest 1984; 74:82.
22. Wong SH, Nestel PH, Trimble RP, Storer BG, Illman RJ, Topping DL. The adaptive effects of dietary fish and safflower oil on lipid and lipoprotein metabolism in perfused rat liver. Biochem Biophys Acta 1983; 792:103.
23. Wong S, Reardon M, Nestel P. Reduced triglyceride formation from long chain polyenoic fatty acids in rat hepatocytes. Metabolism 1985; 34:900–905.
24. Benner KG, Sasaki A, Gowen DR, Weaver A, Connor WE. The differential effect of eicosapentaenoic acid and oleic acid on lipid synthesis and VLDL secretion in rabbit hepatocytes. Lipids 1990; 25:534–540.
25. Illingworth DR, Harris WS, Connor WE. Inhibition of low density lipoprotein synthesis by dietary omega-3 fatty acids in humans. Arteriosclerosis 1984; 4:270–275.

26. Ventura MA, Woollett LA, Spady DK. Dietary fish oil stimulates hepatic low density lipoprotein transport in the rat. J Clin Invest 1989; 84:528–537.

27. Connor WE, Prince MJ, Ullman D, Riddle M, Hatcher L, Smith FE, Wilson D. The hypotriglyceridemic effect of fish oil in adult-onset diabetes without adverse glucose control. Ann NY Acad Sci 1993; 683:337–440.

28. Schmidt EB, Kristensen SD, DeCaterina R, Illingworth DR. The effects of n-3 fatty acids on plasma lipids and lipoproteins and other cardiovascular risk factors in patients with hyperlipidemia. Atherosclerosis 1993; 103:107–121.

29. Huff MW, Telford DE. Dietary fish oil increases the conversion of very low density lipoprotein B to low density lipoprotein. Arteriosclerosis 1989; 9:58–66.

30. Heine RJ. Dietary fish oil and insulin action in humans. Ann NY Acad Sci 1993; 683:110–121.

31. Connor WE. Diabetes, fish oil and vascular disease. Ann Int Med 1995; 123:950–952.

32. Toft I, Bonaa KH, Ingebretsen OC, Nordoy A, and Jenssen T. Effects of n-3 polyunsaturated fatty acids on glucose homeostasis and blood pressure in essential hypertension. A randomized, controlled trial. Ann Intern. Med 1995; 123:950–952.

33. Bonaa KH, Bjerve KS, Straumme B, Gram IT, Thelle D. Effect of eicosapentaenoic and docosahexaenoic acids on blood pressure in hypertension: a population-based intervention trial from the Tromso study. New Engl J Med 1990; 322:795–801

34. McLennan PL, Abeywardena MY, Charnock JS. Influence of dietary lipids on arrhythmias and infarction after coronary artery ligation in rats. Can J Physiol Pharmacol 1985; 63:1411–1417.

35. McLennan PL, Abeywardena MY, Charnock JS. Dietary fish oil prevents ventricular fibrillation following coronary artery occlusion and reperfusion. Amer Heart J 1988; 116:706–717.

36. Hallaq H, Sellmayer A, Smith TW, Leaf A. Protective effect of eicosapentaenoic acid on ouabain toxicity in neonatal rat cardiac myocytes. Proc Natl Acad Sci USA 1990; 87:7834–7838.

37. Hallaq H, Smith TW, Leaf A. Modulation of dihydropyridine-sensitive calcium channels in heart cells by fish oil fatty acids. Proc Natl Acad Sci USA 1992; 89:1760–1764.

38. Siscovick DS, Raghunathan TE, King I, Weinmann SO, Wicklund KG, Albright J, et al. Dietary intake and cell membrane levels of long-chain n-3 polyunsaturated fatty acids and the risk of primary cardiac arrest. JAMA 1995; 274:1363–1367.

39. Burr ML, Fehily AM, Gilbert JF, Rogers S, Holliday RM, Sweetnam PM, Elwood PC, Deadman NW. Effects of changes in fat, fish, and fibre intakes on death and myocardial reinfarction: diet and reinfarction trial (DART). Lancet. 1989; 2:757–762.

40. Leaf A, Weber PC. Cardiovascular effects of n-3 fatty acids. New Engl J Med 1988; 318:549–557.

41. Goodnight SH Jr, Harris WS, Connor WE. The effects of dietary omega-3 fatty acids upon platelet composition and function in man: a prospective, controlled study. Blood 1981; 58:880–885.

42. Harker LA, Kelly AB, Hanson SR, Krupski W, Bass A, Osterud B, FitzGerald GA, Goodnight SH, Connor WE. Interruption of vascular thrombus formation and vascular lesion formation by dietary n-3 fatty acids in fish oil in non human primates. Circulation. 1993; 87:1017–1029.

43. DeCaterina R, Giannessi D, Mazzone A, Bernini W, Lazzerini G, Maffei S, Cerri M, Salvatore L, Weksler B. Vascular prostacyclin is increased in patients ingesting ω-3 polyunsaturated fatty acids before coronary artery bypass graft surgery. Circulation 1990; 82:428–438.

44. Shimokawa H, Vanhoutte PM. Dietary omega-3 fatty acids and endothelium-dependent relaxation in porcine coronary arteries. Am J Physiol 1989; 256:H968–H973.

45. Nordoy A, Hatcher L, Goodnight S, FitzGerald GA, Connor WE. Effects of dietary fat content, saturated fatty acids and fish oil on eicosanoid production and hemostatic parameters in normal men. J Lab Clin Med 1994; 123:914–920.

46. Newman WP, Propst MT, Rogers DR, Middaugh JP, Strong JP. Athersclerosis in Alaskan natives. Lancet 1993; 1056,1057.

47. Kromhout D, Bosschieter EB, Coulander C. The inverse relation between fish consumption and 20-year mortality from coronary heart disease. New Engl J Med 1985; 312:1205–1209.

48. Dolecek TA, Grandits G. Dietary polyunsaturated fatty acids and mortality in the Multiple Risk Factor Intervention Trial (MRFIT). World Rev Nutr Diet 1991; 66:205–216.

49. Ascherio A, Rimm EB, Stampfer MJ, Giovannucci EL, Willett WC. Dietary intake of marine n-3 fatty acids, fish intake, and the risk of coronary disease among men. New Engl J Med 1995; 332:977–982.

50. Connor WE, Connor SL. Diet, atherosclerosis and fish oil. In: Advances in Internal Medicine, 35th ed. H. Stollerman, M.D. Siperstein, eds., Chicago, IL: Year Book Publishers, 1989; pp.139–172.

51. Leaf DA, Connor WE, Barstad L, Sexton G. Incorporation of dietary n-3 fatty acids into the fatty acids of human adipose tissue and plasma lipid classes. Am J Clin Nutr 1995; 62:68–73.

PART II
PREVENTION OF MAJOR DISABILITIES

13

The Relationship Between Nutritional Factors and Age-Related Macular Degeneration

Shirley Hung and Johanna M. Seddon

1. INTRODUCTION

Age-related macular degeneration (AMD) is the primary cause of incurable blindness in the United States *(1)*. Among people aged 65 yr and older, approx 25% have signs of age-related maculopathy, including large or confluent drusen, retinal pigmentary changes, geographic atrophy, and exudative disease *(2)*. About 7% of persons 75 yr of age or older have advanced AMD with visual loss *(2)*. We expect to see 1.9 million cases of advanced AMD with visual loss in this age group by the year 2025 *(2,3)*. It is also estimated that 25.7 million people age 45 and older will have signs of either early or late AMD in the year 2025; 23.1 million with signs of early AMD, and 2.6 million with late AMD *(2,3)*. Given the large public health impact of this disease, research focused on causes of this disease is essential.

Treatment for AMD is essentially limited to laser photocoagulation *(4–6)*. This method of treatment is effective for only a small portion of patients. The causes of AMD have not been identified, although the possible role of low intake of antioxidant vitamins and minerals has recently received attention *(7)*. If proven, increased consumption of antioxidant vitamins and minerals could be a method of primary prevention of AMD.

The biologic plausibility of this diet-health hypothesis focuses on the control of oxidative byproducts, in particular the reactive oxygen species (ROS). Current theories on oxidative damage estimate that the body is exposed to 10^{10} ROS mol/d under normal metabolic conditions resulting from endogenous sources alone *(8)*. Oxidative damage from environmental factors, such as exposure to sunlight, is also thought to increase ROS *(9)*. It is plausible that through dietary intervention, increasing intake of antioxidant nutrients could have a major impact on the control of excessive ROS damage.

This chapter reviews current theories on the pathogenesis of AMD and the potential role of specific dietary nutrients in its development or progression. Current epidemiologic and animal experimental evidence regarding nutrition and its relationship with AMD as well as a review of ongoing studies, recommendations for future studies, and possible nutritional interventions to reduce damage as a result of photo-oxidative insults are discussed.

From: *Preventive Nutrition: The Comprehensive Guide for Health Professionals*
Edited by A. Bendich and R. J. Deckelbaum Humana Press Inc., Totowa, NJ

245

Table 1
Reactive Oxygen Species (ROS) Quenching Ability of Specific Antioxidants *(15)*

Reactive species		Antioxidant
$^1O_2$	Singlet oxygen	Vitamins A, C, E, β-carotene *(70,71)*, certain other carotenoids *(14)*
$O_2^{-\cdot}$	Superoxide free radical	Superoxide dismutase, vitamins C, E, β-carotene
ROO·	Peroxyl-free radical	Vitamins C and E
H_2O_2	Hydrogen peroxide	Catalase, glutathione peroxidase
LOOH	Lipid peroxides	Glutathione peroxidase

2. DIET-RELATED THEORIES ASSOCIATED WITH THE DEVELOPMENT OF AMD

2.1. Antioxidant Theory

Since normal physiological processes produce free radicals or ROS *(8)*, the necessity for controlling the damaging effects of ROS is essential for maintaining good health. According to their functions, two types of antioxidants are most relevant to AMD. Protective antioxidants act by reducing the formation of radicals and reactive oxygen species by decomposition of hydrogen peroxide without generating radicals (glutathione peroxidase, glutathione S-transferase, peroxidase, catalase), or by quenching active oxygen (carotenoids, superoxide dismutase) *(9)*. Radical-scavenging antioxidants can either inhibit chain initiation or break chain propagation by trapping a radical before it reaches its cellular target (vitamin C, vitamin E, carotenoids) *(9)*.

The retina may be prone to oxidative damage because of the abundance of long-chain lipids *(10,11)*. The macula, in particular, may be the most prone to oxidative damage because of its increased exposure to blue light and higher concentrations of highly unsaturated long-chain fatty acids *(12)*. The electromagnetic energy carried in a photon of visible blue light (450–500 nm/s) is higher than the energy of a photon of visible light in the red spectrum (650–700 nm/s). In the presence of a photosensitizer (natural cell constituents that absorb light, such as porphyrins, flavins, such as riboflavin *(13)*, ketones, quinone, aromatic molecules, and other compounds) and blue light, molecular oxygen in its ground state—known as triplet oxygen—is converted into its high-energy form, singlet oxygen ($^1O_2$). Singlet oxygen has paired antiparallel electrons, whereas other free radical ROS produced by regular oxidative processes *(14)* have an unpaired electron (molecular oxygen contains two electrons with parallel spin states). The flipping of one of the electrons in singlet oxygen results in a higher energy potential, and thus makes it an oxidative agent capable of causing damage to DNA, proteins, lipids, and carbohydrates in the eye *(14)*.

Several nutrients with antioxidant capacities can quench different types of ROS (*see* Table 1). Carotenoids have been shown to be ideally suited to quench singlet oxygen *(8)*, whereas vitamin E is uniquely suited to stop nonenzymatic peroxidation of lipids *(15)*. It seems reasonable to infer that if dietary intake of several nutrients with antioxidant capacities—carotenoids, vitamin C, vitamin E, zinc, selenium, copper—is less than optimal, the body's ability to regulate ROS may be compromised

(8,15). Just as it has been suggested that antioxidants can inhibit oxidative modification of LDL, thereby preventing or slowing the progression of atherosclerosis *(8)*, we speculate that a similar mechanism may also exist for antioxidants in the eye. Inadequate levels of antioxidants may lead to excess oxidized byproducts accumulating in the retinal pigment epithelium (RPE) *(16)*. It is unknown at which point the process may become irreversible.

2.2. Atherosclerotic Theory

Although the pathogenesis of AMD is still not well understood, an alternative theory suggests that the dietary risk factors associated with atherosclerosis *(17)* are also common to AMD. In the classic diet–heart hypothesis, dietary lipids are primarily responsible for raising or lowering serum lipoproteins *(18)*. The relationship between AMD and dietary fat intake follows from the classic diet–heart hypothesis that high intakes of saturated fats will increase risk of cardiovascular disease as a result of a net increase in serum low density lipoprotein (LDL). The autoimmune response generated against oxidized LDL, found in arteriosclerotic plaques, is hypothesized to be the driving mechanism behind the pathogenesis of arteriosclerosis. One can speculate that this may also be associated with AMD *(8)*. The proposed mechanism is based on susceptibility of lipids to peroxidation by ROS because of insufficient levels of antioxidants. The presence of two compounds, lipofuscin (an age-related pigment found in all older animals) and malondialdehyde (product of autoxidized polyunsaturated fatty acids and a possible intermediate compound of lipofuscin), found in atherosclerotic plaques and in RPE deposits *(17)*, are indigestible by cellular enzymes and are thought to be products of lipid oxidation. The accumulation of these deposits in healthy tissue can result in necrosis or death of functioning tissue *(11,17)*. The limitation of this theory is the lack of evidence linking autoxidation and lipofuscin accumulation in the RPE *(19)*. The key to the understanding of the pathogenesis of AMD may be the inability to effectively prevent or remove nondigestible compounds from healthy eye tissue *(20)*.

3. PROPERTIES OF RELEVANT NUTRIENTS AND THEIR FUNCTIONS

Micronutrient deficiencies have been shown to play critical roles in the etiology of many diseases. This may also be the case for AMD. Although genetic susceptibility may be an important risk factor, low intake of key nutrients during the critical period of disease initiation may have just as much influence in the development and progression of this disease. This has yet to be determined.

3.1. Nutrients Involved in the Antioxidant Theory

3.1.1. NUTRIENT-DEPENDENT ENZYMATIC COMPLEXES

As discussed above, antioxidants fall into two classes: preventive antioxidants and chain-breaking antioxidants. Oxidoreductases are major antioxidant regulators and comprise a broad class of enzymes that include: oxidases, dehydrogenases, hydroperoxidases, and oxygenases *(15)*. A major class of oxygenases are enzymes in the cytochrome P450 system, whose primary function is to detoxify such substance as drugs, pollutants, and chemical carcinogens, (xenobiotics), adding an oxygen atom to the substrate to inactivate them *(15)*. There are three oxidoreductase enzymes that may be relevant to AMD.

3.1.1.1. CATALASE

Catalase is an enzyme that has four heme groups and is found in the cytosol *(15)*. It plays a major role in catalytic splitting of hydrogen peroxide into water and molecular oxygen *(15)*. Catalase activity in human retinal pigment epithelium has been shown to be six times greater than in other ocular tissues *(21)*, suggesting that it is an important component of the RPE antioxidant system *(21)*. Catalase activity also has been observed to decrease with age as degeneration in both macular and peripheral RPE increases *(21)*.

3.1.1.2. SUPEROXIDE DISMUTASE

Superoxide dismutase is a metalloenzyme found in all aerobic cells. It quenches superoxide anion-free radicals produced by cellular respiration *(15)*. Superoxide dismutase generates hydrogen peroxide using two molecules of superoxide and requires both zinc and copper for catalytic function *(15)*. The hydrogen peroxide can then be converted into water and molecular oxygen by catalase or glutathione peroxidase *(15)*. Superoxide dismutase activity has not been shown to decrease with age *(21)*.

3.1.1.3. GLUTATHIONE PEROXIDASE

Also found in the cytosol, glutathione peroxidase provides a second line of defense against hydroperoxides, which can damage membranes and other cell parts *(14)*. Selenium is an essential part of this enzyme *(see* Section 3.1.4.2.). Selenium, as part of glutathione peroxidase, appears to act synergistically with tocopherol, vitamin E, in the regulation of lipid peroxidation *(14)*. In tandem with catalase, glutathione peroxidase degrades hydrogen peroxide to water via glutathione reductase and flavin adenine dehydrogenase (FAD) in the pentose phosphate shunt *(14)*.

3.1.2. VITAMINS

The vitamins of most interest currently in AMD studies are vitamin C, vitamin E, and the carotenoids.

3.1.2.1. VITAMIN C

Ascorbic acid (vitamin C) has antioxidant ability that is well known *(22–24)*. Ascorbate is capable of reacting with a broad category of reactive oxygen species, making it an excellent first line of defense against oxidative damage *(15)*. Ascorbate, as an endogenous antioxidant in plasma, can protect against peroxidative damage caused by aqueous peroxyl radicals and the oxidants released from activated neutrophils *(25)*. Ascorbate in the cytosol has been shown to regenerate oxidized vitamin E found primarily in cellular lipid membranes *(26)*. One study has demonstrated that levels of ascorbic acid can be increased in the lens, aqueous humor, and plasma through dietary supplementation *(27)*.

3.1.2.2. VITAMIN E

Vitamin E is the generic name for a class of fat-soluble compounds called tocopherols *(23,28)*. Major dietary sources of vitamin E are wheat germ, corn, soybean, sunflower, and olive oils *(15,23)*. The requirement for vitamin E increases with increasing polyunsaturated fat intake *(15,23,29,30)*. Vitamin E protects against tissue oxidation *(31)*. It has recently been suggested that a cells' antioxidant ability is dependent on the ratio of glutathione peroxidase to vitamin E *(32)*. As glutathione concentrations become lower, vitamin E is rapidly depleted from the cells *(31)*.

The tocopherols act as chain-breaking antioxidants by transfering a phenolic hydrogen to a peroxyl-free radical of a peroxidized polyunsaturated fatty acid *(28)*. Vitamin E is particularly effective in breaking chain reactions involving nonenzymatic lipid peroxidation *(15)*. The phenoxy-free radicals of tocopherol formed after reacting with a peroxyl radical may react with vitamin C to regenerate tocopherol *(26)*. Alternatively, it may react with other peroxyl-free radicals, resulting in oxidation of the chromane ring and side-chain producing a nonfree-radical product *(15,23)*. This oxidation product is then conjugated with glucuronic acid via the 2-hydroxyl group and excreted in the bile *(28)*.

3.1.2.3. VITAMIN A

Vitamin A encompasses a large group of compounds that includes alcohol (retinol), aldehyde (retinal), acid (retinoic acid), and the active forms of vitamin A. Retinol is an essential precursor of 11-cis-retinaldehyde, a fundamental component of rhodopsin, the primary visual pigment in the retinal rod cells *(33)*. Active forms of vitamin A are found only in animal sources although carotenoid precursors, such as β-carotene, obtained mainly from plant sources, can be converted in the body to form the active compound *(15,28)*. The necessity of vitamin A for ocular health has long been established *(23)*. Deficiencies manifest themselves in the form of xerophthalmia and other degenerative eye diseases *(23)*. Vitamin A itself (retinol, retinal, or retinoic acid), however, has not been shown to be related to AMD.

3.1.3. CAROTENOIDS

There are approx 600 carotenoid pigments documented currently *(34)*. Of these, over 50 can be metabolized to active vitamin A in a variety of animal species *(35)*, although carotenoids with pro-vitamin A activity are not the only ones that are important biologically. Carotenoids are the primary pigments found in red-, yellow-, and orange-colored plant and animal foods *(23)*. Primary dietary sources of these carotenoids are fruits and vegetables *(23,24,36)*. The types of carotenoids found in different foods vary according to their color. Lycopene and cryptoxanthin are found in higher concentrations in bright yellow, orange, and red fruits and vegetables, whereas dark green, leafy vegetables tend to have more lutein and zeaxanthin *(37,38)*.

Carotenoids can function directly by reacting with ROS *(35)*. They show both antioxidant and pro-oxidant activities under certain conditions *(39)*. Four carotenoids, grouped as those with or without pro-vitamin A activity, may play important roles in AMD development.

3.1.3.1. CAROTENOIDS WITH PRO-VITAMIN A ACTIVITY

Beta-carotene is a precursor of the active form of vitamin A, retinol; cleavage between the 9–10 carbons results in the formation of two molecules of retinal *(15)*. Although β-carotene can quench singlet oxygen and prevent lipid peroxidation, it is not as effective an antioxidant in vivo as other carotenoids such as lycopene *(40)*. Alpha-carotene, when cleaved, results in half the amount of active retinol as β-carotene. Alpha-carotene has a similar antioxidant capacity as β-carotene *(40)*.

3.1.3.2. CAROTENOIDS WITH NO PRO-VITAMIN A ACTIVITY

Lutein and zeaxanthin are two carotenoids that have recently sparked growing interest in the field of nutritional AMD research. Recent studies suggest that consumption of foods rich in lutein and zeaxanthin may be highly protective against AMD *(41)*. Lutein and zeaxanthin have no pro-vitamin A activity *(35)*, although they are similar in chemical structure to α- and β-carotene (α-carotene and lutein differ by two hydroxyl groups on the ring structures; the same is true for β-carotene and zeaxanthin).

Both lutein and zeaxanthin are preferentially deposited in the macula. Lutein is found in the peripheral rods and zeaxanthin in the cone cells of the macula. The yellow pigment absorbs in the light spectrum 450–500 nm, and thus, may prevent excessive oxidative damage that could be caused by blue light *(9,42)*. The high concentration of these two carotenoids in the macula suggests an important antioxidant or other protective function for these two compounds.

3.1.4. Minerals as Metalloenzymes

3.1.4.1. ZINC

Zinc is essential trace element of the metalloenzyme retinal dehydrogenase that is involved in the metabolism of vitamin A-containing visual pigments *(15)*. Zinc is also necessary for the synthesis of retinol-binding protein, the primary transport protein of vitamin A throughout the body *(15,28)*. Zinc is an essential cofactor in over 100 enzymes, including carbonic anhydrase, superoxide dismutase, alkaline phosphatase, catalase, and retinol dehydrogenase *(24)*. It is the second most abundant trace element in the body and high concentrations can be found in the RPE and choroid *(23)*. Zinc-binding capacity in the RPE may also be dependent on a low-mol-wt protein called metallothionein *(43)*. Although zinc is known to be necessary for the normal metabolism of the retinochoroidal complex, its exact role in the maintenance of normal retinal function remains undefined *(44)*. Zinc is involved in the synthesis of extracellular matrix molecules and is essential for the stability of cellular membranes as well as for normal immune function *(24)*.

3.1.4.2. SELENIUM

Selenium is an essential component of glutathione peroxidase, a key enzyme in the regulation of ROS *(15)*. Selenium is required for normal pancreatic function, which is necessary for the digestion and absorption of lipids, including vitamin E *(15)*. Selenium's proposed relationship to AMD is in the function of glutathione peroxidase as an antioxidant. Deficiencies in selenium may decrease enzyme activity and may lead to increased lipid peroxidation and accumulation of oxidative byproducts in the RPE *(45)*.

3.1.4.3. OTHER MINERALS

Copper is a metal cofactor in copper-dependent superoxide dismutase. Manganese is another required cofactor in the enzyme superoxide dismutase. Manganese is concentrated in the photoreceptor outer segment membrane of the retina, where it acts as a free radical scavenger *(28)*.

3.2. Atherosclerotic Theory

The pathogenesis of AMD has been linked to several cardiovascular risk factors, such as smoking, cholesterol level, and dietary intake of fats. The relationship between AMD and dietary fat intake is not well understood, although it follows from the classic diet–heart hypothesis that a diet high in saturated fat or cholesterol and low in polyunsaturated fat will raise serum cholesterol levels, promoting development of atheromatous plaques *(18)*. The proposed relationship between lipids and AMD involves not only their susceptibility to oxidation by ROS, but also their net effect on serum cholesterol levels. Three studies report that lipids in the retina form hydroperoxide byproducts, which accumulate with constant exposure to light *(11)*. It has been generally accepted that dietary intake of polyunsaturated fatty acids is associated with lipofuscin accumulation *(46)*. Dietary supplementation of vegetable oils rich in linoleic acid increase both n-6 and n-3 polyunsaturated fatty acids in the retinas of piglets *(47)*.

3.2.1. LIPIDS

Phospholipids, specifically phosphatidyl choline, phosphatidyl ethanolamine, phosphtidyl inositol, and phosphatidyl serine *(48)*, are the major complex lipids found in the retina, RPE, and Bruch's membrane or choroid. The dominant fatty acids found in the retina and the macular area in particular are palmitic (16:0), stearic (18:0), and oleic (18:1) *(48)*.

Inadequate levels of antioxidants in the presence of unsaturated fatty acids may result in an excess of oxidized lipid byproducts that may then accumulate in the RPE and could result in tissue degeneration and death. Although it is generally accepted that polyunsaturated fats are more susceptible to oxidation by oxidative agents, it is unknown if a high polyunsaturated fat intake in the presence of low antioxidant nutrients significantly increases risk for atherosclerotic plaques.

Oxidized lipid byproducts, malondialdehyde, and lipofuscin, indigestible by cellular enzymes, have been found in both atherosclerotic plaques and in eyes with AMD. Accumulation of these deposits in the retina may result in the death of functioning tissue. It is unknown if these oxidized byproducts induce the same type of autoimmune response in the eye that is seen in atherosclerotic plaque formation.

4. REVIEW OF ANIMAL STUDIES ON DIET AND AMD

The animal models supporting the role of antioxidant nutrients in the prevention of retinal tissue degeneration are relatively consistent (Table 2). The nutrients that have been studied include vitamin C, vitamin E, β-carotene, lutein, zeaxanthin, and a few trace minerals.

Many studies have investigated the protective effect of ascorbate against retinal injury caused by excessive exposure to blue light and excessive oxygen *(49–53)*. In addition to vitamin C, β-carotene protected the RPE from damage caused by excessive light in primates *(51)*.

Vitamin E deficiency in primates produced changes in the macula similar to the drusen seen in humans within 3 yr of dietary depletion *(10)*. Similar studies in rats also produced central retinal changes and loss of photoreceptor cells, especially in groups deficient in vitamin E and sulfur-containing amino acids *(45)*. One study using primates showed that dietary depletion of zeaxanthin and lutein inhibited the development of the yellow pigment usually seen in the macula *(54)*. Among one group of free-living primates, aging was associated with retinal changes similar to those seen in early age-related maculopathy *(55,56)*.

5. REVIEW OF EPIDEMIOLOGIC STUDIES ON DIET AND AMD

There have been six observational epidemiologic studies and one small randomized clinical trial examining the relationship between diet and AMD (*see* Table 3). Because

Table 2
Summary of Animal Studies Evaluating Dietary Nutrients and Retinal Changes

Principal author ref.	Animal	Primary exposure	Outcome	Nutrient(s) studied	Results
Hayes, (10)	Monkeys	Deficient diets	Retinal changes	Vitamin E[a]	Deficient diet produced AMD within 2 yr, specifically—ceroid accumulation, retinal degeneration and photoreceptor layer disruption restricted to macula.
				Vitamin A[b]	Clinical symptoms of xerophthalmia after 16, 19, or 20 mo of study.
Katz (45)	Male rats	Antioxidant deficient diets	Effects on RPE and retina	Vitamin E, Selenium (Se), Chromium (Cr), Methionine[c]	More accumulation of autofluorescent pigment[c] in RPE of deficient rats than in rats supplemented with methionine and Cr. Very little autofluroescence found in rats receiving all four antioxidants.
Tripathi (49)	Rabbits	Oxygen	Hyperoxic injury to immature retinal vascular cells	Vitamin E, Gamma-aminobutyric acid (GABA)	Retinal vascular degeneration retarded in groups supplemented with vitamin E and GABA. Immature retinal vascular cells are rapidly and adversely affected by hypoxia compared to mature cells under the same conditions; this suggests protective free radical scavenging enzymes develop with cell maturity.
Tso (50)	Baboons	Light (30 min) on macula	Distribution of vitamin C in retinas with and without photic injury	Vitamin C	Aqueous vitamin C higher in light-exposed eye. Total vitamin C concentration in RPE, choroid decreased significantly ($p < .05$) in light-exposed eyes.
Ham (51)	Macaque monkeys	Blue light, oxygen	Lesions of macaque retina	Beta-carotene (D)[e]	Animals supplemented with beta-carotene have increased threshold for oxygen and light to produce the same minimal lesion in macaque retina. This suggests that β-carotene is protective against free radicals produced by blue light and oxygen

Reference	Species	Condition	Retinal changes	Nutrient	Results
Anderson (11)	Albino rats frogs	Constant light FeSO$_4$		Polyunsaturated fatty acids (PUFA),	Treatments with light and FeSO$_4$ resulted in loss of long-chain PUFA and accumulation of lipid hydroperoxides in isolated outer rod segments. Decrease in 22:6 n-3 in photo-receptor ROS membrane, but concentration of palmitic acid was unchanged.
Li (52)	Rats	Diet	Photoreceptor damage in RPE	Vitamin C[f]	6–13 d after 24 h exposure to light, supplemented rats had significantly less outer segment photoreceptor cells than rats on normal diets.
Organisciak (53)	Rats	Light-dark cycles	Rhodopsin photoreceptor cell nuclei	Vitamin C, docosahexaenoic acid (22:6 n-3)	Rats supplemented with vitamin C had higher concentrations of rhodopsin and 22:6 n-3 than unsupplemented light-exposed rats.
Whitley, '88 (abstract)	Pigs	Diet Ocular changes	Photoreceptor cells, RPE edema,	Zinc	Abnormal migration of photoreceptor cells from outer nuclear layer toward the RPE in animals with zinc-deficient diets. RPE exhibited signs of edema and occasional opaque bodies seen in zinc-deficient rats, suggesting chronic zinc deficiency may be important in AMD.
Feeney-Burns, '88 (abstract)	Monkeys	Semi-purified diet chow (control)	Macular changes	Protein	No macular pigment was observed in animals fed semipurified diets; virtually no plasma carotene or xanthophyll was found. Serial histopathologic sections revealed punctuate window defects to be sites of vacuolated RPE cells, not drusen. No drusen were found in any animal.

(continued)

Table 2 (continued)

Principal author ref.	Animal	Primary exposure	Outcome	Nutrient(s) studied	Results
Samuelson, '90	Sheep	Age	RPE, progression of ovine lipofuscinosis (OCL)	Zinc, iron, copper, phosphate, sulfur, manganese, chromium	Age-related changes in Zn, Fe, Cu associated with lipopigment accumulation in RPE. Decrease in levels of phosphate, S, Mn as photoreceptor cells and their outer segments are lost in the disease process. Levels of metals observed in retina of 1-yr-old sheep with OCL the same as levels in the RPE of 10+yr-old normal sheep.
Hrboticky (47)	Piglets	Diet	Retinal polyunsaturated fatty acid (PUFA) composition	Linoleic acid (18:2 n-6) linolenic acid (18:3 n-3)	Normal accretion of 22:6 n-3 in retinas of piglets deficient in long-chain PUFAs but sufficient in 18:2 n-6, 18:3 n-3.
Hope (55)	Monkeys	Free-living diet	Drusen: natural progression	Free-living diet	The prevalence and severity of drusen are linearly related to increasing age and significantly higher in specific maternal lineage. Percentage of female animals with drusen was twice that of male animals.

[a]Plasma vitamin E <100 μg/dL in deficient group compared with >600 μg/dL in control group.
[b]Plasma vitamin A <5 μg/dL in deficient group compared with >15–20 μg/dL in control group.
[c]Nutrient concentrations determined from liver homogenates.
[d]Autofluroescence pigment in rat RPE is similar to lipofuscin deposits found in human RPE.
[e]64 d dietary source of β-carotene in the form of Solatene mixture prepared by Roche. Plasma β-carotene levels >360 μg/dL.
[f]Vitamin C injection given peritoneally 24 h 0.5 g/k.

of the small sample size and nonsignificant results from the case-control study by Blumenkranz et al., it is presented in the table only and not discussed in the text.

5.1. Antioxidant Theory

Newsome et al. undertook a prospective, randomized, double-masked, placebo-controlled trial involving zinc supplementation of persons with AMD *(57)*. Ninety people were randomized to zinc and 84 to placebo. Ten people were lost to follow-up in the treatment group and 13 in the placebo group. Baseline visual acuity and fundus photographs were taken before and after zinc supplementation. Comparison of macular appearance on photos taken at the last study visit and at the baseline visit showed that more eyes in the zinc-treated group were stable or had less accumulation of visible drusen. However, as a result of the pilot nature of the study, the authors and investigators in general do not recommend widespread use of zinc supplements.

Goldberg et. al., *(58)* in their analysis of 3082 person over 45 yr of age in the first National Health and Nutrition Examination Survey, found a significant inverse association between dietary intake of fruits and vegetables high in pro-vitamin A carotenoids and vitamin C (using consumption less than once per week as reference category) and prevalence of AMD and cataract in persons 45–75 yr of age *(58)*. The inverse association between high fruit and vegetable consumption and prevalence of AMD was observed even after adjustment for age, sex, race, systolic blood pressure, cerebral vascular disease, and refractive error. No association was found between AMD and frequency of consumption of fruits and vegetable rich in vitamin A (> 7 times/wk compared to < once per week). Since "wet" (neovascular, advanced AMD) and "dry" (mostly early stage) AMD cases were not specified, it is unknown if results differed for specific types of AMD.

The Eye Disease Case-Control Study (EDCCS) involved 421 cases and 615 controls from five ophthalmologic centers in the United States. All cases were "wet" AMD, the more advanced stage of disease. Higher serum carotenoid levels were inversely associated with advanced AMD (OR = 0.4, CI 95%: 0.2–0.6). Individually, serum levels of vitamins E (OR = 0.6, CI 95%: 0.4–1.04), vitamin C (OR = 0.7, CI 95%: 0.5–1.2), and selenium (OR = 1.3, CI 95%: 0.8–2.1) were not significantly associated with AMD. When all serum values for carotenoids, vitamins C, E, and selenium were combined into an antioxidant index, the association was protective (OR = 0.3, CI 95%: 0.1–0.7) *(59)*. In another EDCCS study investigating risk factors for neovascular age-related macular degeneration, serum zinc levels were not associated with risk for AMD, for both those taking supplements and those who did not (OR = 1.3, CI 95%: 0.7–2.2 no supplement, and OR = 1.4 CI 95%: 0.7–2.8 with supplements) *(60)*.

In the Baltimore Longitudinal Study of Aging (BLSA), West et al., used data from 976 participants who had lens and macular photos taken twice a year from January 1988 through January 1, 1990, of which 85% had fundus photos taken and 82% had plasma nutrient data available. They reported a protective effect for AMD among those with higher fasting serum α-tocopherol (OR = 0.43, CI 95%: 0.25–0.73) after adjusting for age, sex, and nuclear opacity in a multiple logistic model *(61)*. Using an antioxidant index for fasting serum levels of ascorbate, α-tocopherol, and β-carotene, they also found a protective effect on AMD (OR = 0.43, CI 95%: 0.26–0.70) *(61)*.

Seddon et al., investigated the dietary intake of 356 cases of wet AMD and 520 controls in five ophthalmology centers in the United States—the multicenter EDCCS. Nu-

Table 3
Summary of Epidemiological Studies Evaluating Dietary Antioxidants and AMD

Principal author ref.	Design	Subjects, n	AMD outcome			Nutrient(s) studied	OR for multivariate model
			Wet	Dry	Total		
Blumenkranz, '86	Case-control	26 cases 23 controls (spouses)	NA[a]	NA	26	Vitamins A, C, E	Not significant
Newsome (57)	Prospective randomized trial	80 treatment (T) 71 placebo (P)	15 (T) 8 (P)	65 63	80 71	Zinc supplement	Less drusen in supplement group and decreased vision loss
Goldberg (58) (NHANES1)	Cross-sectional	178 cases	NA	NA	178	Vitamin A (S)[b] Vitamin C (S)	0.59 (0.37, 0.99) 0.98 (0.79–1.23)
Eye Disease Case Control study (60)	Case-control	421 cases 615 controls	421	0	421	Vitamin C (s)[b] Vitamin E (s) Selenium (s) Carotenoids (s)[c] Antioxidant index[d]	0.70 (0.5–1.2) 0.60 (0.4–1.04) 1.30 (0.8, 2.1) 0.30 (0.2, 0.6) 0.40 (0.2, 0.6)
Sanders (64)	Matched case-control	65 cases 65 controls	9	56	65	Vitamin A (s)[b] Vitamin E (s) β-carotene (s) α-carotene (s) Lutein (s) Lycopene (s) β-cryptoxanthin (s)	1.20 (0.67, 2.14) 0.85 (0.48, 1.50) 0.50 (0.20, 1.20) 0.85 (0.48, 1.50) 1.37 (0.57, 3.38) 1.00 (0.40, 2.57) 1.35 (0.58, 3.28)

256

Study	Design	Cases/Controls	NA			Nutrient	OR (95% CI)
West (61) Longitudinal Study on Aging	Cross-sectional	226 cases	11	215	226	Vitamin A (s)[b]	1.01 (0.6–1.8)
						Vitamin C (s)	0.70 (0.5, 1.2)
						Vitamin E (s)	0.43 (0.3–0.7)
						β-carotene (s)	0.62 (0.41–1.1)
						Antioxidant index[d]	0.43 (0.3, 0.7)
Seddon (68)	Case-control	356 cases 520 controls	356	0	356	Carotenoids (d)[e]	0.57 (0.4–0.9)
						Lutein/zeaxanthin (d)	0.44 (0.2, 0.8)
						Vitamin A (d)[g]	0.57 (0.4–0.9)
						Vitamin C (d)	0.83 (0.5–1.3)
						Vitamin E (d)	1.46 (0.9–2.4)

[a]NA = number of cases not specified.
[b]Nutrients derived from serum.
[c]Serum carotenoids included lutein/zeaxanthin, β-carotein, α-carotene, cryptoxanthin, lycopene.
[d]Antioxidant index includes nutrients listed singly.
[e]Nutrients obtained from a semiquantitative food frequency questionnaire (SFFQ).
[f]Energy-adjusted, two-nutrient multivariate model comparing highest to lowest quintiles.
[g]Preformed vitamin A or retinal estimated from SFFQ.

trients were assessed using a validated semiquantitative food frequency questionnaire. They found that a higher dietary intake of carotenoids was associated with lower risk of AMD *(41)*. Adjusting for other risk factors, they found that those in the highest quintile of dietary carotenoid intake had a 43% lower risk for AMD compared with those in the lowest quintile (OR = 0.57, CI 95%: 0.35–0.92) *(41)*. Among specific carotenoids, lutein and zeaxanthin, found primarily in dark green leafy vegetables, were most strongly protective *(41)*. Higher consumption of spinach or collard greens, specifically, was associated with a strong protective effect against AMD (*p* for trend < 0.001) *(41)*. Dietary intake of preformed vitamin A, or vitamins C, and E were not associated with statistically significant reduction in risk of AMD *(41)*. Use of vitamin supplements in general was not protective, although a small beneficial effect of multivitamin use could not be ruled out.

5.2. Similar Risk Factors for Atherosclerosis and AMD Epidemiology

Verhoeff et al. were possibly the first to propose the relationship between atherosclerotic risk factors and AMD *(62)*. There are several epidemiologic studies that have examined this relationship (Table 4).

Hyman and colleagues reported an increased prevalence of AMD among those with a history of cardiovascular disease *(63)*. This matched a case-control study of 162 cases and 175 controls that investigated the history of one or more cardiovascular diseases, smoking and other variables, such as chemical exposures, family history of macular disease, blue or medium pigmented eyes, decreased hand grip strength, and hyperopia. The risk of AMD was significant for those with a history of one or more cardiovascular and disease (OR = 1.7, CI 95%: 1.1–2.7) and among male smokers (OR = 2.6, CI 95%: 1.15–5.75).

Sanders et al. also conducted a matched case-control study of 65 cases of AMD (nine wet and 59 dry). They investigated the relationship between plasma retinol, α-tocopherol, such carotenoids as lutein, β-cryptoxanthin, α- and β-carotene, cholesterol concentration, polyunsaturated fatty acid content of plasma and erythrocyte phospholipids, and AMD *(64)*. Overall, they found no significant associations. An interesting point to note is that when plasma carotenoid concentrations between smoking and nonsmoking subjects were compared, after adjusting for age and sex, nonsmokers had significantly higher carotenoid levels than smokers. Lutein was significantly lower for smokers than nonsmokers at *p* < 0.001 level. Beta-carotene and β-cryptoxanthin, another nonpro-vitamin A carotenoid, were significantly lower for smokers than nonsmokers at the *p* < 0.05 level.

The EDCCS study found that current use of postmenopausal exogenous estrogens among women was inversely associated with AMD (OR = 0.3, CI 95%: 0.1–0.6) *(60)*. Cigaret smoking and higher serum cholesterol levels *(60)* were associated with increased risk for neovascular AMD. These observations are consistent with the hypothesis linking risk factors for cardiovascular disease with AMD *(60)*.

Klein et al. also examined the relationship between AMD and cardiovascular disease and smoking *(65,66)* in a cross-sectional study. This population-based prevalence study of 492 persons aged 43–86 in Beaver Dam, WI, showed an inverse association between serum lipids and early AMD. Higher hematocrit levels and leukocyte counts were also associated with exudative AMD *(65)*. Although no association between smoking status and early AMD was found, exudative AMD was more common in current smokers compared to those who never smoked *(66)*.

Seddon et al. conducted a prospective analysis to examine the relationship between smoking and AMD in a cohort of women from the Nurses' Health Study. There were 223 incident cases of AMD confirmed by medical records. An independent review of fundus photographs was also performed on a sample of cases. They observed that both current and past smokers had a higher risk of developing AMD with visual loss of 20/30 or worse, compared to those who had never smoked. These multivariate models controlled for age, body mass index, history of hypertension, alcohol consumption, and energy-adjusted carotene intake *(67)*.

Using the EDCCS case-control study group to examine the relationship between different types of dietary fat and AMD among 356 cases of wet AMD *(68)*, Seddon et al. found that total fat and vegetable fats were significantly and adversely associated with risk for AMD. Only fish oils were found to be protective. Animal fats were not significantly associated with AMD.

Finally, Mares-Perlman et al. also looked at the relationship between dietary fat and AMD among residents participating in the Beaver Dam Eye Study. There were 314 cases of early AMD and 30 cases of wet AMD *(69)*. Saturated fat, linoleic acid, and cholesterol (reported in mg/4200 kJ) were associated with increased risk for early AMD. Total fat, as percent kilojoules, and oleic acid were not significantly associated with risk for early AMD.

6. CONCLUSIONS

Animal research suggests that higher levels of vitamin C, vitamin E, and β-carotene are protective against the damaging effects of excess oxygen and light exposure on the retina. Primate models show that two dietary carotenoids, lutein and zeaxanthin, are components of the yellow pigment seen in the macula and may prevent the development of drusen-like bodies. No animal studies to date have directly examined the relationship between cardiovascular risk factors and AMD. A limitation of animal studies is that the retinal changes observed do not include all of the signs of AMD, including neovascularization and atrophy, found in humans. There are currently no animal models for AMD that completely reflect the human disease.

Studies of AMD in humans have also provided evidence for a protective effect of antioxidant nutrients, mainly the carotenoids lutein and zeaxanthin. One cross-sectional and three case-control studies *(41,58,59,61)* have shown protective effects of different antioxidant nutrients measured from serum or from dietary intake. Only one clinical trial examined zinc supplementation and AMD. However, a limitation of this study is its small sample size and methodological issues in the assessment of visual acuity and definition of AMD. Furthermore, no support for a protective effect of zinc was found in a large case-control study of exudative AMD *(60)*.

Several epidemiologic studies that evaluated cardiovascular risk factors and AMD indicate that higher serum cholesterol levels *(60,65)*. cigarette smoking (both past and current) *(60,67)*, and higher hematocrit and leukocyte levels are positively associated with AMD *(65)*. Current use of postmenopausal estrogens (compared to never and past users) among women was inversely associated with neovascular AMD *(60)*. Two studies investigating the relationship between dietary fat and AMD found significant asso-

Table 4
Summary of Epidemiological Studies Evaluating Cardiovascular Risk Factors and AMD

Principal author ref.	Design	Subjects, n	AMD outcome			Parameters studied	OR for multivariate model
			Wet	Dry	Total		
Hyman (63)	Matched[a] Case-control	162 cases 175 controls	NA	NA	162	≥1 CVD[b] Smoke, men Smoke, women	1.7 (1.1, 2.7) 2.6 (1.15, 5.75) 0.84 (0.48, 1.47)
Eye Disease Case-control Study Group (60)	Case-control	421 cases	421	0	421	Total cholesterol Smoking Estrogen use	4.1 (12.3, 7.3) 2.2 (1.3, 3.5) 0.3 (0.1, 0.8)
Klein (65)	Cross-sectional	803 cases	59	744	803	Cholesterol, women[c] Cholesterol, men[c] Hematocrit[d] Leukocyte[d]	0.89 (0.80, 0.98) 0.89 (0.84, 0.96) 1.09 (1.00, 1.19) 1.10 (1.00, 1.19)
Sanders (64)	Matched[a] Case-control	65 cases 65 controls	9	56	65	Plasma cholesterol 18:2n-6 plasma[e] 18:2n-6 erythrocyte[e] 22:6n-3 plasma[e] 22:6n-3 erythrocyte[e]	1.00 (0.40, 2.48) 0.62 (0.26, 1.46) 0.9 (0.37, 2.18) 0.82 (0.35, 1.93) 0.92 (0.37, 2.32)
Klein (65)	Cross-sectional	871 cases	41 W[f] 56 M[f]	422 W 352 M	463 W 408 M	Smoke (female, early AMD) Smoke (male, early AMD) Smoke (female, wet AMD) Smoke (male, wet AMD)	1.29 (0.98, 1.70)[g] 1.02 (0.81, 1.29)[g] 2.06 (1.03, 4.10) 2.50 (1.01, 6.20)

Study	Design	Cases/Controls				Variable	OR (95% CI)
Seddon (68) (abstract)	Case control	356 cases 520 controls	356	0	356[h]	Total fat	1.71 (1.02–2.8)
						Vegetable fat	1.99 (1.2–3.3)
						Animal fat	0.84 (0.5–1.9)
						Ω-3 fatty acids	0.59 (0.5–0.9)
Seddon (67) (abstract)	Prospective	223 cases	NA	NA	223	Smoke 1–14 cigarettes[i]	1.05 (0.56, 1.94)
						Smoke 15–24 cigarettes	1.38 (0.81, 2.25)
						Smoke ≥ 25 cigarettes	1.99 (1.18, 1.71)
Vingerling	Cross-sectional	104 cases	NA	NA	104	Plaques in carotid bifurcation	4.7 (1.8, 12.2)
						Plaques carotid artery	2.5 (1.4, 4.5)
						Plaques lower extremity	2.5 (1.4, 4.5)
Mares-Perlman (69)	Case control	167 cases 167 controls	30	314	344	Total fat (%kJ)	1.30 (0.90, 1.90)[j]
						Saturated fat	1.80 (1.20, 2.70)
						18:2 oleate	1.20 (0.80, 1.80)
						18:3 linoleate	1.10 (1.10, 2.40)
						Cholesterol (mg/4200 kJ)	1.60 (1.10, 2.40)

[a]Matched on age and sex.
[b]Cardiovascular disease includes myocardial infarction, angina, other heart problems, arteriosclerosis, hypertension, stroke, circulatory problems and/or transient ischemia.
[c]Cholesterol in mmol/L; OR using early AMD as dichotomous outcome.
[d]OR using exudative AMD as dichotomous outcome.
[e]Phospholipids.
[f]W denotes women 43–86 yr of age, M denotes men 43–86 yr of age.
[g]Ever smokers compared to never smokers measured in pack years (total number cigarettes smoked per day divided by 20).
[h]AMD with visual loss ≥20/30.
[i]Current vs never smokers with a significant dose-dependent test for trend (p < 0.05).
[j]Adjusted odds ratios for early AMD only; odds ratios for late AMD were in similar directions, but all nonsignificant at p < 0.10 level.

261

ciations with advanced AMD for vegetable fat (adverse) and Ω-3 acids (protective) *(68)*, and between saturated fat, cholesterol, and linoleic acid (adverse) and early AMD *(69)*.

Randomized clinical trials would provide the most conclusive data about the effect of antioxidant nutrients in the eye *(7)*. More prospective studies and randomized clinical trials are needed to clarify the association between diet and AMD, particularly for vitamin E, vitamin C, selenium, and the carotenoids—lutein, zeaxanthin, β-carotene, and dietary lipids. Further studies are also needed to further clarify the roles of such nutrients as selenium, manganese, zinc, copper, and riboflavin. Additional basic research is needed to further define the mechanism of oxidation and its effect on the eye, and the extent to which oxidative effects occur in vivo. Better markers of oxidative stress may be helpful to identify people at higher risk who may possibly benefit from antioxidants.

6.1. Current Research in Progress

Ongoing large-scale randomized trials should provide valuable data on which to base public health recommendations. The Age-Related Eye Disease Study (AREDS) is a multicenter randomized clinical trial sponsored by the National Eye Institute. The study has approx 5000 patients enrolled at 11 centers across the country to examine the effects of supplemental vitamin C, vitamin E, β-carotene, zinc, and copper. Patients at lower risk for developing visual loss caused by AMD have been randomized into two groups: high-dose antioxidant vitamins and minerals or placebo. Patients at higher risk of developing visual loss as a result of AMD have been randomized into four groups in a factorial design: antioxidant vitamins; zinc and copper; antioxidant vitamins, zinc and copper, or placebo. Other large randomized trials that focus on cancer and heart disease outcomes may also provide additional information.

Several prospective observational studies are also in progress. These data are valuable because they include dietary information (estimated from food frequencies or serum), cardiovascular risk factors, and other environmental risk factors related to AMD development. Dietary data from women in the Nurses' Health Study (NHS) are being evaluated to examine the relationship between high and low lifetime intakes of foods rich in lutein, zeaxanthin, and other nutrients and incidence of AMD. The Health Professional's Follow-up Study, having similar data as the NHS, is a valuable resource for similar analyses among men. The Beaver Dam Eye Study, a cohort of men and women in Wisconsin, is also still ongoing. All of these studies will provide valuable information regarding the potential role of diet and supplements in preventing AMD or slowing its progression. Large sample sizes in these studies will permit investigators to address these and other questions that may be relevant to AMD development.

6.2. Dietary Recommendations

The data at present are insufficient to support a clinical recommendation for vitamin and mineral supplement use for AMD prevention since effectiveness, appropriate dose, and duration are still unknown. The 1989 Recommended Dietary Allowances (RDA) can be used as the minimum level to be consumed by all individuals, regardless of AMD status *(24)*. The RDA's may not, however, represent optimal intakes to prevent retinal disease *(24)* and may be lower than what is needed for optimal ocular health. Nutrient-dense foods, especially carotenoid (β-carotene, lutein, zeaxanthin)-rich vegetables (broccoli, collard greens, kale, or spinach), should be encouraged, since the most consistent epidemiologic evidence to date supports a strong inverse association between serum carotenoid levels or dietary carotenoid intake and AMD. Even though it is biologically plausible that the intake of antioxidant-rich foods is protective, the benefit may be because of other compounds in these foods and not the antioxidant nutrients themselves. If this is the case, it is easily understood why antioxidant supplements containing only certain nutrients may not be helpful in AMD prevention.

Recommendations regarding cholesterol and dietary fat intake should follow current guidelines for decreasing cardiovascular risk. Data are insufficient to support recommendations to change intake of specific dietary fats, although the potential benefit of Ω-3 fatty acids on AMD *(68)* should be further explored.

In summary, until more data become available, a diet that is high in fruits and vegetables, rich in carotenoids and low in saturated and processed fats, is a reasonable goal. Following the current National Cancer Institute and National Academy of Sciences' recommendations to eat at least five servings of fruit and/or vegetables every day to reduce risk for developing heart disease and some types of cancers may yield additional benefits to patients at risk for developing AMD.

REFERENCES

1. National Advisory Eye Council Report of the Retinal and Choroidal Diseases Panel: Vision Research: A National Plan: 1983–1987. Washington DC: US Dept of Health and Human Services, 1984.
2. Klein R, Klein B, Linton KLP. Prevalence of age-related maculopathy: the Beaver Dam Study. Ophthalmology 1992; 99:933–943.
3. U.S. Department of Commerce. Statistical Abstract of the United States 1995. September, 1995, US Bureau of the Census, Current Population Reports, pp. 25–1104.
4. Macular Photocoagulation Study Group. Argon laser photocoagulation for neovascular maculopathy. Arch Ophthalmol 1986; 104:694–701.
5. Macular Photocoagulation Study Group. Persistent and recurrent neovascularization after krypton laser photocoagulation for neovascular lesions of age-related macular degeneration. Arch Ophthalmol 1990; 108:825–831.
6. Macular Photocoagulation Study Group. Krypton laser photocoagulation for neovascular lesions of age-related macular degeneration. Arch Ophthalmol 1990; 108:816–824.
7. Seddon JM, Hennekens CH. Vitamins, minerals, and macular degeneration: promising but unproven hypotheses. Arch Ophthalmol 1994; 112(2):176–179.
8. Frei B. Reactive oxygen species and antioxidant vitamins: mechanisms of action. Am J Med 1994; 97(3A):5S–14S.
9. Young RW. Solar radiation and age-related macular degeneration. Surv Ophthalmol 1988; 32:252–269.
10. Hayes KC. Retinal degeneration in monkeys induced by deficiencies of vitamin E or A. Invest Ophthalmol 1974; 13:499–510.
11. Anderson RE, Rapp LM, Wiegand RD. Lipid peroxidation and retinal degeneration. Curr Eye Res 1984; 3(1):181–191.
12. Gottsch JD, Bynoe LA, Harlan JB, Rencs EV, Green WR. Light-induced deposits in Bruch's membrane of protoporphyric mice. Arch Ophthalmol 1993; 111:126–129.
13. Eckhert CD, Hsu MH, Pang N. Photoreceptor damage following exposure to excess riboflavin. Experimentia 1993; 49:1084–1087.
14. Foote CS. Detection and characterization of Singlet Oxygen, in. Reactive Oxygen Species in Chemistry, Biology and Medicine, Quintanilha A, New York: Plenum, published in cooperation with NATO Scientific Affairs Division, 1988.
15. Murray RK, Granner DK, Mayes PA, Rodwell VW. Harper's Biochemistry, 23rd ed. A Lange Medical Book, Norwalk, CT: Appleton & Lange, 1993.
16. Vanderhagen AM, Yolton DP, Kaminski MS, Yolton RL. Free radicals and antioxidant supplementation: a review of their roles in age-related macular degeneration. J Am Optom Assoc 1993; 64(12):871–878.
17. Young RW. Pathophysiology of age-related macular degeneration. Survey Ophthalmol 1987; 31:291–306.

18. Willett W, Churchill. Nutritional epidemiology. In: Monographs in Epidemiology and Biostatistics. Mac Mahon, B, ed. vol 15. New York: Oxford University Press, 1990;

19. Katz ML, Robison Jr G. Nutritional influences on autoxidation, lipofuscin accumulation and aging. In: Free Radicals, Aging and Degenerative Diseases. Johnson J, Walford R, Armon D, Miquel J, eds. New York, Liss, 1986; 221–259.

20. Holz FG, Seraidah G, Pauleikhoff D, Bird AC. Analysis of lipid deposits extracted from human macular and peripheral Bruch's membrane. Arch Ophthalmol 1994; 112:402–406.

21. Liles MR, Newsome DA, Oliver PD. Antioxidant enzymes in the aging human retinal pigment epithelium. Arch Ophthalmol 1991; 109:1285–1288.

22. Frei B. Ascorbic acid protects lipids in human plasma and low-denstiy lipoprotein against oxidative damage. Am J Clin Nutr 1991; 54:1113S–1118S.

23. International Life Sciences Foundation. Present Knowledge in Nutrition, 6th ed. Brown ML, ed. Washington, DC: International Life Sciences Institute—Nutrition Foundation, 1990; 532.

24. National, Research and Council. Recommended Dietary Allowances. 10th ed. Washington, DC: National Academy Press, 1989.

25. Roberfroid M, Calderon PB. Free Radicals and Oxidation Phenomena in Biological Systems. New York: Marcel Dekker, 1995.

26. Niki E, Saito T, Kawakami A, Kamiya Y. Inhibition of oxidation of methyl linoleate in solution by vitamin E and vitamin C. J Biol Chem 1984; 259:4177–4182.

27. Taylor A, Jacques PF, Nadler D, Morrow F, Sulsky SI, Shepard D. Relationship in humans between ascorbic acid consumption and levels of total and reduced ascorbic acid in lens, aqueous humor, and plasma. Current Eye Res 1991; 10:751–759.

28. Linder MC. Nutritional Biochemistry and Metabolism with Clinical Applications, 2nd ed. New York: Elsevier, 1991.

29. Horwitt MK. Vitamin E and lipid metabolism in man. Am J Clin Nutr 1962; 8:451–461.

30. Horwitt MK. Status of human requirements for vitamin E. Am J Clin Nutr 1974; 27:1182–1193.

31. Machlin LJ, Bendich A. Free radical tissue damage: protective role of antioxidant nutrients. FASEB J 1987; 1:441–445.

32. Tirmenstein M, Reed DJ. Effects of glutathione on the alpha-tocopherol-dependent inhibition of nuclear lipid peroxidation. J Lipid Res 1989; 30:959–965.

33. Stryer L. Biochemistry, 2nd ed. New York: Freeman, 1981.

34. Stroub O. Key to Carotenoids, 2nd ed. Basel, Birkhauser Verlag, 1987; 1–296.

35. Krinsky NI. Antioxidant functions of carotenoids. Free Radical Biol Med 1989; 7:617–635.

36. Briggs GM, Calloway DH. Nutrition and Physical Fitness, 11th ed. New York: Holt, Rinehart and Winston, 1979; 380.

37. Mangels AR, Holden JM, Beecher GR, Forman MR, Lanza E. Carotenoid content of fruits and vegetables: an evaluation of analytic data. J Am Diet Assoc 1993; 93:284–296.

38. Chug-Ahuja JK, Holden JM, Forman MR, Mangels R, Beecher GR, Lanza E. The development and application of a carotenoid database for fruits, vegetables, and selected multicomponent foods. J Am Diet Assoc 1993; 93:318–323.

39. Olson J, Allen, Krinsky NI. Introduction: the colorful, fascinating world of the carotenoids: important physiologic modulators. FASEB J 1995; 9:1547–1550.

40. DiMascio P, Kaiser S, Sies H. Ranking carotenoids as singlet oxygen quenchers: lycopene as the most efficient biological carotenoid singlet oxygen quencher. Arch Biochem Biophys 1989; 274(2):532–538.

41. Seddon JM, Ajani UA, Sperduto RD, Hiller R, Blair N, Burton TC, et al., Dietary carotenoids, vitamins A, C, and E, and advanced age-related macular degeneration. Eye disease case-control study group. JAMA 1994; 292(18):1413–1420.

42. Schalch W, ed. Carotenoids in the retina—a review of their possible role in preventing or limiting damage caused by light and oxygen. In: Free Radicals and Aging. Emerit I, and BC, eds, Basel, Switzerland: Birkhauser Verlag, 1994; 290–298.

43. Oliver PD, Tate DJ, Newsome DA. Metallothionein in human retinal pigment epithelial cells: expression, induction and zinc uptake. Current Eye Res 1992; 11(2):183–188.

44. Newsome DA, Oliver PD, Deupree DM, Miceli MV, Diamond JG. Zinc uptake by primate RPE and choroid. Current Eye Res 1992; 11(3):213–217.

45. Katz ML, Parker KR, Handelman GJ, Bramel TL, Dratz EA. Effects of antioxidant nutrient deficiency on the retina and retinal pigment epithelium of albino rats: a light an delectron microscopic study. Exp Eye Res 1982; 34:339–369.

46. Katz ML, Robison G. Nutrition influences on autoxidation, lipofuscin accumulation, and aging. In: Modern Aging Research Johnson J Jr, Walford R, Harmon D, Miquel J, eds. New York: Liss, 1986; 221–259.
47. Hrboticky N, MacKinnon MJ, Innis SM. Retina fatty acid composition of piglets fed from birth with a linoleic acid-rich vegetable-oil formula for infants. Am J Clin Nutr 1991; 53:483–490.
48. Gülcan HG, Alvarez RA, Maude MB, Anderson RE. Lipids of human retina, retinal pigment epithelium, and Bruch's membrane/choroid: comparison of macular and peripheral regions. Invest Ophthalmol Vis Sci 1993; 34:3187–3193.
49. Tripathi BJ, Tripathi RC. Cellular and subcellular events in retinopathy of oxygen toxicity with a preliminary report on the preventive role of vitamin E and gamma-aminobutyric acid: a study in vitro. Curr Eye Res 1984; 3(1):193–208.
50. Tso MO, M, Woodford BJ, Lam KW. Distribution of ascorbate in normal primate retina and after photic injury: a biochemical, morphological study. Curr Eye Res 1984; 3:181–191.
51. Ham WT, Mueller HA, Ruffolo JJ, Millen JE, Cleary SF, Guerry RK, et al. Basic mechanisms underlying the production of photochemical lesions in the mammalian retina. Curr Eye Res 1984; 1:165–174.
52. Li ZY, Tso MO, M, Woodford BJ, Wang HM, Organisciak DT. Amerlioration of photic injury in rat retina by ascorbic acid. Invest Ophthalmol Vis Sci 1984; 25(Suppl):90.
53. Organisciak DT, Wang H, Li ZY, Tso MO, M. The protective effect of ascorbate in the retinal light damage of rats. Invest Ophthalmol Vis Sci 1985; 26:1580–1588.
54. Gerster H. Review: antioxidant protection of the aging macula. Age Aging 1991; 20:60–90.
55. Hope GM, Dawson WW, Engel HM, Ulshafer RJ, Kessler MJ, Sherwood MB. A primate model for age related macular drusen. Br J Ophthalmol 1992; 76:11–16.
56. Borges J, Li ZY, Tso MO. Effects of repeated photic exposures on the monkey macula. Arch Ophthalmol 1990; 108(5):727–733.
57. Newsome DA, Swartz M, Leone N, Elston RD, Miller E. Oral zinc in macular degeneration. Arch Ophthalmol 1988; 106:192–198.
58. Goldberg J, Flowerdew G, Smith E, Brody JA, Tso MO, M. Factors associated with age-related macular degeneration: an anlysis of data from the First National Health and Nutrition Examination Survey. Am J Epidemiol 1988; 128:700–710.
59. The Eye Disease Case-Control Group. Antioxidant status and neovascular age-related macular degeneration. Arch Ophthalmol 1993; 111:104–109.
60. The Eye Disease Case-Control Group. Risk factors for neovascular age-related macular degeneration. Arch Ophthalmol 1992; 110(12):1701–1708.
61. West S, Vitale S, Hallfrisch J, Munoz B, Muller D, Bressler S, et al. Are antioxidants or supplements protective for age-related macular degeneration? Arch Ophthalmol 1994; 112:222–227.
62. Verhoeff FH, Grossman HP. Pathogenesis of disciform degeneration of the macula. Arch Ophthalmol 1937; 18:561–585.
63. Hyman L, Lilienfeld Abraham M, Ferris FL, III, Fine SL. Senile macular degeneration: a case-control study. Amer J Epidemiol 1983; 118(2):213–227.
64. Sanders T, AB, Haines AP, Wormald R, Wright LA, Obeid O. Essential fatty acids, plasma cholesterol, and fat-soluble vitamins in subjects with age-related maculopathy and matched control subjects. Am J Clin Nutr 1993; 57:428–433.
65. Klein R, Klein BE, Franke T. The relationship of cardiovascular disease and its risk factors to age-related maculopathy. The Beaver Dam Eye Study. Ophthalmology 1993; 100(3):406–414.
66. Klein R, Klein BE, Linton KL, DeMets DL. The Beaver Dam Eye Study: the relation of age-related maculopathy to smoking. Am J Epidemiol 1993; 137(2):190–200.
67. Seddon JM, Hankinson S, Speizer F, Willett WC. A prospective study of smoking and age-related macular degeneration. Am J Epidemiol 1995; SER S34 (Abstract).
68. Seddon JM, Ujani U, Sperduto R, Yannuzzi L, Burton T, Haller J, et al. Dietary fat intake and age-related macular degeneration. Invest Ophthalmol Vis Sci 1994; 35(4):2003.
69. Mares-Perlman AJ, Brady EW, Klein R, VandenLangenberg MG, Klein EB, Palta M. Dietary fat and age-related maculopathy. Arch Ophthalmol 1995; 113:743–748.
70. Stahl W, Sies H. Physical quenching of singlet oxygen and cis-trans isomerization of carotenoids. Ann NY Acad Sci 1993;
71. Liebler DC. Antioxidant reactions of carotenoids. Ann NY Acad Sci 1993; 691:20–31.

14   Antioxidant Status and Risk for Cataract

Allen Taylor and Paul F. Jacques

1. INTRODUCTION

Although the number of associations between nutriture and age-related eye diseases have burgeoned in the last decade, early studies regarding antioxidant properties of nutrients were performed virtually immediately after the discovery of ascorbate in the early part of the century. Studies regarding the etiology of cataract now include laboratory and epidemiological investigations. This chapter briefly reviews available data, as well as intervention trials, regarding associations between antioxidant nutrients and eye lens cataract in humans. Readers can refer to other recent reviews *(1–4)* for more thorough treatments, particularly with respect to animal studies. Much of the rich body of pioneering work is, of necessity, given limited coverage here *(5–7)*.

The primary function of the eye lens is to collect and focus light on the retina (Fig. 1). To do so it must remain clear throughout life. The lens is located posterior to the cornea and iris and receives nutriture from the aqueous humor. Although the lens appears to be free of structure it is exquisitely designed. A single layer of epithelial cells is found directly under the anterior surface of the collagenous membrane in which it is encapsulated (Fig. 2). The epithelial cells at the germinative region divide, migrate posteriorly, and differentiate into lens fibers. The fibers elaborate as their primary gene produces the predominant proteins of the lens, called crystallins. They also lose their organelles. New cells are formed throughout life but older cells are usually not lost. Instead, they are compressed into the center or nucleus of the lens. There is a coincident dehydration of the proteins and the lens itself. Together with modifications of the protein (noted below) and other constituents, these changes result in a less flexible lens on aging.

As the lens ages the proteins are photo-oxidatively damaged, aggregate, and accumulate in lens opacities. Dysfunction of the lens as a result of opacification is called cataract. The term "age-related cataract" is used to distinguish lens opacification associated with old age from opacification associated with other causes, such as congenital and metabolic disorders *(8)*.

2. PUBLIC HEALTH ISSUES REGARDING CATARACT

Cataract is one of the major causes of blindness throughout the world *(9–11)*. In the United States, the prevalence of visually significant cataract increases from approx 5% at age 65 to about 40% for persons older than 75 yr *(12–14)*. In less developed coun-

From: *Preventive Nutrition: The Comprehensive Guide for Health Professionals*
Edited by A. Bendich and R. J. Deckelbaum Humana Press Inc., Totowa, NJ

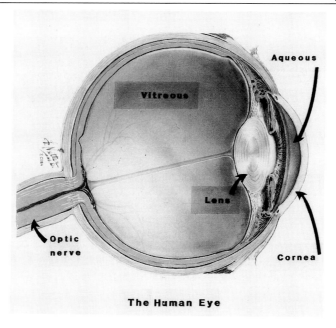

Fig. 1. Cross-section of the eye.

tries, such as India *(15)*, China *(16)*, and Kenya *(17)*, cataracts are more common and develop earlier in life than in more developed countries. For example, by age 60 cataract with low vision or aphakia (i.e., absence of the lens, which is usually the result of cataract extraction) is approximately five times more common in India than in the United States *(14,15)*. The impact of cataract on impaired vision is much greater in less developed countries, where >90% of the cases of blindness and visual impairment are found *(11,18–21)* and where there is a dearth of ophthalmologists to perform lens extractions *(22,23)*. Such surgery is routinely successful in restoring sight.

Given both the extent of disability caused by age-related cataract and its costs, $5 billion/yr* in the United States, it is urgent that we elucidate causes of cataract and identify strategies to slow the development of this disorder. It is estimated that a delay in cataract formation of about 10 yr would reduce the prevalence of visually disabling cataract by about 45% *(9)*. Such a delay would enhance the quality of life for much of the world's older population and substantially reduce both the economic burden because of disability and surgery related to cataract.

3. CLINICAL FEATURES OF CATARACT

There are several systems for evaluating and grading cataracts. Most of these employ an assessment of extent or density and location of the opacity *(24)*. Coloration or brunescence is also quantified, since these diminish visual function *(25,26)*. Usually evaluated are opacities in the posterior subcapsular (PSC), nuclear (Nuc), cortical (Cort), and multiple (mixed) locations (Fig. 2 and Table 1).

---

*Congressional Testimony of S.J. Ryan, May 5, 1993.

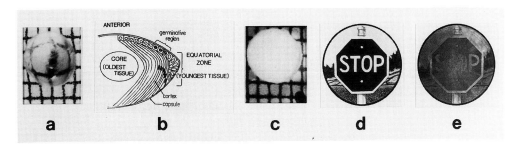

Fig. 2. Clear and cataractous lens. (**A**) Clear lens allows an unobstructed view of the wire grid placed behind it. (**B**) Cartoon of the structure of the lens. The anterior surface of the lens has a unicellular layer of epithelial cells (youngest tissue). Cells at the anterior equatorial region divide and migrate to the cortex as they are overlaid by less mature cells. These cells produce a majority of the crystallins. As development and maturation proceed, the cells denucleate and elongate. Tissue originally found in the embryonic lens is found in the core (oldest tissue). (**C**) The cataractous lens prohibits viewing the wire grid behind it. (**D**) Artist's view through a clear uncolored young lens. The image is clear and crisp. (**E**) Artist's view through a lens with developing cataract. The image is partially obscured, and the field is darkened as a result of browning of the lens that accompanies aging.

Table 1
Cataract Risk Ratio[a]: High vs Low Intake and Plasma Levels for Vitamin C

| Reference[b] and number of subjects | Nutrient source | Cataract type | | | | | |
		Mixed	Cortical	Posterior Subcapsular	Nuclear	Any	Advanced
Robertson (41) n = 304	Supplement	—	—	—	—	—	0.30*
Jacques and Chylack (27) n = 112	Intake	—	0.27	0.09*	—	0.25	—
	Plasma		0.27	0.09**		0.29	
Leske et al. (42) n = 1380	Intake	0.72	0.80	0.73	0.48*	—	—
Jacques et al. n = 294	Supplement	—	0.63	—	.18*,c	0.22*,c	0.17*,c
Mares-Perlman et al. (42) n = 1980	Supplement	—	1.8*	—	0.7*	—	—
Mohan et al. (44) n = 1990	Plasma	1.87*	—	—	—	—	—
Vitale et al. (46) n = 671	Plasma	—	1.01	—	1.31	—	—

*$p \leq 0.05$.
**$p \leq 0.1$.
[a]Risk ratio represents the prevalence odds ratio for all studies.
[b]Studies reporting estimates of odds ratio or relative risk.
[c]For persons who consumed ascorbate supplements > 10 yr., this is the only study in which long-term nutrient intake was assessed, Jacques et al., manuscript submitted; any ≥ grade 1, advanced ≥ grade 2.

4. OXIDATION AND CATARACT FORMATION

The solid mass of the lens is about 98% protein. Because these proteins undergo minimal turnover as the lens ages, they are subject to the chronic stresses of exposure to light and oxygen. Consequently, it is not surprising that these proteins are extensively damaged in the aged lens. Lens opacities develop as the damaged proteins aggregate and precipitate (1). Fiber cell membrane lipid damage is also associated with lens opacities (3,27,28). Smoking and ultraviolet light, which appear to induce oxidative stress (29,30), are also associated with elevated cataract risk (31–38), as well as with depletion of plasma ascorbate and carotenoid levels (29,39,43).

In young lenses, damaged proteins are usually maintained at harmless levels by defense systems. Primary defenses that directly protect the lens against the initial oxidative insult include small molecule antioxidants (e.g., vitamins C and E and carotenoids) and antioxidant enzyme systems (e.g., superoxide dismutase, catalase, and the glutathione redox cycle) (47–51). The lens also has secondary defense systems, which include proteolytic enzymes that selectively identify and remove damaged or obsolete proteins (1,52–58). Accumulation of (photo-)oxidized (and/or otherwise modified) proteins in older lenses indicates that protective systems are not keeping pace with the insults that damage lens proteins. This occurs in part because like bulk proteins, enzymes that comprise some of the protective systems are damaged by photo-oxidation (1,6,58). Interactions between the primary and secondary antioxidant defense systems and putative ramifications of these relationships on cataract risk are summarized in Fig. 3.

5. ASSOCIATIONS BETWEEN ANTIOXIDANTS AND CATARACT

Many cell-free, in vitro, and animal studies addressed putative roles for antioxidants in maintenance of lens and retina function. These were reviewed recently and inspired the epidemiological work described below (1,3). In order to fully appreciate the data presented, readers should be aware that the various studies used different lens classification schemes, different definitions of high and low levels of nutrients, and different age groups of subjects.

More than ten epidemiological studies examined the associations between cataract and antioxidant nutrients (23,27,41–46,59–61). Seven of the studies were retrospective case-control studies comparing the nutrient levels of cataract patients with that of similarly aged individuals with clear lenses (27,41–44,46,61). Our ability to interpret data from retrospective studies such as these is limited by the concurrent assessment of lens status and nutrient levels. Prior diagnosis of cataract might influence behavior of cases including diet and it might also bias reporting of usual diet. Three other studies assessed nutrient levels and/or supplement use and then followed individuals with intact lenses for 8 (45,60), and 5 yr (23), respectively. Prospective studies such as these are less prone to bias because assessment of exposure is performed before the outcome is present. These latter studies did not directly assess lens status, but used cataract extraction or reported diagnosis of cataract as a measure of cataract risk. Extraction may not be a good measure of cataract incidence (development of new cataract), because it incorporates components of both incidence and progression in severity of existing cataract. However, extraction is the result of visually disabling cataract and is the endpoint that we wish to prevent. Although Hankinson et al. (45) measured nutrient intake over a 4-yr pe-

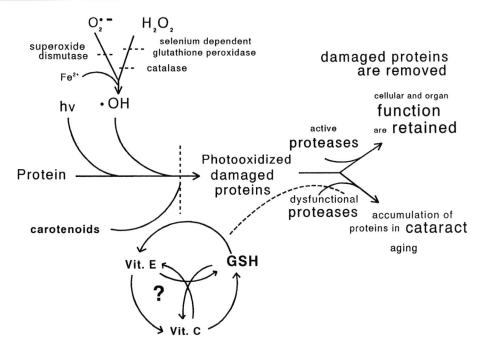

Fig. 3. Schematic showing proposed interactions among lens constituents, oxidants, light, antioxidants, antioxidant enzymes, and proteases. The constituent proteins in the lens are extremely long lived. In both lens and retina they are subject to damage by light and various forms of oxygen. Such damage is limited by antioxidant enzymes (superoxide dismutase, catalase, glutathione reductase/peroxidase) that convert active oxygen to less damaging species. Direct protection may also be offered by antioxidants (vitamin C, vitamin E, carotenoids, and glutathione [GSH]). Levels of reduced forms of some, but not all, of these molecules may be determined by interactions between them and with the environment *(82–84)*. On aging, antioxidant levels in some eye tissues (lens) are diminished and the antioxidant enzymes may be at reduced catalytic competence, resulting in increased levels of damage. Proteins that are obsolete or damaged are reduced to their constituent amino acids if proteolytic activity is sufficient. If proteolytic activity is insufficient, damaged proteins may accumulate, aggregate, and precipitate in cataracts in the lens. Older tissues frequently show lower levels of proteolytic activities. H_2O_2, hydrogen peroxide; O2., superoxide radical; HO., hydroxyl radical; the dashed lines indicate sites where antioxidants might protect against damage to proteins and proteases.

riod, Knekt et al. *(60)* used only one measure of serum antioxidant status, and Seddon et al. *(23)* used only one measure of supplement use. One measure may not provide an accurate assessment of usual, long-term nutrient levels. Multiple measures may be the best nutritional correlate of cataract *(62)*. Another study *(n=367)*, which monitored cataract in vivo and cataract extraction but did not find associations between nutriture and cataract, is not further described because the cataract classifications do not match those shown in Table 1 *(38)*.

5.1. Vitamin C

Vitamin C is probably the most effective, least toxic water-soluble antioxidant identified in mammalian systems *(63,64)*. Lens concentrations of vitamin C (~mM) are many fold higher than in plasma or other tissues *(65)*. However, vitamin C concentrations are compromised on aging and/or cataractogenesis *(22,52)*. Interest in the utility of vitamin C has been fueled by observations that eye tissue levels of this vitamin are related to dietary intake in humans *(65)* and animals *(22,52)* and the concentration of vitamin C in the lens was increased with dietary supplements beyond levels achieved in persons who already consumed more than two times the RDA (60 mg/d) for vitamin C *(65)*. Although biochemically plausible, there are no data to demonstrate that vitamin C induces damage in the lens in vitro *(6,66,67)*.

Vitamin C was considered in eight published studies *(27,41–46,61)* and one preliminary report *(59)* and observed to be inversely associated with at least one type of cataract in seven of these studies (Table 1). Jacques and Chylack *(27)* observed that persons with high plasma vitamin C levels >90 μ*M* had less than one-third the prevalence of early cataract as persons with low plasma vitamin C <40 μ*M*, although this difference was not statistically significant (risk ratio [RR]:0.29; confidence interval 95% [CI]:0.06–1.32) after adjustment for age, sex, race, and history of diabetes. They observed similar relationships between intake of vitamin C and cataract prevalence. Among persons with higher vitamin C intakes (>490 mg/d), the prevalence of cataract was 25% of the prevalence among persons with lower intakes (<125 mg/d) (RR:0.25; CI:0.06–1.09) *(27)*.

This relationship is corroborated by data from other studies. Robertson and coworkers *(41)* compared cases (with cataracts that impaired vision) to age- and sex-matched controls who were either free of cataract or had minimal opacities that did not impair vision. Results indicated that the prevalence of cataract in persons who consumed daily vitamin C supplements of >300mg/d was approximately one-third the prevalence in persons who did not consume vitamin C supplements (RR:0.30; CI:0.24–0.77). Leske and coworkers *(42)* observed that persons with vitamin C intake in the highest 20% of their population group had a 52% lower prevalence for nuclear cataract (RR:0.48; CI:0.24–0.99) compared with persons who had intakes among the lowest 20% after controlling for age and sex. Weaker inverse associations were noted for other types of cataract. After controlling for nine potential confounders, including age, diabetes, smoking, and energy intake, Hankinson and coworkers *(45)* did not observe an association between total vitamin C intake and rate of cataract surgery (RR:0.98; CI:0.72–1.32) in a large prospective study when they compared women with high intakes (median = 705 mg/d) to women with low intakes (median = 70 mg/d) (Table 2). However, they did note that women who consumed vitamin C supplements for >10 yr had a 45% reduction in rate of cataract surgery (RR:0.55; CI:0.32–0.96). Age-adjusted analyses (Jacques et al., manuscript submitted, Table 1) based on 165 women with high vitamin C intake (mean = 294 mg/d) and 136 women with low vitamin C intake (mean = 77 mg/d) demonstrated that the women who took vitamin C supplements ≥10 yr had >70% lower prevalence of early opacities (RR:0.27; CI:0.11–0.67) and >80% lower risk of advanced opacities (RR:0.19; CI:0.05–0.80) at any site compared with women who did not use vitamin C supplements.

In comparison to the data noted above, Mares-Perlman and coworkers *(43)* report that past use of supplements containing vitamin C was associated with a reduced prevalence of nuclear cataract (RR:0.7; CI:0.5–1.0), but an increased prevalence of cortical cataract (adjusted RR:1.8; CI:1.2–2.9) after controlling for age, sex, smoking, and history of heavy alcohol consumption (Table 1). Mohan et al. *(44)* also noted an 87%

Table 2
Risk Ratio for Cataract Extraction in Persons with High vs Low Nutrient Status

| | Nutrient | | | | | | | |
| | Vitamin C | | Vitamin E | | Carotenoids | | Nutrient index | |
Study	Plasma	Intake	Plasma	Intake	Plasma	Intake	Plasma	Intake
Hankinson et al. (45) n = 50,828	—	98 55[a]	—	0.88	—	0.73* 0.61[b]	—	0.60* —
Knekt et al. (60) n = 1419	—	—	0.53	—	0.59[c]	—	0.38*	—
Seddon et al. (23) n = 17,744	—	—	—	—	—	—	—	0.79[d]

*$P \leq 0.05$.
[a]There was a 45% reduction in rate of cataract surgery for women who used vitamin C supplements for ≥ 10 yr.
[b]Assessed as total vitamin A.
[c]β-carotene.
[d]For multivitamin supplement users.

(RR:1.87; CI:1.29–2.69) increased prevalence of mixed cataract with posterior subcapsular and nuclear involvement for each standard deviation increase in plasma vitamin C levels. Vitale and coworkers (46) observed that persons with plasma levels >80 μM and <60 μM had similar prevalences of both nuclear (RR:1.31; CI:0.61–2.39) and cortical (RR:1.01; CI:0.45–2.26) cataract after controlling for age, sex, and diabetes. Similarly, no differences in cataract prevalence were observed between persons with high (>261 mg/d) and low (<115 mg/d) vitamin C intakes. One other study (61) failed to observe any association between prevalence of cataract and vitamin C intake.

5.2. Vitamin E

Vitamin E, a natural lipid-soluble antioxidant, can inhibit lipid peroxidation (68) and appears to stabilize lens cell membranes (69). Vitamin E may be affected by ascorbate (see legend to Fig. 3), and also enhances glutathione recycling, perhaps helping to maintain reduced glutathione levels in the lens and aqueous humor (70).

Three studies assessing plasma vitamin E levels also reported significant inverse associations with cataract (Table 3). Knekt and coworkers (60) followed a cohort of 1419 Finns for 15 yr and identified 47 patients admitted to ophthalmological wards for mature cataract. They selected two controls per patient matched for age, sex, and municipality. These investigators reported that persons with serum vitamin E concentrations above approx 20 μM had about one-half the rate of subsequent cataract surgery (RR:0.53; CI:0.24–1.1) compared with persons with vitamin E concentrations below this concentration. Vitale and coworkers (46) observed the age-, sex-, and diabetes-adjusted prevalence of nuclear cataract to be about 50% less (RR:0.52; CI:0.27–0.99) among persons with plasma vitamin E concentrations >29.7 μM compared to persons with levels <18.6 μM. A similar comparison showed that the prevalence of cortical cataract did not differ between those with high and low plasma vitamin E levels

Table 3
Cataract Risk Ratio[a]: High vs Low Intake and Plasma Levels for Vitamin E

Reference[b] and number of subjects	Nutrient source	Cataract type					
		Mixed	Cortical	Posterior subcapsular	Nuclear	Any	Advanced
Robertson et al. (41) n = 304	Supplement	—	—	—	—	—	0.44*
Jacques and Chylack (27) n = 112	Intake	—	0.37	0.40	—	0.45	—
	Plasma		0.84	0.33		0.83	
	Supplement					0.33[d]	
Leske et al. (42) n = 1380	Intake	0.58*	0.59*	1.18	0.66	—	—
Vitale et al. (46) n = 671	Plasma	—	0.96	—	0.52*	—	—
Mares-Perlman et al. (43) n = 1980	Supplement	—	1.2	—	0.9	—	—
Mares-Perlman (40) n = 400	Serum α-Tocopherol						
	Men	—	3.94	—	3.74	3.95	—
	Women	—	2.11	—	1.47	3.19	—
	Serum γ-Tocopherol						
	Men	—	1.30	—	0.53	1.05	—
	Women	—	2.06	—	0.59	1.25	—
	Intake						
	Men	—	—	—	0.85	—	—
	Women	—	—	—	1.89	—	—

*$p = \leq 0.05$.
[a]Risk ratio represents the prevalence odds ratio for all studies.
[b]Studies reporting estimates of odds ratio or relative risk.
[c]Jacques et al., unpublished.

(RR:0.96; CI:0.52–1.78). Jacques and Chylack (27) also observed the prevalence of posterior subcapsular cataract to be 67% (RR:0.33; CI:0.03–4.13) lower among persons with plasma vitamin E levels above 35 μM relative to persons with levels below 21 μM after adjustment for age, sex, race, and diabetes; however, the effect was not statistically significant. Prevalence of any early cataract (RR:0.83; CI:0.20–3.40) or cortical cataract (RR:0.84; CI:0.20–3.60) did not differ between those with high and low plasma levels. Plasma vitamin E was also inversely associated with prevalence of cataract in a large Italian study after adjusting for age and sex, but the relationship was no longer statistically significant after adjusting for other factors, such as education, sunlight exposure, and family history of cataract (61). One other study failed to observe any association between cataract and plasma vitamin E levels (44). Mares-Perlman et al. (40) completed a recent study in which they observed an inverse (nonsignificant) relationship (RR:0.61; CI:0.32–1.19) between serum γ-tocopherol (which has lower biological vitamin E activity compared to α-tocopherol) and severity of nuclear sclerosis but a positive, significant relationship between elevated serum α-tocopherol levels and severity of nuclear cataract (RR:2.13; CI:1.05–4.34).

Vitamin E intake was inversely correlated with cataract risk in two studies (Table 3). Robertson and coworkers *(41)* found among age- and sex-matched cases and controls that the prevalence of cataract was 56% lower (RR:0.44; CI:0.24–0.77) in persons who consumed vitamin E supplements (>400 IU/d) than in persons not consuming supplements. Jacques and Chylack (unpublished) also observed a 67% (RR:0.33; CI:0.12–0.96) reduction in prevalence of cataract for vitamin E supplement users after adjusting for age, sex, race, and diabetes. In contrast, these investigators observed a nonsignificant inverse association when they related total vitamin E intake (combined dietary and supplemental intake) to cataract prevalence *(27)*. Persons with vitamin E intake >35.7 mg/d had a 55% lower prevalence of early cataract (RR:0.45; CI:0.12–1.79) than did persons with intakes <84 mg/d. Leske and colleagues *(42)* also observed that vitamin E intake was inversely associated with prevalence of cataract after controlling for age and sex. Persons with vitamin E intakes among the highest 20% had an approx 40% lower prevalence of cortical (RR:0.59; CI:0.36–0.97) and mixed (RR:0.58; CI:0.37–0.93) cataract relative to persons with intakes among the lowest 20%.

In contrast with the studies noted above, Mares-Perlman and coworkers *(43)* observed only weak, nonsignificant associations between vitamin E supplement use and nuclear (RR:0.9; CI:0.6–1.5) and cortical (RR:1.2; CI:0.6–2.3) cataract. Hankinson et al. (45) found no association between vitamin E intake and cataract surgery. Women with high vitamin E intakes (median= 210 mg/d) had a similar rate of cataract surgery (RR:0.96; CI:0.72–1.29) as women with low intakes (median = 3.3 mg/d). In partial contrast with their positive correlations between serum α-tocopherol levels and cataract, Mares-Perlman et al. *(40)* found that dietary vitamin E was associated with diminished risk for nuclear cataract in men, but not in women *(40)*.

5.3. *Carotenoids*

The carotenoids, like vitamin E, are natural lipid-soluble antioxidants *(68)*. β-carotene is the best known carotenoid because of its importance as a vitamin A precursor. It exhibits particularly strong antioxidant activity at low partial pressures of oxygen (15 torr) *(73)*. Partial pressure of oxygen in the core of the lens is approx 20 torr *(74)*. However, it is only one of ≈400 naturally occurring carotenoids *(75)* and other carotenoids may have similar or greater antioxidant potential *(76,77)*. In addition to β-carotene, α-carotene, lutein, and lycopene are important carotenoid components of the human diet *(78)*. Carotenoids have been identified in the lens in ≈10 ng/g wet weight concentrations *(79,80)*, but there are no laboratory data relating carotenoids to cataract formation.

Jacques and Chylack *(27)* observed that persons with high-plasma total carotenoid concentrations (>3.3 μM) had less than one-fifth the prevalence of cataract compared to persons with low plasma carotenoid levels (<1.7 μM) (RR:0.18; CI:0.03–1.03) after adjustment for age, sex, race, and diabetes (Table 4). However, they were unable to observe an association between carotene intake and cataract prevalence *(27)*. Persons with carotene intakes above 18,700 IU/d had the same prevalence of cataract as those with intakes below 5677 IU/d (RR:0.91; CI:0.23–3.78). Knekt and coworkers *(60)* reported

Table 4

Cataract Risk Ratio[a]: High vs Low Intake and Plasma Levels of Carotenoids

Study[b]	Nutrient source	Mixed	Cortical	Posterior subcapsular	Nuclear	Any	Advanced
Jacques and Chylack (27) n = 112	Intake	—	1.00	0.71	—	0.91	
	Plasma[c]	—	0.14*	0.18	—	0.18	—
Vitale et al. (46) n = 671	Plasma[d]	—	0.72	—	1.57	—	
Mares-Perlman[e,f] n = 400 (40)	Total carotenoids Serum						
	Women	—	3.26*	—	3.95*	4.41*	—
	Men	—	0.62	—	0.55	0.35	—
	Intake						
	Women	—	—	—	1.72	—	—
	Men	—	0.62	—	0.41	—	—
	α-Carotene Serum						
	Women	—	0.87	—	2.62	1.61	—
	Men	—	0.82	—	0.60	0.45	—
	Intake						
	Women	—	—	—	2.09	—	—
	Men	—	—	—	0.3*	—	—
	β-Carotene Serum						
	Women	—	2.00	—	2.80	3.53	—
	Men	—	0.28*	—	0.86	0.33*	—
	Intake						
	Women	—	—	—	1.31	—	—
	Men	—	—	—	0.44	—	—
	Lycopene Serum						
	Women	—	3.21	—	2.26*	2.63	—
	Men	—	0.37	—	1.69	0.48	—
	Intake						
	Women	—	—	—	1.21	—	—
	Men	—	—	—	0.62	—	—
	β-Cryptoxanthan Serum						
	Women	—	1.45	—	1.56	1.41	—
	Men	—	0.54	—	0.56	0.38	—
	Intake						
	Women	—	—	—	4.10*	—	—
	Men	—	—	—	1.07	—	—
	Lutein Serum						
	Women	—	1.75	—	4.09	3.30	—
	Men	—	4.84	—	0.71	1.50	0.006
	Intake						
	Women	—	—	—	1.43	—	—
	Men	—	—	—	0.77	—	—

*p= ≤0.05.

[a]Risk ratio represents the prevalence odds ratio for all studies.

[b]Studies reporting estimates of odds ratio or relative risk.

[c]Total carotenoids.

[d]β-Carotene.

[e]Risk ratio is given for the entire cohort, and when significant, for the appropriate gender group.

[f]Subjects did not fast prior to the blood draw.

that among age- and sex-matched cases and controls, persons with serum β-carotene concentrations above approx 0.1 μ*M* had a 40% reduction in the rate of cataract surgery compared with persons with concentrations below this level (RR:0.59; CI:0.26–1.25). Hankinson and coworkers *(45)* reported that the multivariate-adjusted rate of cataract surgery was about 30% lower (RR:0.73; CI:0.55–0.97) for women with high carotene intakes (median = 14,558 IU/d) compared with women with low intakes of this nutrient (median = 2935 IU/d). However, although cataract surgery was inversely associated with total carotene intake, it was not strongly associated with consumption of carotene-rich foods, such as carrots. Rather, cataract surgery was associated with lower intakes of such foods as spinach that are rich in lutein and zeaxanthin carotenoids, rather than β-carotene. The most recent study that correlated serum carotenoids and severity of nuclear and cortical opacities *(40)* indicates that higher levels of individual or total carotenoids in the serum were not associated with less severe nuclear or cortical cataract overall. However, associations differed between men and women. A significant trend for lower-risk ratio for either opacity with measuring serum levels of β-carotene was observed in men. A marginally significant trend for lower risk of cortical opacities with higher levels of β-carotene was also noted for men. Higher serum levels of α-carotene, β-cryptoxanthan, and lutein were significantly related to lower risk for nuclear sclerosis only in men who smoked. In contrast, higher levels of some carotenoids were often directly associated with elevated nuclear sclerosis and cortical cataract, particularly in women. Vitale and colleagues *(46)* also examined the relationships between plasma β-carotene levels and age-, sex-, and diabetes-adjusted prevalence of cortical and nuclear cataract. Although the data suggested a weak inverse association between plasma β-carotene and cortical cataract and a weak positive association between this nutrient and nuclear cataract, neither association was statistically significant. Persons with plasma β-carotene concentrations above 0.88 μ*M* had a 28% lower prevalence of cortical cataract (RR:0.72; CI:0.37–1.42) and a 57% (RR:1.57; CI:0.84–2.93) higher prevalence of nuclear cataract compared to persons with levels below 0.33 μ*M*.

5.4. Smoking, Antioxidants, and Cataracts

Smoking is associated with diminished carotenoid *(39)* and ascorbate status *(29)*. Smoking is also associated with enhanced risk for cataract *(35,36)*. Of interest are recent observations that for male smokers there appears to be an inverse relationship between serum levels of α-carotene, β-cryptoxanthan, lutein, and severity of nuclear sclerosis *(40)* (the reverse may be true for women) and diminished risk for cataract in smokers who use multivitamins *(23)*.

5.5. Antioxidant Nutrient Combinations

Combinations of multiple antioxidant nutrients were also considered (Table 5) because of possible synergistic effects of the antioxidant nutrients on cataract risk (Fig. 3). The first, and perhaps most important, study in terms of revealing the utility of diet indicates a significant fivefold decrease in risk ratio for cataract between persons consuming ≥1.5 servings of fruits and/or vegetables *(27)*. Jacques and Chylack *(27)* also found that the adjusted prevalence of all types of cataract was 40% (RR:0.62; CI:0.12–1.77) and 80% (RR:0.16; CI:0.04–0.82) lower for persons with moderate and high-antioxidant index scores (based on combined plasma vitamin C, vitamin E, and carotenoid levels), as compared with persons with low scores. Using a similar index based on combined antioxidant nutrient intakes (vitamin C, vitamin E, and carotene, as well as riboflavin), Leske and coworkers *(42)* found that persons with high scores had 60% lower adjusted prevalence of cortical (RR:0.42; CI:0.18–0.97) and mixed (RR:0.39; CI:0.19–0.80) cataract compared to those who had low scores. However, Robertson and coworkers *(41)* found no enhanced benefit to persons taking both vitamin E and vitamin C supplements compared with persons who only took either vitamin C or vitamin E. Mohan and coworkers *(44)* constructed a somewhat more complex antioxidant scale that included red blood cell levels of glutathione peroxidase, glucose-6-phosphate dehydrogenase, and plasma levels of vitamin C and vitamin E. Even though they failed to see any protective associations with any of these individual factors, and even reported a positive association between plasma vitamin C and prevalence of cataract, they found that persons with high-antioxidant index scores had a substantially lower prevalence of cataracts involving the posterior subcapsular region (RR:0.23, CI:0.06–0.88) or mixed cataract with posterior subcapsular and nuclear components (RR:0.12; CI:0.03–0.56) after multivariate adjustment. Hankinson and coworkers *(45)* calculated an antioxidant score based on intakes of carotene, vitamin C, vitamin E, and riboflavin and observed a 24% reduction in the adjusted rate of cataract surgery among women with high-antioxidant scores relative to women with low scores (RR:0.76; CI:0.57–1.03). Knekt and coworkers *(60)* observed that the rate of cataract surgery for persons with high levels of both serum vitamin E and β-carotene concentrations appeared lower than the rate for persons with either high vitamin E or high β-carotene levels. Persons with high serum levels of either nutrient had a rate of cataract surgery that was 40% less than persons with low levels of both nutrients (RR:0.38; CI:0.15–1.0). Vitale and coworkers *(46)* also examined the relationship between antioxidant scores (based on plasma concentrations of vitamin C, vitamin E, and β-carotene) and prevalence of cataract, but did not see evidence of any association. The age-, sex-, and diabetes-adjusted risk ratios were close to one for both nuclear (RR:0.96; CI:0.54–1.70) and cortical (RR:1.17; CI:0.62–2.20) cataract. Relationships between multiple antioxidant nutrients and cataract risk are further supported by multivitamin use data. Leske and coworkers *(42)* found that use of multivitamin supplements was associated with decreased prevalence for each type of cataract: 60%, 48%, 45%, and 30%, respectively, for posterior subcapsular (RR:0.40; CI:0.21–0.77), cortical (RR:0.52; CI:0.36–0.72), nuclear (RR:0.55; CI:0.33–0.92), and mixed (RR:0.70; CI:0.51–0.97) cataracts. Seddon and coworkers *(23)* also observed a reduced risk for incident cataract for users of multivitamins (RR:0.73; CI:0.54–0.99).

5.6. Intervention Trials

To date only one intervention trial designed to assess the effect of vitamin supplements on cataract risk has been completed. Sperduto and coworkers *(81)* took advantage of two ongoing, randomized, double-blinded vitamin and cancer trials to assess the impact of vitamin supplements on cataract prevalence. The trials were conducted among almost 4000 participants aged 45–74 yr from rural communes in Linxian, China. Participants in one trial received either a multinutrient supplement or placebo. In the second trial, a more complex factorial design was used to evaluate the effects of four different vitamin/mineral combinations: retinol (5000 IU) and zinc (22 mg); riboflavin (3 mg) and niacin (40 mg); vitamin C (120 mg) and molybdenum (30 μg); and vitamin E (30 mg), β-carotene (15 mg), and selenium (50 μg). At the end of the 5–6-yr

Table 5
Cataract Risk Ratio[a]: High vs Low Intake and Plasma Nutrient Index Using Multiple Antioxidant Nutrients

		Cataract type					
Ref.[b]	Nutrient source	Mixed	Cortical	Posterior subcapsular	Nuclear	Any	Advanced
Robertson et al. (41) n = 304	Supplement	—	—	—	—	0.32*	—
Jacques and Chylack (27) n = 112	Intake	—	0.37	0.33	—	0.45	—
	Plasma	—	0.16*	0.00*	—	0.17*	—
	Fruits and vegetables[d] Intake	—	0.20*	0.08*	—	0.18*	—
Leske et al. (42) n = 1380	Supplement[c]	0.39*	0.42*	0.89	0.52	—	—
		0.70*	0.52*	0.40*	0.55*	—	—
Mohan et al. (44) n = 1990	Plasma	0.12*	—	0.23*	—	—	—
Mares-Perlman et al. (40) n = 1980	Supplement[d]	—	1.6*	0.8	0.6*	—	—
Vitale et al. (46) n = 671	Plasma	—	1.17	—	0.96	—	—
Seddon et al. (23) n = 17,744	Supplement[c]	—	—	—	—	0.73*	—

*$p = \leq 0.05$.
[a]Risk ratio represents the prevalence odds ratio for all studies.
[b]Studies reporting estimates of odds ratio or relative risk.
[c]For multivitamin supplement users.
[d]For persons who consume at least 3.5 servings of fruits and vegetables per day.

follow-up, the investigators conducted eye examinations to determine the prevalence of cataract.

In the first trial there was a significant 43% reduction in the prevalence of nuclear cataract for persons aged 65–74 yr for persons receiving the multinutrient supplement (RR:0.57; CI:0.36–0.90, Table 6). The second trial demonstrated a significantly reduced prevalence of nuclear cataract in persons receiving the riboflavin/niacin supplement relative to those persons not receiving this supplement (RR:0.59; CI:0.45–0.79). The effect was strongest in those aged 65–74 yr (RR:0.45; CI:0.31–0.64). However, the riboflavin/niacin supplement appeared to increase the risk of posterior subcapsular cataract (RR:2.64; CI:1.31–5.35). The results further suggested a protective effect of the retinol/zinc supplement (RR:0.77; CI:0.58–1.02) and the vitamin C/molybdenum supplement (RR:0.78; CI:0.59–1.04) on prevalence of nuclear cataract.

Table 6
Cataract Risk Ratio—Intervention Trials

Study	Nutrient source	Mixed	Cortical	Posterior subcapsular	Nuclear	Any	Advanced
Sperduto (81) n = 4000	Multivitamin	—	1.05	1.41	0.80	—	—
			—	—	0.57[a],*	—	—
	Riboflavin	—	1.08	2.64*	0.59*		
	Niacin	—	—	—	0.45[a],*	—	—
	Retinol, Zn^{2+}	—	1.08	0.59	0.77	—	—
	Vit. C, Mo	—	0.92	1.25	0.78	—	—
	Se, Vit. E, β-carotene	—	0.96	1.56	1.19	—	—

*$p \leq 0.05$.
[a]subjects 65–74 yr of age.

6. CONCLUSIONS AND RECOMMENDATIONS

Age-related eye diseases can be devastating in terms of quality of life of our most frail and with respect to national public health and economics. Although it is too early to declare that increased consumption or intake of specific levels of nutrients is associated with diminished risk of cataract at any one location in the eye, the impression one gets from examining the work done to date is that nutrient intake can be optimized to delay cataract. Optimization of nutriture can be achieved through better diets and, perhaps, with the aid of supplements once appropriate levels of specifically beneficial nutrients are defined. Appropriate contemporary questions with respect to decreased risk for cataract might be: how much of a nutrient is the optimal intake and for how long or when would intake of the nutrient be useful? The answer to these questions is almost at hand. Two studies indicated that persons who consumed supplements of ascorbate for over 10 yr have decreased risk for cataract or cataract extraction. However, these results should be corroborated by other research, including quantitative information regarding the quantity and the term of intake of other nutrients as well. The epidemiological data also indicate that it is imperative to execute longitudinal studies and possibly intervention trials. Monitoring correlations between nutrient status and intermediate markers of cataract (when they are defined) may allow anticipation of relationships between nutrient status and cataract.

7. ACKNOWLEDGMENTS

We acknowledge the assistance of Thomas Nowell in the preparation of figures.

REFERENCES

1. Taylor A, Jacques PF, Dorey CK. Oxidation and aging: impact on vision. J Toxicol Indust Health 1993; 9:349–371.
2. Bunce GE, Kinoshita J, Horwitz J. Nutritional factors in cataract. Ann Rev Nutr 1990; 10:233–254.
3. Jacques PF, Chylack LT Jr, Taylor A. Relationships between natural antioxidants and cataract formation. In: Natural Antioxidants in Human Health and Disease. Frei B, ed. Orlando: Academic Press, 1994; 513–533.

4. Taylor A. Vitamin C. In: Nutrition in the Elderly: The Boston Nutritional Status Survey. Hartz SC, Russell M, Rosenberg, IH, eds. London: Smith Gordon Limited, 1992; 147–50.

5. Taylor A. Cataract: relationships between nutrition and oxidation. J Am Coll Nutr 1993; 12:138–146.

6. Blondin J, Taylor A. Measures of leucine aminopeptidase can be used to anticipate UV-induced age-related damage to lens proteins: ascorbate can delay this damage. Mech Aging Dev 1987; 41:39–46.

7. Blondin J, Baragi VJ, Schwartz E, Sadowski J, Taylor A. Delay of UV-induced eye lens protein damage in guinea pigs by dietary ascorbate. Free Radic Biol Med 1986; 2:275–281.

8. Jacques PF, Taylor A. Micronutrients and age-related cataracts. In: Micronutrients in Health and in Disease Prevention. Bendich A, Butterworth CE, eds. New York: Marcel Dekker Inc, 1991; 359–379.

9. Kupfer C. The conquest of cataract: a global challenge. Trans Ophthalmol Soc UK 1984; 104:1–10.

10. Schwab L. Cataract blindness in developing nations. Internat Ophthalmol Clinics 1990; 30:16–18.

11. World Health Organization. Use of intraocular lenses in cataract surgery in developing countries. Bull WHO 1991; 69:657–666.

12. Klein BEK, Klein R, Linton KLP. Prevalence of age-related lens opacities in a population: the Beaver Dam Eye Study. Ophthalmology 1992; 99:546–552.

13. Klein R, Klein BE, Linton KL, DeMets DL. The Beaver Dam Eye Study: the relation of age-related maculopathy to smoking. Am J Epidemiol 1993; 137:190–200.

14. Leibowitz H, Krueger D, Maunder C, et al. The Framingham Eye Study Monograph. Surv Ophthalmol (Suppl), 1980; 24:335–610.

15. Chatterjee A, Milton RC, Thyle S. Prevalence and etiology of cataract in Punjab. Br J Ophthalmol 1982; 66:35–42.

16. Wang G-M, Spector A, Luo C-Q, et al. Prevalence of age-related cataract in Ganzi and Shanghai. The Epidemiological Study Group. Chin Med J 1990; 103:945–951.

17. Whitfield R, Schwab L, Ross-Degnan D, Steinkuller P, Swartwood J. Blindness and eye disease in Kenya: ocular status survey results from the Kenya Rural Blindness Prevention Project. Br J Ophthalmol 1990; 74:333–340.

18. Chan CW, Billson FA. Visual disability and major causes of blindness in NSW: a study of people aged 50 and over attending the Royal Blind Society 1984 to 1989. Aust NZ J Ophthalmol 1991; 19:321–325.

19. Dana MR, Tielsch JM, Enger C, Joyce E, Santoli JM, Taylor HR. Visual impairment in a rural Appalachian community: prevalence and causes. JAMA 1990; 264:2400–2405.

20. Salive ME, Guralnik J, Christian W, Glynn RJ, Colsher P, Ostfeld AM. Functional blindness and visual impairment in older adults from three communities. Ophthalmology 1992; 99:1840–1847.

21. Wormald RPL, Wright LA, Courtney P, Beaumont B, Haines AP. Visual problems in the elderly population and implications for services. Br Med J 1992; 304:1226–1229.

22. Berger J, Shepard D, Morrow F, Taylor A. Relationship between dietary intake and tissue levels of reduced and total vitamin C in the guinea pig. J Nutr 1989; 119:1–7.

23. Seddon JM, Christen WG, Manson JE, et al. The use of vitamin supplements and the risk of cataract among US male physicians. Am J Public Health 1994; 84:788–92.

24. Chylack LT Jr, Wolfe JK, Singer DM, et al. The lens opacities classification system III. Arch Ophthalmol 1993; 111:831–836.

25. Chylack LT Jr, Wolfe JK, Friend J, Singer DM, Wu SY, Leske MC. Nuclear cataract: relative contributions to vision loss of opalescence and brunescence. Invest Ophthalmol Vis Sci 1994; 35:4,2632 (Abstract).

26. Wolfe JK, Chylack LT Jr, Leske MC, Wu SY, LSC Group. Lens nuclear color and visual function. Invest Ophthalmol Vis Sci 1993; 34:4,2550 (Abstract).

27. Jacques PF, Chylack LT Jr. Epidemiologic evidence of a role for the antioxidant vitamins and carotenoids in cataract prevention. Am J Clin Nutr 1991; 53:352S–355S.

28. Berman ER. Biochemistry of the eye. New York: Plenum, 1991; 210–308.

29. Schectman G, Byrd JC, Gruchow HW. The influence of smoking on vitamin C status in adults. Am J Health 1989; 79:158–162.

30. Zigman S. Effects of near ultraviolet radiation on the lens and retina. Doc Ophthalmol 1983; 55:375–391.

31. Brilliant LB, Grasset NC, Pokhrel RP, et al. Associations among cataract prevalence, sunlight hours, and altitude in the Himalayas. Am J Epidemiol 1983; 118:250–264.

32. Christen WG, Manson JE, Seddon JM, et al. A prospective study of cigarette smoking and risk of cataract in men. JAMA 1992; 268:989–993.

33. Hankinson SE, Willett WC, Colditz GA, et al. A prospective study of cigarette smoking and risk of cataract surgery in women. JAMA 1992; 268:994–998.

34. Taylor HR, West SK, Rosenthal FS, et al. Effect of ultraviolet radiation on cataract formation. New Engl J Med 1988; 319:1429–1433.

35. West SK, Munoz B, Emmett EA, Taylor HR. Cigarette smoking and risk of nuclear cataracts. Arch Ophthalmol 1989; 107:1166–1169.

36. West S. Does smoke get in your eyes? JAMA 1992; 268:1025–1026.

37. Zigman S, Datiles M, Torczynski E. Sunlight and human cataract. Invest Ophthalmol Vis Sci 1979; 18:462–467.

38. Wong L, Ho SC, Coggon D, Cruddas AM, et al. J Epidemiol Commun Health 1993; 47:46–49.

39. Russell-Briefel R, Bates MW, Kuller LH. The relationship of plasma carotenoids to health and biochemical factors in middle-aged men. Am J Epidemiol 1985; 122:741–749.

40. Mares-Perlman JA, Brady WE, Klein BEK, Klein R, Palta M, Bowen P, Stacewicz-Sapuntzakis M. Invest Ophthalmol Vis Sci 1995; 36:276–288.

41. Robertson JMcD, Donner AP, Trevithick JR. Vitamin E intake and risk for cataracts in humans. Ann NY Acad Sci 1989; 570:372–382.

42. Leske MC, Chylack LT Jr, Wu S. The lens opacities case-control study risk factors for cataract. Arch Ophthalmol 1991; 109:244–251.

43. Mares-Perlman JA, Klein BEK, Klein R, Ritter LL. Relationship between lens opacities and vitamin and mineral supplement use. Ophthalmology 1994; 101:315–325.

44. Mohan M, Sperduto RD, Angra SK, et al. India-US case-control study of age-related cataracts. Arch Ophthalmol 1989; 107:670–676.

45. Hankinson SE, Stampfer MJ, Seddon JM, et al. Nutrient intake and cataract extraction in women: a prospective study. Br Med J 1992; 305:335–339.

46. Vitale S, West S, Hallfrisch J, et al. Plasma antioxidants and risk of cortical and nuclear cataract. Epidemiology 1994; 4:195–203.

47. Fridovich I. Oxygen: aspects of its toxicity and elements of defense. Curr Eye Res 1984; 3:1–2.

48. Giblin FJ, McReady JP, Reddy VN. The role of glutathione metabolism in detoxification of H_2O_2 in rabbit lens. Invest Ophthalmol Vis Sci 1992; 22:330–335.

49. Rathbun WB, Holleschau AM, Murray DL, Buchanan A, Sawaguchi S, Tao RV. Glutathione synthesis and glutathione redox pathways in naphthalene cataract in the rat. Curr Eye Res 1990; 9:45–53.

50. Varma SD, Chand O, Sharma YR, Kuck JF, Richards KD. Oxidative stress on lens and cataract formation. Role of light and oxygen. Curr Eye Res 1984; 3:35–57.

51. Zigler JS, Goosey JD. Singlet oxygen as a possible factor in human senile nuclear cataract development. Curr Eye Res 1984; 3:59–65.

52. Berger J, Shepard D, Morrow F, Sadowski J, Haire T, Taylor A. Reduced and total ascorbate in guinea pig eye tissues in response to dietary intake. Curr Eye Res 1988; 7:681–686.

53. Shang F, Taylor A. Oxidative stress and recovery from oxidative stress are associated with altered ubiquitin conjugating and proteolytic activities in bovine lens epithelial cells. Biochem J 1995; 307:297–303.

54. Huang LL, Jahngen-Hodge J, Taylor A. Bovine lens epithelial cells have a ubiquitin-dependent proteolysis system. Biochem Biophys Acta 1993; 1175:181–187.

55. Jahngen-Hodge J, Laxman E, Zuliani A, Taylor A. Evidence for ATP ubiquitin-dependent degradation of proteins in cultured bovine lens epithelial cells. Exp Eye Res 1991; 52:341–347.

56. Jahngen-Hodge J, Cyr D, Laxman E, Taylor A. Ubiquitin and ubiquitin conjugates in human lens. Exp Eye Res 1992; 55:897–902.

57. Obin MS, Nowell T, Taylor A. The photoreceptor G-protein transducin (G_t) is a substrate for ubiquitin-dependent proteolysis. Biochem Biophys Res Comm 1994; 200:1169–1176.

58. Taylor A, Davies KJA. Protein oxidation and loss of protease activity may lead to cataract formation in the aged lens. Free Radic Biol Med 1987; 3:371–377.

59. Jacques PF, Lahav M, Willett WC, Taylor A. Relationship between long-term vitamin C intake and prevalence of cataract and macular degeneration. Exp Eye Res (Suppl. 1) 1992; 55:S152 (Abstract).

60. Knekt P, Heliovaara M, Rissanen A, Aromaa A, Aaran R. Serum antioxidant vitamins and risk of cataract. Br Med J 1992; 305:1392–1394.

61. The Italian-American Cataract Study Group. Risk factors for age-related cortical, nuclear, and posterior subcapsular cataracts. Am J Epidemiol 1991; 133:541–553.

62. Taylor A, Jacques P, Lahav M, Hankinson S, Lee Y, Willett W. Relationship between long-term dietary and supplement ascorbate intake and risk of cataract. Exp Eye Res Suppl 1 1994; 59:S133 (Abstract).

63. Frei B, Stocker R, Ames BN. Antioxidant defenses and lipid peroxidation in human blood plasma. Proc Natl Acad Sci USA 1988; 85:9748–9752.

64. Levine M. New concepts in the biology and biochemistry of ascorbic acid. New Engl J Med 1986; 314:892–902.

65. Taylor A, Jacques PF, Nadler D, Morrow F, Sulsky SI, Shepard D. Relationship in humans between ascorbic acid consumption and levels of total and reduced ascorbic acid in lens, aqueous humor, and plasma. Curr Eye Res 1991;10:751–759.

66. Garland DD. Ascorbic acid and the eye. Am J Clin Nutr 1991; 54:1198S–1202S.

67. Naraj RM, Monnier VM. Isolation and characterization of a blue fluorophore from human eye lens crystallins: in vitro formation from Maillard reaction with ascorbate and ribose. Biochem Biophys Acta 1992; 1116:34–42.

68. Machlin LJ, Bendich A. Free radical tissue damage: protective role of antioxidant nutrients. FASEB J 1987; 1:441–445.

69. Libondi T, Menzione M, Auricchio G. In vitro effect of alpha-tocopherol on lysophosphatidylcholine-induced lens damage. Exp Eye Res 1985; 40:661–666.

70. Costagliola C, Iuliano G, Menzione M, Rinaldi E, Vito P, Auricchio G. Effect of vitamin E on glutathione content in red blood cells, aqueous humor and lens of humans and other species. Exp Eye Res 1986; 43:905–914.

71. Organisciak DT, Berman ER, Wang H, Feeney-Burns L. Vitamin E in human neural retina and retinal pigment epithelium: effect of age. Curr Eye Res 1987; 6:1051–1055.

72. Organisciak DT, Feeney-Burns L, Bridges CD. On the measurement of vitamin E in human ocular tissues (letter). Curr Eye Res 1987; 6:1487–1488.

73. Burton W, Ingold KU. Beta-carotene: an unusual type of lipid antioxidant. Science 1984; 224:569–573.

74. Kwan M, Niinikoski J, Hunt TK. In vivo measurement of oxygen tension in the cornea, aqueous humor, and the anterior lens of the open eye. Invest Ophthalmol 1972; 11:108–114.

75. Erdman J. The physiologic chemistry of carotenes in man. Clin Nutr 1988; 7:101–106.

76. Di Mascio P, Murphy ME, Sies H. Antioxidant defense systems: the role of carotenoids, tocopherols and thiols. Am J Clin Nutr 1991; 53:194S–200S.

77. Krinsky NI, Deneke SS. Interaction of oxygen and oxy-radicals with carotenoids. J Natl Cancer Inst 1982; 69:205–210.

78. Micozzi MS, Beecher GR, Taylor PR, Khachik F. Carotenoid analyses of selected raw and cooked foods associated with a lower risk for cancer. J Natl Cancer Inst 1990; 82:282–285.

79. Daicker B, Schiedt K, Adnet JJ, Bermond P. Canthaxamin retinopathy. An investigation by light and electron microscopy and physiochemical analyses. Graefe's Arch Clin Exp Ophthalmol 1987; 225:189–197.

80. Yeum K-J, Taylor A, Tang G, Russell RM. Measurement of carotenoids, retinoids, and tocopherols in human lenses. Invest Ophthalmol Vis Sci 1995; 36:2756–2761.

81. Sperduto RD, Hu T-S, Milton, RC, et al. The Linxian Cataract Studies: Two nutrition intervention trials. Arch Ophthalmol 1993; 111:1246–1253.

82. Burton GW, Wronska U, Stone L, Foster DO, Ingold KU. Biokinetics of dietary RRR-α-tocopherol in the male guinea pig at three dietary levels of vitamin C and two levels of vitamin E. Evidence that vitamin C does not "spare" vitamin E in vivo. Lipids 1990; 25:199–210.

83. Meister A. Glutathione-ascorbic acid antioxidant system in animals. J Biol Chem 1994; 269:9397–9400.

84. Wefers H, Sies H. The protection by ascorbate and glutathione against microsomal lipid peroxidation is dependent on vitamin E. FEBS Lett. 1988; 174:353–357.

15   Osteoporosis

Vitamins, Minerals, and Other Micronutrients

Robert P. Heaney

1. INTRODUCTION

1.1. Nutrition in the Osteoporotic Fracture Context

Osteoporosis is a condition of skeletal fragility as a result of decreased bone mass and microarchitectural deterioration of bone tissue, with consequent increased risk of fracture. The condition is multifactorial in pathogenesis. Nutrition affects bone health in two distinct ways. First, bone tissue deposition, maintenance, and repair are the result of cellular processes that are as dependent on nutrition as are the corresponding processes of any other tissue. The production of bone matrix, for example, requires the synthesis and posttranslational modification of collagen and an array of other proteins. Nutrients involved in these cellular activities include vitamins C, D, and K and the minerals phosphorus, copper, manganese, and zinc. Additionally, the regulation of calcium homeostasis requires normal magnesium nutrition. Second, the skeleton serves as a very large nutrient reserve for two minerals, calcium and phosphorus, and the size of that reserve (in other words, the strength of the skeletal structures) will be dependent in part on the daily balance between absorbed intake and excretory loss of these two minerals.

Strength in bone, as in most engineering structures, is dependent not only on its mass density but also on the arrangement of its material in space and on the intrinsic strength of its component material (particularly, in bone, as that strength is influenced over long periods of use by the accumulation of unrepaired fatigue damage). All three factors play a role in most low trauma fractures and it is not possible to say which may be the most important in any given case.

Bone mass and density are themselves influenced by many factors. The three most commonly found to be limiting in industrialized nations are physical activity, gonadal hormones, and nutrition. In adults of these nations the nutrients most apt to be in short supply are calcium and vitamin D. Calcium intake, specifically, may be inadequate for the straightforward reason that it is low; however, even when statistically "normal," it may still be inadequate because of subnormal absorption *(1)* or greater than normal excretory loss *(2,3)*. Other nutrients are also essential for building a healthy skeleton, but, except for calcium, their effects are usually seen most clearly during growth.

Although much of the following discussion will focus on calcium, it is necessary to stress at the outset that calcium is a nutrient, not a drug, and hence its beneficial effects will be confined to individuals whose intake of calcium is insufficient. Also, calcium is

From: *Preventive Nutrition: The Comprehensive Guide for Health Professionals*
Edited by A. Bendich and R. J. Deckelbaum Humana Press Inc., Totowa, NJ

not an isolated nutrient; it occurs in foods along with other nutrients, and it has been shown that diets low in calcium tend also to be nutritionally poor in other respects *(4)*. Thus, although it is necessary to deal with nutrients one at a time in an analysis such as this, the disorders in our patients are likely to be more complex.

2. CALCIUM

2.1. The Requirement for Calcium

The primitive function of the skeleton is to serve as a source and as a sink for calcium and phosphorus; that is, as a reserve to offset shortages and as a place for safely storing surpluses. We see this reserve feature of skeletal function expressed, for example, in laboratory animals, such as cats, rats, and dogs, which, when placed on low-calcium intakes, will reduce bone mass as needed to maintain near constancy of calcium levels in the extracellular fluid *(5)*. This activity is mediated by parathyroid hormone (PTH) *(6)* and involves actual bone destruction, not leaching of calcium from bone.

Along the path of evolution, bone in the higher, terrestrial vertebrates acquired a second role, namely internal stiffening and rigidity—what is today the most apparent feature of the skeleton. Calcium and phosphorus are the only nutrients with a reserve that possesses such a secondary function. Reserves, of their nature, are designed to tide us over external shortages. When intake is inadequate, the reserve is first depleted. With most nutrients this has no detectable impact on the health or functioning of the organism. Only after the reserve is exhausted and the metabolic pool begins to be depleted does clinical disease express itself. For some nutrients (e.g., vitamin A, energy), the reserve can be quite large and the latent period may last many months. For others (e.g., the water-soluble vitamins), however, the reserve may be very small and detectable dysfunction develops quickly when intake drops.

With calcium, by contrast, the reserve is vast relative to the cellular and extracellular metabolic pools of calcium. As a result, dietary insufficiency virtually never impairs tissue functions that are dependent on calcium, at least in ways we now recognize. However, since bone strength is a function of bone mass, it follows inexorably that any decrease whatsoever in the size of the calcium reserve—any decrease in bone mass—will produce a corresponding decrease in bone strength. We literally walk about on our calcium reserve. It is this unique feature of calcium nutriture that is the basis for the linkage of calcium and bone status.

2.2. Ascertaining the Requirement for Calcium

Calcium functions as a threshold nutrient, much as does iron. This means that below some critical value the effect (bone mass for calcium or hemoglobin mass for iron) will be limited by available supplies, whereas above that value, i.e., the "threshold," no further benefit will accrue from additional increases in intake. This biphasic relationship is illustrated in Fig. 1, in which the intake-effect relationship is depicted first schematically (Fig. 1A), and then as exemplified by data derived from a growing animal model (Fig. 1B). The requirement can be defined as the intake at which the curve becomes flat. In Fig. 1B the effect of the nutrient is expressed directly as the amount of bone calcium an animal is able to accumulate from any given intake. However, if "effect" is broadened to mean "any change whatsoever," then the diagram fits mature adults as well, and the best representation of the requirement at all ages is the intake value just at or above the effect threshold of Fig. 1.

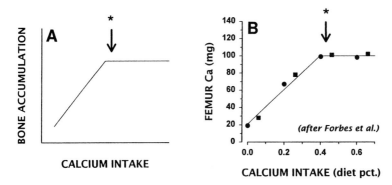

Fig. 1. Threshold behavior of calcium intake. (**A**) Theoretical relationship of bone accumulation to intake. Below a certain value—the threshold—bone accumulation is a linear function of intake (the ascending line); in other words, the amount of bone that can be accumulated is limited by the amount of calcium ingested. Above the threshold (the horizontal line), bone accumulation is limited by other factors and is no longer related to changes in calcium intake. (**B**) Actual data from two experiments in growing rats, showing how bone accumulation does, in fact, exhibit a threshold pattern. (Redrawn from data in Forbes RM et al., J Nutr 1979; 109:1652–1660. *(7)*) (Copyright Robert P. Heaney, 1992. reproduced with permission.)

There has been much uncertainty and confusion in recent years about what that intake may be for various ages and physiological states. With the 1994 Consensus Development Conference on Optimal Calcium Intake *(8)*, the bulk of that confusion has been resolved. The evidence for the intakes recommended by the consensus panel is summarized both in the Conference report and in recent reviews of the relationship of nutrition and osteoporosis *(9)*, and only the highlights will be mentioned in ensuing sections of this chapter.

It is worth noting, however, that the recommendations of the Consensus Conference, although expressed in quantitative terms, were basically qualitative: Contemporary calcium intakes in the United States, by both men and women, are too low for optimal bone health. The most persuasive of the evidence leading to this conclusion came in the form of several randomized controlled trials showing both reduction in age-related bone loss and reduction in fractures following augmentation of prevailing calcium intakes *(10–17)*. For technical reasons relating to bone remodeling biology *(8)*, randomized controlled trials are not well suited to dose ranging. Hence, although the panel was persuaded that prevailing intakes were too low, their recommended levels in several cases involved ranges and were clearly prudential judgments, centered of necessity on intakes employed in the trials concerned. The panel's recommendations and the corresponding 1989 RDAs *(19)* are set forth in Table 1.

2.3. Primary Prevention: The Acquisition of Genetically Programmed Bone Mass

The human skeleton contains at birth approx 25 g calcium and, at maturity in women, 1000–1200 g. All of this difference must come in by way of the diet. Further, unlike other structural nutrients, such as protein, the amount of calcium retained is always substantially less than the amount ingested. This is both because absorption efficiency is relatively low, even during growth, and because calcium is lost daily through shed skin,

Table 1
Various Estimates of the Calcium Requirement in Women

Age	1989 RDA	NIH[a]
1–5	800	800
6–10	800	800–1200
11–24	1200	1200–1500
Pregnancy/lactation	1200	1200–1500
24–50/65	800	1000
65–	800	1500

[a]Recommendations for women as proposed by the Consensus Development Conference on Optimal Calcium Intake (8)

nails, hair, and sweat, as well as in urine and nonreabsorbed digestive secretions. Only about 4–8% of ingested calcium is retained. This inefficient retention is not so much because ability to build bone is limited, but because the primitive calcium intake to which our physiologies are adapted was high. An absorptive barrier is a protection against calcium surfeit, and inefficient retention reflects primitive environmental abundance.

When ingested calcium is less than optimal, the balance between formation and resorption, normally positive during growth, falls towards zero. This occurs because PTH augments bone resorption at the endosteal-trabecular surface in order to sustain the level of ionized calcium in the extracellular fluid. When the demands of mineralization at the periosteum and growth plates exceed the amount of calcium absorbed from the diet and released from growth-related bone modeling, more PTH is secreted and resorption increases still further, until balance becomes zero or even negative. Growth in bone size continues, however, and a limited quantity of mineral now has to be redistributed over an ever larger volume.

Net bone accumulation will be greater as calcium intake increases, but only to the point where endosteal-trabecular resorption is solely because of the genetic program governing growth, and is not being driven by body needs for calcium. Above that level, as seen in Fig. 1, further increases in calcium intake will produce no further bone accumulation. The intake required to achieve the full genetic program, and thus to assure peak bone mass, is the intake that corresponds to the beginning of the plateau region in Fig. 1. This value will be different for different stages of growth, in part because growth rates are not constant and also because, as body size increases, obligatory calcium losses through skin and excreta increase as well.

When the many published reports of calcium balance studies during growth are combined, it is possible to make out in humans the pattern of plateau behavior found in laboratory animals and then, from the aggregated data, to estimate the intake values that correspond to the threshold (20). Figure 2 represents one example of the relationship between intake and retention, combining the results of many published studies of calcium balance derived from a subset of the adolescents whose balances were assembled by Matkovic (21). It clearly shows the plateau type of behavior that both animal studies and theoretical considerations predict. It also shows that, at intakes less than the plateau threshold, daily storage is less than optimal, i.e., accumulation of bone is being limited by intake. Any such limiting intake must be considered inadequate.

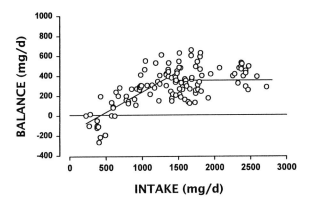

Fig. 2. The relationship of calcium intake, on the horizontal axis, to calcium retention (balance), on the vertical axis, for a subset of the adolescents described by Matkovic and Heaney *(20)*. Note that despite the "noisiness" that is inevitable in measurements of balance in humans, there is clear evidence of an intake plateau, as observed in the animal experiments of Fig. 1. Note also that, for this age, the threshold of the plateau occurs at about 1500 mg Ca/d. (Copyright Robert P. Heaney, 1992. Reproduced with permission.)

As can be seen, the threshold value for adolescents is about 1500 mg. Best available estimates for the value of this threshold at other stages of growth are 1400 mg in children and 1000 mg in young adults out to age 30 *(see below)*.

These values, based on retrospective analysis of balance data, are buttressed by three randomized controlled trials of calcium supplementation in children and adolescents *(13,14,22)* and by a longitudinal observational study in young adults *(23)*. The controlled trials demonstrated that bone gain during growth was greater when intake was elevated above the RDA. This suggests that the current RDAs lie on the ascending portion of the threshold curves of Fig. 2 rather than on the plateau, as they should.

The longitudinal study of young adults *(23)* showed prospectively that bone augmentation continues into the third decade. Bone mass gains in this study ranged from 0.5%/yr for the forearm to 1.25%/yr for total body bone mineral. The single most important correlate of the rate of bone accumulation in the subjects of this study was calcium intake. The rate of bone accumulation was inversely proportional to age, with the best estimate of the age at which the rate reached zero being approx 29–30 yr. Thus, the window of opportunity to achieve the full genetic program appears to remain at least partly open until about age 30.

2.4. Secondary Prevention: The Conservation of Acquired Bone Mass

Studies of calcium requirement in mature, but still premenopausal women have, in general, yielded results compatible with the NIH recommendations of Table 1. Welten et al. *(24)*, in a meta-analysis of studies in this age group, concluded that calcium intake was positively associated with bone mass. Heaney et al. *(25)*, in a study of estrogen-replete women ingesting their habitual calcium intakes, found a mean intake for zero balance of slightly under 1000 mg/d, and Nordin et al. *(2)* a figure closer to 600 mg/d. Recker et al. *(26)*, in a prospective study of bone mass in premenopausal women, found no detectable bone loss over a 2-yr period on an estimated mean calcium intake of 651 mg.

In conclusion, although there may be other health reasons for maintaining an even higher calcium intake during the mature years, bone health seems to be supported adequately by an intake in the range of 800–1000 mg/d; however, lower intakes may lead to premenopausal bone loss or failure to achieve peak mass, or both.

2.5. Menopause

Estrogen seems to adjust the bending setpoint of the mechanical feedback loop that regulates bone mass. Accordingly, whenever women lose ovarian hormones, either naturally at menopause or earlier as a result of anorexia nervosa or athletic amenorrhea, the skeleton appears to sense that it has more bone than it needs, and hence allows resorption to carry away more bone than formation replaces. (Precisely the same change occurs when men lose testosterone for any reason.) This is equivalent to raising the setpoint of the feedback loop that functions to maintain bone bending under load within safe limits. Although varying somewhat from site-to-site across the skeleton, the downward adjustment in bone mass because of gonadal hormone lack amounts to approx 15% of the bone a woman had prior to menopause (27).

The importance of this phenomenon in a discussion of nutrient effects is to distinguish menopausal bone loss from nutrient deficiency loss and to stress that menopausal loss, which is mainly because of absence of gonadal hormones, not because of nutrient deficiency, cannot be substantially influenced by diet. Almost all of the published studies of calcium supplementation within 5 yr following menopause failed to prevent bone loss. Even Elders et al., who employed a calcium intake in excess of 3100 mg/d succeeded only in slowing menopausal loss, not in preventing it (28). Only Aloia's report (17) contains clear evidence for a benefit of a high calcium intake at this life stage, and even here, estrogen produced a greater effect. Nevertheless, one can find in many of the published reports evidence of small calcium effects at even this life stage, and it may be that in any group of early menopausal women there are some whose calcium intake is so inadequate that they are losing bone for two reasons (estrogen lack *plus* calcium insufficiency).

As important as menopausal bone loss is, it is only a one-time downward adjustment, and, if nutrition is adequate, the loss continues for only a few years, after which the skeleton comes into a new steady state (although at a 15% lower bone mass). It is in this context that the importance of achieving a high peak skeletal mass during growth becomes apparent. One standard deviation for lumbar spine bone mineral content in normal women is about 15% of the young adult mean, and for total body bone mineral, about 12%. Hence, a woman at least one standard deviation above the mean can sustain the 15% menopausal loss and still end up with about as much bone as the average woman has before menopause. By contrast, a woman at or under one standard deviation below the young adult mean premenopausally drops to two standard deviations below the mean as she crosses menopause and is therefore, by the WHO criteria (29), already osteopenic and verging on frankly osteoporotic.

As noted, the menopausal bone mass adjustment theoretically stops with a loss of about 15%, but this is true only so long as calcium intake is adequate. In this regard, it is important to note that estrogen has nonskeletal effects as well, i.e., it improves intestinal absorption and renal conservation (24,30,31). As a result, an estrogen-deficient woman has a higher calcium requirement, and unless she raises her calcium intake after menopause, she will continue to lose bone after the estrogen-dependent quantum has

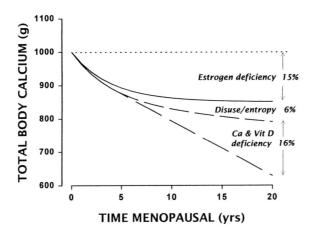

Fig. 3. Partition of age-related bone loss in a typical postmenopausal woman with an inadequate calcium intake. Based on a model described in detail elsewhere *(27)*. (Copyright Robert P. Heaney, 1990. Reproduced with permission.)

been lost, even if the same diet would have been adequate to maintain her skeleton before menopause. In other words, early in the menopausal period, her bone loss is mainly (or entirely) because of estrogen withdrawal, whereas later it will be because of inadequate calcium intake. Figure 3 assembles schematically the set of factors contributing to bone loss in the postmenopausal period. The figure shows both the self-limiting character of the loss as a result of estrogen deficiency and the usually slower, but continuing loss because of nutritional deficiency (if present). Unlike the estrogen-related loss, which mostly plays itself out in 3–6 yr, an ongoing calcium deficiency loss will continue to deplete the skeleton indefinitely for the remainder of a woman's life; that is, unless calcium intake is raised to a level sufficient to stop it. Furthermore, since both absorption efficiency *(30)* and calcium intake *(32)* decline with age, the degree of calcium shortfall actually tends to worsen with age.

Thus, it is important for a woman to increase her calcium intake after menopause. Both the 1984 NIH consensus conference on osteoporosis and the 1994 Consensus Conference on Optimal Calcium Intake *(8)* recommended intakes of 1500 mg/d for estrogen-deprived postmenopausal women. It may be that the optimal intake is somewhat higher still *(see below)*, but median intakes in the United States for women of this age are in the range of 500–600 mg/day *(32,33)*, and if the bulk of them could be raised even to 1500 mg/d, the impact on skeletal health would be considerable.

2.6. Senescence

Age-related bone loss occurs in both sexes, regardless of gonadal hormone levels, generally starting at about age 50. However, it is obscured in the years immediately following menopause in women by the substantially larger effect of estrogen withdrawal *(see* Fig. 3). It probably occurs, however, even in estrogen-treated women, at about the same rate as in men. This rate is generally reported to be on the order of 0.5–1.0%/yr during the sixth and seventh decades, and probably accelerates with advancing age. For example, loss from the hip in the control subjects of the study by Chapuy et al. *(11)*, at an average age of 84, was 3%/yr. Age-related loss involves both cortical and trabecular bone and can come about by several mechanisms: disuse, remodeling errors, and nutritional deficiency, as summarized in Fig. 3.

Although nutrient deficiency is clearly only a part of the total problem, it is common. That the 3% loss in the control subjects of Chapuy et al. was related to their calcium intakes is indicated by the fact that this loss was completely obliterated in the supplemented women. Intestinal calcium absorption efficiency declines with age (30), at the same time as nutrient intake itself generally declines (32); the result is that the diet of aging individuals becomes more and more inadequate. McKane et al. (34) have recently shown that the high PTH levels and abnormal PTH secretory dynamics typically found in elderly women are a result of calcium deficiency, and that PTH function can be entirely normalized by calcium intakes of 2400 mg/d.

It is also in this age group that the most dramatic and persuasive evidence for fracture prevention by high calcium intakes has been produced in recent years. This is partly because most fragility fractures rise in frequency with age, and hence the opportunity to see a fracture benefit (if one exists) is greater then. Chapuy et al. (11) showed a reduction in hip fracture risk of 43% by 18 mo after starting supplementation with calcium plus vitamin D, and a 32% reduction in other extremity fractures. Chevalley et al. (15), in another study in elderly women, showed that even when vitamin D was given to both groups, extra calcium reduced femoral bone loss *and* vertebral fracture incidence. More recently, Recker et al. (35) in a 4-yr, randomized controlled trial in elderly women (mean age 73), demonstrated that a calcium supplement reduced both age-related bone loss and incident vertebral fractures. Their subjects had all received a multivitamin supplement containing 400 IU of vitamin D, as had the subjects of Chevalley et al.; hence, the effect in the calcium-supplemented groups of both studies can be attributed to the calcium alone.

These findings do not mean that vitamin D is unimportant in this age group *(see* Section 3.). It is likely that intakes of both calcium and vitamin D are inadequate in the elderly, and the unrecognized prevalence of combined deficiency has made it difficult to study the actual requirements of either nutrient in this age group.

The calcium intake achieved in the Chapuy study was about 1700 mg/d, 1400 mg/d in the Chevalley study, and about 1600 mg/d in the Recker study. These values are in the range of the intake earlier found by Heaney et al. (24) to be the mean requirement for healthy estrogen-deprived older women (1500–1700 mg/d). All these studies are, therefore, consistent with the NIH recommendation of 1500 mg/d (Table 1).

An important feature of these controlled trials in already elderly individuals was that bone mass was low in both treated and control groups at the start of the study, and although a significant difference in fracture rate was produced by calcium supplementation, even the supplemented groups would have to be considered as having an unacceptably high fracture rate. What these studies do not establish is how much lower the fracture rate might have been if a high calcium intake had been provided for the preceding 20–30 years of these women's lives. The studies of Matkovic et al. (36) and Holbrook et al. (37), although not randomized trials, strongly suggest that the effect may be larger than has been found with treatment started in the eighth and ninth decades of life. Both of these observational studies reported a hip fracture rate that was roughly 60% lower in elderly whose habitual calcium intakes had been high. Although findings from observational studies such as these had not been considered persuasive in the absence of

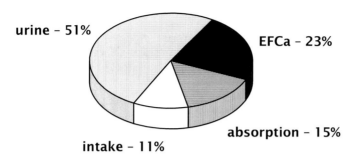

Fig. 4. Partition of variance in calcium balance in normal women among the input-output processes involved in calculation of balance. EFC: endogenous fecal calcium. (Copyright Robert P. Heaney, 1994. Reproduced with permission.)

proof from controlled trials, the Chapuy, Chevalley, and Recker studies have now met that need.

Together the aggregate of available studies underscores the importance of achieving at least the 1500 mg target figure of the NIH recommendations for the elderly. At the same time it must be stressed, once again, that osteoporosis is a multifactorial condition, and that removing one of the pathogenic factors (i.e., insuring an adequate calcium intake) cannot be expected to eradicate all osteoporotic fractures.

2.6. Nutrient-Nutrient Interactions: Factors that Influence the Requirement

There are several nutritional factors that influence or have been proposed to influence the calcium requirement. The principal interacting nutrients are sodium, protein, caffeine, and fiber. Fiber and caffeine influence calcium absorption *(38–40)* and typically exert relatively minor effects, whereas sodium and protein influence urinary excretion of calcium *(40,41)*, and can be of much greater significance for the calcium economy. The effects of phosphorus and fat in humans are minor to nonexistent.

The basis for the importance of nutritional influences on absorption and excretion of calcium is illustrated in Fig. 4, which partitions the variance in calcium balance observed in 560 balances in healthy middle-aged women studied in the author's laboratory. As Fig. 4 shows, only 11% of the variance in balance among these women is explained by differences in their actual calcium intakes. By contrast, absorption efficiency explains about 15%, whereas urinary losses explain more than half.

2.6.1. Influences on Intestinal Absorption of Calcium

2.6.1.1. Fiber

The effect of fiber is variable, and generally small. Many kinds of fiber have no influence at all on absorption, such as the fiber in green, leafy vegetables *(9)*. The fiber in wheat bran, by contrast, reduces absorption of coingested calcium, although except for extremes of fiber intake *(42)*, the effect is generally relatively small. Often lumped together with fiber are such associated food constituents as phytate and oxalate. Both can reduce the availability of any calcium contained in the same food, but, unlike bran, generally do not affect coingested calcium from other foods. For example, for equal ingested loads, the calcium of beans is only about half as available as the calcium of milk

(43), whereas the calcium of spinach and rhubarb is nearly totally unavailable *(44)*. For spinach and rhubarb, the inhibition is mostly because of oxalate. For common beans, phytate is responsible for about half the interference, and oxalate the other half. Even so, the effects of phytate and oxalate are highly variable. There is a sufficient quantity of both antiabsorbers in beans to complex all the calcium also present, and yet absorptive interference is only half what might be expected.

2.6.1.2. CAFFEINE

Often considered to have a deleterious effect on the calcium economy, caffeine actually has the smallest effect of the known interacting nutrients. A single cup of brewed coffee causes deterioration in calcium balance of ~3 mg *(39,40,45)*, mainly by reducing absorption of calcium *(39)*. The effect is probably on active transport, although this is not known for certain. This small effect is more than adequately offset by a tablespoon or two of milk *(39,45)*.

2.6.2. INFLUENCES ON RENAL CONSERVATION OF CALCIUM

2.6.2.1. PROTEIN AND SODIUM

As noted, the effects of protein and of sodium are substantial *(2,3,40)*. Both nutrients increase urinary calcium loss across the full range of their own intakes, from very low to very high—so it is not a question of harmful effects of an *excess* of these nutrients. Sodium and calcium share the same transport system in the proximal tubule, and every 2300 mg of sodium excreted by the kidney pulls 20–60 mg of calcium out with it. Also, every gram of protein metabolized in adults causes an increment in urine calcium loss of about 1 mg. This latter effect is probably a result of excretion of the sulfate load produced in the metabolism of sulfur-containing amino acids (and is thus a kind of endogenous analog of the acid-rain problem). For diets high in calcium, as would have been the case for our hunter-gatherer ancestors, high protein and possibly high sodium intakes could have been handled by the body perfectly well. These nutrients create problems for the calcium economy of contemporary adult humans mainly because we typically have calcium intakes that are low relative to those of preagricultural humans, and sodium intakes that are high.

At low sodium and protein intakes, the calcium requirement for an adult female may be as little as 450 mg/d *(41)*, whereas if her intake of both nutrients is high, she may require as much as 2000 mg/d to maintain calcium balance. A forceful illustration of the importance of sodium intake is provided by the report of Matkovic et al. *(46)* that urine calcium remains high in adolescent girls on calcium intakes too low to permit bone gain. The principal determinant of urinary calcium in such young women is sodium intake *(47)*, not calcium intake.

Differences in protein and sodium intake from one national group to another are part of the explanation why studies in different countries have shown sometimes strikingly different calcium requirements. At the same time, one usually finds a positive correlation between calcium intake and bone mass within the national range of intakes *(48)*. Hence, although sodium (and protein) intake differences between cultures obscure the calcium effect, they do not obliterate it.

2.6.2.2. ACID ASH RESIDUE

The acid/alkaline ash characteristic of the diet is also important, although the quantitative relationship of this diet feature to the calcium requirement has been less fully explored to date. Nevertheless, it has clearly been shown that substitution of metabolizable anions (e.g., bicarbonate or acetate) for fixed anions (e.g., chloride) in various test diets will lower obligatory urinary calcium loss substantially *(49,50)*. This suggests that primarily vegetarian diets create a lower calcium requirement, and provides a further explanation for the seemingly lower requirement in many nonindustrialized populations. However, it is not yet clear whether, within a population, vegetarians have higher bone mass values than omnivores.

2.6.2.3. PHOSPHORUS

Phosphorus is commonly believed to reduce calcium absorption, but the evidence for that effect is scant to nonexistent, and there is much contrary evidence. Spencer has shown no effect of even large increments in phosphate intake on overall calcium balance at low, normal, and high intakes of calcium *(51)*. In adults, Ca:P ratios ranging from 0.2 to above 2.0 are without effect on calcium balance, at least so long as adjustments are made for calcium intake. What phosphorus does is depress urinary calcium loss and elevate digestive juice secretion of calcium, by approximately equal amounts, with no net effect on balance *(52)*. Although it is true that stoichiometric excesses of phosphate will tend to form complexes with calcium in the chyme, various calcium phosphate salts have been shown to exhibit absorbability similar to other calcium salts, and phosphate is, of course, a principal anion of the major food source of calcium (dairy products). In any case, phosphate itself is more readily absorbed than calcium (by a factor of at least 2×), and at intakes of both nutrients in the range of their respective RDAs, absorption will leave a stoichiometric excess of calcium in the ileum, not the other way around. This explains the seeming paradox that high calcium intakes can block phosphate absorption (as in management of end-stage renal disease), whereas achievably high phosphate intakes have little or no effect on calcium absorption.

2.6.2.4. ALUMINUM

Although not in any proper sense a nutrient, aluminum, in the form of Al-containing antacids, also exerts significant effects on obligatory calcium loss in the urine *(53)*. By binding phosphate in the gut, these substances reduce phosphate absorption, lower integrated 24-h serum phosphate levels, and thereby elevate urinary calcium loss. (This is the opposite of the more familiar hypocalciuric effect of oral phosphate supplements.) Therapeutic doses of Al-containing antacids can elevate urine calcium by 50 mg/d or more.

2.7. Calcium Sources

The best calcium sources are, of course, foods. In a modern, Western diet, food items that provide more than 100 mg of calcium per serving are limited to dairy products (with the exception of cottage cheese), greens of the mustard family (collards, kale, mustard), calcium-set tofu, sardines, and a few nuts (especially hazelnuts and almonds). Smaller amounts of calcium are ubiquitous in many leafy vegetables, but with the exception of shellfish, calcium levels are low in most meats, poultry, or fish. As noted earlier, the calcium of beans is only about half as available as the calcium of milk, and the calcium of high oxalate vegetables (such as spinach and rhubarb) is almost completely unavailable.

In general, most diets without dairy products have gross calcium nutrient densities under 20 mg Ca/100 kcal, and available calcium densities lower still. Since total energy intake for adult American women is in the range of 1400–1600 kcal/d, it follows that most diets low in dairy products will be low in calcium—probably 300 mg Ca/d or less—far short of levels currently recommended as optimal.

In part as a response to this dilemma, the Surgeon General, in his 1988 report on Nutrition and Health *(54)*, recommended judicious, low-level calcium fortification of many items in the food chain. An increasing number of fortified foods is becoming available each year—ranging from fruit juice, to bread, to potato chips, to rice. Where bioavailability of the calcium in these foods has been ensured, they should be useful adjuncts in the attempt to improve calcium intake at the population level.

The principal supplement on the US market is calcium carbonate, available as such, or as oyster shell or dolomite. When the tablet is competently formulated, so that it disintegrates in gastric juice, or when the supplement is chewed (as with TUMS or Os-Cal chewables), the carbonate is quite well absorbed and generally very well tolerated. There is no requirement for gastric acid so long as the carbonate salt is taken with meals. Calcium citrate and calcium phosphate are also good sources, but they tend to be more expensive. In the rare case in which the carbonate is not well tolerated, these other sources provide useful alternatives.

Divided doses enhance absorption from both supplements and foods, since absorption fraction is an inverse function of load size. All calcium sources (including food) interfere with iron absorption when the two nutrients are ingested at the same meal. Hence, if a person is iron-deficient and is taking an iron supplement, it is best if that meal not contain a large amount of calcium (food or supplement).

3. VITAMIN D

Vitamin D facilitates active transport of calcium across the intestinal mucosa, at least partly by inducing the formation of a calcium-binding transport protein in intestinal mucosal cells. This function is particularly important for adaptation to low calcium intakes. Absorption also occurs passively, probably mainly by way of paracellular diffusion. This route is not dependent on vitamin D, and is not as well studied. The proportion of absorption by the three mechanisms varies with intake and is not well characterized in humans; at high calcium intakes (above 2000 mg/d) absorption fraction approaches 10–15% of intake. Under these circumstances it is likely that active transport contributes relatively little to the total absorbed load. Nevertheless, it is generally considered that vitamin D status influences absorptive performance and that it thereby influences the calcium requirement.

A principal storage form of the vitamin is 25-hydroxyvitamin D [25(OH)D], and its plasma level is generally regarded as the best clinical indicator of vitamin D status. Although usually considered to be about three orders of magnitude less potent than calcitriol in promoting active transport in animal receptor assays, there is growing evidence that it may possess physiological functions in its own right *(55)*, and in the only human dose-response studies performed to date, 25(OH)D was found to have a molar potency in the range of 1/125 to 1/400 that of $1,25(OH)D_3$ *(56)*, not the 1/2000 figure usually considered to reflect relative 25(OH)D activity.

Vitamin D status commonly deteriorates in the elderly, whose plasma 25(OH)D levels are generally lower than in young adults *(57)*. This difference is partly because of decreased solar exposure, partly because of decreased efficiency of skin vitamin D synthesis, and partly because of decreased intake of milk, the principal dietary source of the vitamin. Moreover, the elderly exhibit other abnormalities of the vitamin D endocrine system that may further impair their ability to adapt to reduced calcium intake. These include decreased responsiveness of the renal 1-α-hydroxylase to parathyroid hormone *(58)* and decreased mucosal responsiveness to calcitriol *(59)*.

For all these reasons there is a growing body of opinion that the requirement for vitamin D rises with age *(60)*, and a body of data that strongly suggests that relative vitamin D deficiency plays a role in several components of the osteoporosis syndrome. Perhaps most persuasive of all is the finding by Heikinheimo et al. *(60)*, in a randomized, controlled trial, of substantial reduction in all fractures in an elderly Finnish population given a single injection of 150,000–300,000 IU vitamin D each fall.

The foregoing studies (as well as others) lead inexorably to the conclusion that vitamin D insufficiency is prevalent in the middle-aged and elderly of Northern Europe and North America. Moreover, in virtually none of these studies was frank osteomalacia a significant feature of the problem. This old criterion for true vitamin D deficiency may well be much too insensitive to be nutritionally useful today. How the vitamin D requirement ought to be defined is another matter. Holick has shown that it takes an intake of ~600 IU/d, from all sources to sustain serum 25(OH)D levels *(61)*, and the doses of vitamin D used in the studies summarized above also suggest that an intake in the range of 500–800 IU/d is required for full expression of the known effects of vitamin D in adults. This is substantially above the current RDA of only 200 IU for adults *(19)*

4. VITAMIN K

The chemistry and physiology of vitamin K have been extensively reviewed elsewhere *(62,63)*. In brief, vitamin K is necessary for the gamma-carboxylation of glutamic acid residues in a large number of proteins. Most familiar are those related to coagulation, in which seven vitamin K-dependent proteins are involved in one way or another. The gamma-carboxyglutamic acid residues in the peptide chain bind calcium, either free or on the surface layers of crystals, and have been thought to function in varying ways including catalysis of the coagulation cascade, inhibition of mineralization (as in urine), and generation of osteoclast chemotactic signals.

Three vitamin K-dependent proteins are found in bone matrix: osteocalcin (bone gla protein [BGP]), matrix gla-protein, and protein S. Only BGP is unique to bone. There is also a kidney gla protein (nephrocalcin), which may be involved in renal conservation of calcium. BGP binds avidly to hydroxyapatite and is chemotactic for bone-resorbing cells. Roughly 30% of the synthesized BGP is not incorporated into matrix, but is released instead into the circulation, where, like alkaline phosphatase, it can be measured and used as an indicator of bone turnover. In vitamin K deficiency, such as would occur with coumarin anticoagulants, serum BGP levels decline and the degree of carboxylation of the circulating BGP falls dramatically. Although it would seem, therefore, that vitamin K deficiency would have detectable skeletal effects, they have been very hard to find. Rats reared and sustained to adult life under near total suppression of BGP γ carboxylation show only minor skeletal defects, mostly related to abnormalities in the growth apparatus *(62)*. In aging humans, the problem of detecting skeletal abnormalities is compounded by the fact that the bulk of the skeleton was formed prior to the onset of any deficiency, and thus tends to be an insensitive indicator of current nutritional stresses.

Various vitamin K-related abnormalities have been described in association with osteoporosis, but their significance to skeletal status remains unclear. Circulating vitamin K and menaquinone levels are low in hip fracture patients *(64)*. BGP is under-carboxylated in osteoporotics, and this defect responds to relatively small doses of vitamin K. Finally, urine calcium has been reported to be high in osteoporotics and to fall on administering vitamin K *(65)*.

Whether or not vitamin K is important for bone health, serum vitamin K levels are indicators of general nutritional status, and it may simply be that the observation of low vitamin K levels in osteoporotics, especially in those with hip fracture, is mainly a reflection of the often poor nutrition of these individuals.

5. MAGNESIUM

The adult female RDA for magnesium is 280 mg/d *(19)*. Only about 25% of adult US females achieve this level of intake. Average intakes tend to be in the range of 70–80% of the RDA. Although severe magnesium deficiency is a well-described syndrome *(66)*, interfering both with PTH secretion and PTH action on bone, it is uncertain whether mild departures from the RDA have any adverse effect, or even whether the RDA needs to be as high as it is now set. There is, as well, a widespread popular belief that magnesium is necessary for optimal calcium absorption. However, the many studies establishing the benefit of supplemental calcium described earlier achieved their effect without adding magnesium to the diets of their subjects. Furthermore, Spencer, in a series of careful metabolic studies, showed that major increases in magnesium intake had no significant effect on absorption efficiency for calcium *(67)*, Thus, there is no known justification for supplemental magnesium in prevention or treatment of osteoporosis. Moreover, magnesium salts, when used as a component of a combined supplement tablet (e.g., as in dolomite), displace calcium and make it more difficult (i.e., more pills are required) to get sufficient calcium by this route.

6. TRACE MINERALS

Several trace minerals, notably zinc, manganese, and copper, are essential metallic cofactors for enzymes involved in synthesis of various bone matrix constituents. Ascorbic acid (along with zinc) is needed for collagen crosslinkage. In growing animals, diets deficient in these nutrients produce definite skeletal abnormalities *(68)*. Additionally, zinc deficiency is well known to produce growth retardation and other abnormalities in humans. However, it is not known whether significant deficiencies of these elements develop in previously healthy adults, or at least, if they do, whether such deficiencies contribute detectably to the osteoporosis problem. Copper deficiency is reported to be associated with osteoporotic lesions in sheep, cattle, and rats *(69)*. Copper has not been much studied in connection with human osteoporosis, but in one study in which serum copper was measured, levels were negatively correlated with lumbar spine BMD, even after adjusting for body weight and dietary calcium intake *(70)*.

In one four-way, randomized trial, copper, as a part of a trace mineral cocktail including also zinc and manganese, slowed bone mineral loss in postmenopausal women when given either with or without supplemental calcium *(71)*. There appeared to be a small additional benefit from the extra trace minerals; however, the only statistically significant effect in this study was associated with the calcium supplement. This could mean that trace mineral deficiency plays no role in osteoporosis, but it could also mean that not all of the women treated suffered from such deficiency. In fact, since both osteoporotic and age-related bone loss are multifactorial, and since there is no known way to select subjects for inclusion on the basis of presumed trace mineral need, one would presume that only some of the subjects in such a study might be deficient. Thus, the suggestive findings of this study have to be considered grounds for further exploration of this issue.

7. NUTRITION AND HIP FRACTURE

Nutrition enters into the hip fracture problem in two ways: in predisposing to fracture and in recovery from the assault of the injury and its repair. Fractures in the old elderly, and particularly hip fractures, are concentrated in institutionalized persons with multiple disabilities. The osteoporotic elderly, generally, are known to have depleted lean body mass and fat mass, and, when studied, have been found to have low circulating values for several key nutritional indicator variables, from serum albumin to ferritin and vitamin A *(72)*. Survival two years after injury is four times higher in patients with serum albumin values above 3.5 g/dL than in patients with values below 3.0 *(72)*. Additionally, patients with hip fracture often have low calcium intakes, and in the majority of studies evaluating the matter, dietary calcium earlier in life is inversely associated with hip fracture risk. In brief, hip fracture is a problem concentrated in multiply compromised individuals, and the prospect of successfully intervening to reduce risk has proved daunting even to contemplate.

However, one aspect of the problem is partly amenable to control. The relative malnutrition of patients suffering hip fracture and coming to the hospital for repair contributes significantly to the often unsatisfactory outcomes for this common fracture (i.e., 15–20% excess mortality; 50% institutionalization of the survivors). Delmi et al. *(72)*, in a randomized trial of a protein-based nutrient supplement given to patients newly hospitalized for hip fracture, found that only 26% of unsupplemented individuals had outcomes classified as good at 6 mo after injury, whereas nearly 60% of supplemented individuals had good outcomes. The investigators noted that the hospital diets offered the unsupplemented individuals were nutritionally adequate, but were frequently unconsumed, whereas the investigators ensured the ingestion of the supplement. This is not an isolated observation; others *(73)* had earlier found qualitatively similar benefit from nutritional supplementation in such patients, and thus, the consistency of these findings constitutes a challenge to the health professions to apply these basic nutritional principles in the management of their patients.

8. RECOMMENDATION

Calcium intake should be high throughout life: 1500 mg/d during growth and at least that much in the elderly. Foods are the best sources, but given caloric restriction, that means fat-free milk and yogurt, for the most part, as well as the widespread availability of calcium-fortified foods. Supplements are convenient and often necessary, but should not be a substitute for a national nutritional policy or for a good diet. The elderly are commonly vitamin D-deficient as well as calcium-deprived. Conscious efforts must be made to ensure a daily intake of 600–800 IU. The old elderly often suffer some degree of global undernutrition in addition to their specific deficiencies of calcium and vitamin

D. Given the common isolation of elderly living alone, this is not an easy problem to solve. At least we can mount an effort to feed them when they develop fractures.

REFERENCES

1. Heaney RP, Recker RR. Distribution of calcium absorption in middle-aged women. Am J Clin Nutr 1986; 43:299–305.
2. Nordin BEC, Polley KJ, Need AG, Morris HA, Marshall D. The problem of calcium requirement. Am J Clin Nutr 1987; 45:1295–1304.
3. Nordin BEC, Need AG, Morris HA, Horowitz M. Sodium, calcium and osteoporosis. In: Nutritional Aspects of Osteoporosis. Burckhardt P, Heaney RP, eds. New York: Raven, 1991; 85:279–295.
4. Barger-Lux MJ, Heaney RP, Packard PT, Lappe JM, Recker RR. Nutritional correlates of low calcium intake. Clin in Appl Nutr 1992; 2:39–44.
5. Jowsey J, Gershon-Cohen J. The relationship of dietary calcium to osteoporosis. Metabolism 1964; 13:221–226.
6. Jowsey J, Raisz LG. Experimental osteoporosis and parathyroid activity. Endocrinology 1968; 82: 384–396.
7. Forbes RM, Weingartner KE, Parker HM, Bell RR, Erdman JW Jr. Bioavailability to rats of zinc, magnesium and calcium in casein-, egg- and soy protein-containing diets. J Nutr 1979; 109:1652–1660.
8. NIH Consensus Conference: optimal calcium intake. JAMA 1994; 272:1942–1948.
9. Heaney RP. Nutritional factors in osteoporosis. Ann Rev Nutr 1993; 13:287–316.
10. Dawson-Hughes B, Dallal GE, Krall EA, Sadowski L, Sahyoun N, Tannenbaum S. A controlled trial of the effect of calcium supplementation on bone density in postmenopausal women. New Engl J Med 1990; 323:878–883.
11. Chapuy MC, Arlot ME, Duboeuf F, et al. Vitamin D_3 and calcium to prevent hip fractures in elderly women. New Engl J Med 1992; 327:1637–1642.
12. Reid IR, Ames RW, Evans MC, Gamble GD, Sharpe SJ. Effect of calcium supplementation on bone loss in postmenopausal women. New Engl J Med 1993; 328:460–464.
13. Johnston CC Jr, Miller JZ, Slemenda CW, et al. Calcium supplementation and increases in bone mineral density in children. New Engl J Med 1992; 327:82–87.
14. Lloyd T, Andon MB, Rollings N, et al. Calcium supplementation and bone mineral density in adolescent girls. JAMA 1993; 270:841–844.
15. Chevalley T, Rizzoli R, Nydegger V, et al. Effects of calcium supplements on femoral bone mineral density and vertebral fracture rate in vitamin D-replete elderly patients. Osteoporosis Int 1994; 4:245–252.
16. Reid IR, Ames RW, Evans MC, Sharpe SJ, Gamble GD. Determinants of the rate of bone loss in normal postmenopausal women—the importance of fat mass and renal calcium handling. Am J Med 1995; 98:331–335.
17. Aloia JF, Vaswani A, Yeh JK, Ross PL, Flaster E, Dilmanian FA. Calcium supplementation with and without hormone replacement therapy to prevent postmenopausal bone loss. Ann Intern Med 1994; 120:97–103.
18. Heaney RP. The bone remodeling transient: implications for the interpretation of clinical studies of bone mass change. J Bone Miner Res 1994; 9:1515–1523.
19. Recommended Dietary Allowances, 10th edition. Washington, DC, National Acad. Press, 1989.
20. Matkovic V, Heaney RP, Calcium balance during human growth. Evidence for threshold behavior. Am J Clin Nutr 1992; 55:992–996 .
21. Matkovic V. Calcium metabolism and calcium requirements during skeletal modeling and consolidation of bone mass. Am J Clin Nutr 1991; 54:245S–260S.
22. Chan GM, Hoffman K, McMurray M. The effect of dietary calcium supplementation on pubertal girls' growth and bone mineral status. J Bone Miner Res 1991; 6:S240.
23. Recker RR, Davies KM, Hinders SM, Heaney RP, Stegman MR, Kimmel DB. Bone gain in young adult women. JAMA 1992; 268:2403–2408.
24. Welten DC, Kemper HCG, Post GB, van Staveren WA. A meta-analysis of the effect of calcium intake on bone mass in females and males. J Nutr 1995; 125:2802–2813.
25. Heaney RP, Recker RR, Saville PD. Menopausal changes in calcium balance performance. J Lab Clin Med 1978; 92:953–963.
26. Recker RR, Lappe JM, Davies KM, Kimmel DB. Change in bone mass immediately before menopause. J Bone Miner Res 1992; 7:857–862.

27. Heaney RP. Estrogen-calcium interactions in the postmenopause: a quantitative description. Bone Miner 1990; 11:67–84.
28. Elders PJM, Netelenbos JC, Lips P, et al. Calcium supplementation reduces vertebral bone loss in perimenopausal women: a controlled trial in 248 women between 46 and 55 years of age. J Clin Endocrinol Metab 1991; 73:533–540.
29. Kanis JA, Melton LJ III, Christiansen C, Johnston CC, Khaltaev N. The diagnosis of osteoporosis. J Bone Miner Res 1994; 9:1137–1141.
30. Heaney RP, Recker RR, Stegman MR, Moy AJ. Calcium absorption in women: relationships to calcium intake, estrogen status, and age. J Bone Min Res 1989; 4:469–475.
31. Nordin BEC, Need AG, Morris HA, Horowitz M, Robertson WG. Evidence for a renal calcium leak in postmenopausal women. J Clin Endocrinol Metab 1991; 72:401–407.
32. Carroll MD, Abraham S, Dresser CM. Dietary intake source data: US, 1976–80. Vital & Health Statistics, Serv. 11-NO. 231, DHHS. Publ. No. (PHS) 83-PHS, March 1983. Washington DC, Gov. Printing Office.
33. Alaimo K, McDowell MA, Briefel RR, et al. Dietary intake of vitamins, minerals, and fiber of persons ages 2 months and over in the United States: Third National Health and Nutrition Examination Survgey, Phase 1, 1988–1991. Advance data from vital and health statistics; no. 258. Hyattsville, MD, National Center for Health Statistics. 1994.
34. McKane WR, Khosla S, Egan KS, Robins SP, Burritt MF, Riggs BL. Role of calcium intake in modulating age-related increases in parathyroid function and bone resorption. J Clin Endocrinol Metab 1996; 81:1699–1703.
35. Recker RR, Hinders S, Davies KM. Correcting calcium nutritional deficiency prevents spine fractures in elderly women. Am J Med 1995; submitted.
36. Matkovic V, Kostial K, Simonovic I, Buzina R, Brodarec A, Nordin BEC. Bone status and fracture rates in two regions of Yugoslavia. Am J Clin Nutr 1979; 32:540–549.
37. Holbrook TL, Barrett-Connor E, Wingard DL. Dietary calcium and risk of hip fracture: 14-year prospective population study. Lancet 1988; 2:1046–1049.
38. Pilch SM, ed. Physiological effects and health consequences of dietary fiber. Prepared for the Center for Food Safety and Applied Nutrition, Food and Drug Administration under Contract No. FDA 223–84–2059 by the Life Sciences Research Office, Federation of American Societies for Experimental Biology. Available from FASEB Special Publications Office, Bethesda, MD, 1987.
39. Barger-Lux MJ, Heaney RP. Caffeine and the calcium economy revisited. Osteoporosis Int 1995; 5:97–102.
40. Heaney RP, Recker RR. Effects of nitrogen, phosphorus, and caffeine on calcium balance in women. J Lab Clin Med 1982; 99:46–55.
41. Nordin BEC, Need AG, Morris HA, Horowitz M. The nature and significance of the relationship between urinary sodium and urinary calcium in women. J Nutr 1993; 123:1615–1622.
42. Weaver CM, Heaney RP, Martin BR, Fitzsimmons ML. Human calcium absorption from whole wheat products. J Nutr 1991; 121:1769–1775.
43. Weaver CM, Heaney RP, Proulx WR, Hinders SM, Packard PT. Absorbability of calcium from common beans. J Food Sci 1993; 58:1401–1403.
44. Heaney RP, Weaver CM. Oxalate in vegetables. Effect on calcium absorbability. J Bone Miner Res 1993; 8:S333.
45. Barrett-Connor E, Chang JC, Edelstein SL. Coffee-associated osteoporosis offset by daily milk consumption. JAMA 1994; 271:280–283.
46. Matkovic V, Fontana D, Tominac C, Goel P, Chesnut CH III. Factors that influence peak bone mass formation: a study of calcium balance and the inheritance of bone mass in adolescent females. Am J Clin Nutr 1990; 52:878–888.
47. Matkovic V, Ilich JZ, Andon MB, et al. Urinary calcium, sodium, and bone mass of young females. Am J Clin Nutr 1995; 62:417–425.
48. Lau EMC, Cooper C, Woo J. Calcium deficiency—a major cause of osteoporosis in Hong Kong Chinese. In: Nutritional Aspects of Osteoporosis. Burckhardt P, Heaney RP, eds. New York: Raven, 1991; 85:175–180.
49. Berkelhammer CH, Wood RJ, Sitrin MD. Acetate and hypercalciuria during total parenteral nutrition. Am J Clin Nutr 1988; 48:1482–1489.
50. Sebastian A, Harris ST, Ottaway JH, et al. Improved mineral balance and skeletal metabolism in postmenopausal women treated with potassium bicarbonate. New Engl J Med 1994; 330: 1776–1781.
51. Spencer H, Kramer L, Osis D, Norris C. Effect of phosphorus on the absorption of calcium and on the calcium balance in man. J Nutr 1978; 108:447–457.

52. Heaney RP, Recker RR. Determinants of endogenous fecal calcium in healthy women. J Bone Miner Res 1994; 9:1621–1627.

53. Spencer H, Kramer L, Norris C, Osis D. Effect of small doses of aluminum-containing antacids on calcium and phosphorus metabolism. Am J Clin Nutr 1982; 36:32–40.

54. The Surgeon General's Report on Nutrition and Health. DHHS (PHS) Publication No. 88–50211, 1988.

55. Barger-Lux MJ, Heaney RP, Lanspa SJ, Healy JC, DeLuca HF. An investigation of sources of variation in calcium absorption physiology. J Clin Endocrinol Metab 1995; 80:406–411.

56. Colodro IH, Brickman AS, Coburn JW, Osborn TW, Norman AW. Effect of 25-hydroxy-vitamin D3 on intestinal absorption of calcium in normal man and patients with renal failure. Metabolism 1978; 27:745–753.

57. Francis RM, Peacock M, Storer JH, Davies AEJ, Brown WB, Nordin BEC. Calcium malabsorption in the elderly: the effect of treatment with oral 25-hydroxyvitamin D$_3$). Eur J Clin Invest 1983; 13:391–196.

58. Slovik DM, Adams JS, Neer RM, Holick MF, Potts JT Jr. Deficient production of 1,25-dihydroxyvitamin D in elderly osteoporotic patients. New Engl J Med 1981; 305:372–374.

59. Francis RM, Peacock M, Taylor GA, Storer JH, Nordin BEC. Calcium malabsorption in elderly women with vertebral fractures: evidence for resistance to the action of vitamin D metabolites on the bowel. Clin Sci 1984; 66:103–107.

60. Heikinheimo RJ, Inkovaara JA, Harju EJ, et al. Annual injection of vitamin D and fractures of aged bones. Calcif Tissue Int 1992; 51:105–110.

61. Holick MF. Sources of vitamin D: diet and sunlight. In: Challenges of Modern Medicine, Nutritional Aspects of Osteoporosis (Proceedings of 2nd International Symposium on Osteoporosis, Lausanne, May 1994). Burckhardt P, Heaney RP, eds. Rome, Italy: Ares-Serono Symposia Publications, 1995; 7:289–309.

62. Price PA. Role of vitamin-K-dependent proteins in bone metabolism. Ann Rev Nutr 1988; 8:565–583.

63. Szulc P, Delmas PD. Is there a role for vitamin K deficiency in osteoporosis? In: Challenges of Modern Medicine, Nutritional Aspects of Osteoporosis (Proceedings of 2nd International Symposium on Osteoporosis, Lausanne, May 1994). Burckhardt P, Heaney RP, eds. Rome, Italy: Ares-Serono Publications, 1995; 7:357–366.

64. Hodges SJ, Pilkington MJ, Stamp TCB, et al. Depressed levels of circulating menaquinones in patients with osteoporotic fractures of the spine and femoral neck. Bone 1991; 12:387–389.

65. Knapen MHJ, Hamulyak K, Vermeer C. The effect of vitamin K supplementation on circulating osteocalcin (bone gla protein) and urinary calcium excretion. Ann Int Med 1989; 111:1001–1005.

66. Shils ME. Magnesium. In: Modern Nutrition in Health and Disease, 8 ed., Vol. 1. Shils ME, Olson JA, Shike, M, eds. Philadelphia, PA; Lea & Febiger, 1994; 165–184.

67. Spencer H, Fuller H, Norris C, Williams D. Effect of magnesium on the intestinal absorption of calcium in man. J Am College Nutr 1994; 13:485–492.

68. Mertz W, ed. Trace Elements in Human and Animal Nutrition, 5th edition. San Diego, CA: Academic 1987

69. Strain JJ. A reassessment of diet and osteoporosis—possible role for copper. Med Hypotheses 1988; 27:333–338.

70. Howard G, Andon M, Bracker M, Saltman P, Strause L. Low serum copper, a risk factor additional to low dietary calcium in postmenopausal bone loss. J Trace Elements Ex Med 1992; 5:23–31.

71. Strause L, Saltman P, Smith K, Andon M. The role of trace elements in bone metabolism. In: Nutritional Aspects of Osteoporosis, Serono Symposia Publication vol. 85. Burckhardt P, Heaney RP, eds. New York: Raven, 1991; 223–233.

72. Delmi M, Rapin C-H, Bengoa J-M, Delmas PD, Vasey H, Bonjour J-P. Dietary supplementation in elderly patients with fractured neck of the femur. Lancet 1990; 335:1013–1016.

73. Bastow MD, Rawlings J, Allison SP. Benefits of supplementary tube feeding after fractured neck of femur. Br Med J 1983; 287:1589–1592.

16 Antioxidant Nutrients and Prevention of Oxidant-Mediated, Smoking-Related Diseases

Ronald Anderson

1. INTRODUCTION

Certain high-risk occupations, adverse socioeconomic and sociocultural circumstances, and unhealthy, avoidable aspects of lifestyle may, individually or collectively, result in heightened levels of oxidative stress, predisposing the individual to future development of oxidant-mediated organ dysfunction and disease *(1,2)*. Outdated and/or poorly regulated industrial practices, unacceptably high levels of vehicle exhaust emissions, overpopulation associated with overcrowded, poorly ventilated, nonelectrified dwellings and poor dispersal of atmospheric pollutants because of unfavorable climatic conditions and/or topography are problems commonly encountered in, but not limited to, many developing countries *(3,4)*. In these circumstances, chronic exposure to excessive levels of atmospheric pollution in the workplace, environment, and home is accompanied by increased oxidative stress. Unhealthy lifestyles, such as poor dietary habits, especially low intake of fresh fruits and vegetables *(5)*, cigarette smoking *(2)*, and in some cases excessive exposure to ultraviolet radiation *(6)*, also accelerate the onset of those degenerative diseases (cataracts, cardiovascular diseases, cancer, pulmonary dysfunction, and emphysema), which have a suspected oxidant-mediated etiology *(1,2)*.

Cigarette smoking is the most common and eminently avoidable cause of lifestyle-related oxidative stress associated with accelerated onset of degenerative disease and premature death. Moreover, the toxicology of cigarette smoke inhalation is probably broadly similar to that of many other inhaled, pro-oxidative irritants. For these reasons I have focused primarily on cigarette smoking to review the relationships that exist among atmospheric pollution, nutrition, and oxidant-mediated diseases.

2. CIGARETTE SMOKING

The magnitude of the ongoing, and apparently increasing, threat posed to public health by cigarette smoking is emphasized by the following recently published comment *(7)*.

> *Smoking represents a great failure in public health; more than 40 years after the hazards were first established, cigarettes are still responsible for 30% of deaths in middle age in Britain and the United States, and worldwide sales are increasing (7).*

From: *Preventive Nutrition: The Comprehensive Guide for Health Professionals*
Edited by A. Bendich and R. J. Deckelbaum Humana Press Inc., Totowa, NJ

This statement is based on data derived from an epidemiological study designed to investigate mortality in relation to smoking over a 40-yr period in male British doctors *(8)*. Alarmingly, the results of this study demonstrate that the hazards of long-term use of tobacco were substantially underestimated in previous studies conducted over shorter periods; a revised estimate is that about half of all regular cigarette smokers will eventually be killed by their habit *(8)*. The average decrease in life expectancy of smokers relative to nonsmokers is 8 yr *(8)*. If current smoking trends persist, it is predicted that smoking will be one of the largest causes of premature death in the world *(7)*.

2.1. Origins of Oxidants During Smoke Exposure

There are two major sources of oxidative stress in smoke-exposed individuals. First, the gas and tar phases of cigarette smoke contain extremely high levels of organic radicals, the respective, approximate concentrations being 10^{15}/puff and 10^{17}/g. Secondly, inhalation of cigarette smoke has a profoundly irritant effect on the phagocytic cells of the immune system, causing an increase in both the numbers and oxidant-generating activities of these cells *(9–12)*. Consequently, chronic exposure of the smoker to high levels of reactive oxidants is accompanied by an increased risk of oxidant-mediated diseases. These events are summarized in Fig. 1.

2.2. Proinflammatory Effects of Cigarette Smoking

Cigarette smoking causes an acute localized inflammatory reaction that is characterized by the accumulation of phagocytes (neutrophils and macrophages) in the membranous bronchioles and alveoli of the lungs, leading to destruction of the peribronchiolar alveolar attachments and pulmonary dysfunction *(13,14)*. These inflammatory events are not confined to the lung, however, and systemic, proinflammatory effects of cigarette smoking have also been demonstrated in numerous studies. Compared to nonsmokers, cigarette smokers have significantly increased circulating leukocyte counts, which are inversely correlated with the degree of airflow limitation *(9,15)*. In addition, the decline in forced expiratory flow in 1 s (FEV_1), an important measure of pulmonary function, is inversely correlated with both the initial peripheral leukocyte count *(16)* and the change in leukocyte count over time, independently of the smoking habit *(17)*. The normal tempo of neutrophil production in the bone marrow is about $0.5–1.5 \times 10^9$/kg of body weight daily. These short-lived phagocytes are released into the circulation and account for up to 70% of the circulating leukocyte population. The normal range for circulating leukocyte counts in apparently healthy adult humans is $4–11 \times 10^6$ per mL of blood, which is an underestimation since approx 50% of the circulating neutrophil pool is adherent to vascular endothelium. On average, cigarette smoking increases the numbers of circulating leukocytes (mainly neutrophils and monocytes) by 20–30%, but in some cases the increase may exceed 100%. Cigarette smoking not only increases the numbers of circulating and pulmonary phagocytes, but also enhances the pro-oxidative and adhesive properties of these cells. Phagocytes from cigarette smokers are sensitized for increased production of reactive oxidants *(11,12,18)*, which is attributable, at least in part, to increased content of the pro-oxidative enzyme myeloperoxidase (MPO) *(19)* and is closely correlated with the degree of pulmonary dysfunction *(20)*. Cigarette smoke-mediated activation of neutrophils in vivo causes delayed transit of these cells through the pulmonary microcirculation *(21,22)*, which is probably because of oxidant-mediated adhesion of these cells to vascular endothelium *(23,24)*, altered

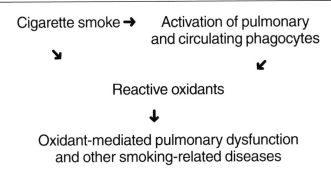

Fig. 1. Events leading to pulmonary dysfunction in smokers.

Table 1
Mechanisms Involved in the Etiology of Oxidant-Mediated Disorders

Disease	Pro-oxidative mechanism
Cancer	Oxidative damage to DNA Inactivation of DNA repair enzymes
Pulmonary emphysema and tissue damage in autoimmune diseases, such as rheumatoid arthritis	Potentiation of the proteolytic activity of phagocyte-derived proteases
Cardiovascular disease	Oxidative modification of LDL Adhesion of phagocytes to vascular endothelium
Acquired immunosuppression	Oxidative inactivation of the protective activities of B- and T-lymphocytes, as well as NK cells

expression of cellular adhesion molecules *(25)*, intravascular aggregation of neutrophils and platelets *(23,26)*, and increased release of MPO and elastase *(22,27)*.

3. HARMFUL ACTIVITIES OF OXIDANTS

Phagocyte-derived reactive oxidants, as well as those present in cigarette smoke, have a range of harmful activities. These oxidants have been reported to be cytotoxic for a wide variety of eukaryotic cells *(28,29)* and are also immunosuppressive, carcinogenic, proproteolytic, proadhesive, and proatherogenic. The biochemical mechanisms involved in the etiology of oxidant-mediated disorders are summarized in Table 1. Although the relative contributions of oxidants derived directly from cigarette smoke and those from smoke-activated phagocytes to the oxidative events involved in the pathogenesis of smoking-related diseases are unknown, the combined assault from these two sources is unremitting and difficult to counteract.

3.1. Oxidants as Carcinogens

Given the complexity and range of reactive oxidants that it contains, it is hardly surprising that several pro-oxidative mechanisms have been proposed to account for the observed direct DNA-damaging effects of cigarette smoke *(2,29,30)*. Polyhydroxy aromatic compounds present in tar have been proposed to bind to the genetic material, leading to generation of hydrogen peroxide (H_2O_2), which in turn causes DNA strand breaks by a hydroxyl radical ($\cdot OH$)-dependent mechanism *(30)*.

The association among chronic inflammation, phagocyte-derived oxidants, and development of epithelial cancers is well-recognized *(31)*. Activated phagocyte products have been identified as potential carcinogens since they oxidatively damage DNA and promote malignant transformation in bystander cells in tissue culture *(22)*. Hydrogen peroxide is the oxidant primarily responsible for phagocyte-mediated DNA damage to neighboring cells. This permeant oxidant interacts with intracellular transition metals to generate $\cdot OH$ in close proximity to DNA, leading to oxidative damage to adenine, guanine, thymine, and cytosine, and DNA strand breaks *(31)*. Although DNA damage in living cells is subject to cellular repair, it may occasionally escape repair, or repair may be incorrect. In such cases unrepaired or misrepaired DNA could have deleterious consequences, leading to gene modifications that may ultimately promote cellular transformation *(32)*. Ominously, it has also been reported that the permeant, phagocyte-derived reactive oxidant, hypochlorous acid (HOCl), oxidatively inactivates the DNA repair enzyme poly(ADP ribose)polymerase in bystander cells exposed to activated neutrophils *(33)*, indicating that phagocyte-derived oxidants not only damage DNA, but also compromise DNA repair mechanisms (*see* Chapter 20).

3.2. Proteolytic Activities of Oxidants

Reactive oxidants present in cigarette smoke, as well as those released by activated phagocytes, have been reported to potentiate the activity of neutrophil-derived proteolytic enzymes. Neutrophil granules contain a large family of over 20 enzymes, but four proteolytic enzymes, the neutral serine proteases, elastase and proteinase 3, and the two metalloproteinases, collagenase and gelatinase, seem to have the greatest potential to act as mediators of tissue injury *(34)*. These proteases are released extracellularly by activated neutrophils *(27)*, and each cleaves key components of the extracellular matrix, which is composed of a complex mix of collagens, elastin, proteoglycans, and glycoproteins that lies under epithelia and surrounds connective tissue cells *(34)*. Extracellular release of proteases and generation of reactive oxidants by activated neutrophils are concomitant and interrelated events. Reactive oxidants, especially phagocyte-derived HOCl *(34)*, as well as poorly defined oxidants present in cigarette smoke *(2)*, dramatically potentiate the proteolytic activity of these neutrophil proteases by direct and indirect mechanisms. In the case of elastase and proteinase 3, HOCl and cigarette smoke promote the oxidative inactivation of α-1-protease inhibitor (API), the major plasma and tissue inhibitor of these enzymes. Collagenase and gelatinase, on the other hand, are secreted in a latent form by neutrophils and undergo oxidative activation on exposure to HOCl *(34,35)*. When oxidatively activated, collagenase and gelatinase potentiate the activity of elastase and proteinase 3 by cleaving API within its active site loop, causing irreversible inactivation of this protease inhibitor *(34,35)*. The consequence is uncontrolled elastolysis in the lungs of cigarette smokers, leading to pulmonary dysfunction and emphysema.

3.3. Pro-Atherogenic Properties of Oxidants

Reactive oxidants are thought to be intimately involved in the pathogenesis of atherosclerosis by promoting oxidative modification of low density lipoproteins (LDLs), which then accumulate in the arterial intima and appear to be the major contributors to the formation of the atherosclerotic lesion *(36)*. Oxidized LDLs are selectively chemotactic for monocytes/macrophages and, unlike native LDLs, are taken up by these cells, resulting in the formation of cytokine-producing foam cells *(36)*. Interestingly, oxidized LDL has recently been described to be immunogenic, initiating the formation of autoantibodies against neo-epitopes on the oxidatively modified molecule *(36,37)*. The nature of the involvement (i.e., primary or secondary) of these autoantibodies in the etiology and progression of atherosclerosis remains to be established.

There are several possible mechanisms by which inhalation of cigarette smoke may promote oxidative modification of LDL, including direct oxidation of this molecule by smoke-derived oxidants. Since plasma contains high concentrations of antioxidants, however, it seems improbable that meaningful oxidation of LDL would occur in the circulation. Alternatively, cigarette smoking may predispose to atherosclerosis as a secondary consequence of accelerated consumption of circulating nutritional antioxidants, such as ascorbate and β-carotene, rendering LDL vulnerable to phagocyte- and endothelial cell-derived reactive oxidants as it passes through the artery wall *(36,38)* (*see* Chapter 9).

3.4. Proadhesive Activity of Oxidants

Exposure of vascular endothelium to superoxide (O_2^-) • or H_2O_2 in vitro induces prolonged expression of the adhesion molecules P- and E-selectins on endothelial cells with resultant adherence of neutrophils *(36,37)*. Oxidant-mediated activation of neutrophil adhesion to vascular endothelium is probably intimately involved in the pathogenesis of postischemic vascular injury. In this setting, however, the proadhesive oxidants originate primarily from the endothelial cells. Ischemia and hypoxia promote the proteolytic conversion of xanthine dehydrogenase to the superoxide-generating enzyme xanthine oxidase in endothelial cells. Subsequent activation of this enzyme during reperfusion/reoxygenation leads to generation of O_2^- • and H_2O_2:

$$\text{xanthine} \xrightarrow{\textit{xanthine oxidase}} \text{urate} + O_2^- \bullet \tag{1}$$

These oxidants (O_2^- and H_2O_2) not only cause direct vascular injury, but also upregulate expression of P- and E-selectins on vascular endothelium, leading to adherence and activation of neutrophils, which contribute to vascular damage by pro-oxidative mechanisms. These events may explain the involvement of neutrophils in the exacerbation of myocardial damage that accompanies restoration of circulation and reoxygenation during the postinfarct period.

An additional mechanism of oxidant-mediated proadhesive activity has recently been described in smoke-exposed rodents. Using a dorsal skinfold chamber combined with intravital fluorescence microscopy to study the microcirculation in fine striated skin muscle, Lehr and colleagues have demonstrated that exposure of hamsters to cigarette smoke results in rapid adhesion of leukocytes to the endothelium of postcapillary venules and aterioles, as well as the formation of intravascular aggregates of leukocytes and platelets *(8)*. Although the exact mechanisms of these smoke-induced adhesive interactions between circulating leukocytes and vascular endothelium were not established, it was suggested that reactive oxidants present in cigarette smoke may upregulate expression of P-selectin on endothelial cells *(8)*. These proadhesive events are probably mechanistically involved in the etiology of smoking-related pulmonary and cardiovascular diseases.

3.5. Immunosuppressive Properties of Oxidants

Reactive oxidants are also potent antiproliferative agents. Permeant oxidants, such as H_2O_2 and HOCl, inhibit the proliferative activity and functions of B-lymphocytes, T-lymphocytes, and natural killer (NK) cells in vitro, probably by interfering with the activity of several enzymes involved in cellular energy metabolism *(39,40)*. Smoking-related pro-oxidative events may compromise pulmonary defense mechanisms since smokers have decreased antibody responses to inhaled microbial antigens *(41)* as well as abnormal NK function *(42)*. However, the precise mechanisms and relative contributions of smoke- and phagocyte-derived oxidants to smoking-related immunosuppression remain to be established.

4. ANTIOXIDANT NUTRIENTS AND SMOKING-RELATED DISEASES

It is abundantly clear that radical and nonradical reactive oxidants are intimately involved in the etiology of smoking-related pulmonary dysfunction, bronchial carcinoma, and cardiovascular disorders. The rate at which these diseases develop in individual smokers probably involves a dynamic interplay between oxidants and other toxins present in cigarette smoke, the numbers and pro-oxidative activities of circulating and resident pulmonary phagocytes, and the efficiency of the smoker's antioxidant defenses.

Smoking-induced oxidative stress is associated with increased turnover of the antioxidative nutrients vitamin C *(43)*, β-carotene *(44)*, and vitamin E *(45)* in the circulation and lungs, and with activation of genes encoding antioxidant enzymes in the lungs of cigarette smokers *(46)*. Oral administration of combinations of vitamin C, vitamin E, and β-carotene to cigarette smokers pre-empts the activation of genes coding for the antioxidant enzymes glutathione peroxidase and superoxide dismutase in bronchoalveolar lavage cells, suggesting that inadequate intake of these nutrients may be a determinant of susceptibility to development of smoking-related diseases.

4.1. Vitamin C

The negative impact of cigarette smoking on plasma vitamin C levels is well-recognized *(43)* and because of, at least in part, increased turnover of the vitamin, explains the observed dose-response relationship between cigarettes smoked per day and the decline in plasma vitamin C *(46,47)*. Neutralization of oxidants present in cigarette smoke *(43)*, as well as those released by smoke-activated phagocytes *(48)*, are the probable mechanisms of accelerated consumption of the vitamin. Since vitamin C has been demonstrated to protect α-1-protease inhibitor against oxidative inactivation by both cigarette smoke *(49)* and activated phagocytes *(50)* in vitro, and to prevent activation of latent metalloproteinases *(51)*, as well as cigarette smoke-mediated adhesion of leukocytes to vascular endothelium in hamsters *(23)*, this vitamin is probably critically involved in protecting the lungs against oxidant-inflicted damage and dysfunction. Indeed, data from a recently published epidemiological study have highlighted a clear and significant positive correlation between dietary intake of vitamin C and pulmonary competence *(52)*. Interestingly and importantly, the association between vitamin C and pulmonary function persisted after adjustment for cigarette smoking, indicating that this protective activity of the vitamin is not limited to smoke-mediated oxidative stress *(52)*.

4.2. Vitamin E and β-Carotene

Vitamin E has also been reported to regulate both the production and reactivity of ROS by activated neutrophils in vitro and ex vivo *(53–55)*, whereas β-carotene is a scavenger of phagocyte-derived singlet oxygen *(56)* and HOCl *(54)*. Neither of these antioxidants, however, appears to be an efficient scavenger of smoke-derived oxidants *(38)*. Nevertheless, dietary intake of vitamin E and β-carotene, like that of vitamin C, may be a determinant of pulmonary competence in cigarette smokers by protecting the lungs against the destructive effects of smoke-activated phagocytes. This contention is supported by data from a recently conducted study that described significant positive correlations between plasma levels of β-carotene and several spirometric parameters in asymptomatic, male cigarette smokers, but not in nonsmokers *(57)*.

Distinct relationships between plasma levels of vitamin E and pulmonary function have also been reported in both smokers and nonsmokers *(58)*. In nonsmoking males plasma vitamin E was positively and significantly correlated with pulmonary competence, whereas, somewhat surprisingly, inverse correlations were observed between these parameters in a matched group of cigarette smokers *(58)*. It was proposed that in the physiological setting, typified by nonsmokers, maintenance of vitamin E homeostasis is probably adequate to protect the lungs against routine, environmental, and endogenous oxidative stress, accounting for the positive relationship with pulmonary function. However, sustained and excessive oxidative stress may necessitate mobilization of tissue stores of the vitamin and diversion to the lungs, which would explain the apparent inverse association between plasma vitamin E and pulmonary competence in smokers *(58)*. This type of mobilization of vitamin E to the lungs has been described in rats experimentally exposed to cigarette smoke *(59)* and ozone *(60)*.

4.3. Antioxidant Nutrients and Cardiovascular Disease

An association between adequate dietary intake of β-carotene and the antioxidant vitamins, particularly vitamin E, and reduced incidence of, and mortality from, cardiovascular disease, has been demonstrated in a number of large epidemiological studies *(61–64)*. Although smoking has been identified as a major risk for development of cardiovascular disease, these associations persisted after adjustment for smoking status, demonstrating the predisposing role of additional factors, especially low dietary intake of these antioxidant nutrients. Moreover, physiologic levels of vitamin C have been reported to inhibit the oxidative modification of LDL in vitro *(65)*, whereas short-term oral administration of relatively high doses of this vitamin or of vitamin E prevent *(66)* or retard *(36)* peroxidative alteration of LDL ex vivo. Identification of autoantibodies to oxidized LDL in individuals with atherosclerosis and the possible involvement of these in the etiology of this condition *(67a)* suggests that antioxidant nutrient status may determine the susceptibility of LDL to oxidative, autoantigenic modification. In support of this, we have recently detected increased levels of circulating autoantibodies to both oxidized LDL and cardiolipin in asymptomatic cigarette smokers aged over 30 yr. The levels of these autoantibodies were significantly and inversely correlated with plasma levels of vitamin C, indicating that intake of this antioxidant nutrient may be a determinant of development of atheresclerosis in smokers *(67b)*.

4.4. Antioxidant Nutrients and Cancer

Decreased dietary intake and/or accelerated consumption of the antioxidant vitamins and β-carotene during sustained oxidative stress is probably a common cause of cancer *(68)*. Cigarette smoking is the primary cause of lung cancer and is also associated with the development of cancer at several other sites (mouth, larynx, esophagus, bladder, pancreas) *(7)*. Significant inverse correlations between the dietary intake and/or plasma levels of the antioxidant nutrients and development of cancer at various sites have been reported in numerous epidemiological studies. The consistency of these reports in conjunction with corroborative laboratory studies has prompted calls for the implementation of nutrient-based, preventive public health strategies *(5,68)*. These laboratory and epidemiological studies have not, however, been supported by data from some of the recently completed antioxidant nutrient intervention studies *(69,70)*. Although aspects of the design of these intervention studies may have inadvertently obscured the possible preventive effects of vitamin C, vitamin E, and β-carotene, it is clear that definitive answers about the anti-cancer properties of these agents await the outcome of large-scale ongoing studies (*see* Chapter 6).

5. PREDICTORS OF OXIDANT-MEDIATED DISEASE

Although cigarette smoking has been used in this chapter as the prototype cause of lifestyle-related oxidative stress, the mechanisms of smoking-associated, oxidant-mediated tissue damage and disease are probably broadly operative in other settings, including environmental and occupational exposure to excessive levels of atmospheric pollution. Even in these settings, however, active *(71)* and passive *(72)* exposure to cigarette smoke may often be the primary offender.

Interestingly, the inverse relationships between dietary intake and/or plasma levels of the antioxidant nutrients vitamin C, vitamin E, and β-carotene and future development of degenerative disease and cancer described in major epidemiological studies remain after adjustment for smoking history. There must, therefore, be a common mechanism operative in both smokers and nonsmokers, but clearly exacerbated by cigarette smoking, that determines susceptibility to oxidant-mediated disease. This mechanism may involve a dynamic interplay between dietary intake of antioxidant nutrients and the numbers and reactivities of the abundant, highly aggressive, oxidant-generating phagocytic cells of the immune system. Although critically involved in host defense against microbial pathogens, the sheer numbers of these cells and the undiscerning nature of their arsenal of toxic antimicrobial oxidants constitutes an unrelenting threat to other host cells and tissues. Coexistence between the host and the phagocytic cells of his or her immune system is probably fragile and minor imbalances may compromise the containment (damage limitation) functions of vitamin C, vitamin E, and β-carotene, creating the potential hazard of phagocyte-inflicted oxidative damage.

Such imbalances may be caused by several common, often avoidable, aspects of lifestyle that disrupt oxidant/antioxidant homeostasis. Poor dietary habits may impair antioxidant defenses through decreased intake of the antioxidant vitamins and β-carotene, whereas cigarette smoking, occupational and environmental atmospheric pollution, as well as excessive exposure to ultraviolet radiation *(6)* may cause a futile, potentially harmful increase in the numbers and pro-oxidative activities of resident and circulating phagocytes.

5.1. Phagocytes, Antioxidants, and Degenerative Disorders

The health threat posed by sustained, relatively moderate increases in the numbers of circulating phagocytes is emphasized by evidence from numerous epidemiological studies that have consistently shown that the circulating leukocyte count, and the neutrophil count in particular, measured well before the onset of manifest clinical disease is an *independent* predictor of decline in pulmonary function *(17)*, development of several cardiovascular conditions, including myocardial infarction, sudden cardiac death, all coronary heart disease (CHD) combined, stroke and essential hypertension *(73–75)*, as well as lung cancer incidence and mortality, possibly cancer at all sites *(76,77)*, and death from all causes *(78)*. For each decrease in the circulating leukocyte count of 1000/mL blood, the risk of CHD death decreased by 14% *(73)*, whereas the relative odds for a 2000/mL difference in leukocyte count for development of lung cancer ranged from 1.20–1.58 in three different populations *(76)*. The circulating leukocyte count was found to be superior to systolic blood pressure, cholesterol levels, and smoking history, and second only to age as a predictor of mortality *(78)*. It must be emphasized that the increments in circulating leukocyte counts that seemingly predispose to degenerative disease and cancer are relatively modest, being within the normal range for apparently healthy adults.

It is interesting, and probably not coincidental, that clinical disorders for which elevated circulating leukocyte counts are predictive are essentially the same as those that have been demonstrated in epidemiological studies to be associated with decreased dietary intake and/or plasma levels of the antioxidant nutrients. This implied mechanistic relationship by which sustained, albeit modest, increases in the numbers and pro-oxidative activities of circulating leukocytes cause depletion of nutritional antioxidants and accelerated onset of degenerative diseases and cancer, as well as decline in pulmonary function, remains to be established. Nevertheless, such a relationship is supported by recent observations that plasma levels of vitamin C are inversely related to circulating total leukocyte and neutrophil counts in smokers and nonsmokers, and positively correlated with plasma vitamin E *(48)*. Plasma levels of β-carotene have been reported to correlate inversely with circulating neutrophil counts in young, asymptomatic cigarette smokers, but not in nonsmokers *(79)*.

In the setting of sustained increases in the circulating leukocyte count, chronic, excessive production of reactive oxidants by phagocytes may be linked to pulmonary and cardiovascular damage, as well as carcinogenesis. Increased destruction of antioxidants as a result of elevated numbers and activities of leukocytes may also increase the vulnerability of LDL and DNA to oxidative damage by other cell types simply by depleting blood and tissues of these protective agents. The circulating leukocyte count, which has surprising predictive power for future development of degenerative diseases and cancer, may, therefore, be a primary determinant of optimum intake of antioxidant nutrients.

6. CIRCULATING LEUKOCYTE COUNTS AND RECOMMENDED DAILY INTAKE OF VITAMINS C AND E AND β-CAROTENE

The proposed dynamic, inverse association between the levels of the antioxidant nutrients and the circulating leukocyte count remains to be conclusively established. However, if the relationship is substantiated, it may be possible to use the circulating leukocyte count to formulate optimum intakes of vitamin C, vitamin E, and β-carotene. We have used data from a recently completed study conducted on asymptomatic, young male cigarette smokers to calculate "optimum" daily intake of these antioxidant nutrients based on the numbers and pro-oxidative activities of circulating leukocytes. The average increase in the circulating leukocyte count of smokers in our study was 2×10^6/mL (6.2×10^6/mL and 8.2×10^6/mL for 85 male nonsmokers and 100 age- and sex-matched cigarette smokers, respectively). The average increase in the smoking-related, phagocyte-mediated oxidant burden was calculated to be 71% (because of increased numbers and pro-oxidative activities of circulating leukocytes). Based on this increase in the oxidant burden and on RDAs of 60 and 15 mg/d for vitamin C and vitamin E, respectively, and a proposed intake of 6 mg/d for β-carotene, the estimated increases in the daily intakes (above the RDA levels) for each increment of 1×10^6/mL in the circulating leukocyte count above 6.2×10^6/mL are 20 mg vitamin C, 5 mg vitamin E, and 2 mg β-carotene. Given that the upper limit of the normal range for circulating leukocyte counts for apparently healthy adult humans is approx 11×10^6/mL, the estimated daily intakes of the antioxidant nutrients required to protect *all* individuals with leukocyte counts less than or equal to this value are 160, 40, and 16 mg for vitamin C, vitamin E, and β-carotene respectively. Admittedly there are several flaws in the calculation, such as: it is based on RDAs that may or may not be optimal, in vitro activation of phagocytes may not be representative of the in vivo situation, and it may not be necessary to increase the daily intake of all three antioxidants proportionately. In spite of these limitations, however, it is noteworthy that these values are in good agreement with intake estimates based on data from metabolic *(80)*, experimental *(8)*, and epidemiological studies *(43)*.

7. CONCLUSIONS

Lipoproteins and extracellular matrix proteins, such as elastin, and many cellular molecules, including DNA, membrane lipids, and enzymes involved in DNA repair and energy production, are extremely vulnerable to oxidant-mediated damage. Certain avoidable and unavoidable aspects of lifestyle, because they are associated with accelerated destruction and/or decreased intake of antioxidant nutrients, may, therefore, predispose to development of acquired immune dysfunction, cancer, and degenerative diseases, such as atherosclerosis, cataracts, and pulmonary emphysema.

8. RECOMMENDATIONS

Avoidance of unhealthy aspects of lifestyle, such as low intake of fresh fruits and vegetables, cigarette smoking, and excessive exposure to sunlight, are essential for maintenance of antioxidant homeostasis and prevention of oxidant-mediated diseases. Since even in affluent societies some of these objectives are difficult to achieve *(82)*, modest supplementation with antioxidant nutrients represents a potentially efficient and inexpensive strategy to counteract the potential threat of oxidant-inflicted diseases. Daily intakes of about 200 mg, 40 mg, and 6–16 mg of vitamin C, vitamin E, and β-carotene, respectively, would seem appropriate.

REFERENCES

1. Fulton M, Thomson M, Elton RA, Brown S, Wood DA, Oliver MF. Cigarette smoking, social class and nutrient intake: relevance to coronary heart disease. Eur J Clin Nutr 1988; 42:797–803.

2. Pryor WA, Stone K. Oxidants in cigarette smoke. Ann NY Acad Sci 1993; 686:12–28.

3. Godlee R. Air pollution I. From pea soup to photochemical smog. Br Med J 1991; 303:1459–1461.

4. Melia RJ, Florey C de V, Altman DG, Swan AV. Association between gas cooking and respiratory disease in children. Br Med J 1977; 2:149–152.

5. Block G. Micronutrients and cancer: time for action? J Natl Cancer Inst USA 1993; 85:846–848.

6. Savage JE, Theron AJ, Anderson R. Activation of neutrophil membrane-associated oxidative metabolism by ultraviolet radiation. J Invest Dermatol 1993; 101:532–536.

7. Peto R. Smoking and death: the past 40 years and the next 40. Br Med J 1994; 309:937–939.

8. Doll R, Peto R, Wheatley K, Gray R, Sutherland I. Mortality in relation to smoking: 40 years' observations on male British doctors. Br Med J 1994; 309:901–911.

9. Corré F, Lellouch J, Schwartz D. Smoking and leucocyte counts. Lancet 1971; 2:632–634.

10. Hoidal JR, Niewoehner DE. Lung Phagocyte recruitment and metabolic deterioration induced by cigarette smoke in humans and hamsters. Am Rev Resp Dis 1982; 126:548–552.

11. Anderson R, Rabson AR, Sher R, Koornhof HJ. The NBT test in cigarette smokers. Am J Clin Pathol 1974; 61:879.

12. Hoidal JR, Fox RB, Lemarbe PA, Perri R, Repine JE. Altered oxidative metabolic responses *in vivo* of alveolar macrophages from asymptomatic cigarette smokers. Am Rev Respir Dis 1981; 123:85–87.

13. Wright JL, Hobson JE, Wiggs B, Pare PD, Hogg JC. Airway inflammation and peribronchiolar attachments in the lungs of non-smokers, current and ex-smokers. Lung 1988; 166:277–286.

14. Ludwig PW, Schwartz BA, Hoidal JR, Niewoehner DE. Cigarette smoking causes accumulation of polymorphonuclear leukocytes in alveolar septum. Am Rev Respir Dis 1985; 131:828–830.

15. Chan-Yeung M, Dy Buncio A. Leukocyte count, smoking and lung function. Am J Med 1984; 76:31–37.

16. Chan-Yeung M, Abbound R, Dy Buncio A, Vedal S. Peripheral leukocyte count and longitudinal decline in lung function. Thorax 1988; 43:462–466.

17. Sparrow D, Glynn RJ, Cohen M, Weiss ST. The relationship of the peripheral leukocyte count and cigarette smoking to pulmonary function among adult men. Chest 1984; 86:383–386.

18. Ludwig RW, Hoidal JR. Alterations in leukocyte oxidative metabolism in cigarette smokers. Am Rev Respir Dis 1982; 126:977–980.

19. Bridges RB, Fu MC, Rehm SR. Increased neutrophil myeloperoxidase activity associated with cigarette smoking. Eur J Resp Dis 1985; 67:84–93.

20. Richards GA, Theron AJ, Van der Merwe CA, Anderson R. Spirometric abnormalities in young smokers correlate with increased chemiluminescence responses of activated blood phagocytes. Am Rev Respir Dis 1989; 139:181–187.

21. MacNee W, Wiggs B, Belzberb AS, Hogg JC. The effect of cigarette smoking on neutrophil kinetics in human lungs. New Engl J Med 1989; 321:924–928.

22. Bosken CH, Doerschuk CM, English D, Hogg JC. Neutrophil kinetics during active cigarette smoking in rabbits. J Appl Physiol 1991; 71:630–637.

23. Lehr H-A, Frei B, Arfors KE. Vitamin C prevents cigarette smoke-induced leukocyte aggregation and adhesion to endothelium *in vivo*. Proc Natl Acad Sci USA 1994; 91:7688–7692.

24. Lehr H-A, Kress E, Menger MD, et al. Cigarette smoke elicits leukocyte adhesion to endothelium in hamsters: inhibition by Cu-Zn SOD. Free Radic Biol Med 1993; 14:573–581.

25. Klut ME, Doerschuk CM, Van Eeden SF, Burns AR, Hogg JC. Activation of neutrophils within pulmonary microvessels of rabbits exposed to cigarette smoke. Am J Resp Cell Mol Biol 1993; 9:82–89.

26. Bridges AB, Hill A, Belch JJF. Cigarette smoking increases white blood cell aggregation in whole blood. J Royal Soc Med 1993; 86:139–141.

27. Hind CRK, Joyce H, Tennent GA, Pepys MB, Pride NB. Plasma leucocyte elastase concentrations in smokers. J Clin Pathol 1991; 44:232–235.

28. Babior BM. Oxidants from phagocytes: agents of defense and destruction. Blood 1984; 64:959–964.

29. Leanderson P. Cigarette smoke-induced DNA damage in cultured human lung cells. Ann NY Acad Sci 1993; 686:249–261.

30. Borish ET, Cosgrove JP, Church DF, Deutsch WA, Pryor WA. Cigarette tar causes single strand breaks in DNA. Biochem Biophys Res Comm 1985; 133:780–786.

31. Weitzman SA, Gordon LI. Inflammation and cancer: role of phagocyte-generated oxidants in carcinogenesis. Blood 1990; 76:655–663.

32. Jackson JH, Gajewski E, Schraufstatter U, et al. Damage to the bases in DNA induced by stimulated human neutrophils. J Clin Invest 1989; 84:1644–1649.

33. Van Rensburg CEJ, Van Staden AM, Anderson R. Inactivation of poly(ADP-ribose)polymerase by hypochlorous acid. Free Radic Biol Med 1991; 11:285–291.

34. Weiss SJ. Tissue destruction by neutrophils. New Engl J Med 1989; 320:365–376.

35. Desrochers PE, Mookhtiar K, Van Wart HE, Hasty KA, Weiss SJ. Proteolytic inactivation of α_1-proteinase inhibitor and α_1-chymotrypsin by oxidatively activated human neutrophil metalloproteinases. J Biol Chem 1992; 267: 5005–5012.

36. Witztum JL. The oxidation hypothesis of atherosclerosis. Lancet 1994; 344:793–795.

37. Lopes-Virella MF, Virella G. Atherosclerosis and autoimmunity. Clin Immunol Immunopathol 1994; 73:155–167.

38. Cross CE, O'Neill CA, Reznick AZ, et al. Cigarette smoke oxidation of human plasma constituents. Ann NY Acad Sci 1993; 686:72–90.

39. El-Hag A, Lipsky PE, Bennett M, Clark RA. Immunomodulation by neutrophil meyloperoxidase and hydrogen peroxide: differential susceptibility of human lymphocyte functions. J Immunol 1987; 139:2406–2413.

40. Anderson R, Smit MJ, Jooné GK, Van Staden AM. Vitamin C and cellular immune functions: protection against hypochlorous acid-mediated inactivation of glyceraldehyde-3-phosphate dehydrogenase and ATP generation in human leukocytes as a possible mechanism of ascorbate-mediated immunostimulation. Ann NY Acad Sci 1990; 587:34–48.

41. McSharry C, Wilkinson PC. Cigarette smoking and the antibody response to inhaled antigens. Immunol Today 1986; 7:98.

42. Ferson M, Edwards A, Lind A, Milton GW, Hersey P. Low natural killer cell activity and immunoglobulin levels associated with smoking in human subjects. Int J Cancer 1979; 23:603–609.

43. Schectman G. Estimating ascorbic acid requirements for cigarette smokers. Ann NY Acad Sci 1993; 686:335–346.

44. Bridges RB, Chow CK, Rehm SR. Micronutrient status and immune function in smokers. Ann NY Acad Sci 1990; 587:218–231.

45. Pacht ER, Kaseki H, Mohammed JR, Cornwell DG, Davis WB. Deficiency of vitamin E in the alveolar fluid of cigarette smokers. J Clin Invest 1986; 77:789–796.

46. Tribble DL, Guiliano L, Fortmann SP. Reduced plasma ascorbic acid concentrations in nonsmokers regularly exposed to environmental tobacco smoke. Am J Clin Nutr 1993; 58:886–890.

47. Van Antwerpen VL, Theron AJ, Richards GA, Anderson R. Plasma vitamin C in male smokers. J Smoking-Related Dis 1994; 5:167–170.

48. Van Antwerpen VL, Theron AJ, Myer MS, et al. Cigarette smoke-mediated oxidative stress, phagocytes, vitamin C, vitamin E and tissue injury. Ann NY Acad Sci 1993; 686:53–65.

49. Pryor WA, Dooley MM. Inactivation of human alpha-1-proteinase inhibitor by cigarette smoke: effect of smoke phase and buffer. Am Rev Resp Dis 1983; 131:941–943.

50. Theron AJ, Anderson R. Investigation of the protective effects of the anti-oxidants ascorbate, cysteine and dapsone on the phagocyte-mediated oxidative inactivation of human alpha-1-protease inhibitor in vitro. Am Rev Respir Dis 1985; 132:1049–1054.

51. Suomalainen K, Sorsa T, Lindy O, Saari H, Konttinen YT, Uitto VJ. Hypochlorous acid activation of human neutrophil and gingival crevicular fluid collagenase can be inhibited by ascorbate. Scand J Dent Res 1991; 99:397–405.

52. Schwartz J, Weiss ST. Relationship between dietary vitamin C and pulmonary function in the First National Health and Nutrition Examination Survey (NHANES 1). Am J Clin Nutr 1994; 59:110–114.

53. Baehner RL, Boxer LA, Ingraham LM, Buetterick C, Haak RA. The influence of vitamin E on human polymorphonuclear cell metabolism and function. Ann NY Acad Sci 1982; 293:237–250.

54. Richards GA, Theron AJ, Van Rensburg CEJ, et al. Investigation of the effects of oral administration of vitamin E and beta-carotene on the chemiluminescence responses and the frequency of sister chromatid exchanges in circulating leukocytes from cigarette smokers. Am Rev Resp Dis 1990; 142:648–654.

55. Anderson R, Theron AJ, Myer MS, Richards GA, Savage JE. Vitamin E is a potent inhibitor of superoxide generation by neutrophils activated with soluble, but not particulate stimuli of membrane-associated oxidative metabolism. J Nutr Immunol 1992; 1:43–63.

56. Steinbeck MJ, Khan AU, Karnovsky MJ. Intracellular singlet oxygen generation by phagocytosing neutrophils in response to particles coated with a chemical trap. J Biol Chem 1992; 267:13,425–13,433.

57. Van Antwerpen VL, Theron AJ, Richards GA, Van der Merwe CA, Van der Walt R, Anderson R. Relationship between the plasma levels of beta-carotene and lung functions in cigarette smokers. Int J Vit Nutr Res 1995; 65:231–235.

58. Van Antwerpen VL, Theron AJ, Richards CA, et al. Vitamin E, pulmonary functions and phagocyte-mediated oxidative stress in smokers and non-smokers. Free Radic Biol Med 1995; 18:935–941.

59. Chow CK, Airriess GR, Changchit C. Increased vitamin E content in the lungs of chronic cigarette-smoked rats. Ann NY Acad Sci 1989; 570:425–427.

60. Elsayed NM. Mobilization of vitamin E to the lung under oxidative stress. Ann NY Acad Sci 1989; 570:439,440.

61. Trout DL. Vitamin C and cardiovascular risk factors. Am J Clin Nutr 1991; 53:322S–325S.

62. Hallfrisch J, Singh VN, Muller DC, Baldwin H, Bannon ME, Andres R. High plasma vitamin C associated with high plasma HDL- and HDL_2 cholesterol. Am J Clin Nutr 1994; 60:100–105.

63. Gey KF, Puska P, Jordan P, Moser UK. Inverse correlation between plasma vitamin E and mortality from ischemic heart disease in cross-cultural epidemiology. Am J Clin Nutr 1991; 53:326S–334S.

64. Riemersma RA, Wood DA, MacIntyre CCA, Elton RA, Gey KF, Oliver MF. Risk of angina pectoris and plasma concentrations of vitamins A, C and E and carotene. Lancet 1991; 337:1–5.

65. Jailal I, Veg GL, Grundy SM. Physiologic levels of ascorbate inhibit the oxidative modification of low density lipoprotein. Atherosclerosis 1990; 82:185–191.

66. Harats D, Ben-Naim M, Dabach Y, et al. Effect of vitamin C and vitamin E supplementation on susceptibility of plasma lipoproteins to peroxidation induced by acute smoking. Atherosclerosis 1990; 85:47–54.

67a. Salonen JT, Ylä-Herttuala S, Yamamoto R, et al. Autoantibody against oxidised LDL and progression of carotid atherosclerosis. Lancet 1992; 339:883–887.

67b. Fickl H, Van Antwerpen VL, Richards GA, Van der Westhuyzen DR, Davies N, Van der Walt R, Van der Merwe CA, Anderson R. Increased levels of autoantibodies to cardiolipin and oxidised low density lipoprotein are inversely associated with plasma vitamim C in cigarette smokers. Atherosclerosis 1996; 124:75–81.

68. Packer L. Health effects of nutritional antioxidants. Free Radic Biol Med 1993; 15:685–686.

69. The Alpha-Tocopherol and Beta-Carotene Cancer Prevention Study Group. The effect of vitamin E and beta-carotene on the incidence of lung cancer and other cancers in male smokers. New Engl J Med 1994; 330:1029–1035.

70. Greenberg ER, Baron JA, Tosteson TD, et al. A clinical trial of antioxidant vitamins to prevent colorectal adenoma. New Engl J Med 1994; 331:141–147.

71. Theron AJ, Richards GA, Myer MS, et al. Investigation of the relative contributions of cigarette smoking and mineral dust exposure to activation of circulating phagocytes, alterations in plasma concentrations of vitamin C, vitamin E and beta-carotene, and pulmonary dysfunction in South African gold miners. Occ Environ Med 1994; 51:564–567.

72. Richards GA, Terblanche APS, Theron AJ, et al. Health effects of passive smoking in adolescent children. S Afr Med J 1996; 86:143–147.

73. Grimm RH Jr, Neaton JD, Ludwig W. Prognostic importance of the white blood cell count for coronary, cancer and all-cause mortality. JAMA 1985; 254:1932–1937.

74. Phillips AN, Neaton JD, Cook DG, Grimm RH, Shaper AG. Leukocyte count and risk of major coronary heart disease events. Am J Epidemiol 1992; 136:59–70.

75. Friedman GD, Selby JV, Quesenberry CP Jr. The leukocyte count: a predictor of hypertension. J Clin Epidemiol 1990; 43:907–911.

76. Phillips AN, Neaton JD, Cook DG, Grimm RH, Shaper AG. The leukocyte count and risk of lung cancer. Cancer 1992; 69:680–684.

77. Friedman GD, Fireman BH. The leukocyte count and cancer mortality. Am J Epidemiol 1991; 133:376–380.

78. De Labry LO, Campion EW, Glynn RJ, Vokonas PS. White blood cell count as a predictor of mortality: results over 18 years from the normative aging study. J Clin Epidemiol 1990; 43:153–157.

79. Van Antwerpen VL, Theron AJ, Richards GA, et al. Plasma levels of beta-carotene are inversely correlated with circulating neutrophil counts in young male cigarette smokers. Inflammation 1995; 19:405–414.

80. Kallner AB, Hartmann D, Hornig DH. On the requirements of ascorbic acid in man: steady-state turnover and body pool in smokers. Am J Clin Nutr 1981; 34:1347–1355.

81. Frei B, England L, Ames BN. Ascorbic acid is an outstanding anti-oxidant in blood plasma. Proc Natl Acad Sci USA 1989; 86:6377–6381.

82. Block G. Micronutrients and cancer: time for action? J Natl Cancer Inst (USA) 1993; 85:846–848.

17 Micronutrients and Immunity in Older People

John D. Bogden and Donald B. Louria

1. INTRODUCTION

Aging has been described as a group of processes that promotes vulnerability to challenges, thereby increasing the likelihood of death. Since there is evidence that depressed immunity can increase the risk of death, it is likely that changes in immunity with age are a key factor in the aging process.

There are a considerable number of theories of aging. These include the free-radical, programmed senescence, and immunologic theories *(1,2)*. Evidence for the immunologic theory of aging is based largely on the well-described changes that occur in all species that have been studied, including humans, and on observations from cross-sectional studies that demonstrate an association between maintenance of good immune function and longevity *(1,3)*. A limitation of this theory is that it lacks the universality of other theories, such as the free radical theory of aging, since it is not applicable to lower organisms that do not have well-developed immune systems. Of course, the complexity of aging may require the use of more than one theory to understand it, and the various theories are not necessarily independent of one another. For example, recent evidence demonstrates that antioxidant nutrients that reduce free radical damage can improve immunity in older people *(4)*, suggesting that the free radical and immunologic theories may overlap.

2. IMMUNITY/AGING RELATIONSHIPS

2.1. General Changes in Immunity with Aging

Changes in immunity with aging include inhibited T-lymphocyte functions, decreased antibody production and responses, increased autoimmune activity with compromised self/non-self discrimination, and greater heterogeneity in immunologic responses *(5–7)*. With regard to the latter, depressed T-cell function is the most common and may begin as early as the sixth decade. However, T-cell dysfunction is neither inevitable nor predictable. For example, we *(8)* measured delayed hypersensitivity skin-test responses in 100 people aged 60–89. We found that although 41% were anergic to a panel of seven skin-test antigens and an additional 29% were "relatively anergic," responding to only one of the seven antigens, the remaining 30% were reactive, responding to two or more of the skin-test antigens, often with sizable reactions.

The above general changes in immunity are based on data from numerous studies of

From: *Preventive Nutrition: The Comprehensive Guide for Health Professionals*
Edited by A. Bendich and R. J. Deckelbaum Humana Press Inc., Totowa, NJ

specific aspects or measures of immunity that change with age, including altered lymphocyte subpopulation percentages, thymic involution and decreased thymic hormone concentrations, decreased suppressor activity of T-cells, reduced IL-2 secretion, impaired delayed hypersensitivity responses, decreased in vitro lymphocyte proliferative responses to mitogens, reduced antibody titers after vaccination, increased serum autoantibodies, and increased soluble serum interleukin-2 receptors (sIL-2R) *(9)*.

2.2. Specific Changes in Immunity with Aging

2.2.1. INVOLUTION OF THE THYMUS

The most striking changes in immunity with increasing age are inhibited T-cell functions. These are likely related to the well-known involution of the thymus *(10)*. The differentiation process by which stem cells become T-lymphocytes occurs in this organ. It is a two-lobed structure in mammals, located in the thorax above the heart.

There are several stages in the process by which immature stem cells (pre-T-cells) become mature T-cells. These are migration to the thymus, where some cells are stimulated to grow and others die; differentiation, in which the mature phenotype of T-cells develops in the thymus, including surface expression of accessory molecules; positive selection, in which self major histocompatibility complex (MHC)-restricted T-cells are selected and other cells rejected; and negative selection, which ensures that surviving mature T-cells are self-tolerant. The selective survival or death of cells results in a self-MHC-restricted, self antigen-tolerant, mature T-cell population *(10)*.

The thymus is the principal site of T-cell maturation. Involution with age causes it to be undetectable in people after puberty. Since some maturation of T-cells continues throughout adult life, it is likely that a remnant of the thymus or some other tissue continues to effect T-cell maturation *(10)*. However, since memory T-cells have a long lifespan (20 yr or more) *(10)*, the involution of the thymus does not cause compromised immunity in young adults, but is likely to contribute to depressed immunity as the time since thymic involution becomes longer.

The involution of the thymus prior to the peak reproductive years suggests that this process may provide an evolutionary advantage. One hypothesis is that involution provides a net benefit, since it reduces the danger of autoimmune reactions *(11)*. According to this theory, the increased risk of cancer or infectious diseases as a result of depressed cellular immunity is a detriment that is offset by a reduced risk of autoimmune disease that accompanies thymic involution. Although attractive, this theory of immunologic "trade-offs" as an adaptation to aging requires additional supporting evidence.

An alternative hypothesis has been proposed by Siskind *(12)*, who suggests that adaptation to environmental pathogens occurs early in life, and thereafter relative constancy of immune function rather than adaptability may be most beneficial. He further speculates that efforts to modify cellular immunity in later life, e.g., by pharmacologic or nutritional means, may do more harm than good. Although interesting, this hypothesis is not widely supported and not consistent with the known association between good cellular immunity and reduced morbidity and mortality in older people.

2.2.2. T-LYMPHOCYTE FUNCTIONS

Changes in T-lymphocytes with aging include a shift in relative percentages of subpopulations, and qualitative changes in cell surface receptors of individual cells *(13)*. In comparison to T-cells from younger people, cells of the elderly are deficient in in vitro

Table 1
Some Specific Changes in Immunity with Increased Age

Involution of the thymus
Decreased thymic hormone concentrations
Decreased delayed hypersensitivity skin test responses
Decreased IL-2 secretion
Decreased lymphocyte proliferative responses to mitogens
Lower antibody titers after vaccination
Increased serum autoantibodies
Increased soluble IL-2 receptors
Reduced phagocytosis by polymorphonuclear leukocytes

production of certain T-cell growth factors, such as IL-2, and have a decreased ability to bind and respond to it *(14–17)*. McMurray *(15)* has outlined evidence that implicates nutrient-mediated effects at virtually every step in the development and expression of T-cell immunity, from direct effects on the thymus and thymic hormone production through T-cell maturation and distribution, antigen reactivity, lymphokine production, and even composition of the T-cell membrane.

Delayed hypersensitivity skin test (DHST) responses involve T-lymphocyte proliferation, production of IL-2 and other lymphokines, and infiltration of the test site with mononuclear cells resulting 24–72 h later in induration and erythema; it is the T-cell parameter that is most consistently and profoundly affected by nutritional status *(15)*. Reduced DHST is also the immune parameter most consistently associated in older people with increased infectious disease morbidity and mortality from all causes, as found by Meakins et al. *(18);* and Christou et al. *(19)* for surgery patients; and by Wayne et al. *(20)* and Roberts-Thomson et al. *(21)* for initially healthy people aged 60 or older.

In their investigation, Christou et al. *(19)* studied the relationship between presurgery DHST responses and postsurgical sepsis-related death in 245 subjects with a median age of 67 yr and a range of 24–98 yr. Anergic subjects experienced significantly more post-surgical mortality than those who were reactive. Since all the subjects had gastrointestinal cancers that required surgery, it could be argued that the initial severity of the disease increased both the incidence of anergy and the risk of dying postoperatively. Thus, initial disease severity could explain the apparent strong relationship between preoperative DHST responses and postsurgical mortality. However, the study of Wayne et al. *(20)* did not have this confounder since they looked prospectively at healthy adults over a 10-yr time period. In this investigation, the authors followed 273 initially healthy subjects age 60 or older with no history of serious medical problems. DHST responses were measured at enrollment. Anergy (failure to respond to any of four skin-test antigens) at enrollment in the study was associated with a significantly increased risk of dying in the 10-yr follow-up period (Fig. 1). For example, at the end of 10 yr, 89% of the initially reactive subjects were still alive, but 22% of the anergic subjects had died. The study demonstrates that anergy to skin-test antigens, even when present in healthy older people, is associated with subsequent increased all-cause mortality. The authors also found a 2½-fold increase in cancer mortality in the initially anergic group in comparison to the reactive group. However, this was not statistically significant because of the relatively small number of cancer deaths observed.

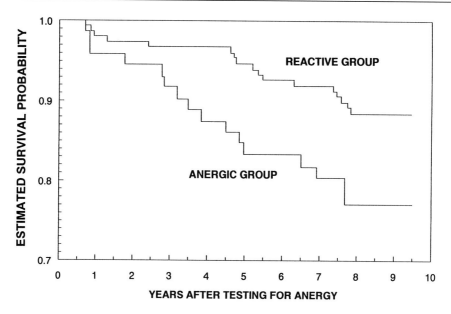

Fig. 1. Kaplan-Meier curves of all-cause mortality for initially anergic and reactive older people during a 10-yr follow-up period. Subjects (*n* = 273) were aged 60 or older and apparently healthy at enrollment. Participants were considered anergic if their responses to each of four skin test antigens were < 5 mm of induration. Most of the excess mortality in the anergic group occurred within 5 yr of enrollment. Adapted from Wayne et al. *(20).*

Evidence for the decline in T-cell function with age includes a considerable number of studies that demonstrate reduced lymphocyte proliferative responses (LPR) to mitogens or antigens, as well as depressed delayed hypersensitivity responses to recall antigens *(7,16–23).* Indeed, these two measures of T-cell function have been the most widely studied functional tests done in conjunction with assessment of the effects of nutritional intervention on immunity. A problem with lymphocyte proliferative responses to mitogens is the considerable variability of these assays, even in laboratories with rigid quality control procedures.

There is some evidence for changes in T-lymphocyte subsets with aging, in particular decreases in CD4+, increases in CD8+ cells, and decreases in the CD4+/CD8+ ratio *(9).* There is also evidence that lymphocyte subsets are altered in older people who are ill. For example, Markewitz et al. *(24)* have found that immunosuppression in cardiopulmonary bypass surgery patients aged 55 or older is associated with decreased CD4+ T-cells and increases in CD8+ T-cells. Higa et al. *(25)* have found that increases in CD8+ T-cells predict a longer period of recovery after onset of acute herpetic pain during herpes zoster infection. The increased incidence of this disease in older people is thought to be the result of the depressed cellular immunity that occurs with age *(14).*

Measurement of lymphocyte subsets is a key component in evaluation of immune function *(26,27).* Knowledge of lymphocyte subset numbers (cells/mL and percent of total) allows determination of relationships between immune functions and the number and percentage of cells responsible for these functions. This can permit distinguishing between effects as a result of increased numbers of a particular subgroup of cells vs enhanced activity by the same number of cells. The latter could be related to antigen binding capacity per cell. Indeed, changes in antigen binding capacity per cell could be a mechanism by which micronutrients influence immune functions. However, the role that changes in antigen binding capacity per cell may play in declining immunity with age is largely unexplored.

2.2.3. OTHER IMMUNE SYSTEM CHANGES WITH AGING

There is some evidence for a decline in B-cell functions with age, although it is likely related at least in part to the T-cell dependence of B-cell functions. Older people vaccinated with tetanus toxoid, varicella-zoster, or hepatitis B antigens demonstrate reduced antibody production as well as a greater percentage of nonresponders. This may also be true after pneumococcal and influenza virus immunization, although the evidence is not as convincing (28).

Perskin and Cronstein (29) have reported that aging produces alterations in neutrophil plasma membrane viscosity that may result in compromised neutrophil function and increased susceptibility to infection with pyogenic bacteria. This is consistent with studies of Nagel et al. (30), Shoham-Kesare and Gershon (31), and Corberand et al. (32) that suggest compromised in vitro activity of neutrophils from older people.

A review by Makinodan et al. (33) suggests that although antigen-responsive cells, such as B-cells, monocytes, and killer cells, are vulnerable to aging, T-cells are clearly the most vulnerable. This is the reason that most studies of nutrition, immunity, and aging have focused on T-cell functions.

Sen et al. (28) have published an insightful review that distinguishes between an increased incidence vs greater severity of infectious diseases in older people. For example, they report an increased case-fatality ratio for bacterial meningitis and pneumococcal pneumonia in older people and an increased incidence of such diseases as urinary tract infections and varicella zoster. Other diseases, such as influenza virus infection and gram-negative sepsis, are both more frequent and more severe in older people. They suggest that in addition to changes in immunity with age, local urinary tract, respiratory tract, and neurologic changes may contribute to the increase in infectious disease morbidity and mortality in older people.

Relationships among the interleukins, their receptors, and immunity have been widely discussed in the recent immunology literature. Of particular interest in the elderly is interleukin-2(IL-2), since its production is decreased in older people (9). Interestingly, soluble IL-2R levels are higher in older than in younger adults (34) and it has been suggested that this may be a factor in the decline of cellular immunity with age, since high serum concentrations of soluble IL-2R may compete with and decrease IL-2 binding to T-cell IL-2 receptors and thereby compromise immunity (35,36). We have previously found that serum IL-2R concentrations are lower in physically active older people and that exercise/physical activity habits and multivitamin supplementation may interact to influence soluble serum IL-2R concentrations (37). We have also verified the higher levels of soluble IL-2R in older people and found that increased soluble IL-2R concentrations are significantly associated with lower DHST responses (unpublished data).

There may be a "survivor" aspect to the relationship between advanced age and immune capacity. The oldest people, including centenarians studied by Sansoni et al. (38), tend to have well-preserved immune functions, such as natural killer cell activity, that are often better than those of 50–80-y olds. In addition, those above age 90 tend to have lower serum autoantibody concentrations than those in the 60–80 yr range *(14,39)*. Thus, enhanced immunity and reduced autoimmunity appear to be associated with the ability to live to age 90 and beyond.

3. MICRONUTRIENT NUTRITION AND IMMUNITY

3.1. Nutrition, Immunity, and Aging

One key question is whether the decline in immunity with aging is the result, at least in part, of nutritional deficiencies and/or increased requirements. Another possibility is that micronutrient supplementation might improve immunity even in the absence of an underlying deficiency. However, relatively few studies have simultaneously investigated nutrition and immune functions in older people.

Human studies of protein-calorie malnutrition (PCM) in underdeveloped countries or in hospitalized adults demonstrate a causal association between undernutrition and secondary immunodepression that results in diminished resistance to infectious diseases *(14,15,40,41)*. This association is consistent enough to permit the use of DHST in medical and surgical patients as a predictor of clinical prognosis *(19)*. Thus, there appears to be little doubt that severe malnutrition has a major impact on resistance to disease that is mediated in part through the immune system. There is also evidence that moderate to marginal undernutrition may compromise immunity *(42,43)*. However, the impact of moderate and marginal undernutrition on immune functions is not as well defined *(15)*.

McMurray *(15)* has noted that dietary deficiencies, both moderate and severe, of specific nutrients profoundly alter cell-mediated immune responses in humans and experimental animals. Diets with inadequate contents of calories, protein, vitamin A, pyridoxine, biotin, or zinc can result in depressed production of thymic hormones critical for T-lymphocyte differentiation. Reduced numbers and depressed in vitro function of T-cells have also been reported in experimental deficiencies of zinc, copper, iron, and vitamins A and E. Depressed DHST responses are a consistent result of dietary inadequacies of protein, pyridoxine, folate, iron, zinc, and vitamins A and C.

The classic review by Beisel *(44)* extensively examined the literature up to 1982 on single nutrients and immunity. The water-soluble vitamins that appear to be most critical for maintaining immunity are vitamin B6, folate, vitamin B12, and vitamin C. Among the lipid soluble micronutrients, vitamins A and E appear to exert the most significant impacts. Recent studies have shown that vitamin D is also an important immune modulator *(45)*. Trace metals that exert substantial influences on immune functions are iron, zinc, selenium, and copper *(15,44)*.

Since the variability in immune responses increases with aging, subgroups that have impaired immunity because of nutrient deficiencies are more likely to be observed in the elderly than in other age groups. In addition, when episodes of nutritional vulnerability overlap with suboptimal immune function, an adverse synergistic interaction is possible *(15)*. These factors make it more rewarding to study nutrition/immunity relationships in older rather than in younger adults. Beisel *(46)* has noted that individual studies of immunity and nutrition in humans have not been systematic or comprehensive. This is no doubt related to the very considerable expense that would be incurred in studying multiple immune responses in a sizeable number of older people.

3.2. Cross-Sectional Studies on Micronutrient Nutrition and Immunity

Goodwin and Garry *(47)* compared immunological functions of healthy elderly New Mexico residents consuming higher than RDA levels (5 times the RDA or greater) of micronutrients to similar subjects not taking supplements. Micronutrients evaluated were vitamins A, C, D, and E, the B vitamins, iron, calcium, and zinc. There was no significant difference between the two groups in DHST responses or in vitro lymphocyte proliferative responses to mitogens. The authors suggested that the immune-enhancing properties of high doses of vitamins may be the result of a nonspecific adjuvant effect that does not persist with time.

More recently the same authors *(48)* studied 230 healthy older men and women to determine if subclinical micronutrient deficiencies could contribute to the depressed immunity found in many of the elderly. Immune functions studied included DHST responses, in vitro lymphocyte proliferative responses to PHA, lymphocyte counts, and levels of serum autoantibodies. Spearman correlation coefficients were calculated to assess associations between blood micronutrient concentrations and selected immune functions. The authors also compared subjects with the lowest responses to those with the highest. There were no significant associations between low serum micronutrient concentrations and immune functions, and the authors suggested that subtle nutrient differences did not appear to contribute to the immunodeficiency of aging. However, the population sample studied was relatively affluent and people taking prescription drugs or daily over-the-counter medications, as well as those with a serious medical problem, were excluded. Thus, the study may have excluded those subjects who might benefit most from micronutrient supplements.

The above studies were not attempts to intervene by provision of micronutrient supplements, but were assessments of associations between the subjects' usual intakes or blood concentrations and selected immune functions. Variables that cannot be controlled in cross-sectional studies may mask associations between nutritional factors and immunity, especially since immunity is likely to be dependent on a number of factors, only one of which is nutritional status. Such studies are valuable as a way to identify nutrients for more intensive study, but can only provide statistical associations that may not be cause/effect relationships. The latter can be assessed by standard placebo-controlled double-blind clinical trials.

3.3. Clinical Trials of Single Nutrients

Several clinical trials have been conducted in recent years. Jacob et al. *(49)* studied the effects of moderate ascorbate depletion on immunity and other factors in young adult males confined to a metabolic ward. Ascorbate depletion was achieved using daily doses of 5–20 mg/d, whereas repletion was achieved with doses of 60 (the RDA) to 250 mg/d. Although lymphocyte proliferative responses to mitogens were not affected by ascorbate depletion/repletion, DHST responses to a panel of seven recall antigens were markedly depressed by ascorbate depletion. Repletion for 28 d at either 60 or 250 mg/d did not restore the mean antigen score to the predepletion level, although there was some improvement in induration in three of the eight men studied. These results suggest that DHST is more sensitive to ascorbate depletion than mitogen responses. They further suggest that the repletion period was of insufficient duration to produce a return of DHST to baseline levels and/or the repletion doses were not large enough. The latter possibility is supported by another study *(50)* that demonstrates that higher doses of ascorbate can enhance LPR to mitogens. The inconsistency in the results for mitogen responses vs DHST may reflect the different cellular populations involved in these processes, the greater sensitivity of DHST to nutritional factors, the inherent variability of mitogen assays, or artifacts of the in vitro mitogen tests that do not adequately represent the in vivo situation.

Fuller et al. *(51)* studied the effect of β-carotene supplementation on the UV-radiation-induced photosuppression of DHST in 24 young adult males, aged 19–39 yr. They found that exposure to a UV-A/B light source over a 16-d period significantly reduced DHST responses in a control (placebo) group to 39% of the initial values, but did not induce significant reductions in a group given 30 mg β-carotene per day. Since young men were studied, it was not known if these results would occur in young women or in older men and women. Recently, this group repeated this study in an elderly population and found similar effects, although there was more variability in DHST responses in the older people compared to young adults *(52)*.

Watson et al. *(53)* investigated the effects of β-carotene on lymphocyte subpopulations in male and female subjects with a mean age of 56 yr. Beta-carotene was given at doses of 15, 30, 45, or 60 mg/d for 2 mo. Using monoclonal antibodies to identify lymphocyte subsets, they found that the percentages of T-helper and natural killer cells, as well as cells with IL-2 and transferrin receptors, were increased in a dose-related fashion. There were no significant effects of β-carotene on T-suppressor cells. However, the number of subjects in each treatment group was only 3–5; thus, further investigation is needed to confirm these findings. Ringer *(54)* and coworkers found that administration of high doses of β-carotene, up to 300 mg/d, to younger adults for 1 mo did not significantly affect lymphocyte proliferative responses to mitogens or IL-2 production. The contrasting results of these studies may be because of the younger age of the subjects in Ringer's study, or the shorter duration of supplementation. The use of different laboratory tests may also be a factor, since Watson et al. assessed T-cell subpopulations and Ringer et al. performed functional assays. In addition, augmentation of cellular immunity may not be readily achieved nor be desired in younger subjects with well-functioning immune systems.

Talbott et al. *(55)* in a pilot study investigated the impact of pyridoxine supplementation on lymphocyte responses in 15 older (aged 65–81 yr) mostly female subjects and found that administration of 50 mg/d of pyridoxine hydrochloride significantly increased in vitro lymphocyte proliferative responses to phytohemagglutin, pokewood mitogen, and *Staphylococcus aureus*.

Meydani et al. *(56)* have reported that vitamin B6 deficiency impairs IL-2 production and lymphocyte proliferation in older adults. Each of these measurements was reduced by about 50% by depletion, whereas repletion with near RDA levels of B6 eventually increased values to about the baseline levels. Although only eight subjects were studied, this well-designed investigation supports a number of other studies that suggest that vitamin B6 may play a key role in immune responses *(57)*.

Meydani et al. *(58)* also studied the effects of daily supplementation with 800 mg dl-α-tocopheryl acetate or a placebo for 30 d on cell-mediated immunity in healthy subjects, aged 60 yr or older living in a metabolic ward; this dose is more than 50 times the current RDAs for males and females aged 51+. DHST, IL-2 production, and mitogen responses to concanavalin A were significantly increased in the vitamin E-supplemented group. The percentage increases were greatest for IL-2 production (32%

increase) and least for mitogen responses to concanavalin A. Seventy-one percent of the supplemented subjects experienced an increase in DHST responses (induration) with a mean increase of 53%. More recently, this research group studied healthy older subjects consuming their usual diets, and found that DHST was enhanced after 4 mo of administration of vitamin E at doses of 60, 200, or 800 IU/d, but mitogen responses were improved only by the highest dose *(59)*. The latter observation may be related to the well known substantial variability of in vitro mitogen responses. Antibody titers to vaccination were also improved in the vitamin E-supplemented, but not the placebo group.

There has been considerable interest in the potential for zinc to improve immune functions in older people. It is clear that severe zinc deficiency in animals and people, e.g., as found in the disease acrodermatitis enteropathica, can greatly compromise cellular immunity and lead to the development of life-threatening opportunistic infections *(60)*. There are also reports of significant associations between plasma or cellular zinc concentrations and immune functions, such as DHST responses in older people *(8,61)*. However, recent studies of the impact of zinc supplementation on immunity in older people have not been encouraging. They have either demonstrated no beneficial effect of zinc supplements on immunity or an adverse effect even when the supplements contained modest doses of zinc in the range of 15–25 mg/d *(62,63)*. In the absence of an underlying deficiency, use of zinc supplements by older people, especially at doses that exceed the current RDA of 15 mg/d, are more likely to adversely affect immunity than improve it.

3.4. Clinical Trials of Combinations of Micronutrients

The above studies *(49–63)* focused on the effects of relatively large doses of individual micronutrients on immune functions. There have been only five published placebo-controlled trials of the effects of multivitamin/mineral supplements on immune functions in older people.

In the first of these studies, we investigated the effects of zinc given in combination with a multivitamin on immune functions in 63 older people *(64)*. All subjects received a low dose multivitamin/mineral supplement that contained all the essential micronutrients except zinc. In addition, subjects received 15 or 100 mg of zinc, or a placebo. Daily consumption of the multivitamin/mineral supplement for 1 yr was associated with enhanced DHST and mitogen responses, but these effects were reduced and delayed by ingestion of 15 and especially 100 mg of zinc each day. These data suggest that interactions among micronutrients may influence their effects on immunity, and that some individual micronutrients, even at modest doses, may have unexpected adverse effects. The adverse impact of zinc is consistent with other previously cited recent studies that indicate that zinc supplements in healthy older people either do not improve immunity or adversely affect it *(62,63)*.

The second is the study of Chandra *(65)*, who reported the results of 12 mo of daily supplementation of a group of healthy subjects aged 65 or older with a micronutrient formulation containing relatively low doses of nine vitamins and five trace elements and higher levels of the antioxidants vitamin C, vitamin E, and β-carotene. Chandra found that, in comparison to a placebo group, the micronutrient group had higher numbers of some T-cell subsets and natural killer cells, enhanced LPR to mitogens, increased in vitro IL-2 production, higher antibody responses to influenza vaccine, and greater NK cell activity. In addition, supplemented subjects experienced significantly fewer days (23±5) of illness per year because of infectious diseases than subjects in the placebo group (48±7 d). These recent results are consistent with the hypothesis presented in our paper published in 1990 (64) that a low dose micronutrient supplement could improve immune functions in older people. The results of Chandra further suggest that there may be beneficial clinical effects, i.e., a reduced prevalence of infectious diseases, as a result of micronutrient supplementation.

Presupplementation plasma concentrations of retinol, β-carotene, vitamin C, and vitamin B6 were low in some subjects in Chandra's study, with the percentage of subjects with initially low concentrations of each between 12.5 and 22.9%. Most of the low concentrations were corrected by supplementation, so that the percent of subjects with low values of the aforementioned concentrations decreased to 0–4.4%, which was accompanied by the enhanced immune functions that he observed. However, this observation does not prove that the decrease in the percent of subjects with low concentrations was responsible for the improved immune functions found.

Limitations of the study of Chandra include the fact that there was no assessment of dietary micronutrients from food and immune functions were assessed only at baseline and after 1 yr of supplementation. In addition, the occurrence of infectious diseases was reported as the number of days for which subjects were infected per year. The latter is the product of the incidence of infectious diseases and their duration. Thus, a single infection persisting for 30 d is equivalent to six infections of 5 d duration each. It is important to know the effects of micronutrient supplementation on the incidence of new infections, as well as the nature and duration of each type of infection.

Penn et al. (66) studied the effects on immune functions of a supplement containing vitamin C (100 mg), vitamin A (8000 IU), and vitamin E (50 mg); it was given for 28 d to half of the 30 elderly subjects studied. All were patients who had been hospitalized for at least three months. The number and percent of CD4+ and CD8+ T-cells were significantly increased in the supplemented group but not in a placebo group. Proliferative responses of lymphocytes to the mitogen phytohemagglutinin (PHA) were also significantly increased in the supplemented group by 64–283%, but were not affected by the placebo. There was biochemical evidence of deficiencies of vitamins A, C, and/or E in 5–47% of the supplemented subjects at enrollment into the study. Thus, it is possible that the improvement in cellular immunity in these subjects with short-term administration of vitamins A, C, and E was because of correction of underlying deficiencies that are more likely to be present in hospitalized than in independently living older people. These results suggest that this group of micronutrients may be particularly important for enhancement of immune responses in older people.

In the fourth study, Chavance et al. (67) enrolled 218 subjects aged 60 or older who were living independently and had not used any vitamin supplements for at least the prior 3 mo. They were given a low-dose multivitamin or placebo for 4 mo. No clinical or laboratory assessments of immune function were conducted. The authors found no significant effects of supplementation on the incidence of infections; however, effects on the duration of each infection or the total number of days of infection were not assessed. As suggested by the authors, the failure to find any significant effects on the incidence of infections may be because of the short duration of supplementation. This is consistent with our results and those of Chandra (65), which suggest that periods of supplementation of about 6–12 mo are required before improvements in immune functions occur in older people.

More recently we conducted a randomized, placebo-controlled, double-blind trial of the effects of low-dose micronutrient supplementation on plasma vitamin and trace metal concentrations and immune functions in independently living healthy older subjects *(68)*. This study will be described in some detail. The over-the-counter micronutrient supplement used in the study was Theragran M, which contains low to moderate doses of each of the essential micronutrients.

Of the 65 subjects enrolled, 56 (86%) completed the 1-yr study. About two-thirds were females. As expected, there were no statistically significant effects of the placebo on plasma micronutrient concentrations. In contrast, the data for the micronutrient supplement group show statistically significant increases at 6 and/or 12 mo for plasma concentrations of ascorbate, β-carotene, folate, vitamin B6, and α-tocopherol. These data verify that supplementation with low doses of the latter micronutrients can increase their plasma concentrations in older people.

Table 2 contains the data on DHST for all study subjects combined and for males and females separately. For induration in the placebo group, there were no statistically significant differences between the 0- and 6-mo results, 0- and 12-mo results, or 6 and 12 month data. Similar results were obtained for the analyses of the data for the placebo group on the number of positive responses.

For the micronutrient supplement group, there was also no significant difference for the data on induration at 0 and 6 mo. However, there was a statistically significant difference between the 0 and 12-mo induration results ($p=0.005$). There was an increase in induration between 6 and 12 mo, but this did not achieve statistical significance ($p=0.056$). Similar trends were observed for the individual skin-test antigens.

Similar results were also obtained for the number of positive responses in the micronutrient treatment group. The mean number of positive responses in the placebo group increased by only 4.8% between 0 and 12 mo, and induration by 8.0%. In contrast, in the micronutrient supplement group, the mean number of positive responses increased by 64% and induration by 61% between 0 and 12 mo. These data provide strong evidence for the enhancement of DHST after 1 yr of micronutrient supplementation.

The results also suggest that some enhancement of DHST responses occurred sooner (at 6 mo) in the male subjects than in the females (Table 2). The male subjects had significantly greater DHST responses than the females at enrollment; this is consistent with previous data that suggest that DHST responses in males may differ from those in females *(69)*. The diets of the male subjects differed from the females, being higher in energy intake as well as intake of individual micronutrients, and it is possible that this factor may have interacted with micronutrient supplementation to influence DHST responses.

There was an increase between zero and 12 mo in the number of subjects in the placebo group with low blood concentrations of some of the micronutrients measured, specifically β-carotene, retinol, folate, and vitamin B6. This trend differed significantly from the micronutrient group, for which the number of low values changed very little between 0 and 12 mo. Thus, the improvement in skin-test responses in the micronutrient group is not the result of the correction of underlying micronutrient deficiencies for the nine micronutrient concentrations that we determined in blood, at least as defined by current guidelines for low circulating concentrations. The increased number of low values in the placebo group suggests that older people who do not take vitamin supplements for a year may have an increased risk of developing one or more low concentrations, particularly for vitamin B6, folate, and β-carotene.

Table 2
Delayed-Hypersensitivity Skin-Test Responses of Placebo and Micronutrient Groups[a]

Subgroup and response type	Placebo group			Micronutrient group		
	0 mo	6 mo	12 mo	0 mo	6 mo	12 mo
All subjects						
Positive responses	1.65 ± 0.30	1.42 ± 0.25	1.73 ± 0.29	1.45 ± 0.25^b	$1.76 \pm 0.27^{b,c}$	2.38 ± 0.33^c
Total induration, mm	5.37 ± 1.02	4.76 ± 0.93	5.80 ± 0.95	5.21 ± 0.98^b	$5.73 \pm 0.94^{b,c}$	8.40 ± 1.25^c
Males						
Positive responses	2.93 ± 0.60	1.93 ± 0.30	2.50 ± 0.78	1.64 ± 0.33^b	$2.59 \pm 0.43^{b,c}$	2.86 ± 0.53^c
Total induration, mm	8.86 ± 1.91	6.36 ± 1.29	8.88 ± 2.51	6.23 ± 1.15	8.85 ± 1.58	10.91 ± 2.08
Females						
Positive responses	1.18 ± 0.29	1.24 ± 0.31	1.45 ± 0.27	1.33 ± 0.36^b	$1.25 \pm 0.29^{b,c}$	2.08 ± 0.42^c
Total induration, mm	4.08 ± 1.09	4.17 ± 1.16	4.67 ± 0.83	4.58 ± 1.41^b	3.83 ± 0.95^b	6.86 ± 1.49^c

[a]Mean ± SE; $n = 26$ for placebo group (7 males, 19 females), $n = 29$ for micronutrient group (11 males, 18 females). Positive responses are the mean number of antigens eliciting a response from a total of seven antigens. Total induration is the sum of the indurations of all positive responses. Within groups, values in the same row with different letter superscripts are significantly different, $P < 0.05$ (Wilcoxon signed-rank test).

There were no significant correlations between DHST responses and serum vitamin concentrations, consistent with the observations of Goodwin and Garry in their cross-sectional studies (48). There were, however, statistically significant correlations between the changes in skin test responses between 0 and 12 mo and the corresponding changes in blood micronutrient concentrations for four serum micronutrients: ascorbate, β-carotene, α-tocopherol, and folate (r=0.27–0.33). These data suggest that future studies of micronutrient nutrition and immunity could focus on the aforementioned four micronutrients. The data further suggest that the absence of associations prior to supplementation between DHST responses and serum vitamin concentrations does not preclude the finding of such associations between changes in DHST responses and serum concentrations after supplementation. Of course, such associations are not proof of a causal relationship.

Our data and that of Chandra (65) suggest that enhancement of immune functions in older subjects by low-dose micronutrient supplementation takes approx 1 yr. These results also suggest that the diets of older people are inadequate in one or more micronutrients and/or that the current RDAs for one or more micronutrients may be too low to support optimal immunity in older adults.

It could be argued that a 60% increase in DHST responses over a 1-yr period is only a mean increase of about 5%/mo. However, this increase far exceeds the decline in DHST responses per year that occurs with aging, and thus may completely prevent it. These results suggest that older subjects who take a "one-a-day" type multivitamin supplement faithfully for at least 6–12 mo may experience a substantial improvement in measures of cellular immunity, such as DHST responses. It is possible that more rapid and/or larger increases in DHST responses would occur if higher doses of micronutrients were used.

3.5. Need for Additional Investigations of Micronutrient/Immunity Relationships

It could be argued that the above studies (64–68) that focused on the effects of multivitamins on immune functions, in combination with the short-term higher dose single nutrient studies, such as those of Meydani (58,59), Watson (53), and Talbott (55), provide sufficient information about the relationships among micronutrient supplementation, immunity, and the occurrence of infectious diseases, and that no new studies are needed. However, despite the evidence provided by these studies, we do not know if long-term daily use of multivitamin/mineral supplements will enhance immune functions and reduce the incidence and severity of infectious and other diseases in older people beyond the 1-yr duration of the longest studies done to date. This is an unfortunate gap in our knowledge, because millions of older Americans currently consume a multivitamin/mineral supplement daily, either alone or in combination with one or more single nutrients at higher doses (70,71). This situation is in part the result of the limited objectives of all previously completed studies. All of the single-nutrient studies have been of short duration, usually using high doses of one micronutrient, given to a relatively small number of subjects. None of these studies has assessed the impact of single nutrient supplementation on the incidence of infectious diseases and other illnesses, a limitation related to the small number of subjects enrolled in these studies and their short duration, with a consequent lack of statistical power to assess disease incidence. Although valuable, the five studies on multivitamin supplements also have limitations:

1. The study of Chavance et al. *(67)* was of only 4 mo duration. Although this study assessed the impact of multivitamin supplementation on the incidence of infectious diseases, it did not include any measures of immune function.
2. The study of Penn *(66)* was of only 1 mo duration and included only older people who had been hospitalized for at least three mo.
3. Our studies *(64,68)* assessed DHST responses, lymphocyte proliferative responses to mitogens, and NK cell activity, but we could not examine other measures of immunity or clinical outcomes and confined the period of supplementation to 1 yr.
4. The study of Chandra *(65)* was also of only 1 yr duration, did not include assessment of dietary micronutrients, did not distinguish between the incidence and duration of infectious illnesses, and assessed selected immune functions only once after initiating supplementation.

Thus, additional clinical studies of micronutrient/immunity relationships are warranted.

4. FACTORS THAT CAN INFLUENCE MICRONUTRIENT/IMMUNITY RELATIONSHIPS

Factors that may influence micronutrient/immunity relationships in older people include gender, stress, disease, physical activity and exercise, obesity, and food choices. In our recent study *(68)* of the effects of low-dose micronutrient supplements on immunity in older people, improvements in DHST responses occurred sooner in the males than the females. Although the reason for this is not known, one possibility is that the higher intake of micronutrients from food in the men results in a larger total micronutrient intake. Thus, this effect may be a consequence of the generally greater energy and micronutrient intake of males.

There are a considerable number of reports that psychological and physiological stress in experimental animals and people can depress cellular immune functions *(72,73)*, although it is beyond the scope of this chapter to assess these studies in any detail. As an example, death of a spouse has been associated with depressed immune functions *(73)*. However, virtually all studies of relationships between stress and immunity have not adequately assessed nutritional factors that may be altered by stress, and in many cases have completely ignored nutrition. Physical and psychological stress can modify food intake in animals and people, and thus studies of stress/immunity relationships are usually confounded by nutritional factors that have not been adequately evaluated.

There is considerable evidence that physical activity/exercise patterns can influence immunity *(74–78)*. In general, the data suggest that very strenuous exercise can acutely depress immunity. For example, various studies have found that participants in marathons have a significantly increased risk to experience respiratory infections in the 1–2-wk period following the race *(77,78)*. Chronic overtraining has also been associated with depressed immunity *(76)*. In contrast, regular moderate exercise appears to enhance immune functions *(76)*. One hypothesis is that regular exercise contributes to the maintenance of muscle mass, and muscle is the source of a key nutrient, glutamine, required by lymphocytes *(79)*. In addition, alterations in cytokine levels as a result of regular exercise may be a factor *(80,81)*.

Stallone *(82)* has recently outlined studies that indicate that excess body weight in humans or experimental animals is associated with impairments in host defense mechanisms. Definitive studies have not been done, but there are data suggesting both beneficial and detrimental effects of weight loss on immunity. In experimental animals, it is well-known that chronically reduced energy intake without malnutrition can profoundly ameliorate the detrimental effects of aging on immunity and can increase mean and maximum lifespan *(83)*. The well-established importance of some micronutrients in the maintenance of immune function suggests that choices of foods high in these micronutrients may be beneficial, but this has not been validated in well-controlled studies.

Goodwin *(84)* has suggested that the relationship between depressed cellular immune function and subsequently increased mortality may be a result of compromised immunity being a marker for clinically latent diseases or poor overall physiologic function. Impaired immunity may also contribute to a reduced ability to defend against infections, cancers, and perhaps CHD. Each of these possibilities may contribute to the increased morbidity and mortality associated with depressed immunity in healthy older people.

5. RESEARCH NEEDED ON MICRONUTRIENT NUTRITION AND IMMUNITY

Several cross-sectional studies that assess relationships between micronutrient nutrition and immunity have been done in the past 12 yr *(47,48)* as previously discussed. In general, significant associations between serum micronutrient concentrations or use of micronutrient supplements and various measures of immunity were not found. However, these studies compared micronutrient supplement users with nonusers, but did not evaluate use of specific supplements, and it is likely that some individual or combinations of micronutrients can improve immunity and others cannot.

The clinical trials of micronutrient supplementation and immunity done to date have usually involved healthy older subjects consuming their usual diets. In the case of some single nutrient studies, subjects lived in metabolic units and consumed standardized meals that contained about the RDA of all essential micronutrients. It is possible that the improvements in immunity found in some studies are because of correction of underlying deficiencies. However, it is also likely that micronutrient supplements enhance immunity even in the absence of underlying deficiencies, at least based on current concepts of "deficiency." This should not be surprising, since optimal immune function was not a factor in establishment of the current RDAs, or in defining laboratory normal ranges for circulating micronutrient concentrations. In fact, daily intakes that optimize immunity may differ from both the current RDAs and intakes that may prevent chronic diseases. For example, the current RDA for vitamin E (8–10 mg α-tocopherol equivalents for adult females and males, respectively) is likely to be substantially less than amounts that optimize immune functions or prevent CHD *(58,59,85,86)*. Similarly, the current RDA for vitamin C is adequate to prevent development of scorbutic lesions, but appears to be less than the intake that could optimize immunity or reduce cataract formation *(4,87)*. Recommendations for an optimal intake of any micronutrient will need to balance the impact of that nutrient on various health outcomes as well as consider possible adverse effects of relatively high doses. There is considerable evidence that patterns of physical activity and exercise can influence immunity both acutely and chronically, but no studies have addressed interactions among physical activity, immunity, and micronutrient nutrition.

It should be emphasized that the potential of micronutrient supplements to improve immunity or exert other beneficial effects must be considered in relation to their consumption from food. This is especially true for low to moderate dose supplements, for which the intake from food and supplements may be similar. Clearly, supplement use should be encouraged in conjunction with a sound diet that emphasizes fruits, vegetables, whole grains, and other sources of micronutrients and limits the intake of saturated fats. However, it is likely that beneficial intakes of some nutrients, such as vitamin E, may not be possible from a good diet in the absence of supplement use.

The promising results of studies done to date suggest continued research on micronutrient nutrition and immunity, especially in older people. Such efforts should include:

1. A focus on long-term placebo-controlled double-blind clinical trials and prospective epidemiologic studies.
2. Study of interactions among physical activity/exercise patterns, immunity, and micronutrient nutrition.
3. Evaluation of effects of micronutrient nutrition on both humoral (e.g., antibody responses to vaccination) and cellular (e.g., DHST responses) immunity using clinically relevant assays and on clinical outcomes, e.g., infectious disease incidence, duration, and severity.
4. Evaluation of dietary modification alone or in combination with low doses of micronutrients. Studies of older people consuming their usual diets are also needed.
5. Long-term studies that address the persistence of the effects of micronutrients on immunity both during and subsequent to micronutrient supplementation.
6. Use of appropriate inclusion and exclusion criteria in identification of subjects for study.
7. Study of both single micronutrients and multivitamin/minerals, with a focus on the antioxidant micronutrients and other widely used single or multiple micronutrient supplements.
8. Identification of host-specific factors (e.g., gender, age range) that influence micronutrient/immunity interactions and the basis for these effects.
9. Identification of the molecular mechanisms that determine the effects of micronutrients on immunity.

About 100 million Americans (approx 40% of the population) take multivitamin/mineral supplements, either alone or in combination with higher doses of the antioxidant vitamins *(70,71)*. Well-designed studies that assess the health impacts of this practice are urgently needed and should include evaluation of effects on the immune system.

6. SUMMARY

We still have much to learn about the effects of micronutrients on immunity. Nevertheless, the results of the above and other studies suggest that:

1. Placebo-controlled clinical trials are the best approach for studying effects of micronutrients on immunity;
2. High doses of some single nutrients may improve immunity in relatively short time periods—weeks to months, but the persistence of these effects is not known at this time. High doses of other micronutrients may adversely affect immunity;
3. Some micronutrients may interfere with the beneficial effects of other micronutrients on immunity; this effect will depend on relative doses;

4. Low- to moderate-dose multivitamin/mineral supplements may require considerable time (6 mo to a year or more) before they enhance immune functions and reduce susceptibility to infectious diseases, and the timing of their effects may differ in men and women; and

5. High- and even low-dose micronutrient supplements may enhance immunity even in the absence of evidence of underlying deficiencies.

7. RECOMMENDATIONS

Physicians and other health care providers should advise their patients to eat diets low in saturated fat and high in fruits and vegetables. This can ensure consumption of significant amounts of the micronutrients (and other phytochemicals) that can favorably affect immunity. In addition, older subjects, especially those with poor diets, should be encouraged to take a low-dose multivitamin/mineral supplement. Higher but safe doses of the antioxidant micronutrients vitamin C, β-carotene, and vitamin E may also be appropriate for many people. Taking high doses of other micronutrients that can adversely affect immunity, for example zinc, should be persuasively discouraged.

The favorable effects of regular exercise on immunity should also be mentioned to patients. Most of this advice (low fat diet, high intake of fruits and vegetables, regular exercise, and supplemental vitamins) may not only promote optimal immunity, but is also likely to reduce the risk of CHD and some cancers.

REFERENCES

1. Warner HR, Butler RN, Sprott RL, Schneider EL. Modern Biological Theories of Aging. New York: Raven, 1987.
2. Schneider EL. Theories of aging; a perspective. In: Modern Biological Theories of Aging. Warner HR, Butler RN, Sprott RL, Schneider EL, eds. New York: Raven, 1987; pp. 1–3.
3. Hayflick L. The aging process: current theories. Drug-Nutrient Interact 1985; 4:13–33.
4. Bendich A. Antioxidant micronutrients and immune responses. Ann NY Acad Sci 1990; 587:168–180.
5. Ben-Yehuda A, Weksler ME. Immune senescence: mechanisms and clinical implications. Cancer Invest 1992; 10:525–531.
6. Makinodan T. Patterns of age-related immunologic changes. Nutr Rev 1995; 53:S27–S34.
7. Effros RB, Walford RL. Infection and immunity in relation to aging. In: Aging and the Immune Response. Goidl EA, ed. New York: Marcel-Dekker, 1987; 45–65.
8. Bogden JD, Oleske JM, Munves EM, et al. Zinc and immunocompetence in the elderly: baseline data on zinc nutriture and immunity in unsupplemented subjects. Am J Clin Nutr 1987; 45:101–109.
9. Kuvibidilia S, Yu L. Ode D, Warrier RP. The immune response in protein-energy malnutrition and single nutrient deficiencies. In: Nutrition and Immunology. Klurfeld DM, ed. New York: Plenum, 1993:121–155.
10. Abbas AK, Lichtman AH, Pober JS. Cellular and molecular immunology. Philadelphia: Saunders, 1994; 166–186.
11. Aronson M. Involution of the thymus revisited: immunological trade-offs as an adaptation to aging. Mech Ageing Dev 1993; 72:49–55.
12. Siskind GW. Aging and the immune system. In: Modern Biological Theories of Aging. Warner HR, Butler RN, Sprott RL, Schneider EL, eds. New York: Raven, 1987; 235–242.
13. Makinodan T, Kay MB. Age influence on the immune system. Adv Immunol 1980; 29:287–330.
14. Weksler ME. The senescence of the immune system. Hospital Practice 1981; 16:53–64.
15. McMurray DN. Cell-mediated immunity in nutritional deficiency. Prog Food Nutr Sci 1984; 8:193–228.
16. Schwab R, Weksler ME. Cell biology of the impaired proliferation of T cells from elderly humans. In: Aging and the Immune Response. Goidl EA, ed. New York: Marcel Dekker, 1987; 67–80.
17. James SJ, Makinodan T. Nutritional intervention during immunologic aging: past and present. In: Nutritional Intervention in the Aging Process. Armbrecht HJ, Prendergast JM, Coe RM, eds. New York: Springer-Verlag, 1984; 209–227.

18. Meakins JL, Pietsch JB, Bubenick O, et al. Delayed hypersensitivity: indicator of acquired failure of host defenses in sepsis and trauma. Ann Surg 1977; 186:241–250.
19. Christou NV, Tellado-Rodriguez J, Chartrand L, et al. Estimating mortality risk in preoperative patients using immunologic, nutritional, and acute-phase response variables. Ann Surg 1989; 210:69–77.
20. Wayne SJ, Rhyne RL, Garry PJ, Goodwin JS. Cell-mediated immunity as a predictor of morbidity and mortality in subjects over 60. J Gerontol 1990; 45:M45–48.
21. Roberts-Thomson IC, Whittingham S, Youngchaiyud U, McKay IR. Aging, immune response, and mortality. Lancet 1974; 2:368–370.
22. Hicks MJ, Jones JF, Thies AC, Weigle KA, Minnich LL. Age-related changes in mitogen-induced lymphocyte function from birth to old age. Am J Clin Pathol 1983; 80:159–163.
23. Murasko DM, Nelson BJ, Silver R, Matour D, Kaye D. Immunologic response in an elderly population with a mean age of 85. Am J Med 1986; 81:612–618.
24. Markewitz A, Faist E, Lang S, et al. Successful restoration of cell-mediated immune response after cardiopulmonary bypass by immunomodulation. J Thorac Cardiovas Surg 1993; 105:15–24.
25. Higa K, Noda B, Manabe H, Sato S, Dan K. T-lymphocyte subsets in otherwise healthy patients with herpes zoster and relationships to the duration of acute herpetic pain. Pain 1992; 51:111–118.
26. Stites DP. Clinical laboratory methods for detection of cellular immunity. In: Basic and Clinical Immunology, 7th ed. Stites DP, Terr AI, eds. Norwalk, CT: Appleton & Lange 1991; 263–283.
27. Giorgi JV. Lymphocyte subset measurements: significance in clinical medicine. In: Manual of Clinical Laboratory Immunology, 3rd ed. Rose NR, Friedman H, Fahey JL, eds. Washington, DC, American Society for Microbiology, 1986; 236–246.
28. Sen P, Middleton JR, Perez G, et al. Host defense abnormalities and infection in older persons. Infect in Med 1994; 11:364–370.
29. Perskin MH, Cornstein BN. Age-related changes in neutrophil structure and function. Mech Ageing Dev 1992; 64:303–313.
30. Nagel JE, Han K, Coon PJ, Adler WH, Bender BS. Age differences in phagocytosis by polymorphonuclear leukocytes measured by flow cytometry. J Leukocyte Biol 1986; 39:399–407.
31. Shoham-Kesari H, Gershon H. Impaired reactivity to inflammatory stimuli of neutrophils from elderly donors. Aging Immunol Infect Dis 1992; 3:169–183.
32. Corberand J, Ngyen F, Laharrague P, et al. Polymorphonuclear functions and aging in humans. J Am Geriatr Soc 1981; 29:391–397.
33. Makinodan T, Lubinski J, Fong TC. Cellular, biochemical, and molecular basis of T-cell senescence. Arch Pathol Lab Med 1987; 111:910–914.
34. Rubin LA, Nelson DL. The soluble interleukin-2 receptor: biology, function, and clinical application. Ann Intern Med 1990; 113:619–627.
35. Manoussakis MN, Papadopoulos GK, Drosos AA, Moutsopoulos HM. Soluble interleukin-2 receptor molecules in the serum of patients with autoimmune diseases. Clin Immunol Immunopathol 1989; 50:321–332.
36. Lahat N, Shtiller R, Zlotnick AY, Merin G. Early IL-2/sIL-2R surge following surgery leads to temporary immune refractoriness. Clin Exp Immunol 1993; 92:482–486.
37. Bogden JD, Kemp FW, Liberatore BL, et al. Serum interleukin-2 receptor concentrations, physical activity, and micronutrient nutrition in older people. J Cell Biochem 1993; 17B:86.
38. Sansoni P, Brianti V, Fagnoni F. NK cell activity and T-lymphocyte proliferation in healthy centenarians. Ann NY Acad Sci 1992; 663:505–507.
39. Mariotti S, Sansoni P, Barbesino G, et al. Thyroid and other organ-specific autoantibodies in healthy centenarians. Lancet 1992; 339:1506–1508.
40. Chandra RK. Nutrition and immunity. Contemp Nut 1986; 11:1–4.
41. Chandra RK. Immunodeficiency in undernutrition and overnutrition. Nutr Rev 1981; 39:225–231.
42. McMurray DN, Loomis SA, Casazza LJ, Rey H, Miranda R. Development of impaired cell-mediated immunity in mild and moderate malnutrition. Am J Clin Nutr 1981; 34:68–77.
43. Dowd PS, Heatley RV. The influence of undernutrition on immunity. Clin Sci 1984; 66:241–248.
44. Beisel WR. Single nutrients and immunity. Am J Clin Nutr 1982; 35:417–468.
45. Yoder MC, Manolagas SC. Vitamin D and its role in immune function. Clin Appl Nutr 1991; 1:35–41.
46. Beisel WR. Nutrition and infection. In: Nutritional Biochemistry and Metabolism. Linder MC, ed. New York: Elsevier, 1985; 369–394.
47. Goodwin JS, Garry PJ. Relationships between megadose vitamin supplementation and immunological function in a healthy elderly population. Clin Exp Immunol 1983; 51:647–653.
48. Goodwin JS, Garry PJ. Lack of correlation between indices of nutritional status and immunologic function in elderly humans. J Gerontol 1988; 43:M46–49.

49. Jacob RA, Kelley DS, Pianalto FS, et al. Immunocompetence and oxidant defense during ascorbate depletion of healthy men. Am J Clin Nutr 1991; 54:1302S–1309S.

50. Anderson R, Oosthuizen R, Maritz R, Theron A, Van Rensburg AJ. The effects of increasing weekly doses of ascorbate on certain cellular and humoral immune functions in normal volunteers. Am J Clin Nutr 1980; 33:71–76.

51. Fuller CJ, Faulkner H, Bendich A, Parker RS, Roe DA. Effect of beta-carotene supplementation on photo-suppression of delayed-type hypersensitivity in normal young men. Am J Clin Nutr 1992; 56:684–690.

52. Herraiz L, Rahman A, Paker R, Roe D. The role of beta-carotene supplementation in prevention of photo-suppression of cellular immunity in elderly men. FASEB J 1994; 8:A423.

53. Watson RR, Prabhala RH, Plezia PM, Alberts DS. Effect of beta-carotene on lymphocyte subpopulations in elderly humans: evidence for a dose-response relationship. Am J Clin Nutr 1991; 53:90–94.

54. Ringer TV, DeLoof MJ, Winterrowd GE, et al. Beta-carotene's effects on serum lipoprotein and immunologic indices in humans. Am J Clin Nutr 1991; 53:688–694.

55. Talbott MC, Miller LT, Kerkvliet NI. Pyridoxine supplementation: effect on lymphocyte responses in elderly persons. Am J Clin Nutr 1987; 46:659–664.

56. Meydani SN, Ribaya-Mercado JD, Russell RN, et al. Vitamin B-6 deficiency impairs interleukin 2 production and lymphocyte proliferation in elderly adults. Am J Clin Nutr 1991; 53:1275–1280.

57. Rall LC, Meydani SN. Vitamin B6 and immune competence. Nutr Rev 1993; 51:217–225.

58. Meydani SN, Barklund MP, Liu S, et al. Vitamin E supplementation enhances cell-mediated immunity in healthy elderly subjects. Am J Clin Nutr 1990; 52:557–563.

59. Meydani SN, Leka L. Loszewski R. Long-term vitamin E supplementation enhances immune response in healthy elderly. FASEB J 1994; 8:A272.

60. Oleske JM, Westphal ML, Shore S, et al. Correction with zinc therapy of depressed cellular immunity in acrodermatitis enteropathica. Am J Dis Child 1979; 133:915–918.

61. Fraker PJ, Gershwin ME, Good RA, Prasad A. Interrelationships between zinc and immune function. Fed Proc 1986; 45:1474–1479.

62. Bogden JD, Oleske JM, Lavenhar MA, et al. Zinc and immunocompetence in elderly people: effects of zinc supplementation for 3 months. Am J Clin Nutr 1988; 48:655–663.

63. Chandra RK, Hambreaus L, Puri S, Au B, Kutty KM. Immune responses of healthy volunteers given supplements of zinc or selenium. FASEB J 1993; 7:A723.

64. Bogden JD, Oleske JM, Lavenhar MA, et al. Effects of one year of supplementation with zinc and other micronutrients on cellular immunity in the elderly. J Am College Nutr 1990; 9:214–225.

65. Chandra RK. Effect of vitamin and trace-element supplementation on immune responses and infection in elderly subjects. Lancet 1992; 340:1124–1127.

66. Penn ND, Purkins L. Kelleher J, et al. The effect of dietary supplementation with vitamins A, C, and E on cell-mediated immune function in elderly long-stay patients: a randomized controlled trial. Age Ageing 1991; 20:169–174.

67. Chavance M, Herbeth B, Lemoine A, Zhu BP. Does multivitamin supplementation prevent infections in healthy elderly subjects? A controlled trial. Int J Vitam Nutr Res 1993; 63:11–16.

68. Bogden JD, Bendich A, Kemp FW, et al. Daily micronutrient supplements enhance delayed-hypersensitivity skin test responses in older people. Am J Clin Nutr 1994; 60:437–447.

69. Kniker WT, Anderson CT, McBryde JL, Roumiantzeff M, Lesourd B. Multitest CMI for standardized measurement of delayed cutaneous hypersensitivity and cell-mediated immunity. Normal values and proposed scoring system for healthy adults in the USA. Ann Allergy 1984; 52:75–82.

70. Park YK, Kim I, Yetley EA. Characteristics of vitamin and mineral supplement products in the United States. Amer J Clin Nutr 1991; 54:750–759.

71. Block G, Cox C, Madans J, et al. Vitamin supplement use, by demographic characteristics. Am J Epidemiol 1988; 127:297–309.

72. Cooper EL. Stress, Immunity, and Aging. New York: Marcel-Dekker, 1984.

73. Solomon GF. Emotions, immunity, and disease. In: Stress, Immunity and Aging. Copper EL, ed. New York: Marcel Dekker, 1984; 1–10.

74. Watson RR, Eisinger M. Exercise and Disease. Boca Raton: CRC, 1992; 71–178.

75. Keast D, Cameron K, Morton AR. Exercise and the immune response. Sports Med 1988; 5:248–267.

76. Fry RW, Morton AR, Keast D. Overtraining in athletes. Sports Med 1991; 12:32–65.

77. Nieman DC, Johanssen LM, Lee JW, Arabatzis K. Infectious episodes in runners before and after the Los Angeles marathon. J Sports Med Phys Fitness 1990; 30:316–328.

78. Peters EM, Bateman ED. Ultramarathon running and upper respiratory tract infections. S Afric Med J 1983; 64:582–584.

79. Barry-Billings M, Blomstrand E, McAndrew N, Newsholme EA. A communication link between skeletal muscle, brain, and cells of the immune system. Int J Sports Med 1990; 11:S122–S128.
80. Rubenoff R, Rall LC. Humoral mediation of changing body composition during aging and chronic inflammation. Nutr Rev 1993; 51:1–11.
81. Meydani S. Dietary modulation of cytokine production and biologic functions. Nutr Rev 1990; 48:361–368.
82. Stallone DD. The influence of obesity and its treatment on the immune system. Nutr Rev 1994; 52:37–50.
83. Spear-Hartley A, Sherman AR. Food restriction and the immune system. J Nutr Immunol 1994; 3:27–50.
84. Goodwin JS. Decreased immunity and increased morbidity in the elderly. Nutr Rev 1995; 53:S41–S46.
85. Rimm EB, Stampfer MJ, Ascherio A, et al. Vitamin E consumption and the risk of coronary heart disease in men. New Engl J Med 1993; 328:1450–1456.
86. Stampfer MJ, Hennekens CB, Manson JE, et al. Vitamin E consumption and the risk of coronary disease in women. New Engl J Med 1993; 328:1444–1449.
87. Bendich A, Langseth L. Health effects of vitamin C supplementation: a review. J Am Coll Nutr 1995; 14:124–136.

18   Impact of Vitamin A on Immunity and Infection in Developing Countries

Richard D. Semba

1. INTRODUCTION

The prevention of vitamin A deficiency has emerged as one of the most important public health efforts of this century. The observation that vitamin A supplementation reduces child morbidity and mortality in developing countries *(1)* has led to programs and new directions of research. Vitamin A capsules have entered the armamentarium for child survival, along with vaccines, oral rehydration, and the promotion of breast-feeding. Vitamin A plays an important role in immune function and resistance to disease. Improving vitamin A intake, whether through improved diet, fortification of foods, or periodic supplementation, is expected to reduce morbidity and mortality for millions of children *(2)*, and there may be many other therapeutic applications for vitamin A that have not yet been realized. The purpose of this chapter is to provide health professionals with a concise review of epidemiological, immunological, and clinical studies of vitamin A, and to present the current recommendations regarding treatment and prevention of vitamin A deficiency in populations in developing countries.

2. METABOLISM OF VITAMIN A

2.1. Absorption of Vitamin A

Vitamin A is a fat-soluble substance found in animal foods and dairy products. Vitamin A is available as preformed vitamin A, contained in liver, cod liver oil, butter, or eggs, or as pro-vitamin A carotenoids, as found in dark green leafy vegetables, carrots, papaya, and mangos. Retinol is esterified in the intestinal mucosa, packaged into chylomicra, and carried to the liver via the lymphatic circulation *(3)*. Pro-vitamin A carotenoids, such as β-carotene, may be converted to retinaldehyde through cleavage by carotenoid-15,15′-dioxygenase or by an excentric cleavage pathway. Approximately 50 of over 600 carotenoids found in nature may be converted to vitamin A *(4)*. The bioavailability of pro-vitamin A carotenoids is much less that of preformed vitamin A because of a variety of factors, including differences in efficacy of absorption and biochemical conversion. Although carotenoids, such as β-carotene, and vitamin A are often popularly regarded to be equivalent, there may large differences in biological functions of these two nutrients, especially in regard to antioxidant properties, since vitamin A is a less potent antioxidant than β-carotene.

From: *Preventive Nutrition: The Comprehensive Guide for Health Professionals*
Edited by A. Bendich and R. J. Deckelbaum Humana Press Inc., Totowa, NJ

2.2. Storage and Transport of Vitamin A

Approximately 90% of the vitamin A in the body is stored in the liver as retinyl esters *(5)*. The liver has the capacity to store enough vitamin A to last for several months, with longer storage capacity among adults than children. Periodic high doses of vitamin A are largely effective in preventing vitamin A deficiency for long periods because of the liver's ability to store vitamin A *(6)*. Retinol is released from the liver in combination with plasma retinol-binding protein (RBP) and transthyretin (TTR). Retinol is poorly soluble in water and is carried in the blood sequestered inside the carrier proteins, RBP and TTR. Retinol seems to enter cells via specific receptors, although it is unclear whether all cells contain these receptors *(7)*.

2.3. The Retinoid Receptors

Vitamin A exerts its effects through retinoid receptors, which are found in the nucleus of the cell. These receptors resemble steroid and thyroid hormone receptors, and support the idea that vitamin A acts much like a hormone *(8)*. In the cell, retinol is converted to its active metabolite, all-*trans*-retinoic acid. Retinoic acid can control genes through specific receptors that belong to the superfamily of thyroid and steroid receptors *(9,10)*. Retinoic acid receptors act as transcriptional activators for specific target genes. The retinoic acid receptor (RAR) is expressed as several isoforms, referred to as RAR α, β, and γ, for which all-*trans*-retinoic acid acts as a ligand, and retinoid-x receptors (RXR) referred to as RXR α, β, and γ, for which 9-*cis* retinoic acid acts as a ligand. 9-*cis*-retinoic acid seems to be functionally distinct from all-*trans*-retinoic acid, and interconversion may exist between the two isomers. Each RAR and RXR has a specific DNA-binding domain, a retinoic acid response element (RARE) by which these nuclear receptors may affect retinoic acid transcriptional activity. RAR and RXR receptors form heterodimers that bind to DNA and control gene activity. In addition, RXR receptors also can form heterodimers with vitamin D and thyroid hormone receptors *(11)*. The metabolic pathway of vitamin A is shown in Fig. 1. The number of genes regulated by retinoids that have been described in the literature is growing rapidly *(10)*, and the system of regulation is complex.

3. EFFECTS OF VITAMIN A DEFICIENCY

3.1. Immunity

3.1.1. INFECTIOUS DISEASES

Vitamin A deficiency is associated with a variety of infectious diseases, including diarrhea, pneumonia, measles, and human immunodeficiency virus type 1 (HIV-1) infection (Table 1) *(12–25)*. Serum retinol levels may drop during infection because of decreased intake and absorption of dietary vitamin A caused by diarrhea or intestinal pathogens, decreased mobilization of hepatic reserves of retinol, accelerated utilization by target tissues, and increased urinary losses of vitamin A during the acute phase response *(12,26,27)*. Overall, episodes of infection seem to hasten the depletion of vitamin A stores *(12)* Low serum vitamin A levels during infection may have detrimental effects on the immune response, given the close relationship between immune effector cell function and the availability of vitamin A.

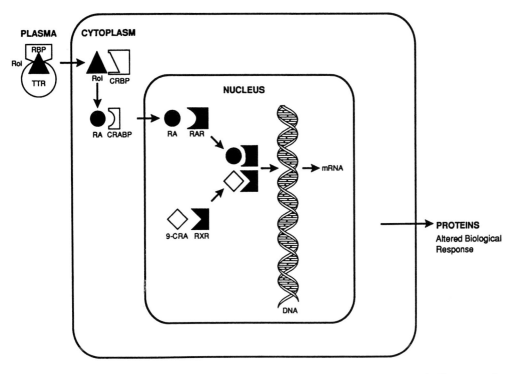

Fig. 1. Metabolic pathway for vitamin A. Rol=retinol, RBP=retinol binding protein, TTR=transthyretin, CRBP=cellular retinol binding protein, RA=retinoic acid, CRABP=cellular retinoic acid binding protein, RAR=retinoic acid receptor, 9-CRA=9-*cis* retinoic acid, RXR=retinoid x receptor. Thyroid hormone and vitamin D may also bind with RXR.

Table 1
Infectious Diseases Associated with Vitamin A Deficiency

Disease	Subjects	Ref.
Chicken pox	Children	*(12)*
Dengue fever	Children	(Semba, et al., unpublished)
Diarrhea	Children, adults	*(13)*
Endometritis	Adults	*(14)*
Human immunodeficiency virus type 1	Children, adults	*(15)*
Leprosy	Adults	*(16)*
Malaria	Children, adults	*(17)*
Measles	Children	*(18)*
Meningococcal disease	Children	*(19a)*
Otitis media	Children	*(19b)*
Pneumonia	Children, adults	*(20)*
Respiratory syncytial virus	Children	*(21)*
Rheumatic fever	Children	*(22)*
Tuberculosis	Children	*(23)*
Schistosomiasis	Adults	*(24)*
Whooping cough	Children	*(25)*

3.1.2. INCREASED MORTALITY

The biological consequences of vitamin A deficiency during infection include increased morbidity and mortality. High mortality rates for children with corneal xerophthalmia were described in Europe around the turn of the century *(13)*. High mortality rates might be expected, since corneal xerophthalmia and keratomalacia, the most severe ocular manifestations of vitamin A deficiency, were usually accompanied by protein-energy malnutrition and a precipitating infection, such as diarrhea, respiratory disease, or measles. With improvements in socioeconomic conditions and diet, vitamin A deficiency became less common in developed countries. In the late 1970s it was noted that children with mild degrees of vitamin A deficiency, i.e., nightblindness and Bitot's spots, had increased mortality *(28)*. These longitudinal studies in Indonesia showed that the mortality rate for children with mild xerophthalmia was four times greater than age-matched controls. The higher mortality was apparent even after accounting for differences in concurrent illnesses and protein-energy status. In addition, children with pre-existing xerophthalmia had higher rates of subsequent diarrhea and respiratory disease, whereas children who developed diarrhea and respiratory disease were at increased risk of subsequently developing xerophthalmia *(29,30)*. Thus, vitamin A status and infection seem to be related in a vicious cycle *(31)*.

Other studies soon confirmed the association between mild vitamin A deficiency and increased morbidity in children *(32,33)*. It is now becoming apparent that even subclinical vitamin A deficiency is associated with higher morbidity and mortality. In a large series of children with acute measles in Zaire, children with the lowest vitamin A levels had the highest mortality *(18)*. Adults with vitamin A deficiency during HIV-1 infection have decreased survival, and the risk of mortality is more than four times greater *(15,34)*.

3.1.3. MUCOSAL IMMUNITY

Vitamin A deficiency may cause a breakdown in mucosal immunity through pathological changes in the epithelia of respiratory, gastrointestinal, and urinary systems. This includes keratinizing metaplasia and loss of goblet cells and mucus *(27)*. Loss of intestinal brush border and goblet cells and squamous metaplasia and destruction of ciliated epithelia in the respiratory system have been reported in vitamin A-deficient animals. Decreased levels of secretory IgA in saliva have been reported in vitamin A-deficient children. Mucosal immunity, the "front line" of the body's immune defenses, may be compromised during vitamin A deficiency.

3.1.4. CELLULAR IMMUNITY

Atrophy of the thymus, spleen, and lymphoid tissues has been observed in children who died with vitamin A deficiency *(27)*. Mild vitamin A deficiency is associated with underlying alterations in circulating T-cell subpopulations, such as decreased CD4+CD45RA+ T-cells, or "naive" CD4 T-cells, and decreased CD4/CD8 ratios. During HIV-1 infection, vitamin A-deficient adults had lower circulating numbers of CD4 T-cells compared to adults with normal vitamin A levels. Vitamin A deficiency is also associated with pathologic alterations of T-cell subpopulations during acute meningococcal infection in children and during HIV-1 infection in adults *(19a)*.

Vitamin A and its metabolites are essential for immune effector cell function, including T-cells of the thymus, lymphocytes in lymphoid tissue, and peripheral blood lymphocytes *(27)*. Retinoic acid is involved in the expression of IL-2 receptor on T-cells. Retinol is essential for growth and differentiation of B-cells and the production of antibodies *(35,36)*. Retinoic acid may enhance immunoglobulin synthesis by cord blood mononuclear cells through increased T-cell help, i.e., modulation of cytokines, which induce B-cells to differentiate into greater numbers of immunoglobulin-secreting cells *(37)*. In-vitro studies suggest that vitamin A modulates growth and function of T and B-cells, either directly or through its active metabolite, all-*trans* retinoic acid.

Vitamin A and β-carotene supplementation are associated with changes in lymphocyte numbers and T-cell subpopulations *(27)*. The depression in circulating lymphocytes following surgery can be reversed by administration of high-dose vitamin A to adults. Children with clinical and subclinical vitamin A deficiency who received vitamin A had increases in circulating CD4 T-cells, especially CD4CD45RA, or "naive" T-cells, and an increase in CD4/CD8 ratio 5 wk after dosing. Measles infection is characterized by immune suppression, leukopenia, and decreased circulating CD4 T-cells. Administration of high-dose vitamin A to children with measles has been shown to increase total circulating lymphocytes as well as enhance IgG responses to measles *(38)*. High doses of β-carotene, a provitamin A carotenoid, have been shown to increase circulating CD4 T-cells in normal adults and adults with HIV-1 infection *(27)*. Thus, vitamin A or β-carotene seem to increase both numbers and proportions of CD4 T-cells in the circulation. Vitamin A and related metabolites are potent enhancers of cellular differentiation, and a possible mechanism for the increase in CD4 T-cells may be vitamin A-related differentation of lymphocytes.

3.1.5. ANTIBODY RESPONSES

A hallmark of vitamin A deficiency is the impaired ability to mount an antibody response against T-cell-dependent protein antigens *(27,39,40)*. Other types of immune responses may be unaffected by vitamin A deficiency. The antibody response to immunization with tetanus toxoid or other antigens has been used to examine immune competence. Vitamin A-deficient children in Indonesia had reduced antibody responses to tetanus toxoid *(41)*. Supplementation with high-dose vitamin A (200,000 IU) was associated with more than twofold enhancement of both primary and secondary IgG responses to tetanus toxoid compared to children who received placebo. Vitamin A potentiated IgG_1 subclass responses to tetanus toxoid, which is the subclass that is usually involved in the protective antibody response to tetanus *(27)*. The simultaneous administration of vitamin A supplements with tetanus-diphtheria-pertussis vaccine at 6, 10, and 14 wk of age in infants has recently been shown to enhance IgG responses to tetanus toxoid (Semba RD, et al., unpublished data). These findings suggest that the ability to mount an IgG response to T-cell-dependent antigens is improved by administration of vitamin A or related retinoids.

3.2. Growth

Vitamin A deficiency is characterized by both stunting and wasting *(42)*. Such a relationship might be expected because the gene for growth hormone is activated by retinoic acid *(43)*. However, the reported effects of vitamin A supplementation on child growth are not consistent *(42)*. A randomized controlled clinical trial involving over 2000 preschool children in Indonesia demonstrated that vitamin A supplementation had a selective effect on ponderal growth in boys but not girls *(44)*. Improved linear growth among both boys and girls was noted in a controlled trial of vitamin A-fortified monosodium glutamate involving over 1600 children *(45)*. A recent trial of vitamin A supplementation showed no effect on growth in 592 preschool children, but this small sample size may have lacked sufficient power to examine the impact of vitamin A on growth *(46)*.

3.3. Reproduction and Pregnancy

Vitamin A is essential for normal reproduction *(47)*. Animals deficient in vitamin A are unable to produce sperm, and vitamin A deficiency may affect fertility in the female. In both humans and animal models, vitamin A deficiency is associated with increased placental infections *(14)*. Vitamin A deficiency in HIV-infected pregnant women is associated with increased mother-to-child transmission of HIV, and increased placental infections, such as chorioamnionitis, may facilitate transmission of HIV *(48)*. Pregnancy increases the risk of vitamin A deficiency for both mother and newborn. Epidemics of nightblindness among pregnant women were well known in Europe in the early part of this century *(49)*, and nightblindness is so common in some cultures in developing countries that it has been considered to be a normal associate of pregnancy, as with morning sickness. Maternal vitamin A status may be important to birth outcome, because increased mortality and low birthweight have been reported among HIV-infected pregnant women who are vitamin A-deficient during pregnancy *(48,50)*. It is yet unknown whether vitamin A deficiency in pregnant women (HIV-negative) is associated with increased infant mortality.

3.4. Hematopoiesis

Hematopoietic stem cells are retinoid-dependent, and impaired hematopoiesis, or anemia, is a common associate of vitamin A deficiency in children *(51)*. Anemia may be because of, in part, impaired ability to mobilize iron stores from the liver during vitamin A deficiency. Vitamin A deficiency is associated with low hemoglobin in HIV-infected injection drug users *(15)*. Vitamin A supplementation or fortification has been shown to improve iron status and reduce anemia among children and pregnant women *(52)*. The combination of vitamin A and iron in a single supplement seems to reduce anemia more effectively than either iron or vitamin A alone *(52)*.

3.5. Vision

Vitamin A deficiency is the leading cause of blindness among children worldwide. Xerophthalmia is used to describe the wide spectrum of ophthalmological disease associated with vitamin A deficiency, and keratomalacia refers to the most severe stage in which the cornea undergoes ulceration and often results in blindness *(53)*. Vitamin A is essential for generation of rhodopsin, a visual pigment necessary for vision. The earliest clinical manifestation of vitamin A deficiency is nightblindness *(53)*. Vitamin A deficiency in general has an effect on mucosal epithelia, including the conjunctiva, and cornea. Mild vitamin A deficiency causes squamous metaplasia of the conjunctiva which may be detectable microscopically, or may form a Bitot's spot, a well-demarcated area of keratinizing squamous metaplasia on the temporal or nasal bulbar conjunctiva. Bitot's spots are considered to be pathognomonic for mild vitamin A deficiency. Severe xerophthalmia is characterized by classic, punched-out, full-thickness corneal ulceration; these ulcers may be sterile or may rapidly become secondarily in-

Table 2
Clinical Features of Vitamin A Deficiency

Organ system	Clinical features
Eye	Nightblindness, Bitot's spots, corneal xerosis, corneal ulcers, keratomalacia, blindness
Immune system	Atrophy of thymus, lymph nodes, spleen; depressed antibody and cell-mediated responses, T-cell subset alterations, increased morbidity and mortality
Hematologic	Anemia
Lungs	Loss of ciliated epithelium, squamous metaplasia, loss of goblet cells and mucus; increased pulmonary infections
Gastrointestinal tract	Loss of brush border, atrophy of Peyer's patches, loss of goblet cells and mucus, greater severity of diarrhea
Genitourinary	Squamous metaplasia of bladder epithelium, increased infections
Reproductive	Reproductive failure, low birthweight, placental infections, higher infant mortality
Skin	Increased infections
Growth	Stunting, wasting

fected with melting of the corneal stroma. The ocular manifestations of vitamin A deficiency are described in detail elsewhere (13,53). It was previously estimated that 500,000 new cases of xerophthalmia, half which lead to blindness, occur each year in India, Bangladesh, and the Philippines combined (54). Recent data suggest that vitamin A capsule distribution programs may be effective in reducing xerophthalmia (55,56), and such estimates of blindness may need to be revised.

4. DIAGNOSIS OF VITAMIN A DEFICIENCY

4.1. Eye Signs and Symptoms

Although vitamin A deficiency has a wide spectrum of clinical manifestations (Table 2), the clinical diagnosis in children is most commonly made through recognition of ocular signs and symptoms, including nightblindness, Bitot's spots, corneal xerosis, or corneal ulceration/keratomalacia (53). The detection of nightblindness and/or Bitot's spots is often useful for determining the prevalence of mild xerophthalmia among children in developing countries. Among pregnant women in developing countries, assessment of nightblindness may be a potential screening test for vitamin A deficiency.

4.2. Serum Retinol Levels

Serum vitamin A levels remain the most widely used indicator of vitamin A status (57) and are especially useful in epidemiologic studies and in individuals during infections. Vitamin A levels <0.7 µmol/L in children and <1.05 µmol/L in adults are consistent with vitamin A deficiency. Factors contributing to low serum vitamin A levels include poor intake and absorption, inadequate liver stores, liver disease, increased utilization, and the acute phase response. During the acute phase response, RBP may dissociate from the RBP-transthyretin-retinol complex in circulating blood, allowing abnormal vitamin A losses in the urine and decreased circulating vitamin A levels (26). High urinary losses of vitamin A have been reported in individuals with pneumonia, nephritis, tuberculosis, sepsis, and malaria *(26)* Recent studies suggest that biological function is compromised when serum vitamin A levels are below 1.05 µmol/L *(57,58)*. Low serum vitamin A levels, whether part of the acute phase response or a result of inadequate hepatic reserves of vitamin A, suggest a higher risk of morbidity and death. Individuals with low vitamin A levels have increased risk of morbidity and mortality during measles *(18)*, HIV infection *(15,34)*, respiratory syncytial virus infection *(21)*, and meningococcal disease *(19a)*. Impairment of immune responses during infections may be related to the inability of T- and B-cells to function without adequate levels of retinol *(27)*.

4.3. Other Methods of Diagnosis

Vitamin A status can be measured by other techniques that measure end organ effects of vitamin A (conjunctival impression cytology, dark adaptation) and liver reserves of vitamin A (relative dose response, modified relative dose response). Conjunctival impression cytology is based on cytological examination of cells removed from the conjunctiva of the eye *(59)*. Dark adaptation has been recognized for decades to be useful, in various forms, for measuring vitamin A deficiency *(60)*. Relative dose response (RDR) *(61)* and modified relative dose response (MRDR) *(62)* are indirect measures of hepatic vitamin A stores. In general, abnormal RDR and MRDR responses correlate well with deficient serum vitamin A levels. A new technique that involves the measurement of pupillary diameter has advantages of being simple, rapid, noninvasive, and early results with use of the technique for assessment of vitamin A status are promising *(63)*.

5. VITAMIN A AS A PUBLIC HEALTH INTERVENTION

5.1. Early History

The use of liver extracts as a cure for nightblindness has been known from antiquity, and vitamin A has been used in the treatment of infections for at least 2000 yr. In the late 1920s and early 1930s, Green and Mellanby dubbed vitamin A the "anti-infective" vitamin and conducted a clinical trial of 550 pregnant women in Sheffield, England that demonstrated that a cod-liver oil type of therapy could reduce severe infections associated with pregnancy and delivery *(14)*. In a controlled trial of 600 English children with acute measles, cod-liver oil was shown to reduce mortality by 58% *(64)*. Cod-liver oil was commonly used to prevent infections in children before World War II. With the advent of antibiotics and improvements in diet, vitamin A deficiency largely disappeared as a public health problem in industrialized countries. The use of vitamin A as an "anti-infective" agent was largely forgotten.

5.2. Clinical Trials of Vitamin A for Reducing Infections and Mortality

Vitamin A deficiency and its relationship with child mortality was rediscovered in Indonesia in the 1970s *(28)*. This observation led to a large community-based study that demonstrated that regular vitamin A supplementation reduced childhood mortality by 34% in Indonesia *(65)*. Earlier historical observations would suggest that such a finding might be expected, but the study generated a great deal of controversy. The Indonesian study was followed by a large series of clinical trials in Indonesia, India, Nepal, Sudan, and Ghana *(45,66,72)*. These studies (Table 3) demonstrated that periodic vitamin A

Table 3
Recent Clinical Trials of Vitamin A Supplementation in Developing Countries

Country	Year	Sample size	Results	Ref.
Indonesia	1986	29,236	34% ↓ mortality	65
Indonesia	1988	11,220	46% ↓ mortality	45
India	1990	15,775	6% ↓ mortality	66
India	1990	15,419	54% ↓ mortality	67
Nepal	1991	24,805	30% ↓ mortality	68
Nepal	1992	7,197	29% ↓ mortality	70
Sudan	1992	29,615	No impact on mortality or xerophthalmia	71
Ghana	1993	21,906	19% ↓ mortality	72
Brazil	1994	1,240	20% ↓ reduction in severe diarrhea	77
Tanzania	1987	180	46% ↓ mortality during measles	73
South Africa	1990	189	80% ↓ mortality during measles	74
South Africa	1991	60	↓ Morbidity during measles	75
Kenya	1994	235	↓ Morbidity during measles	76

supplementation or fortification reduced child mortality. The sole exception was the study conducted in the Sudan, which reported that high dose vitamin A capsules had no impact on either child mortality or vitamin A deficiency itself *(71)*.

The impact of vitamin A supplementation on morbidity and mortality during measles is striking. Worldwide, measles affects approx 70 million children/yr and up to 2 million children may die annually from measles and associated complications. In developing countries, case-fatality rates of 10–20% are not uncommon, and a measles episode may result in diarrhea, pneumonia, encephalitis, blindness, and delayed morbidity and mortality after an attack. High-dose vitamin A supplementation to children with acute, complicated measles reduces mortality by approx 50% (Table 3) *(64,73,74)*. Similarly, the morbidity of diarrhea and pneumonia associated with measles is also reduced by vitamin A supplementation *(75–77)*. It is notable in these studies that high-dose vitamin A supplementation was shown to reduce morbidity and mortality in children without any clinical signs of vitamin A deficiency.

Vitamin A supplementation has a dramatic impact on the severity of infectious disease morbidity and childhood mortality, but it seems to have less of a measurable effect on mild to moderate morbidity. Community-based trials of vitamin A supplementation have not demonstrated a consistent effect on the incidence of mild respiratory disease and diarrhea. Morbidity from respiratory infection, fever, and diarrhea, as measured by a history obtained from the mother or father, tends to be subjective and imprecise. Studies that have utilized weekly or even more frequent monitoring of morbidity are unable to address the issue of severe morbidity, since children who are ill have usually been treated. Preschool children in developing countries are constantly being exposed to new pathogens and have high rates of respiratory disease and diarrhea in the first years of life. The dramatic reductions in severe morbidity and mortality noted in hospital and community-based studies of vitamin A may have led to the inflated expectation that vitamin A might reduce the incidence of respiratory disease and diarrhea among children. On an immunological basis, there is little evidence that vitamin A would prevent infection by a pathogen that is new to the host, and thus have a measurable impact on incidence of infection. However, vitamin A-related immune enhancement may result in a vigorous host response, shorter duration of infection, and fewer complications. This is borne out by clinical trials that show that vitamin A supplementation reduces the severity of infectious disease morbidity as well as mortality (1).

5.3. Current Indications for Use of Vitamin A Supplements in Developing Countries

High-dose oral vitamin A supplements are recommended for children in three general situations: in the treatment of xerophthalmia, in the treatment of acute measles, and as periodic supplementation for the prevention of vitamin A deficiency (78,79). For the treatment of xerophthalmia or acute measles, WHO/UNICEF/IVACG suggest a 200,000 IU capsule of vitamin A on diagnosis, the following day, and 1 mo later for children over 1 yr of age, adolescents, and adults (except women of reproductive age). For children under 1 yr of age or children of any age who weigh < 8 kg, the aforementioned guidelines are followed using 100,000 IU capsules. Many developing countries have instituted periodic high dose vitamin A capsule distribution, and these programs generally use 200,000 IU capsules for children 1–6 yr of age, every 3–6 mo.

For women of reproductive age, pregnant or not pregnant, the WHO/UNICEF/ IVACG recommendations are a daily dose of 10,000 IU for 2 wk. Although this is a general recommendation, this dose is often unavailable in many developing countries. The DV for vitamin A for antenatal vitamins in the United States is 8,000 IU/d, and many commercial vitamins contain this dose, as vitamin A, β-carotene, or a combination of both. In general, high-dose vitamin A capsules should not be used for pregnant women or women of reproductive age who are not using reliable contraception, because of concerns regarding the theoretical teratogenicity of vitamin A. It is also important to recognize that there are well-defined therapeutic indications in which vitamin A has been demonstrated to be efficacious, and indiscriminate use of vitamin A supplements should be discouraged. Current research is attempting to determine whether vitamin A supplementation has any therapeutic value during HIV-1 infection and AIDS, for parasitic infections, such as malaria, and for other infections, such as respiratory syncytial virus infections. Until these studies are completed, there is no data to support use of vitamin A supplements under these circumstances. Vitamin A, as an immune enhancer, may be of value in increase the immune response to some vaccines, and studies are in progress to address potential use of high-dose vitamin A given with vaccination (see Chapter 30).

5.4. Prevention of Vitamin A Deficiency

Approaches for the prevention of vitamin A deficiency include food fortification, nutrition education, home gardening, and preservation of vitamin A-containing fruits and vegetables. Fortification of sugar in Guatemala and monosodium glutamate in Indonesia have shown some success (45) and some countries, such as the Cook Islands, have specifically required that certain imported foodstuffs be fortified (80) One question that is often asked is why vitamin A deficiency is common among children in locations with a wealth of plant food sources of vitamin A, such as the island of Java in Indonesia. Young children may not like the bitter taste in many dark green leafy vegetables. Papaya and mango, which may be more palatable to children, are only available seasonally. It remains to be determined whether nutrition education and home gardening will have a significant impact on the vitamin A status of children in developing countries.

6. SUMMARY AND RECOMMENDATIONS

Vitamin A is a potent immune enhancer that has demonstrated efficacy in reducing morbidity and mortality from infectious diseases among children in developing countries. Improved vitamin A nutriture is expected to prevent 1.3–2.5 million deaths annually worldwide, and periodic high-dose vitamin A supplementation is now widely practiced in many developing countries where vitamin A deficiency is endemic *(2)*. High-dose vitamin A supplementation for children with acute, complicated measles may also be expected to contribute to a reduction in child mortality, given the estimated two million deaths from measles each year. A variety of approaches, such as food fortification, supplementation, nutrition education, and home gardening, may be utilized in developing countries to combat vitamin A deficiency and increase resistance to infectious diseases.

7. ACKNOWLEDGMENTS

This work was supported in part by grants from the National Institutes of Health (AI35143, HD30042), the Thrasher Research Fund, the World Health Organization Expanded Programme on Immunization, and the Office of Nutrition, Bureau for Science and Technology, United States Agency for International Development (Cooperative Agreement DAN-0045-A-5094-00).

REFERENCES

1. Beaton GH, Martorell R, L'Abbé KA, et al. Effectiveness of Vitamin A Supplementation in the Control of Young Child Morbidity and Mortality in Developing Countries. Toronto, Canada: University of Toronto, 1992; 1–108.
2. Humphrey JH, West KP Jr, Sommer A. Vitamin A deficiency and attributable mortality among under-5-year-olds. Bull WHO 1992; 70:225–232.
3. Goodman DS. Biosynthesis, absorption, and hepatic metabolism of retinol. In: The Retinoids, vol. 2. Sporn MB, Roberts AB, Goodman DS, eds. New York: Academic; 1984: 1–39.
4. Blaner WS, Olson JA. Retinol and retinoic acid metabolism. In: The Retinoids: Biology, Chemistry, and Medicine, 2nd ed. Sporn MB, Roberts AB, Goodman DS eds. New York: Raven, 1994; pp. 229–255.
5. Olson JA, Gunning DB, Tilton RA. Liver concentrations of vitamin A and carotenoids, as a function of age and other parameters, of American children who died of various causes. Am J Clin Nutr 1984; 39:903–910.
6. West KP Jr, Sommer A. Periodic, large oral doses of vitamin A for the prevention of vitamin A deficiency and xerophthalmia: a summary of experiences. Washington, DC: Nutrition Foundation, 1984; 1–44.
7. Soprano DR, Blaner WS. Plasma retinol-binding protein. In: The Retinoids: Biology, Chemistry, and Medicine, 2nd ed. Sporn MB, Roberts AB, Goodman DS eds. New York: Raven, 1994; 257–281.
8. Ross AC, Ternus ME. Vitamin A as a hormone: recent advances in understanding the actions of retinol, retinoic acid, and beta carotene. J Am Diet Assoc 1993; 93:1285–1290.
9. Evans RM. The steroid and thyroid hormone receptor superfamily. Science 1988; 240:889–895.
10. De Luca LM. Retinoids and their receptors in differentiation, embryogenesis, and neoplasia. FASEB J 1991; 5:2924–2933.
11. Kliewer SA, Umesono K, Mangelsdorf DJ, Evans RM. Retinoid X receptor interacts with nuclear receptors in retinoic acid, thyroid hormone and vitamin D_3 signalling. Nature 1992; 355:446–449.
12. Campos FACS, Flores H, Underwood BA. Effect of an infection on vitamin A status of children as measured by the relative dose response (RDR). Am J Clin Nutr 1987; 46:91–94.
13. Sommer A. Nutritional Blindness. New York: Oxford University Press; 1982; 1–282.
14. Green JM, Pindar D, Davis G, Mellanby E. Diet as a prophylactic agent against puerperal sepsis with specific reference to vitamin A as an anti-infective agent. Br Med J 1931; ii:595–598.

15. Semba RD, Caiaffa WT, Graham NMH, Cohn S, Vlahov D. Vitamin A deficiency and wasting as predictors of mortality in human immunodeficiency virus-infected injection drug users. J Infect Dis 1995; 171:1196–1202.
16. Sher R, Shulman G, Baily P, Politzer WM. Serum trace elements and vitamin A in leprosy subtypes. Am J Clin Nutr 1981; 34:1918–1924.
17. Stürchler D, Tanner M, Hanck A, et al. A longitudinal study on relations of retinol with parasitic infections and the immune response in children of Kikwawila village, Tanzania. Acta Trop 1987; 44:213–227.
18. Markowitz LE, Nzilambi N, Driskell WJ, et al. Vitamin A levels and mortality among hospitalized measles patients, Kinshasa, Zaire. J Trop Pediatr 1989; 35:109–112.
19a. Semba RD, Bulterys M, Munyeshuli V, Gatsinzi T, Saah A, Chao A, Dushimimana A. Vitamin A deficiency and T-cell subpopulations in children with meningococcal disease. J Trop Pediatr, in press.
19b. Lloyd-Puryear M, Humphrey JH, West KP Jr, et al. Vitamin A deficiency and anemia among Micronesian children. Nutr Res 1989; 9:1009–1016.
20. Lindquist T. Untersuchungen über das Vitamin A bei Pneumonie. Klin Wochenschr 1937; 39:1345–1348.
21. Neuzil KM, Gruber WC, Chytil F, Stahlman MT, Engelhardt B, Graham BS. Serum vitamin A levels in respiratory syncytial virus infection. J Pediatr 1994; 124:433–436.
22. Shank RE, Coburn AF, Moore LV, Hoagland CL. The level of vitamin A and carotene in the plasma of rheumatic subjects. J Clin Invest 1944; 23:289–295.
23. Solon FS, Popkin BM, Fernandez TL, Latham MC. Vitamin A deficiency in the Philippines: a study of xerophthalmia in Cebu. Am J Clin Nutr 1978; 31:360–368.
24. Abdelgani SM, Hussein L, Shaaban S. Vitamin A status in different stages of schistosomal cases and the effectiveness of oral vitamin A therapy. Z Ernahrungswiss 1990; 29:249–255.
25. Blegvad O. Xerophthalmia, keratomalacia, and xerosis conjunctivae. Am J Ophthalmol 1924; 7:89–117.
26. Stephensen C, Alvarez J, Kohatsu J, et al. Vitamin A is excreted in the urine during acute infection. Am J Clin Nutr 1994; 60:388–392.
27. Semba RD. Vitamin A, immunity, and infection. Clin Infect Dis 1994; 19:489–499.
28. Sommer A, Tarwotjo I, Hussaini G, Susanto D. Increased mortality in children with mild vitamin A deficiency. Lancet 1983; 2:585–558.
29. Sommer A, Katz J, Tarwotjo I. Increased risk of respiratory disease and diarrhea in children with preexisting mild vitamin A deficiency. Am J Clin Nutr 1984; 40:1090–1095.
30. Sommer A, Tarwotjo I, Katz J. Increased risk of xerophthalmia following diarrhea and respiratory disease. Am J Clin Nutr 1987; 45:977–980.
31. Sommer A. Vitamin A status, resistance to infection, and childhood mortality. Ann NY Acad Sci 1990; 587:17–23.
32. Milton RC, Reddy V, Naidu AN. Mild vitamin A deficiency and childhood morbidity—an Indian experience. Am J Clin Nutr 1987; 46:827–829.
33. Bloem MW, Wedel M, Egger RJ, et al. Mild vitamin A deficiency and risk of respiratory tract diseases and diarrhea in preschool and school children in northeastern Thailand. Am J Epidemiol 1990; 131:332–339.
34. Semba RD, Graham NMH, Caiaffa WT, et al. Increased mortality associated with vitamin A deficiency during human immunodeficiency virus type 1 infection. Arch Intern Med 1993; 153:2149–2154.
35. Buck J, Ritter G, Dannecker L, et al. Retinol is essential for growth of activated human B cells. J Exp Med 1990; 171:1613–1624.
36. Wang W, Napoli JL, Ballow M. The effects of retinol on in vitro immunoglobulin synthesis by cord blood and adult peripheral blood mononuclear cells. Clin Exp Immunol 1993; 92:164–168.
37. Wang W, Ballow M. The effects of retinoic acid on in vitro immunoglobulin synthesis by cord blood and adult peripheral blood mononuclear cells. Cell Immunol 1993; 148:291–300.
38. Coutsoudis A, Kiepiela P, Coovadia HM, Broughton M. Vitamin A supplementation enhances specific IgG antibody levels and total lymphocyte numbers while improving morbidity in measles. Pediatr Infant Dis J 1992; 11:203–209.
39. Nauss KM. Influence of vitamin A status on the immune system. In: Vitamin A Deficiency and Its Control. Bauernfeind JC, ed. Orlando, FL: Academic, 1986; 207–243.
40. Ross AC. Vitamin A status: relationship to immunity and the antibody response. Proc Soc Exp Biol Med 1992; 200:303–320.
41. Semba RD, Muhilal, Scott AL, et al. Depressed immune response to tetanus in children with vitamin A deficiency. J Nutr 1992; 122:101–107.
42. West KP Jr. Dietary vitamin A deficiency: effects on growth, infection, and mortality. Bull Food Nutr 1991; 13:119–131.

43. Bedo G, Santisteban P, Aranda A. Retinoic acid regulates growth hormone expression. Nature 1989; 339:231–234.
44. West KP Jr, Djunaedi E, Pandji A, et al. Vitamin A supplementation and growth: a randomized community trial. Am J Clin Nutr 1988; 48:1257–1264.
45. Muhilal, Permeisih D, Idjradinata YR, et al. Vitamin A-fortified monosodium glutamate and health, growth, and survival of children: a controlled field trial. Am J Clin Nutr 1988; 48:1271–1276.
46. Ramakrishnan U, Latham MC, Abel R. Vitamin A supplementation does not improve growth of preschool children: a randomized, double-blind field trial in South India. J Nutr 1995; 125:202–211.
47. Eskild W, Hansson V. Vitamin A functions in the reproductive organs. In: Vitamin A in Health and Disease. Blomhoff R, ed. New York: Marcel Dekker, 1994; 531–559.
48. Semba RD, Miotti PG, Chiphangwi JD, et al. Maternal vitamin A deficiency and mother-to-child transmission of HIV-1. Lancet 1994; 343:1593–1597.
49. Birnbacher T, Klaften E. Die Hemeralopie der Schwangeren. Z Augenheilk 1923; 51:309–324.
50. Semba RD, Miotti PG, Chiphangwi JD, Liomba G, Yang LP, Saah AJ, Dallabetta GA, Hoover DR. Infant mortality and maternal vitamin A deficiency during human immunodeficiency virus infection. Clin Infect Dis 1995; 21:966–972.
51. Bloem MW, Wedel M, van Agtmaal EJ, et al. Vitamin A intervention: short-term effects of a single, oral, massive dose on iron metabolism. Am J Clin Nutr 1990; 51:469–478.
52. Suharno D, West CE, Muhilal, Karyadi D, Hautvast JGAJ. Supplementation with vitamin A and iron for nutritional anaemia in pregnant women in West Java, Indonesia. Lancet 1993; 342:1325–1328.
53. Sommer A. Field Guide to the Detection and Control of Xerophthalmia. Geneva: World Health Organization; 1982; 1–58.
54. Sommer A, Tarwotjo I, Hussaini G, Susanto D, Soegiharto T. Incidence, prevalence, and scale of blinding malnutrition. Lancet 1981; ii:1407–1408.
55. Muhilal, Tarwotjo I, Kodyat B, et al. Changing prevalence of xerophthalmia in Indonesia, 1977 to 1992. Eur J Clin Nutr 1995; 48:708–714.
56. Semba RD, Susatio B, Muhilal, Natadisastra G. The decline of admissions for xerophthalmia at Cicendo Eye Hospital, Indonesia, 1981–1992. Int Ophthal 1995; 19:39–42.
57. Underwood BA. Methods for assessment of vitamin A status. J Nutr 1990; 120:1459–1463.
58. Pilch SM. Analysis of vitamin A data from the health and nutrition examination surveys. J Nutr 1987; 117:636–640.
59. Keenum DG, Semba RD, Wirasasmita S, et al. Assessment of vitamin A status by a disk applicator for conjunctival impression cytology. Arch Ophthalmol 1990; 108:1436–1441.
60. Edmund C. Some methods of testing dark-vision. Acta Ophthalmol 1926; 3:153–169.
61. Flores H, Campos F, Araújo CRC, Underwood BA. Assessment of marginal vitamin A deficiency in Brazilian children using the relative dose response procedure. Am J Clin Nutr 1987; 46:91–94.
62. Tanumihardjo SA, Muhilal, Yuniar Y, et al. Vitamin A status in preschool-age Indonesian children as assessed by the modified relative dose response (MRDR) assay. Am J Clin Nutr 1990; 52:1068–1072.
63. Congdon N, Sommer A, Severns M, et al. Pupillary and visual thresholds in young children as an index of population vitamin A status. Am J Clin Nutr 1995; 61:1076–1082.
64. Ellison JB. Intensive vitamin therapy in measles. Br Med J 1932; 2:708–711.
65. Sommer A, Tarwotjo I, Djunaedi E, et al. Impact of vitamin A supplementation on childhood mortality: a randomised controlled community trial. Lancet 1986; 1:1169–1173.
66. Vijayaraghavan K, Radhaiah G, Prakasam BS, et al. Effect of massive dose vitamin A on morbidity and mortality in Indian children. Lancet 1990; 336:1342–1345.
67. Rahmathullah L, Underwood BA, Thulasiraj RD, et al. Reduced mortality among children in southern India receiving a small weekly dose of vitamin A. New Engl J Med 1990; 323:929–935.
68. West KP Jr, Pokhrel RP, Katz J, et al. Efficacy of vitamin A in reducing preschool child mortality in Nepal. Lancet 1991; 338:67–71.
69. Kothari G. The effect of vitamin A prophylaxis on morbidity and mortality among children in urban slums in Bombay. J Trop Pediatr 1991; 37:141.
70. Daulaire NMP, Starbuck ES, Houston RM, et al. Childhood mortality after a high dose of vitamin A in a high risk population. Br Med J 1992; 304:207–210.
71. Herrera MG, Nestel P, El Amin A, et al. Vitamin A supplementation and child survival. Lancet 1992; 340:267–271.
72. Ghana VAST Study Team. Vitamin A supplementation in northern Ghana: effects on clinic attendances, hospital admissions, and child mortality. Lancet 1993; 342:7–12.

73. Barclay AJG, Foster A, Sommer A. Vitamin A supplements and mortality related to measles: a randomised clinical trial. Br J Med 1987; 294:294–296.

74. Hussey GD, Klein M. A randomized, controlled trial of vitamin A in children with severe measles. New Engl J Med 1990; 323:160–164.

75. Coutsoudis A, Broughton M, Coovadia HM. Vitamin A supplementation reduces measles morbidity in young African children: a randomized, placebo-controlled, double-blind trial. Am J Clin Nutr 1991; 54:890–895.

76. Ogaro FO, Orinda VA, Onyango FE, Black RE. Effect of vitamin A on diarrheal and respiratory complications of measles. Trop Geogr Med 1993; 45:283–286.

77. Barreto ML, Santos LMP, Assis AMO, et al. Effect of vitamin A supplementation on diarrhea and acute lower-respiratory-tract infections in young children in Brazil. Lancet 1994; 344:228–231.

78. WHO/UNICEF/IVACG Task Force. Vitamin A supplements. A guide to their use in the treatment and prevention of vitamin A deficiency and xerophthalmia. World Health Organization, Geneva, Switzerland, 1988; 1–24.

79. International Vitamin A Consultative Group. Guidelines for the eradication of vitamin A deficiency and xerophthalmia. Washington, DC: Nutrition Foundation, 1988; I1–IV7.

80. Schaumberg DA, Linehan M, Hawley G, et al. Vitamin A deficiency in the South Pacific. Public Health 1995; 109:311–317.

PART III
OPTIMAL BIRTH OUTCOMES

19 Folic Acid-Containing Multivitamins and Primary Prevention of Birth Defects

Andrew E. Czeizel

1. INTRODUCTION

The deficiency or overdosage of certain nutrients may have a role in the origin of birth defects. First, in 1932, Hale *(1)* demonstrated that a vitamin A-free diet during early pregnancy of sows resulted in offspring without eyeballs. Some of the pigs also had other defects, such as oral clefts, accessory ears, malposition of kidney, and defects of hind legs. Hale's conclusion was "the condition is illustrative of the marked effect that a deficiency may have in the disturbance of the internal factors that control the mechanism of development" *(1)*. Further development of experimental teratology became possible when small rodents were introduced for this purpose. Joseph Warkany (1902–1992) *(2)*, one of the founders of teratology, recognized the importance of purified diets and used these to test various vitamin deficiencies for their teratogenic effects. He found that maternal dietary deficiency can induce structural birth defects, i.e., congenital abnormalities (CAs) *(3)*. Marjorie M. Nelson *(4)* introduced the use of antimetabolites, which made possible conversion of longterm nutritional experiments into short-term chemical testing. First, antimetabolites of folic acid were used and folic acid defiency was proved highly teratogenic in pregnant rats *(5–7)*. Later it was confirmed in humans *(8–10)* as well. This research approach also had strong support from the French investigator, Giroud *(11,12)*. These findings highlighted the developmental importance of folic acid *(13,14)*. However, this first phase of history of malnutritional teratology, including folic acid deficiency, was followed by a longer silent period. The second, recent phase is related to the primary prevention of neural-tube defects in the 1980s.

Anencephaly and spina bifida (aperta or cystica) are the major classes of neural-tube defects (NTDs) *(15)*. Although the genetic (polygenic) background of nonsyndromic, i.e., the so-called isolated NTDs (92% of all cases) is obvious because recurrence in first degree relatives is 10 times higher than their occurrence *(16)*, this group of CAs is very sensitive to environmental factors. The latter is indicated by the very wide range (0.5–12/1000) of NTD incidences in different populations, rapid secular changes in their occurrence, seasonal variation of births with NTD, and mainly by their very obvious socioeconomic status dependence *(17)*: The risk of NTDs was found to increase from a low risk in the highest class to an above-average risk in the lowest class in the United Kingdom and some other countries.

From: *Preventive Nutrition: The Comprehensive Guide for Health Professionals*
Edited by A. Bendich and R. J. Deckelbaum Humana Press Inc., Totowa, NJ

The documented start of the second phase of the folic acid story dates back to 1976. Smithells hypothesized that among triggering environmental factors in the origin of NTDs, undernutrition could be the common denominator, and his group tested this hypothesis: A lower concentration of red cell folate and vitamin C was found during the first trimester of pregnancy in women who later gave birth to an infant with an NTD than in matched controls (18). These findings prompted Smithells and his group to organize the first intervention study (19).

2. INTERVENTION STUDIES (TABLE 1)

In general, NTDs occur between postconceptional d 15 and 28 in humans, i.e., at the critical period of NTDs most women are unaware of their pregnancy. Thus, "periconceptional" supplementation of multivitamins or folic acid should commence at least 28 d prior to conception and continue to the date of the second missed menstrual period.

The final results of the Smithells et al. study were published separately for the Yorkshire region of the United Kingdom (20) and Northern Ireland (21). However, the 91 and 83% reduction in NTD recurrence, respectively, were not accepted by some experts because of possible selection bias. Two ethical committees refused to give permission for the original protocol of the study, i.e., for a randomized clinical trial; thus, the control group was made up of women who had had one or more previous infants with NTDs and were already pregnant when referred to the study centers or declined to take part in the trial. The study in Wales performed by Laurence et al. (22) was a randomized, double-blind trial; however, the difference between study and placebo groups was not significant as a result of the small number of women. In the early 1980s, the Medical Research Council (MRC) (23) in the United Kingdom decided to organize a multicenter (43% of participants came from Hungary) double-blind randomized study. This trial indicated that a pharmacological dose (4 mg) of folic acid supplementation alone can reduce NTD recurrence significantly (by 71%). Based on these results, the Centers for Disease Control (CDC) (24) recommended daily supplementation with 4 mg of folic acid under medical supervision in the periconception period for women at high risk (i.e., who had one or more previous offspring with NTD) for the reduction of NTD recurrence.

However, there were two major questions following the publications of the "recurrence" studies and the Hungarian randomized, double-blind controlled trial attempted to provide data to answer these questions. The first question was: "Does folic acid containing-mulvitamin supplementation also reduce the risk of *first* occurrence of NTD?" About 95% of women who deliver infants with NTD have no previous NTD pregnancies. Thus, one of the critical goals of the Hungarian trial was to determine the efficacy of this new primary preventive method in the reduction of first occurrence of NTD (25). The second question was connected with the dose. The pharmacological dose (e.g., 4 mg) of folic acid may have some adverse effects (15); thus, it cannot be recommended for the population at large and/or without medical supervision. The Hungarian intervention trial, therefore, tested the preventive effect of a physiological dose (0.8 mg) of folic acid as one component of a periconceptional multivitamin supplement. The Hungarian trial was launched on February 1, 1984 and the intervention was completed on April 30, 1992. Pregnancy outcomes were evaluated until the end of April 1993 and the postnatal follow-up continued until the end of April 1994. As it can be

Table 1
The Data of Intervention Studies for the Reduction of NTD Recurrences and Occurrences

Type	Method	Country	Supplement	With supplement		Without supplement		Risk reduction (%)
				No.	%	No.	%	
Recurrence	Nonrandomized	Yorkshire (20)	Multivitamin[a]	1/187	0.5	18/320	5.6	91
		Northern Ireland (21)		4/511	0.8	17/353	4.8	83
	Randomized	Wales (22)	Folic acid (4 mg)	2/60	3.3	4/51	7.8	58
		Multicenter MRC (23)	Folic acid (4 mg)	2/298	0.7	13/300	4.3	84
			Folic acid + other vitamins	4/295	1.4	21/602[c]	3.5	71
			Total	6/593	1.0[c]			
			Other vitamins	8/302	2.6			
Occurrence	Randomized	Hungary (25)	Multivitamin[b]	0/2471	0.0	6/2391	0.25	100

[a]Included 0.36 mg folic acid
[b]Included 0.8 mg folic acid
[c]Including cases supplemented with 'other' vitamins

seen in Table 1, no NTD case was found in the multivitamin group, whereas 6 NTD cases occurred in the placebo-like trace-element group ($p = 0.01$). Thus, the Hungarian trial demonstrated that a multivitamin containing 0.8 mg of folic acid prevented the first occurrences of NTD.

Several observational studies also indicated the efficacy of periconceptional folic-acid containing multivitamin supplementation and folate-containing foods in the prevention of NTDs (26). For example, the study of Werler et al. (27) suggested that daily periconception intake of 0.4 mg of folic acid (the dose most commonly contained in over-the-counter multivitamin preparations) reduced the risk of occurrent NTDs by ~60%. Based on the Hungarian intervention (25) and observational studies (26–27) the CDC (28) in September 1992 and the US Public Health Service recommended that "all women of childbearing age who are capable of becoming pregnant should consume 0.4 mg of folic acid per day for the purpose of reducing their risk of having a pregnancy affected with spina bifida or other neural tube defects" This recommendation was subsequently followed by several countries.

At present there are three possibilities to provide appropriate multivitamin/folic acid consumption for women of childbearing age who are capable of becoming pregnant.

1. Consumption of folate-rich and other vitamin-rich diet. McPartlin et al. (29) study suggested that the optimal daily intake of folate in the pre- and postconceptional period is about 0.66 mg. However, the usual daily intake of folate is about 0.18–0.20 mg (30). It is difficult to imagine a 3.3–3.7-fold increase in folate intake every day in anticipation of conception.
2. Periconceptional supplementation would be a simple and useful approach; however, about 50% of pregnancies are unplanned in the United States, Hungary, and many other industrialized countries. (Only the Netherlands have a 90% proportion of planned and/or wanted pregnancies.) In addition, in general, appropriate pre- or periconceptional care is not available for the practical delivery of periconceptional multivitamin/ folic acid supplementation. Hungary is an exception because of the Hungarian Optimal Family Planning Service (31).
3. Food fortification seems to be the most practical means of supplementation and, it is in discussion in some countries, e.g., United States,* United Kingdom, Hungary. This public health action is comparable to the prevention of goiter by the addition of iodine to salt. However, it may not be possible to fortify foods to a level of folic acid that can protect against NTD without exposing other population groups to levels that may complicate the diagnosis of vitamin B_{12} deficiency.

All the three possibilities should be pursued in parallel to provide options for women who are capable of becoming pregnant.

3. PERICONCEPTION CARE: PLANNING FOR PREGNANCY FOR BOTH PARTNERS

The provision of preconception care was included in the National Health Promotion and Disease Prevention Objectives for the year 2000 in the United States (32). In Hun-

---

*In February 1996, the US Department of Health and Human Services ordered food fortification, and staple foods will be fortified starting in 1998.

gary we prefer to use the term periconception instead of preconception because prenatal care usually begins in about the 8–12th wk of pregnancy; thus, the early postconceptional period was previously omitted from medical health service and the fetuses in their most sensitive early period (from the third postconceptional week until the eighth week) are uncared for, thus, in general, unprotected. Therefore, the Hungarian Optimal Family Planning Service (HOFPS) *(31)* begins 3 mo before pregnancy and continues for 2–3 mo in the postconceptional period. The HOFPS was launched in 1984 and includes information-counseling, examinations, and interventions performed or supervised by qualified nurses. The main goal is to provide information and care for prospective parents to protect the health of the mother, to reduce untoward pregnancy outcomes, birth defects, and developmental disabilities, and to increase the potential for infants to be born as healthy as possible.

In the 1990s, the network of the HOFPS includes 32 centers under the coordination of our Family Planning Clinic. Here the 10 yr experience of our coordinating center is summarized. The HOFPS consists of three steps:

1. *Checkup of reproductive health.* A medical checkup as a "preconceptional screening" is an essential component of the HOFPS for risk identification and assessment (Table 2), and referral of couples or persons to appropriate secondary care *(33)*. We have an extra effort to incorporate males into the HOFPS to help in the development of responsible fatherhood that seems to be successful: Of 8837 females, 7600 (86.0%) were accompanied by their husbands or partners in life (*see* Chapter 20).

2. *The 3-mo preparation for conception* (Table 2). The preparation for conception is an appropriate period to stop smoking, alcohol drinking, and unnecessary drugs with hazards to germ cells and later the fetus. This 3-mo preparation period is an optimal time for the launch of periconceptional multivitamin supplementation. All women were supplied with a folic acid-containing multivitamin (Elevit pronatal).

3. *The better protection of early pregnancy.* In the past, pregnancies were diagnosed after the second missed menstrual period; thus, the most sensitive period of early fetal development was not recognized and protected. In the HOFPS after the 3-mo preparation for conception, females are asked to continue the intake of the multivitamin, to achieve conception on the optimal days (one of the first or second days prior to ovulation) and to visit the Family Planning Clinic immediately after the first missed menstrual period. Thus, the goal of the next visit is pregnancy confirmation by a serum or urine pregnancy test. At that time an ultrasound scanning is suggested 2 wk later (nearly all ectopic pregnancies were diagnosed as a result of this examination, such an early phase assessment allowed for conservative treatment instead of surgery). Women with known occupational hazards were exempted and they were informed how to avoid other risks (e.g., heat bathing, exposure to infected cats), and pregnant women were asked to continue multivitamin supplementation and were referred to the prenatal care clinic with the discharge summary of the HOFPS.

The periconception care is appropriate for the detection of infertile couples and to treat them sooner; and to provide a more effective flow of couples with positive family history, case history, and/or STDs to the appropriate secondary care. The HOFPS is optimal for the introduction of periconceptional multivitamin/folic acid supplementation, to improve the diet, and to reduce smoking and alcohol consumption before conception. Obviously, proper preparation for conception is the earliest and probably the most important method of health promotion in general, and particularly for the prevention of birth defects.

Table 2
Three Steps and Different Items of the HOFPS

1. Checkup of reproductive health
   a. Family history of females and males
   b. Case history of females, e.g., epilepsy, diabetes, and so forth
   c. Vaginal and cervical smear examination for the screening of sexually transmitted infections/disorders
   d. Sperm analysis for the detection of subfertility and pyosperm
   e. Psychosexual exploration of couples
   f. Blood examination for the revealing of rubella seronegative women (who are then vaccinated), anemia, and HIV positivity
2. The 3-mo preparation for conception
   a. Necessary further examinations and/or treatments in the disorders of couples detected at the checkup examination
   b. Protection of germ cells: avoidance of smoking, alcohol, and unnecessary drugs
   c. Discontinuation of contraceptive pills to restore the internal hormonal balance of females (condoms are provided)
   d. Occupational history to reveal occupational hazards (to contact occupational doctor)
   e. Evaluation of maternal heart volume in the available X-ray photos
   f. Measurement of basal body temperature for detection of hormonal dysfunction (and treatment, if necessary) and determination of two optimal days of conception
   g. Preconceptional multivitamin supplementation
   h. Suggestion to check dental status
   i. Guidelines for physical exercise
   j. Guidelines for healthy diet
3. The better protection of early pregnancy
   a. Achievement conception on the optimal days
   b. Early pregnancy confirmation
   c. Postconceptional multivitamin supplementation
   d. Avoidance of teratogenic and other risks
   e. Referral of pregnant women to prenatal care clinics

4. OTHER REPRODUCTIVE EFFECTS OF PERICONCEPTIONAL MULTIVITAMIN SUPPLEMENTATION

The Hungarian trial within the HOFPS was appropriate to study other possible effects of periconceptional folic acid-containing multivitamin supplementation. The great majority of the women in the study were healthy and not malnourished *(30)*.

1. During the preconceptional multivitamin supplementation the female cycle became more regular, i.e., the variance was lower *(34)*. Thus, multivitamin supplementation may have a beneficial effect for women with irregular menstrual cycles.
2. There was no difference in the sexual activity (measured by the rate of weekly sexual intercourse) of couples between the multivitamin and the placebo-like trace-element groups in the preconceptional period *(35)*. However, only women were supplemented and sexual activity is often determined by males.
3. A 7% higher rate of conception occurred in women who were treated with periconceptional multivitamin supplementation compared with those who were given trace-

element only. The time taken to become pregnant was slightly but significantly shorter in the multivitamin group *(36)*.

4. The rate of multiple births, namely twins, was about 50% higher after periconceptional multivitamin supplementation *(37)*. The higher rate of twin conceptions could not be explained by maternal factors (age, parity) or by a higher rate of infertility drug use *(38)*.

5. A significantly lower rate of treated morning sickness (nausea and vomiting) occurred in early pregnancy after periconceptional multivitamin supplementation (3 vs 6.6% in the trace-element group) *(39)*.

6. There was no difference in maternal weight gain between the multivitamin and the trace-element groups before and during pregnancy *(40)*.

7. There was no significant difference in pregnancy outcomes of singletons, including four types of fetal deaths (chemical pregnancies, ectopic pregnancies, miscarriages, including the so-called missed abortions or blighted ova, or stillbirths) and three variables of liveborn infants (sex ratio, birth weight, including low birthweight, and gestation age, including preterm birth) *(41)*. However, the rates of all kinds of fetal deaths, low birthweight, and preterm birth were somewhat, but not significantly, higher in the multivitamin group. In addition, the ratio of boys:girls showed a slight girl excess in the multivitamin group, whereas the well-known boy predominance was seen in the trace-element group. Thus, a small change in the pattern of prenatal selection cannot be excluded.

8. Postnatal somatic (body weight, body length, head circumference) and mental (measured by three tests) development did not show any significant differences between the multivitamin and trace-element groups *(42)*. Thus, the previously found higher rate of worrying, fussiness, and fearfulness in girls born after periconceptional multivitamin supplementation *(43)* was not confirmed.

5. PERICONCEPTIONAL MULTIVITAMIN SUPPLEMENTATION PREVENT OTHER MAJOR STRUCTURAL BIRTH DEFECTS

Structural birth defects, i.e., CAs, were differentiated on the basis of three time windows of diagnosis: during pregnancy in the second and third trimesters *(41)*, at birth *(41)* and later, until and in the follow-up examination of infants *(42)* in the final database of the Hungarian trial. In addition, isolated and multiple CAs were separated *(44)*.

The total rate of cases with CAs was 56.3/1000 in the multivitamin and 73.2/1000 in the trace-element group ($p = 0.018$) in the final database *(45)*. After the exclusion of six NTD cases from the trace-element group, the difference was also significant ($p = 0.042$). The dropout was only 0.9% at the evaluation of cases at birth; thus, the first and second time windows with nearly complete ascertainment are evaluated together. The rate of CAs diagnosed during pregnancy and at birth was 11.3/1000 in the multivitamin and 22.2/1000 in the trace-element group ($p = 0.004$). After the exclusion of six cases with NTD, the difference remained significant between the two study groups ($p = 0.019$). Finally mild CAs (mainly deformations) were excluded in another analysis (Table 3). The rate of major CAs was 20.6/1000 in the multivitamin and 40.6/1000 in the trace-element group ($p < 0.0001$) *(46)*. After the exclusion six NTD cases and three familial cases, the difference in the rate of major CAs between the two study groups was very highly significant ($p < 0.0001$), with a relative risk of 0.48 (CI 95%:0.34, 0.68). In conclusion, periconceptional multivitamin supplementation reduced not only the occurrence of NTD but also the rate of other major CAs (Fig. 1).

Table 3
The Number of Cases with Major CAs in the Two Study Groups and the Relative Risk
of Some Major CA Groups After Periconceptional Multivitamin Supplementation

CA-groups	Multivitamin (N=2471) no.	Trace element (N=2391) no.	Relative risk (with 95% confidence limit)
Isolated			
Neural tube defects	0	6	0.059 (0.000, 0.626)
Cardiovascular CAs			
Conotruncal	3	10	} 0.482 (0.225, 1.031)
Others	7	10	
Cleft palate	0	2	0.200 (0.000, 3.359)
Cleft lip ± palate	4	3	1.329 (0.281, 6.550)
Pyloric stenosis	2	8	0.262 (0.037, 0.994)
Renal agenesis	0	2	} 0.121 (0.021, 0.685)
Obstructive CAs of urinary tract	1	6	
Reduction CAs of limb	1	5	0.233 (0.008, 1.345)
Other major CAs	23	34	0.675 (0.377, 1.086)
Multiple CAs	10	12	0.811 (0.360, 0.811)
Total	51	97	0.510 (0.354, 0.685)

The final database of the Hungarian trial indicated a significant reduction in two CA groups *(46)* in addition to NTD. Nine cases with CAs of the urinary tract were found in the trace-element group and only two in the multivitamin group ($\chi^2 = 4.70$; $p = 0.03$; relative risk: 0.22 CI 95%:0.05, 0.99). The difference was most obvious in the obstructive CAs of the urinary tract. In addition, there were two offspring with renal agenesis in the trace-element group (Table 3). The combined rate of the obstructive CA groups of the urinary tract and renal agenesis (1 vs 8) also showed a significant difference between the two study groups ($\chi^2_1 = 5.69$; $p = 0.017$). Renal agenesis and utero-pelvic junction obstruction may have a common pathogenesis *(47)*.

In the 1950s, Monie et al. *(48–49)* were able to produce CAs of the urinary tract in rat embryos by folic acid deficiency. In a recent human study, Li et al. *(50)* also found a highly significant reduction in the rate of urinary tract defects after the first trimester multivitamin use (0.15 CI 95%:0.05, 0.43).

There were 10 infants with cardiovascular CAs in the multivitamin group and 20 in the trace-element group *(46)* (Table 3). The difference was near the level of significance ($\chi^2_1 = 3.69$; $p = 0.055$); relative risk was 0.48 (CI 95%:0.23, 1.03). The presence of cardiovascular CAs was confirmed before 1 yr of age by cardiological consultation (including echocardiography or cardiac catheterization), surgery, or autopsy. One case with aortic stenosis was familial in the multivitamin group; after the exclusion of this case the difference was significant ($\chi^2_1 = 4.57$; $p = 0.032$). The difference of cardiovascular CAs is mainly explained by two cases of ventricular septal defect in the multivitamin group and eight cases in the trace-element group ($\chi^2_1 = 3.81$; $p = 0.051$). The difference in the rate of conotruncal CAs (in the multivitamin group: 2 ventricular septal defects, 1 double outlet right ventricle; in the trace-element group: 8 ventricular septal

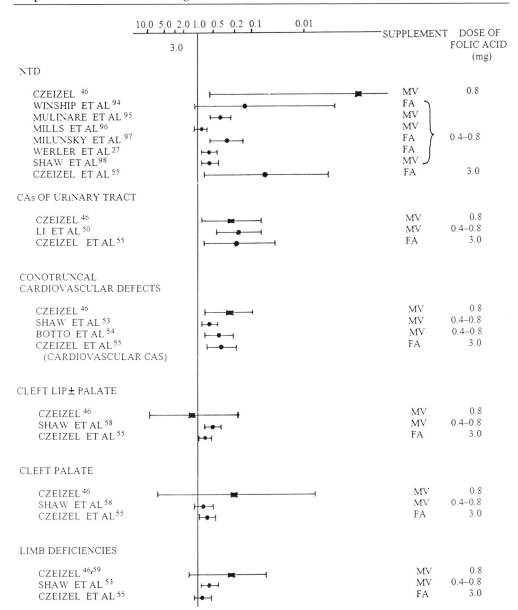

Fig. 1. Summary of "occurrence" studies concerning the candidates of folic acid (FA)—multivitamin (MV) preventable CAs in one randomized trial *(46,59)* (■) and observational studies *(27,50,53–55,58,94–98)* (●). The relative risk estimate (supplemented vs nonsupplemented or users vs nonusers) is shown for each study together with its 95% confidence interval. The dose of folic acid is also shown if data are available.

defects, 1 tetralogy of Fallot, 1 complete transposition) was significant ($\chi_1^2 = 4.01$; $p = 0.045$; relative risk: 0.29 CI 95%:0.08, 1.05).

Cardiovascular CAs were induced by pteroylglutamic acid deficiency during gestation in rat fetuses *(51–52)*. Shaw et al. *(53)* examined whether a woman's reported use of folic acid-containing vitamins was associated with a reduced risk for conotruncal cardiovascular CAs. Data were derived from a population-based case-control study of fetuses and babies among a 1987–1988 cohort of 341,839 births ascertained by the California Birth Defects Monitoring Program. Telephone interviews were conducted with mothers of 239 conotruncal cases (84.2%) and 481 nonmalformed control cases (76.2%). The unadjusted odds ratios for any folic acid-containing vitamin use from 1 mo before conception through 2 mo postconception were 0.65 (CI 95%:0.44, 0.96) for conotruncal CAs. Botto et al. *(54)* also studied the role of periconceptional use of multivitamins in the prevention of conotruncal cardiovascular CAs (transposition of the great arteries, tetralogy of Fallot, and truncus arteriosus) in the population-based Atlanta Birth Defects Case-Control Study. One hundred fifty eight case-infants and 3026 unaffected control-infants born from 1968–1980 were compared. Their results suggested that periconceptional use of multivitamins was associated with a 43% reduction in risk for conotruncal cardiovascular CAs. The effect was strongest for isolated conotruncal CAs (0.41 CI 95%:0.20, 0.84). Among anatomic subgroups of conotruncal CAs, transposition of the great arteries showed the greatest reduction in risk (0.36 (CI 95%:0.15, 0.89(). The protective effect of postconceptional supplementation of pharmacological dose (3 mg) of folic acid for cardiovascular CAs was also seen in the database of the Hungarian Case-Control Surveillance of Congenital Anomalies *(55)*.

In conclusion, at the end of 1995 the available evidence indicated that the rates of three groups of CAs, NTD, certain CA groups of the urinary tract, and cardiovascular CAs, can be reduced significantly by periconceptional multivitamin supplementation. Three other groups of CAs may also have been reduced by periconceptional multivitamin supplementation.

In an animal experimental study in 1955, Nelson et al. *(7)* were able to obtain cleft lip in more than 90% of the rat offspring subjected to a transitory folic acid deficiency as a result of an antimetabolite during d 9–11 of gestation. In the early 1980s Tolarova *(56)* reported a protective effect of multivitamins including folic acid for the recurrence of cleft lips. This database was evaluated recently with similar results by Tolarova and Harris *(57)*. This finding was not confirmed in our Hungarian trial (Table 3). However, in the California Birth Defects Monitoring Program, 1987–1988, Shaw et al. *(58)* investigated whether folic acid-containing vitamin use in the periconceptional period was associated with a reduced risk of oral clefts. Telephone interviews were conducted with mothers of 731 cleft cases (84.7%), and 734 nonmalformed control cases (78.2%). The unadjusted odds ratio for isolated (0.50; CI 95%:0.36, 0.68) and for nonisolated (syndromic) (0.61; CI 95%:0.35, 1.1) cleft lip ± cleft palate, and for isolated (0.73; CI 95%:0.46, 1.2) and nonisolated (0.64; CI 95%:0.35, 1.2) cleft palate was significant in the group of isolated cleft lip ± cleft palate. In conclusion, women who used multivitamins containing folic acid periconceptionally had a 25–50% reduction in risk for offspring with orofacial clefts compared to women who did not use such vitamins. The database of the Hungarian Case-Control Surveillance of Congenital Anomalies also showed a significant reduction in the rate of both isolated cleft lip ± cleft palate and cleft palate after the first and second postconceptional month supplementation with folic acid *(55)*. The explanation for discrepancies in different studies may be the dose. Tolarova *(56)* used a multivitamin that included an extremely high dose of folic acid (10 mg/d). The Hungarian Case-Control Surveillance evaluated the daily use of 3–6 mg of folic acid. In contrast, the Hungarian trial *(25, 46)* used a multivitamin including 0.8 mg of folic acid. It is possible that only a pharmacological dose of folic acid has protective effect on cleft lip.

In the final database of the Hungarian intervention trial there was one case with limb deficiency (terminal transverse) in the multivitamin group and five cases (2 terminal transverse, 2 femur-fibula-ulna complex, 1 split hand and foot) in the trace-element group *(59)*. The difference is not significant ($\chi^2_1 = 2.8$; $p = 0.09$ or Fisher $p = 0.124$). However, the teratogenic effect of folic acid deficiency because of folic acid antagonists, such as aminopterin and methotrexate, caused, among others, limb deficiencies in human embryos *(8–10, 60)*. In addition, Shaw et al. *(53)* examined whether a woman's reported use of a folic acid-containing multivitamin was associated with a reduction in the rate of limb deficiencies. Cases were ascertained from the California Birth Defects Monitoring Program, 1987–1988. Telephone interviews were conducted with mothers of 179 cases with limb deficiency and 481 nonmalformed controls. The unjusted odds ratio for any folic acid-containing multivitamin use from 1 mo before conception through 2 mo postconception were 0.65 (CI 95%:0.43, 0.99) for limb deficiencies.

In the final database of the Hungarian trial *(45, 46)* the number of clinical diagnoses of congenital hypertrophic pyloric stenosis (which is not a typical CA) indicated also some difference (2 vs 8) between the study groups ($\chi^2 = 3.81$; $p = 0.051$). However, one case had no surgery in the trace-element group; thus, it was necessary to exclude this case from the analysis according to our criteria of diagnosis ($\chi^2 = 2.95$; $p = 0.086$).

Obviously, these findings could have major implications in the use of periconceptional folic acid-containing multivitamin supplementation to prevent CAs in general. It is strange, that, although the data concerning the prevention of NTD were accepted with enthusiasm in the international scientific literature in the early 1990s and prompted fast new recommendations for their practical application, the new data concerning the prevention of other CAs have been received with some reservation and without any further recommendations. It may be well to remember that it has taken a long time for the association of folic acid and NTD to be accepted. In addition, it is worth reminding that in the first phase of folic acid history, deficiency resulted in a general teratogenic effect in both animal *(2–7,11–12,48–49,51–52)* and human studies *(8–10,13–14,60)*. In 1964, Hibbard *(13)* reported a higher rate of CAs (3%) in the infants of folate-deficient mothers than in controls (1.6%). It was confirmed by Hibbard and Smithells *(14)* in 1965, who showed a relationship between human embryopathies and a deficiency of folic acid metabolism. Thus, the first human publications also indicated a general teratogenic effect of folic acid deficiency.

On the other hand, we know that different CAs have different etiologies; thus, it is difficult to understand that so many CAs can be prevented by such a simple primary preventive method as periconceptional folic acid-containing multivitamin supplementation. In addition, the aforementioned different CAs have different critical periods (Fig. 2). The latter may explain that postconceptional multivitamin supplementation also seems to be protective for some CAs. Finally, the urinary tract and cardiovascular CAs have a heterogeneous origin; thus, the different subtypes may have different etiological background. However, this is the case in NTDs as well. Thus, it is an important task to understand the biological mechanisms of the preventive effect for CAs achieved by periconceptional multivitamin supplementation.

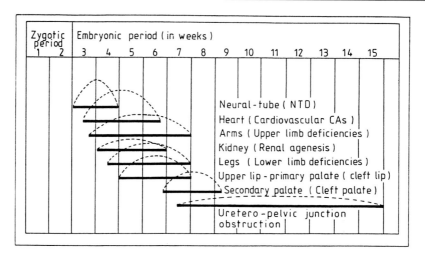

Fig. 2. Critical periods in human developmental fields with very intensive mitoses.

6. THE POSSIBLE MECHANISM OF PREVENTION

The underlying biological mechanisms of folic acid-containing multivitamin supplementation in the prevention of NTDs and other CAs are not fully understood. However, some hypotheses based on available findings seem to be reasonable.

The human organism cannot synthesize folate or folic acid. (The generic term folate describes the many different naturally occuring polyglutamate forms of the vitamin, whereas folic acid is the synthesized monoglutamate form, chemically designated as pteroylglutamic acid). The major dietary sources of folate are fresh and frozen green leafy vegetables (folium is the Latin word for leaf), liver, kidney, asparagus, citrus fruits, and juices, whole wheat bread, and legumes (dry beans). Food folate polyglutamates are converted to monoglutamates by a conjugase in the upper part of the small intestine. Folate conjugase is a zinc metalloenzyme and folate polyglutamates are not well-absorbed by the intestine in zinc-deficient humans *(61)*. After the active and passive absorption of monoglutamates into the intestinal cells, the monoglutamates are fully converted to tetrahydrofolate (THF), which is the parent compound of all biologically active folates. Vitamin C has an important role to prevent the oxidation of THF, thus helping to keep the folate metabolic pool complete *(62)*. 5-methyl-THF is the predominant folate in serum and in tissues. The different stages and relations of folate metabolism are in good agreement with the polygenic inheritance of NTDs and other CAs. The available epidemiological and biochemical evidence suggests that the problem is not primarily the lack of sufficient folate in the diet, but arises from genetically determined changes in the uptake or metabolism, or both in maternal and, particularly, fetal cells *(63–67)*. Thus, an interaction between vitamin dependency (e.g., an inborn error of folate metabolism) and nutrition (such as dietary deficiency) may have a causal role in the origin of NTDs and other CAs. Supplementation with folic acid-containing multivitamins or high doses of folic acid alone may cause an increase in THF concentrations of tissue fluids and it may overcome the failure of local THF supply.

Folic acid may be a key factor in the prevention of NTDs and other CAs because there are two general and important biological effects of THFs *(68,69)*. First, THFs act as a cofactor for enzymes involved in DNA and RNA biosynthesis. Some metabolites of THF provide one-carbon units for the *de novo* synthesis of DNA bases (guanine, adenine, and thymine) because THFs accept single carbons from a variety of donors (mainly serine). Second, THF is involved in the supply of methyl-group to the methylation cycle, because the methyl-group of 5-methyl-THF is used by methionine synthase to recycle homocysteine back to methionine. However, methionine synthase is a vitamin B_{12} dependent enzyme. The study of Schorah et al. *(65)* showed a reduced activity of methionine synthase in placental cytotrophoblast from NTD-affected pregnancies. The conversion of homocysteine to cystathione is directed by cystathione synthase which is a pyridoxine, i.e., vitamin B_6-dependent enzyme. A disturbance in the above processes results in decreased homocysteine remethylation-caused hyperhomocysteinemia and the shortage of methionine; therefore, cells are not able to methylate important compounds, such as proteins, lipids, and myelin. In mothers who gave birth to a child with NTD, homocysteine levels were on average higher compared to controls both before and after an oral methionine-loading test *(70)*. The mean total homocysteine concentration in amniotic fluid of 27 women carrying a fetus with NTD was significantly higher than that of 31 control women carrying a healthy fetus *(71)*. Thus, these findings indicated a defective homocysteine/methionine metabolism in the origin of NTD. Reduced activity of 5,10-methylene-THF reductase (MTHFR) is associated with high plasma homocysteine concentrations *(72)*. The human MTHFR DNA was isolated and its gene was localized to chromosome 1p36.3 *(73)*. A 677C→T mutation was identified in the MTHFR gene resulting in decreased activity, increased thermolability of the enzyme, and raised plasma homocysteine concentrations *(74)*. Van der Put et al. *(75)* studied the frequency of this mutation in the MTHFR gene in 55 patients with spina bifida and parents of such patients. Five percent of 207 controls were homozygous for the 677C→T mutation compared with 16% of mothers, 10% of fathers, and 13% of patients. The mutation was associated with decreased MTHFR activity, low plasma folate, and high plasma homocysteine and low red-cell folate concentrations. The 677C→T mutation should be regarded as a genetic risk factor for spina bifida.* Folate administration may overcome the effect of reduced MTHRF activity; thus, these findings provide a mechanism for the protective role of folate in the reduction of NTD. L-methionine deficiency has been shown to induce NTD in cultured rat embryos *(76–78)* and L-methionine had a preventive effect *(78)*.

There is an increased requirement for folate during pregnancy because of decreased absorption *(79)*, accelerated breakdown of folate to p-aminobenzoylglutamate and its acetylated derivative p-acetamidobenzoylglutamate *(29)*, increased urinary loss, and fetal transfer. The calculated total fetal and placental THF content is 0.8 mg/100 g at term *(80)*; thus, fetal blood has a higher THF level than maternal blood, indicating active placental transfer *(81)*.

The intensity (i.e., "speed") of development, including the activity of mitoses, is extremely active in the postconceptional life, particularly in the first 8 wk. The weight of the fertilized egg, an embryo at the eighth week, a liveborn infant, and a 20-yr old per-

*However, recent papers indicated a more complex pattern (August 1996).

Table 4
Proportion of Preventable CAs by Primary, Secondary, and Tertiary Methods,
Before and After the Introduction of Periconceptional Care, Including Periconceptional
Multivitamin Supplementation

	Preventable CAs, %	
	Before introduction of periconception care	After introduction of periconception care
Primary prevention		
Genetic counseling (and reduction of conception)	0.1	0.2
Care of affected mothers	0.0	0.1
Avoidance of teratogens	1.1	1.2
Multivitamin supplementation	—	11.4
Subtotal	1.2	12.9
Secondary		
Prenatal screening (chromosomal, maternal AFP and triple test, ultrasonography)	8.3	8.4
Neonatal blood screening (PKU, galactosemia, hypothyroidism)	0.6	0.6
Neonatal orthopedic screening	23.6	23.6
Specific postnatal treatment (in undescended testis and patent ductus arteriosus)	2.2	2.2
Subtotal	34.7	34.8
Tertiary; early pediatric surgery	24.0	21.1
Total	60.0	68.8

son is 0.001, 4, 3200, and 65,000 g, respectively. The postnatal increase is only 20 times, whereas it is 800 (26.7/wk) times between the eighth and 38th week of fetal development. However, weight increases 4000 (500/wk) times during organogenesis when the different organs develop. Thus, the requirement of 'bricks' for body building and the mode of genetic regulation (e.g., growth factors) are significantly different between pre- and postnatal life. In addition, cell division is exceptionally rapid at critical stages of specific developmental fields in the embryo (*see* Fig. 2). The cell's ability to increase the synthesis of nucleic acids and to methylate important compounds (e.g., a need for L-methionine) would be compromised by deficiency of folate and other vitamins, resulting in impaired cell function, mitosis, and subsequently CAs.

7. BIRTH DEFECTS ARE PREVENTABLE

At present, 20–25% of infant mortality is caused by CAs in industrialized countries. However, CAs are among the leading causes of death, with a high number of life years lost and impaired life *(82)*. Another important feature of CAs is that they represent a defect condition, because it is difficult to achieve a complete recovery. Thus, prevention is considered the only optimal solution.

In the late 1980s we attempted to estimate the preventable proportion of CAs *(83)* and were able to prove that the widespread pessimistic view concerning the low chance of CA prevention was incorrect: A considerable part (about 60%) of CAs were preventable (Table 4). However, our analysis showed that primary preventive methods played only a small part in the prevention of CAs, whereas the efficacy of secondary prevention is growing and considerable. This is explained by the increasing effectiveness of prenatal examinations as a result of the improvement of diagnostic methods (e.g., ultrasonography) and new approaches (e.g., DNA probes). Thus, we have to do our best to develop and to introduce primary preventive methods instead of the secondary one, i.e., selective abortion. The history of NTD offers a good example to demonstrate the feasibility of this concept.

At present, both primary and secondary preventive methods are available for NTD. The prenatal screening for the detection of NTD fetuses is based on the measurement of the maternal serum α-fetoprotein (MS-AFP) and/or ultrasonography. The MS-AFP is measured between 16 and 18 wk of gestation after the determination of gestational age by ultrasound examination. The latter is appropriate to immediately diagnose anencephalic fetuses. Values of MS-AFP > 2.0–2.5 MoM (multiples of median) for the gestational age are considered suspect. The proportion of abnormal high MS-AFP that can be confirmed by ultrasonographic examinations varied between 1.2 and 3.9% of pregnant women (84). If it is negative, generally it is recommended to repeat MS-AFP. If the second result is also abnormal and a high-resolution ultrasonographic examination cannot detect NTD or other causes of a high MS-AFP (multiple fetuses, fetal death, other CAs, maternal diabetes mellitus), amniocentesis is offered to women because amniotic-AFP and amniotic fluid acetylcholinesterase are confirmatory for the diagnosis of NTD. Fetal death as a result of amniocentesis is about 0.5–1.0%. In general (i.e., low-risk) populations the detection rate (i.e., sensitivity) of MS-AFP testing for open NTD varies from 72–91% and the specificity from 96.2–98.7% (84).

Periconceptional folic acid-containing multivitamin supplementation as a primary preventive method offers an appropriate alternative with the same efficacy. The evaluation of adverse effects shows obviously a better picture for multivitamin supplementation. Very rare adverse effects may occur only after the use of a pharmacological dose of folic acid; such a dose is not recommended. The cost is much lower in the primary prevention compared to secondary one. The main advantage is the lack of pregnancy termination in primary prevention.

If we consider the results of the Hungarian trial, periconceptional multivitamin supplementation resulted in 30.8% reduction in the rate of CAs. Thus, the candidates of preventable CAs by this primary preventive method and periconceptional care can be redistributed in Table 4. In this case, 68.8% of CAs are preventable and there is a significant increase in the proportion of primary prevention (1.2–12.9%) because of periconceptional folic acid-containing multivitamin supplementation.

However, there are some theoretical and technical problems with the use of periconceptional vitamin supplementation. The previously mentioned recommendations for reduction NTD risk include only the supplementation of 0.4 mg folic acid. These recommendations are difficult to accept because there is no direct evidence from a randomized controlled study that 0.4 mg of folic acid alone can reduce the first occurrence of NTDs. The Hungarian trial used 0.8 mg of folic acid in a multivitamin (25). In addition, it is well known that both folate and vitamin B_{12} are involved in DNA synthesis. Recent papers suggest that vitamin B_{12} may be an independent risk factor in the origin of NTD (85,86) because an abnormality in homocysteine metabolism apparently related to methionine synthase is present in many women who give birth to children with

NTD. Vitamin B_{12} completely abolished the embryotoxicity of L-homocysteine in rat embryos, which was shown to be mediated by catalysis of the spontaneous oxidation of L-homocysteine to the less toxic L-homocystine (78). Thus, a hypothesis was developed that L-homocysteine embryotoxicity is explained by the inhibition of transmethylation reactions by increased embryonic 5-adenosylhomocysteine level. In conclusion, a multivitamin containing folic acid and at least vitamin B_{12} (although vitamin B_6, C, and zinc are also advisable) seems to be the optimal for the prevention not only of NTD but other CAs as well.

Recommendations concerning the reduction of NTD recurrence is based on the pharmacological dose (4 mg) of folic acid. However, there is a strong evidence from the Smithells et al. (19–21) study that a multivitamin containing 0.36 mg of folic acid can significantly reduce NTD recurrences. It is not possible to compare directly the data of nonrandomized and randomized studies (Table 1), nevertheless, the efficacy of recurrence risk reduction was more impressive after multivitamin use. Finally, and most importantly, physicians should be aware that daily 4 mg of folic acid may mask the hematologic manifestations of vitamin B_{12} deficiency without preventing its neurologic consequences (87) and may precipitate convulsions in epileptic women whose seizures are well-controlled with phenytoin (89,90), although these findings were not confirmed in other studies (91,92). In addition, after a high dose of supplemental folic acid, more of the unmetabolized vitamin (it may amount to >25% of the dose administrated) appears in the urine (29). The embryo could be exposed to the excess unmetabolized folic acid, a form of the vitamin that an embryo would not encounter normally. Thus, it would seem to be better to use a multivitamin supplement including a physiologic dose (0.4–0.8 mg) of folic acid for the reduction of both occurrence and recurrence of NTDs.

The Hungarian trial and other recent studies indicated a preventive effect not only for NTDs but for some other CA groups, and it seems to be a great breakthrough in the primary prevention of major CAs. However, it was achieved by a folic acid-containing multivitamin. These findings were confirmed by observational studies, all of them based on the intake of multivitamins. Thus, periconceptional folic acid-containing multivitamin supplementation seems to be the most effective method for the prevention of NTD and some other major Cas. In conclusion, periconception care that includes folic acid-containing multivitamin supplementation is a significant finding for the prevention of CAs both quantitatively (an extra 30%) and qualitatively (primary instead of secondary prevention).

8. RECOMMENDATIONS FOR NUTRITIONAL INTERVENTIONS TO REDUCE BIRTH DEFECT RISKS

The history of NTDs shows that we can modify our destiny by the help of science. Before the 1960s nearly all NTD births were fatal. In the 1960s physicians introduced very early complex medical intervention and the lives were saved in the majority of spina bifida cases. In the 1970s the selective criteria of surgical intervention was introduced to reduce the production of multiply handicapped children. In the 1980s prenatal screening was introduced, resulting in a significant drop in the birth of NTD fetuses; however, it increased the number of pregnancy terminations. Finally, in the 1990s, we have a chance to reduce the maldevelopment of neural-tube (and other organs) because of the intentional modification (supplementation) of the diet at least in a certain (periconceptional) period of life. Our hope is that the extension of healthy diet for the whole life will help us to prevent other diseases and to promote our health significantly *(93)*.

Recommendations defined here are based on findings and hypotheses presented in this chapter.

1. Proper preparation for conception is the earliest and probably the most important method of health promotion in general, and particularly for the prevention of birth defects. The establishment of periconception care is feasible and, on the basis of available experience, is reasonable. This network provides an appropriate forum for nutritional interventions as well.
2. The preconceptional period is an appropriate time to change the dietary habit and to improve the lifestyle of prospective parents because their desire to have a healthy baby can ensure compliance. It is an important task to advise all women to have a folate and other vitamin-rich diet from the preconceptional time.
3. Good evidence is available to advise all women capable of becoming pregnant to have periconceptional (i.e., at least 1 mo before until 3 mo after conception) multivitamin (including 0.4–0.8 mg of folic acid) supplementation to reduce the occurrence of major CAs. Beyond folic acid there is growing evidence to include vitamins B_{12}, B_6, C, and zinc. The latter including 0.4–0.8 mg of folic acid appears to be the most effective practical way to reduce the recurrence of NTD as well.
4. Fortification of food (flour, special products of bakery, juice) with folic acid, vitamin B_{12} and possibly some other vitamins would be appropriate to reach the large proportion of women with unplanned pregnancies and low income/poorly educated women, who have difficulty buying nutritious food and supplements to meet the aforementioned standard.
5. There is evidence that appropriate nutritional status of pregnant women can promote the postnatal, including adult, health of offspring. The origin of many common complex diseases (hypertension, coronary heart disease, diabetes mellitus, obesity) may be related to the quality of fetal and infant life *(93)*.
6. Appropriately prepared parents for pregnancy can educate their children from the earliest time (i.e., birth) of their life for a healthy diet and lifestyle. There is a good chance that these habits will then be fixed for their later life.

REFERENCES

1. Hale F. Pigs born without eyeballs. J. Hered 1932; 24:105–109.
2. Warkany J. Congenital malformations induced by maternal dietary deficiency: experiments and their interpretation. Harvey Lecture, 1952–1953. 1971; 18:89.
3. Warkany J. Congenital Malformations. Notes and Comments. Chicago, IL: Year Book Medical Publications, 1971.
4. Nelson MM. Mammalian fetal development and antimetabolities. In: Rhoads EP, ed. Antimetabolites and Cancer. American Association for the Advancement of Science Monograph. Washington, DC, 1955.
5. Evans HM, Nelson MM, Asling CV. Multiple congenital abnormalities resulting from acute folic acid deficiency during gestation. Science 1951; 114:479.
6. Nelson MM, Asling CW, Evans HM. Production of multiple congenital abnormalities in young by maternal pteroylglutamic acid deficiency during gestation. J Nut, 1952; 48:61–79.
7. Nelson MM, Wright HV, Asling CW, Evans HM. Multiple congenital abnormalities resulting from transitory deficiency of pteroylglutamic acid during gestation in the rat. J Nutr, 1955; 56:349–369.
8. Thiersch JB. Therapeutic abortions with a folic acid antagonist, 4-aminopteroylglutamic acid (4-amino PGA) administered by the oral route. Am J Obstet Gynecol 1952; 63:1298–1304.
9. Meltzer HJ. Congenital anomalies due to attempted abortion with 4-aminopteroglutamic acid. JAMA 1956; 161:1253.

10. Warkany J, Beaudry PH, Hornstein S. Attempted abortion with 4-aminopteroglutamic acid (aminopterin): malformations of the child. Am J Dis Child 1959; 97:274–281.

11. Giroud A, Lefevbres-Boisselot J. Influence tératogéne de la carence en acide folique. Compt Rend Soc Biol 1951; 145:526–529.

12. Giroud A. The Nutrition of the Embryo. Charles C. Thomas, Springfield, IL, 1970.

13. Hibbard BM. The role of folic acid in pregnancy with particular reference to anaemia, abruption and abortion. J Obstet Gynecol 1964; 71:529–542.

14. Hibbard ED, Smithells RW. Folic acid metabolism and human embryopathy. Lancet 1965; 1:1254.

15. Czeizel AE. Folic acid in the prevention of neural tube defects. J Pediat Gastroenter Nutr 1995; 20:4–16.

16. Czeizel AE, Tusnády G. Aetiological Studies of Isolated Common Congenital Abnormalities in Hungary. Akadémiai Kiadó, Budapest, 1984.

17. Elwood JM, Little J, Elwood JH. Epidemiology and Control of Neural Tube Defects. Oxford University, Oxford, 1992.

18. Smithells RW, Sheppard S, Schorah CJ. Vitamin deficiencies and neural tube defects. Arch Dis Child 1976; 51:944–949.

19. Smithells RW, Sheppard S, Schorah CJ, Seller MJ, Nevin NC, Harris R. Possible prevention of neural tube defects by periconceptional vitamin supplementation. Lancet 1980; 1:339,340.

20. Smithells RW, Sheppard S, Wild J, Schorah CJ. Prevention of neural tube defect recurrences in Yorkshire: final report. Lancet 1989; 2: 498,499.

21. Nevin NC, Seller MJ. Prevention of neural tube defect recurrences. Lancet 1990; 1:178–179.

22. Laurence KM, James N, Miller MH, Tennant GB, Campbell H. Double-blind randomised controlled trial of folate treatment before conception to prevent recurrence of neural-tube defects. Br Med J 1981; 282:1509–1511.

23. MRC Vitamin Study Research Group. Prevention of neural tube defects: results of the Medical Research Council vitamin study. Lancet 1991; 338:131–137.

24. CDC. Use of folic acid for prevention of spina bifida and other neural tube defects. JAMA 1991; 266:1191,1192.

25. Czeizel AE, Dudás I. Prevention of the first occurrence of neural-tube defects by periconceptional vitamin supplementation. New Engl J Med 1992; 327:1832–1835.

26. Wald N. Folic acid and the prevention of neural tube defects. Ann NY Acad Sci 1993; 678:112–129.

27. Werler MM, Shapiro S, Mitchell AA. Periconceptional folic acid exposure and risk of occurrent neural tube defects. JAMA 1993; 269:1257–1261.

28. CDC. Recommendations for the use of folic acid to reduce the number of cases of spina bifida and other neural tube defects. MMWR 1992; 41:1233–1238.

29. McPartlin J, Halligan A, Scott JM, Darling M, Weir DG. Accelerated folate breakdown in pregnancy. Lancet, 1993; 341:148–149.

30. Czeizel AE, Susánszky E. Diet intake and vitamin supplement use of Hungarian women during the preconceptional period. Int J Vitam Nutr Res 1994; 64:300–305.

31. Czeizel AE. Primary prevention of birth defects by periconceptional care including multivitamin supplementation. Bailliére's Clin Obstet Gynaecol 1995; 9:417–430.

32. Healthy People 2000. National health population and disease prevention objectives. US Department of Health and Human Services. Public Health Service. DHHS Publ. No. 91–502. 13.

33. Czeizel AE, Dudás I, Fritz G. The check-up of reproductive health and genetic counseling. Genet Counseling 1992; 3:61–66.

34. Dudás I, Rockenbauer M, Czeizel AE. The effect of preconceptional multivitamin supplementation on the menstrual cycle. Arch Gynecol Obstet 1995; 256:115–123.

35. Czeizel AE, Rockenbauer M, Susánszky E. No change in sexual activity during periconceptional multivitamin supplementation. Brit J Obstet Gynecol 1996; 103:569–573.

36. Czeizel AE, Métneki J, Dudás I. The effect of preconceptional multivitamin supplementation on fertility. Int J Vitam Nutr Res 1996; 66:55–58.

37. Czeizel AE, Métneki J, Dudás I. Higher rate of multiple births after periconceptional multivitamin supplementation. New Engl J Med 1994; 330:1687–1688.

38. Czeizel AE, Métneki J, Dudás I. The higher rate of multiple births after periconceptional multivitamin supplementation: an analysis of causes. Acta Genet Gemmellol 1994; 43:175–184.

39. Czeizel AE, Dudás I, Fritz G, Técsõi A, Hanck A, Kunovits G. The effect of periconceptional multivitamin-mineral supplementation on vertigo, nausea and vomiting in the first trimester of pregnancy. Arch Gynecol Obstet 1992; 251:181–185.

40. Czeizel AE. Randomized, controlled trial of the effect of periconceptional multivitamin supplementation on pregnancy outcome. In: Wharton BA, ed. Maternal-Child Issues in Nutrition Wyeth-Ayerst Nutritional Seminar Series. Excerpta Medica, Princeton, NJ, 1993; pp. 13–24.

41. Czeizel AE, Dudás I, Métneki J. Pregnancy outcomes in a randomised controlled trial of periconceptional multivitamin supplementation. Final report. Arch Gynecol Obstet 1994; 255:131–139.

42. Czeizel AE, Dobó M. Postnatal somatic and mental development after periconceptional multivitamin supplementation. Arch Dis Child 1994; 70:229–233.

43. Holmes-Siedle M, Dennis J, Lindenbaum RH, Galliard A. Long-term effects of periconceptional multivitamin supplementation for prevention of neural tube defects: a seven to 10 year follow up. Arch Dis Child 1992; 67:1436–1441.

44. Czeizel AE. Prevention of congenital abnormalities by periconceptional multivitamin supplementation. Brit Med J 1993; 306:1645–1648.

45. Czeizel AE. The final data base of congenital abnormalities in the Hungarian randomized controlled trial of periconceptional multivitamin supplementation. Acta Pediat Hung 1994; 34:19–44.

46. Czeizel AE. Reduction of urinary tract and cardiovascular defects by periconceptional multivitamin supplementation. Am J Med Genet 1996; 62:179–183.

47. Robson WLM, Rogers RC, Leung AKC. Renal agenesis, multicystic dysplasia, and uretero-pelvic junction obstruction—a common pathogenesis. Amer J Med Genet 1994; 53:302.

48. Monie IW, Nelson MM, Evans HM. Abnormalities of the urinary system of rat embryos resulting from maternal pteroyglutamic acid deficiency. Anat Rec 1954; 120:119–136.

49. Monie IW, Nelson MM, Evans HM. Abnormalities of the urinary system of rat embryos resulting from transitory deficiency of pteroylglutamic acid during gestation in the rat. Anat Rec 1957; 127:711–724.

50. Li D-K, Daling JR, Mueller BA, Hickok DE, Fantel AG, Weiss NS. Periconceptional multivitamin use in relation to the risk of congenital urinary tract anomalies. Epidemiology 1995; 6:212–218.

51. Baird CD, Nelson MM, Monie IW, Evans HM. Congenital cardiovascular anomalies induced by pteroylgutamic acid deficiency during gestation in the rat. Circ Rev 1954; 2:544–548.

52. Monie IW, Nelson MM. Abnormalities of pulmonary and other vessels in rat fetuses from maternal pteroylglutamic acid deficiency. Anat Rec 1963; 147:397–401.

53. Shaw GW, Wasserman CR, O'Malley CD. Periconceptional vitamin use and reduced risk for conotruncal and limb defects in California. Teratology 1994; 49:372 (abstract)..

54. Botto LD, Khoury MJ, Mulinare J, Erickson JD. Periconceptional multivitamin use and the occurrence of conotruncal heart defects. Results from a population-based case-control study. Pediatrics (in press).

55. Czeizel AE, Tóth M, Rockenbauer M. A case-control analysis of folic acid supplementation during pregnancy. Teratology (in press).

56. Tolarova M. Periconceptional supplementation with vitamins and folic acid to prevent recurrence of cleft lip. Lancet 1982; 2:217.

57. Tolarova M, Harris J. Reduced recurrence of orofacial clefts after periconceptional supplementation with high-dose folic acid and multivitamins. Teratology 1995; 51:71–78.

58. Shaw GM, Lammer EJ, Wasserman CR, O'Malley CD, Tolarova MM. Risks of orofacial clefts in children born to women using multivitamins containing folic acid periconceptionally. Lancet 1995; 345:393–396.

59. Czeizel AE. Limb-reduction defects and folic acid supplementation. Lancet 1995; 345:932.

60. Milunsky A, Graet JW, Gaynor MFJr: Methotrexate induced congenital malformations with a review of the literature. J Pediatr 1968; 72:790–795.

61. Tamura T, Shane B, Baer MT, et al. Absorption of mono- and polyglutamyl folates in zinc-depleted man. Am J Clin Nutr 1978; 31:1984–1987.

62. Stokes PL. Folate metabolism in scurvy. Am J Clin Nutr 1975; 28:126–129.

63. Yates RW, Ferguson-Smith MA, Shenkin A, et al. Is disordered folate metabolism the basis for the genetic predisposition to neural tube defects? Clin Genet 1987; 31:279–287.

64. Gardiki-Kouidou P, Seller MJ. Amniotic fluid folate, vitamin B12 and transcobalamins in neural tube defects. Clin Genet 1988; 33:441–448.

65. Schorah CJ, Habibzadeh N, Wild J, Smithells RW. Possible abnormalities of folate and vitamin B12 metabolism associated with neural tube defects. Ann NY Acad Sci 1993; 678:81–91.

66. Bower C, Stanley FJ, Croft M, et al. Absorption of pteroylpolyglutamates in mothers of infants with neural-tube defects. Br J Nutr 1993; 69:827–834.

67. Wild J, Seller MJ, Schorah CJ, Smithells RW. Investigation of folate intake and metabolism in women who have had two pregnancies complicated by neural tube defects. Br J Obstet Gynecol 1994; 101:197–202.

68. Scott J. Catabolism of folates. In: Folates and Pterins. Vol I. Chemistry and Biochemistry of Folates. Blakley RL, Bankovic SJ, eds. New York: Wiley, 1984; pp. 307–327.

69. Scott JM, Weir DG, Malloy A, McPartlin J, Daly L, Kirke P. Folic acid metabolism and mechanisms of neural tube defect. In: Neural tube defects. CIBA Foundation, Wiley, Chichester, 1994; pp. 180–191.

70. Steegers-Theunissen RPM, Boers GHJ, Trijbels FJM, Eskes TKAB. Neural-tube defects and derangement of homocysteine metabolism. New Engl J Med 1991; 324:199–200.

71. Steegers-Theunissen RP, Boers GH, Blom HJ, Nijhuis JG, Thomas CMG, Borm GF, Eskes TK. Neural tube defects and elevated homocysteine levels in amniotic fluid. Am J Obstet Gynecol 1995; 172:1436–1441.

72. Engbersen AMT, Franken DG, Boers GHJ, Stevens EMB, Trijbels FJM, Blom HJ. Thermolabile 5,10-methylenetetrahydrofolate reductase as a cause of mild hyperhomocysteinemia. Am J Hum Genet 1995; 56:142–150.

73. Goyette D, Summer JS, Milos R. Human methylenetetrahydrofolate reductase: isolation of cDNA, mapping and mutation identification. Nature Genet 1994; 7:195–200.

74. Frosst P, Blom HJ, Milos R. A candidate genetic risk-factor for vascular disease: a common mutation in methylenetetrahydrofolate reductase. Nature Genet 1995; 10:111–113.

75. Van der Put NM, Steegers-Theunissen RPM, Frosst P, Trijbels FJM, Eskes TKAB, Van den Heuvel LP, Mariman ECM, den Heyer M, Rozen R, Blom HJ. Mutated methylentetrahydrofolate reductase as a risk factor for spina bifida. Lancet 1995; 346:1070–1071.

76. Coelho CND, Weber JA, Klein NW, et al. Whole rat embryos require methionine for neural tube closure when cultured on low serum. J Nutr 1989; 119:1716–1725.

77. Coelho CND, Klein NW. Methionine and neural tube closure in cultured rat embryos: morphological and biochemical analyses. Teratology 1990; 42:437–451.

78. Van Aerts LAGJM, Blom HJ, Deabreu R, Trijbels FJM, Eskes TKAB, Peereboor JHJ, Stegeman JHJC, Noordhoek J. Prevention of neural tube defects by and toxicity of L-homocysteine in cultured postimplantation rat embryos. Teratology 1994; 50:348–360.

79. Erbe RW, Wang J-C. Folate metabolism in humans. Am J Med Genet 1984; 17:277–287.

80. Iyengar L, Apte SV. Nutrient stores in human foetal livers. Br J Nutr 1972; 27:313–317.

81. Strelling MK. Transfer of folate to the fetus. Dev Med Child Neurol 1976; 28:533–535.

82. Czeizel AE, Sankaranarayanan K. The load of genetic and partially genetic disorders in man. I. Congenital anomalies: estimates of detriment in terms of years of life lost and years of impaired life. Mut Res 1984; 128:499–503.

83. Czeizel AE, Intõdy Zs, Modell B. What proportion of congenital abnormalities can be prevented? Brit Med J 1993; 306:499–503.

84. Canadian Task Force on the Periodic Health Examination. Periodic health examination, 1994 update. 3. Primary and secondary prevention of neural tube defects. Can Med Assoc J 1994; 151:21–28.

85. Kirke PN, Molloy AM, Daly LE, Burke H, Weir DG, Scott JM. Maternal plasma folate and vitamin B12 are independent risk factors for neural tube defects. Q J Med 1993; 86:703–708.

86. Mills JL, McPartlin JM, Kirke PN, Lee YJ, Conley MR, Weir DG. Homocysteine metabolism in pregnancies complicated by neural-tube defects. Lancet 1995; 345:149–151.

87. Schwartz SO, Kaplan SR, Armstrong BE. The long-term evaluation of folic acid treatment of pernicious anemia. J Lab Clin Med 1950; 35:894–898.

88. Chanarin I, Laidlow J, Lughridge LW, Mollin DL. Megaloblastic anaemia due to phenobarbitone. The convulsant action of therapeutic doses of folic acid. Br Med J 1960; 1:1099–1102.

89. Chien LT, Krumdieck CL, Scott CW, Butterworth CI. Harmful effect of megadoses of vitamins: electroencephalogram abnormalities and seizures induced by intravenous folate in drug-treated epileptics. Am J Clin Nutr 1975; 28:51–58.

90. Strauss RG, Bernstein R. Folic acid and dilantin antagonism in pregnancy. Obstet Gynecol 1975; 44:345–348.

91. Dansky LV, Andermann E, Rosenblat D, et al. Anticonvulsants, folate levels and pregnancy outcome: a prospective study. Ann Neurol 1987; 27:176–182.

92. Biale Y, Lewenthal H. Effects of folic acid supplementation on congenital malformations due to anticonvulsive drugs. Eur J Obstet Gynecol Reprod Biol 1984; 18:211–216.

93. Barker DJP, ed. Fetal and Infant Origins of Adult Disease. British Medical Journal Publication, London, England, 1992.

94. Winship KA, Cahal DA, Weber JCP, Griffin JP. Maternal drug histories and central nervous system anomalies. Arch Dis Child 1984; 59:1052–1060.

95. Mulinare J, Cordero JF, Erickson D, Beery RJ. Periconceptional use of multivitamins and the occurrence of neural tube defects. JAMA 1980; 260:3141–3145.

96. Mills JL, Rhoads GG, Simpson JL, et al. The absence of a relation between the periconceptional use of vitamins and neural-tube defects. New Engl J Med 1989; 321:430–435.

97. Milunsky A, Jick H, Jick SS, Bruell CL, MacLaughlin DS, Rothman KJ, Willett W. Multivitamin/folic acid supplementation in early pregnancy reduces the prevalence of neural tube defects. JAMA 1989; 262:2847–2852.

98. Shaw GM, Schaffer D, Velie EM, Morland K, Harris JA. Periconceptional vitamin use, dietary folate, and the occurrence of neural tube defect. Epidemiology 1995; 6:219–226.

20 Nutritional Prevention of DNA Damage to Sperm and Consequent Risk Reduction in Birth Defects and Cancer in Offspring

Alan A. Woodall and Bruce N. Ames

1. INTRODUCTION

The damage produced by endogenously generated oxygen radicals has been proposed as a major contributory factor to aging and the many degenerative processes associated with it, including cancer, heart disease, and cognitive dysfunction *(1)*. Under physiological conditions, endogenous oxidants are produced at a high rate, resulting in extensive oxidative damage to proteins, lipids, and DNA *(2–5)*. Oxidative damage to DNA, based on the urinary excretion of DNA adducts, occurs at an estimated rate of 10^5 hits/cell/d in the rat and about 10^4 hits/cell/d in the human *(6)* Evidence is accumulating to suggest that rates of cellular oxidative damage can also be modulated by exogenous factors. Oxidative insult to tissues is increased by smoking and exposure to ionizing radiation, and decreased by intake of antioxidants, such as ascorbate and tocopherols, that are part of endogenous antioxidant defenses *(7–10)*. Hence, a critical determinant of the rate of cellular damage is the balance between antioxidant defense capacity and the oxidant insult to the tissue. Improved nutrition, increased intake of antioxidants, and cessation of dangerous habits, such as smoking, is critical for lowering individual risk of degenerative disease.

However, although the public is beginning to realize that prevention of degenerative disease to somatic tissues may depend on dietary and social lifestyle, less attention has been given to the effects that these factors may have on the germline tissues, the egg and sperm, and the possible consequences for offspring. It is generally recognized that maternal smoking and ethanol consumption should be avoided during pregnancy to reduce risk of fetal injury, and that a balanced diet containing adequate levels of vitamins and micro- and macronutrients is desirable during gestation. Conversely, little attention has been given to the role that damage to the sperm cells of the father may play in contributing to risk of genetic damage to the infant. Evidence from both biochemical and epidemiological sources suggests that the prospective male parent also requires an adequate intake of certain nutrients and avoidance of deleterious habits, such as smoking, to limit genetic damage to sperm and reduce risk of birth defects and childhood cancer *(11)*. In this chapter we review evidence to support this argument.

From: *Preventive Nutrition: The Comprehensive Guide for Health Professionals*
Edited by A. Bendich and R. J. Deckelbaum Humana Press Inc., Totowa, NJ

2. OXIDANT DAMAGE TO GAMETES: SPERMATOZOA ARE AT INCREASED RISK OF TRANSMITTING HERITABLE MUTATIONS TO OFFSPRING COMPARED TO OOCYTES

Endogenous oxidative damage to germline DNA is likely to lead to heritable muta-tions and increased incidence of birth defects, genetic diseases, and cancer in offspring. Ionizing radiation, an oxidative mutagen, damages gamete DNA, resulting in mutations that are transmitted to the progeny in experimental animals *(12)*. Most, but not all, DNA damage is expected to be repaired, although damaged residues that remain may be con-verted to mutations during the DNA replication that accompanies cell division in sper-matogenesis, oogenesis, and embryogenesis. Studies of genetic abnormalities and can-cers that are believed to arise from germline mutations show these to have a higher frequency of paternal than maternal origin. One example is the increased frequency of paternal origin of germline mutations in the retinoblastoma gene *(13)* This is not sur-prising when one considers the contrasting physiology of gametogenesis in both sexes. Production of female gametes (oogenesis) occurs when the mother is herself *in utero*. The preoocytes are stored in a mitotically inactive state throughout life and only un-dergo further (meiotic) cell division prior to ovulation. This is in marked contrast with the production of male gametes (spermatogenesis), which are produced continuously throughout adulthood. Mature spermatozoa are thus formed from stem cells after a much greater number of mitotic cell divisions than are oocytes, resulting in an increase in the risk for mutation in sperm. Crow has reviewed this area and quotes J. B. S. Hal-dane in 1947:

> The much larger number of cell divisions between zygote and sperm than between zy-gote and egg, the increased age of fathers of children with new dominant mutations, and the greater evolution rate of pseudogenes on the Y chromosome than on autosomes all point to a much higher [germline] mutation rate in males than in females *(14)*.

It is estimated that the number of cell divisions between egg and zygote is 24, whereas for the male, this is highly dependent on age. Hence, at age 13, an estimated 36 cell divisions have occurred between stem cell and spermatozoon, at age 20, 197 cell di-visions, at age 30, 427 cell divisions and at age 45, 772 cell divisions. Spermatogenesis may occur while the male is exposed to environmental fluxes in oxidant production (e.g., by smoking) and ingesting suboptimal intakes of those nutrients (e.g., ascorbate and tocopherol) that protect the tissues against oxidative stress or are required for DNA integrity (e.g., folate). In addition, once spermatogenic cell division is completed, matu-ration of the spermatid into the spermatozoon involves condensation of the DNA ac-companied by the apparent loss of DNA repair activity *(15)* Damaged residues remain-ing in sperm DNA thus may be delivered to the oocyte on fertilization, increasing the possibility of mutations when the zygote divides. Hence, it is apparent that offspring birth defects and childhood cancer are more likely to be associated with genetic damage to the spermatozoon than to the oocyte.

3. PATERNAL SMOKING AND RISK OF MUTATION TO THE GERMLINE

Maternal smoking during pregnancy can cause many problems, such as intrauterine growth retardation leading to increased incidence of spontaneous abortion, premature birth, and low infant birthweight (*see* chapter 21). However, it is pertinent to note that numerous epidemiological studies over several decades in various countries have failed consistently to find a link between maternal cigarette smoking and genetic damage to the fetus. In contrast, the few epidemiological studies on the effects of paternal smoking and risk of birth defects and childhood cancer suggest, but do not prove, increased risk of birth defects in the offspring of smokers as compared to nonsmokers. A review of the epidemiology of paternal smoking and risk of offspring birth defects and childhood cancer incidence is presented below.

3.1. Paternal Smoking and Risk of Birth Defects

Comstock and Lundin found that neonatal death rate among infants of smoking fathers was 17.2/1000 live births compared to 11.9 (adjusted for sex of child and education of father) among infants of nonsmoking fathers and 26.5 among infants born to parents who both smoked *(16)*. Koo et al. found that wives of smoking spouses have more miscarriages and abortions than wives of nonsmoking spouses ($p = 0.06$) *(17)*. Heary et al. observed a significant association ($p < 0.05$) between paternal smoking and increased neural tube defects (NTDs) (4/8 cases vs 1/17 controls) in offspring *(18)*.

Mau and Netter studied the smoking habits of fathers of 5200 newborns *(19)*. The rate of major malformations among nonsmoking fathers was 0.8% and among smoking fathers 2.1%. Maternal smoking had no influence on the rate of birth defects. The most striking increase in birth defects concerned major facial clefts. One-tenth of 1% of infants of nonsmoking fathers had facial clefts, compared to 0.5% of fathers who smoked 1–10 cigarettes/d and 0.7% of fathers who smoked more than 10 cigarettes/d. There was also an increase in perinatal mortality (unrelated to major birth defects) if the father smoked more than 10 cigarettes/d, even if the mother did not smoke (4.3% compared to 2.8%). It is assumed that facial cleft in this study is equivalent to cleft lip/palate.

Savitz et al. analyzed single live births among 14,685 volunteers who participated in child health studies *(20)*. Paternal cigarette smoking was more common among children with cleft lip (with or without cleft palate) (OR = 1.7, CI 95%:0.5–6.0), hydrocephalus (OR = 2.4, CI 95%:0.6–9.3), ventricular septal defect (OR = 2.0, CI 95%:0.9–4.3), and urethral stenosis (OR=2.0, CI 95%:0.6–6.4). However, inverse associations between paternal smoking and birth defects were more common than positive associations. The authors mention specifically genetically altered sperm as a possible cause of birth defects in infants of smoking fathers. They note that several of the anomalies associated with infants of older fathers were also increased among fathers who smoked. The concordance in defects associated with both advanced paternal age and paternal smoking was notable especially for ventricular septal defects and hydrocephalus.

Schmid, in discussing the Mau and Netter study, attributed the effect of paternal smoking on birth defects to passive smoke *(21)*. However, passive smoking is not a probable explanation for the link between paternal smoking and birth defects because the amount of smoke that reaches the embryo is insignificant compared with the amount that reaches the embryo when the mother herself smokes, and maternal smoking does not appear to increase significantly the risk of genetic birth defects.

Schmidt made an argument similar to ours concerning smoking and genetic damage:

Tobacco smoke contains numerous mutagenic substances (22). They reach the male gonads via the blood. They show their mutagenic action here openly much more strongly than on egg-cells because the spermatogenesis continues over the whole male reproductive period whereas the formation of eggs is already completed in the fetal phase.

Seidman provides a table on the incidence of major and minor congenital malformations by paternal and maternal smoking levels *(23)*. There was a nonsignificant increase in the incidence of major and minor malformations in the offspring of smoking fathers who mate with nonsmoking mothers. This author does not break down the malformations by specific defect.

3.2. Paternal Smoking and Childhood Tumors

Gold et al. examined maternal smoking but not paternal smoking *(24)*. Maternal smoking did not seem to influence the risk of brain tumors in children.

Grufferman et al. found that paternal smoking, but not maternal smoking, increased the risk of rhabdomyosarcoma (RMS) in childhood (relative risk of 3.9, $p = 0.003$) *(25)*. RMS is the sixth most common childhood cancer, with an annual incidence of about four cases per million children and a peak incidence at about ages three to four. The authors suggest that a direct carcinogenic effect of paternal cigarette smoke may be introduced in a prezygotic manner.

Grufferman et al. stated that:

In our recent study of childhood rhabdomyosarcoma (RMS) we found an increase in the risk of RMS among children whose fathers smoked cigarettes. However, there was no association between RMS and mothers' smoking. We hypothesize that differential germ cell damage from cigarette smoking underlies our observations and that this risk of germ cell damage from cigarette smoking and from other environmental exposures is greater for men than for women. The increased susceptibility for male germ cells may be due to the number and timing of meiotic and mitotic cell divisions. In males, germ cells undergo large numbers of meiotic and mitotic divisions throughout the reproductive years. In contrast, in females, generally only one oocyte matures and completes meiosis each month of the reproductive years. Thus, there are very large male-female differences in the number of rapidly dividing germ cells during the reproductive years, and it is rapidly proliferating cells which are most susceptible to genetic damage (26).

John et al. found associations with paternal smoking during the 12 mo prior to conception in the absence of maternal smoking during the first trimester for all childhood cancers combined (OR = 1.2, CI 95% 0.8–2.1), acute lymphocytic leukemia (OR=1.4, 95% CI 0.6 - 3.1)), lymphomas (OR = 1.6 CI 95% 0.5–5.4), and brain cancer (OR = 1.6, CI 95% 0.7–3.5) *(27)*. These correlations, however, appear fairly weak and the figures are similar to those for maternal smoking alone. After adjustment for paternal education, maternal smoking during the first trimester of pregnancy, in the absence of paternal smoking, was associated with an increased risk for all cancers combined (OR = 1.3), acute lymphocytic leukemia (OR = 1.9), and lymphomas (OR = 2.3).

Johnston et al. found in their study of children with germ cell tumors that the smoking pattern of fathers was similar for both cases and controls *(28)*. Magnani et al. found that both maternal and paternal smoking up to the child's birth were associated with non-Hodgkin's lymphoma in childhood *(29)*. After adjusting for socioeconomic status, the odds ratio for paternal smoking was 6.7 and for maternal smoking was 1.7. The author states that the odds ratio for paternal smoking was not correlated with number of cigarettes. The study showed no correlation between acute lymphocytic leukemia and parental smoking.

Neutel and Buck's study only took into consideration the effect of maternal smoking on childhood cancer *(30)*. For cancers of all sites, the children of mothers who smoked during pregnancy had a relative risk of 1.3 (CI 95% 0.8–2.2), which was not significant.

Preston-Martin et al. found that there was a possibly significant increase in risk of childhood brain tumors (OR = 1.5, $p = 0.03$) if during pregnancy the mother lived with a smoker *(31)*; "Our finding that maternal smoking itself was not related to disease but that living with a smoker (usually the child's father) may indicate that paternal exposures are important."

Sandler et al. analyzed cancers of all sites, except basal cell cancer of the skin, among people 15–59 yr old *(32)*. Cancer risk was increased 50% among people whose fathers had smoked. In this study paternal smoking was defined as the father having smoked before the child reached 10 yr of age. Increased risk associated with paternal smoking was not explained by demographic factors, social class, or individual smoking habits. There was only a slight increase in overall cancer risk associated with maternal smoking (relative risk of 1.1, CI 95% 0.7–1.6). However, both maternal and paternal smoking were associated with increased risk for hematopoietic cancers, and a dose-response relationship was seen. The relative risk for hematopoietic cancers increased from 1.7 when one parent smoked to 4.6 when both parents smoked (Mantel-Haerzel χ for trend=3.25, $p < 0.001$). However, the study included a wide range of ages and did not give isolated information on the teenage cases. Therefore, the study does not assess the risk of paternal smoking specifically on childhood cancer.

In summary, the epidemiological evidence presented, although sparse, suggests paternal smoking could be a contributory factor to the risk of genetic damage to the child, whereas maternal smoking, although deleterious to the growth of the fetus and increasing the risk of neonatal death, does not contribute significantly to the risk of genetic defect to the offspring. Most interesting is the possible increased risk of cancer in the offspring of fathers who smoked at the time that the child was conceived, whereas maternal smoking had little effect. There was no correlation between social class or other demographic factors and cancer risk in offspring that might explain such differences. Cigarette smoke contains substantial quantities of mutagens that may reach the testes via the bloodstream to promote genetic lesions and also contains high levels of reactive oxygen species that deplete serum antioxidants *(33)*. The depletion of the blood plasma antioxidant pool may lead to depletion of antioxidants in other tissues and body fluids with which it is in equilibrium, including the seminal plasma and testicular antioxidant pools, thus increasing the risk of oxidant damage during spermatogenesis and subsequent sperm storage. The evidence suggests that further epidemiological and intervention studies are needed and education of prospective fathers of their responsibility in prevention of injury to their children by their cessation of smoking appears warranted.

4. PATERNAL NUTRIENT REQUIREMENTS FOR THE REDUCTION OF GENETIC DAMAGE TO SPERM

Spermatogenesis in mammals requires a considerable devotion of nutritional resources that could otherwise be used to maintain somatic tissue viability. Indeed, one of the major arguments for aging is that the somatic tissues undergo degeneration because biological efforts are channeled into maintaining reproductive capacity at the expense of extended lifespan among mammals *(34)*. Some mammals have periods of seasonal reproductive activity when the female comes into estrus for a short period of time, and thus the males of these species, such as the Sika deer, have evolved to channel their biological resources into reproductive activity, including spermatogensis, to coincide with these periods to best conserve biological resources *(35)*. Human females have evolved reproductive activity that is continuous throughout the year but limited to short periods during each month; thus, human male spermatogenic capacity must be maintained continuously to allow success in reproduction. This requires considerable nutrient resources to maintain the high rates of germline cell division with high replicative accuracy. Mutations to the germline can occur by spontaneous error, which is normally kept low, or by oxidative damage and/or limiting resources of certain nutrients essential for accurate DNA replication and protection of the genome (*see* Chapter 1).

4.1. Prevention of Germline Mutations Arising Via Oxidative Damage: Antioxidant Nutrients

Oxidant stress to tissues results in loss of tissue function and reduced accuracy in DNA replication, which can lead to mutations during cell division. The critical importance of preventing oxidative damage to tissues is reflected in the evolution of a multifaceted antioxidant defense based on small-molecule antioxidants and antioxidant proteins to limit oxidative damage to cells *(36)*. Also, there is a considerable array of enzymes that have evolved to repair oxidative lesions to DNA, suggesting that oxidative damage to DNA has a definite deleterious effect on successful DNA replication and reproductive success. The evolution of specific antioxidant proteins allows organisms to limit oxidative damage in a number of ways:

1. Prevent free-radical formation, e.g., chelate transition metals in such proteins as ceruloplasmin, and transferrin;
2. Destroy oxidants catalytically, e.g., superoxide dismutases, catalase, and glutathione reductase;
3. Sacrificial scavengers of oxidants, e.g., albumin; and
4. Remove oxidant-damaged biomolecules, e.g., DNA glycosylases or phospholipase A_2

The evolved antioxidant protein defense is reinforced by endogenous and exogenous small-molecule antioxidants that exist in the aqueous and lipid phases of cells and extracellular fluids. These include ascorbate, glutathione, urate, tocopherols, carotenoids, ubiquinols, and bilirubin *(37–43)*. The low-mol-wt antioxidants are a vital component of the overall antioxidant defense that acts by scavenging oxidants in a sacrificial manner or by chelating transition metal ions. Numerous studies have demonstrated that low nutritional intakes of ascorbate, tocopherols, and carotenoids are associated with increased risk of cancer, cardiovascular disease, cataract, macular degeneration, and arthritis. Hence, there is a nutritional requirement to maintain an adequate antioxidant defense against oxidant injury to tissues. Maintenance of adequate seminal plasma antioxidants that are derived wholly from the diet appears to be crucial in preventing oxidative damage to sperm cell DNA *(44,45)*.

4.1.1. ASCORBIC ACID

The dietary antioxidant ascorbic acid (AA) may play a critical role in protecting spermatozoa against oxidative damage. AA is present at a high concentration in seminal fluid compared to blood plasma (400 vs 60 μM), presumably reflecting an important

Table 1
Dietary AA Intake, Semen AA, and oxo[8]dG in DNA from Sperm of Individuals Maintained
on Controlled Diets Supplemented with Various Amounts of AA

	Baseline	Depletion	Marginal	Repletion
AA intake (mg/d)	250	5	10 or 20	60 or 250
Number of subjects	10	8	6	4
Length, d	7–14	32	28	28
Semen AA (μM)	399 ± 55[a]	203 ± 72[b]	115 ± 25[c]	422 ± 100[a]
Oxo[8]dG (fmol/μg DNA)	34.0 ± 2.4[d]	66.9 ± 8.5[e]	84.4 ± 22.3[e]	53.8 ± 16.8[d,e]

Values expressed are the mean ± SEM. Mean values in the same row with different superscripts are significantly different at $P < 0.01$ (d vs e, a vs c) or $P < 0.05$.

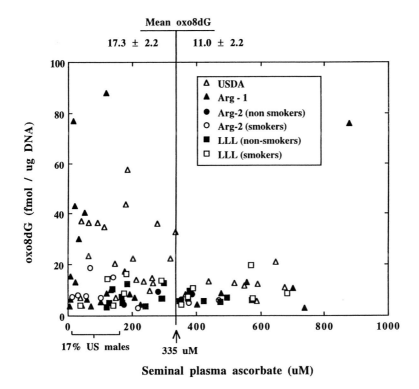

Fig. 1. Relationship between seminal plasma AA and sperm cell oxo[8]dG in male volunteers. Below a seminal plasma AA level of 335 μM, there is a marked increase in the range of sperm cell oxo[8]dG. The key refers to separate studies that were undertaken on samples from collaboration with Argentina (ARG), Lawrence Livermore Laboratory (LLL), or the United States Department of Agriculture Western Human Nutrition Center (USDA). Redrawn from ref. 43.

physiological role for this compound. Depletion of seminal plasma AA in male volunteers on controlled diets significantly increased sperm cell 8-hydroxy-deoxyguanosine (oxo[8]dG) levels, a marker of oxidative damage to DNA (Table 1) 44. The relationship between seminal plasma ascorbate and oxo[8]dG in sperm in free-living individuals also suggests that low levels of seminal plasma AA are associated with increased risk of oxidative damage to sperm DNA (Fig. 1) (44). Ascorbic acid is a powerful antioxidant in

Table 2
Seminal Plasma Ascorbate, α-Tocopherol, and Oxo[8]dG in Sperm Cell DNA
of Smokers vs Nonsmokers

	Nonsmokers	Smokers
No. of cigarettes/d	0	22 ± 1.8
Oxo[8]dG (fmol/μg DNA)	6.7 ± 0.5[b]	10.2 ± 1.1
α-Tocopherol (μM)	0.38 ± 0.05	0.26 ± 0.02[a]
α-Tocopherol/cholesterol[c]	0.73 ± 0.11	0.41 ± 0.06[a]
Ascorbate (μM)	296 ± 24	246 ± 40

Values are mean ± SEM. Means in the same row with superscripts are significantly different
at [a]$P < 0.05$, [b]$P < 0.01$ (see ref. 45).
[c]One α-tocopherol/10[6] cholesterol molecules.

blood plasma and would act in the seminiferous tubules to limit oxidative damage in a
similar manner (46). Thus, the very high level of AA in seminal plasma that is dependent
on diet appears to play a critical role in protecting the paternal genome. Circumstances
that lower the level of seminal plasma AA would thus seem likely to increase risk of oxidative adduct formation in sperm DNA. Low dietary intake of AA is one possibility.
The current US Recommended Daily Allowance (RDA) for AA is 60 mg/d, but this suggested intake is to prevent development of deficiency syndromes (e.g., scurvy) and may
not reflect the intake required for maintenance of an effective antioxidant defense.
Smoking also depletes serum antioxidants, including AA, tocopherols, and carotenoids
(45,47) It is estimated that a smoker needs to consume two- to three-times as much AA
as a nonsmoker to maintain a comparable blood plasma level (48). A recent study has
shown that smokers have lower seminal plasma AA titers and higher oxo[8]dG levels in
sperm DNA than nonsmokers (Table 2) (45). Whether smoking depletes the seminal
plasma AA pool directly, or this is lowered because a consequence of blood plasma AA
depletion is unknown. The latter case seems more likely, as there is some doubt that significant levels of reactive oxygen species from cigarette smoke would reach the testes,
but since the total body AA pool is redistributed rapidly (49), a depletion in blood
plasma AA could account for the lowered seminal plasma AA observed in male smokers. Hence, the combined effects of low fruit and vegetable consumption and smoking
may together depress the seminal AA to such an extent as to increase the level of mutations in sperm cell DNA. Low AA intake also reduces the fertility of the male. Males
with low seminal plasma AA levels have decreased sperm viability, motility, and cell
number, and increased percentage of sperm cell agglutination and abnormal morphol-
ogy compared with volunteers maintained on high AA intakes (50–53). These data suggest that AA plays a vital role in the maintenance of spermatogenic activity and limitation of oxidative lesion formation in sperm cell DNA that could lead to mutation in the
zygote.

4.1.2. α-Tocopherol

Another important dietary antioxidant is α-tocopherol. This is the major lipid-
soluble antioxidant in human blood plasma and together with AA plays a vital role in
limiting oxidative damage to membranes and serum lipoproteins (54). Unlike AA,
which is at higher concentrations in seminal plasma compared with blood plasma,

seminal plasma α-tocopherol (0.38 μM) is much lower than that found in the plasma (typically 15–40 μM) *(45)*. However, smokers have significantly lowered seminal plasma α-tocopherol levels compared with nonsmokers (Table 2). Whether seminal plasma α-tocopherol has a definite role in preventing oxidative damage to sperm or is depressed in the seminal plasma without deleterious effect on sperm genome integrity requires further study. However, the spermatozoan cell membrane contains an unusually high proportion of unsaturated fatty acids that are susceptible to peroxidation. Membrane integrity is vital in maintaining sperm cell viability, and motility and for sperm-egg fusion, so it is possible that α-tocopherol is vital for the protection of the membrane lipid domain of the sperm cell. Limitation of spontaneous lipid peroxidation in sperm cells and seminal plasma is of importance in preventing the production of toxic aldehydes that may have mutagenic properties, and thus α-tocopherol may complement AA in protecting spermatozoa from oxidative damage to the DNA. Further work to establish the role of α-tocopherol, if any, in protection of sperm against oxidative damage is currently underway.

4.1.3. OTHER ANTIOXIDANTS

Carotenoids, ubiquinol-10, uric acid, and bilirubin have all been proposed to be antioxidants in blood plasma. No significant levels of β-carotene or ubiquinol-10 have been reported in seminal plasma (<0.01 μM) *(45)*. It seems unlikely that these compounds are important components that prevent oxidative damage to sperm cells in seminal plasma.

4.2. Prevention of Mutations to Sperm DNA: Role of Nonantioxidant Nutrients

In addition to prevention of oxidative insult to DNA, mutations can arise during DNA replication or repair if inadequate levels of certain nutrients are present. This is seen in the pathophysiological consequences of folate and vitamin B12 deficiency on hemopoiesis, in which increased levels of uracil are erroneously incorporated into DNA *(55)* It is a concern regarding whether similar factors could be important in increasing the number of mutations during spermatogenesis or during zygote division. We discuss those nutrients that we believe may be important in maintaining sperm cell DNA fidelity.

4.2.1. FOLATE

Folate (in the form of tetrahydrofolate) is required as a cofactor during the methylation of deoxyuridylate (dUMP) to deoxythymidylate (dTMP). dTMP is required for the synthesis of deoxythymidine residues, which are essential for DNA replication. Folate (and vitamin B12)-deficient patients have been shown to have high levels of uracil misincorporation into DNA of hemopoietic stems cells required for erythrocyte production *(55,56)*. Uracil misincorporation can lead to chromosomal strand breaks when nicks are formed on opposite strands by uracil glycosylase *(56,57)*. Thus, it appears likely that men with folate-deficient diets may have increased rates of uracil misincorporation into sperm cell DNA. Folate deficiency is the most common vitamin deficiency worldwide because of insufficient fruit and vegetable intake. Chronic alcoholics may particularly be at risk, since in addition to their generally poor diet and consequent low intake of both antioxidant nutrients and other vitamins, the problem is compounded by their decreased absorption of folate across the gastric epithelium *(58)*. Chronic ethanol intake lowers the activity of gastric brush-border folate hydrolase and results in necrosis of the gastric epithelium, both essential for adequate absorption of folate *(59)*. Hence, one concern is that male alcoholics or those on poor diets may be at increased risk of uracil misincorporation in sperm DNA and, thus, increased risk of producing offspring with genetic defects.

4.2.2. ZINC

Zinc is known to be an essential trace element for testicular development and spermatogenesis *(60)*. Zinc concentrations in seminal plasma (about 200 µg/L) are much greater than that in blood plasma (about 6 µg/L), which suggests a specific function for this trace element in spermatogenesis and stability of spermatozoa *(61)*. Zinc concentrations are correlated positively with sperm cell density, and lower zinc concentrations are found in infertile men compared with fertile men *(62)*. A recent study has shown that zinc deficiency leads to increased oxidative damage to testicular cell DNA (as measured by oxo^8dG) and increased protein carbonyl content *(63)*. The mechanistic role of zinc in spermatogenesis is unclear, but it has been suggested that Zn^{2+} enhances the stability of sperm chromatin *(64)*, or is required to maintain sperm function prior to zygote formation *(65)*. Zinc, although a member of the transition metal *d*-block of the periodic table, does not possess any redox activity in the Zn^{2+} state. This means it is unable to participate in oxidant production, as can other transition metal ions, such as those of copper and iron. One possible explanation for such a high Zn^{2+} seminal plasma content would be to occupy sensitive binding sites on proteins and DNA, which would reduce the possibility of redox-active transition metal ion binding to these sites and promote oxidant production. Further research into the mechanisms and function of zinc is required to establish the role that this trace element plays in spermatogenesis and protection of sperm cells against oxidative damage, but it is evident that adequate intakes of zinc are probably required to reduce risk of sperm cell genetic damage in men.

5. RECOMMENDATIONS FOR INTAKES OF NUTRIENTS TO LIMIT SPERM DAMAGE

RDA values are suggested intakes to prevent the occurrence of deficiency disease, rather than the optimal level of a particular nutrient. Other factors, such as whether the individual smokes or consumes large amounts of ethanol, will also affect the intake or amount of vitamins, such as ascorbate, tocopherols, and folate, necessary to maintain adequate levels in the body. Most of the nutrients mentioned in this chapter are obtained in sufficient quantities from a well-balanced omnivorous diet that is high in fresh fruits and vegetables. The current intake of two servings of fruits and three of vegetables per day as recommended by the National Cancer Institute is achieved by only 9% of Americans, and by less of the populace in some European countries (e.g., Scotland). It is estimated that a quarter of the US population is getting insufficient amounts for optimum health *(66,67)*. The cost of fruits and vegetables is one factor that can discourage consumption. People with lower socioeconomic status generally have to spend a higher percentage of their income on food, eat less fruits and vegetables, and are more likely to smoke than are those from the more affluent echelons of society *(68)*. They may be at increased risk of having genetic damage to their offspring. It would be prudent for couples attempting to conceive for the male partner to cease any smoking activity, consume limited amounts of ethanol, and follow a diet high in fresh fruits and vegetables to ameliorate genetic damage to sperm and thus reduce risk of birth defects among children (*see* Chapter 19).

The prospective male parent has a responsibility in preventing genetic injury to his children. The evidence to date suggests that a diet rich in antioxidants, particularly ascorbate, and cessation of smoking is important in reducing oxidative damage to sperm and risk of subsequent genetic malformation of offspring. Further research into the area of paternal dietary, smoking, and alcohol consumption effects on sperm damage is required to be able to provide the necessary public health advice to the general population, especially those planning a family.

REFERENCES

1. Ames BN, Shigenaga MK, Hagen TM. Oxidants, antioxidants and the degenerative diseases of aging. Proc Natl Acad Sci USA 1993; 90:7915–7922.
2. Shigenaga MK, Park JW, Cundy KC, Gimeno CJ, Ames BN. In vivo oxidative DNA damage: measurement of 8-hydroxy-2'-deoxyguanosine in DNA and urine by high-performance liquid chromatography with electrochemical detection. Methods Enzymol 1990; 186:521–530.
3. Fraga CG, Shigenaga MK, Park JW, Degan P, Ames BN. Oxidative damage to DNA during aging: 8-hydroxy-2'-deoxyguanosine in rat organ DNA and urine. Proc Natl Acad Sci USA 1990; 87:4533–4537.
4. Rodriguez-Martinez MA, Ruiz-Torres A. Homeostasis between lipid peroxidation and antioxidant enzyme activities in healthy human aging. MechAgeDev 1992; 66:213–222.
5. Stadtman ER. Protein oxidation and aging. Science 1992; 257:1220–1224.
6. Ames BN, Shigenaga MK. Oxidants are a major contributor to aging. Ann NY Acad Sci 1992; 663:85–96.
7. Morrow JD, Frei B, Longmire AW, Gaziano JM, Lynch SM, Shyr Y, Strauss WE, Oates JA, Roberts LJ. Increase in circulating products of lipid peroxidation (F2-isoprostanes) in smokers. Smoking as a cause of oxidative damage. New Engl J Med 1995; 332:1198–1203.
8. Riley PA. Free radicals in biology: oxidative stress and the effects of ionizing radiation. Int J Radiat Biol 1994; 65:27–33.
9. Mezzetti A, Lapenna D, Pierdomenico SD, Calafiore AM, Costantini F, Riario-Sforza G, Imbastaro T, Neri M, Cuccurullo F. Vitamins E, C and lipid peroxidation in plasma and arterial tissue of smokers and nonsmokers. Atherosclerosis 1995; 112:91–99.
10. Frei B. Reactive oxygen species and antioxidant vitamins: mechanisms of action. Am J Med 1994; 97:5S–13S.
11. Ames BN, Motchnik P, Fraga CG, Shigenaga MK, Hagen TM. Antioxidant prevention of birth defects and cancer. In: Male-mediated Developmental Toxicity. Mattison DR, Olshan A, eds. New York, NY: Plenum, 1994.
12. National Research Council. Health Effects of Exposure to Low Levels of Ionizing Radiation, BEIR V National Academy Press, Washington.
13. Dryja TP, Shizuo M, Petersen R, Rapaport JM, Walton D, Yandell DW. Parental origin of mutations of the retinoblastoma gene. Nature 1989; 339:556–558.
14. Crow J. How much do we know about spontaneous human mutation rates? Environ Mol Mutagen 1993; 21:122–129.
15. Matsuda Y, Seki N, Utsugi-Takeduchi T, Tobari I. X-ray- and mitomycin C (MMC)-induced chromosome aberrations in spermogenic germ cells and the repair capacity of mouse eggs for the X-ray and MMC damage. Mutat Res 1989; 211:65–75.
16. Comstock GW, Lundin FEJ. Parental smoking and perinatal mortality. Am J Obst Gynec 1967; 98:708–718.
17. Koo LC, Ho J, Rylander R. Life-history correlates of environmental tobacco smoke: A study on nonsmoking Hong Kong Chinese wives with smoking versus non-smoking husbands. Soc Sci Med 1988; 26:751–760.
18. Hearey CD, Harris JA, Usatin MS, Epstein DM, Ury HK, Neutra RR. Investigation of a cluster of anencephaly and spina bifida. Am J Epidemiol 1984; 120:559–564.
19. Mau G, Netter P. Die auswirkungen des vaeterlichen zigarettenconsums auf die perinatale sterblichkeit und die missbildungshaeufigkeit. Dtsch Med Wochenschr 1974; 99:1113.

20. Savitz DA, Schwingl P, Keels MA. Influence of paternal age, smoking and alcohol consumption on congential abnormalities. Teratology 1991; 44:429–440.
21. Schmid J. Rauchen, pille und schwangershaft. Schweiz Rundshau Med 1989; 78:100–103.
22. Schmidt F. Rauchen schaedigt die maennliche Zeugungsfaehigkeit. Andrologia 1986; 18:445–454.
23. Seidman DS, Ever-Hadani P, Gale R. Effect of maternal smoking and age on congenital anomalies. Obstet Gynecol 1990; 76:1046–1050.
24. Gold LS, Slone TH, Stern BR, Manley NB, Ames BN. Rodent carcinogens: setting priorities. Science 1992; 258:261–265.
25. Grufferman S, Wang HH, DeLong ER, Kimm SYS, Delzell ES, Falletta JM. Environmental factors in the etiology of rhabdomyosarcoma in childhood. J Natl Cancer Inst 1982; 68:107–113.
26. Grufferman S, Delzell ES, Maile MC, Michalopoulous G. Parents' cigarette smoking and childhood cancer. Med Hypotheses 1983; 12:17–20.
27. John EM, Savitz DA, Sandler DP. Prenatal exposure to parents' smoking and childhood cancer. Am J Epidemiol 1991; 133:123–132.
28. Johnston HE, Mann JR, Williams J, Waterhouse JAH, Birch JM, Cartwright RA, Draper GJ, Hartley AL, Hopton PA, Stiller CA. The inter-regional, epidemiological study of childhood cancer (IREESCC): case-control study in children with germ cell tumours. Carcinogenesis 1986; 7:717–722.
29. Magnani C, Pastore G, Luzzatto L, Terracini B. Parental occupation and other environmental factors in the etiology of leukemias and non-Hodgkin's lymphomas in childhood: a case-control study. Tumori 1990; 76:413–419.
30. Neutel CI, Buch C. Effect of smoking during pregnancy on the risk of cancer in children. J Natl Cancer Inst 1971; 47:59–63.
31. Preston-Martin S, Yu MC, Benton B, Henderson BE. Nitroso compounds and childhood brain tumours: a case-control study. Cancer Res 1982; 42:5240–5245.
32. Sandler EP, Everson RB, Wildox AJ. Cancer risk in adulthood from early life exposure to parents' smoking. Am J Public Health 1985; 75:487.
33. van Antwerpen L, Theron AJ, Myer MS, Richards GA, Wolmarans L, Booysen U, van der Merwe CA, Sluis-Cremer GK, Anderson R. Cigarette smoke-mediated oxidant stress, phagocytes, vitamin C, vitamin E, and tissue injury. Ann NY Acad Sci 1993; 686:53–65.
34. Kirkwood TB. Comparative life spans of species: why do species have the life spans they do? Am J Clin Nutr 1992; 55:1191S–1195S.
35. Suzuki M, Kaji K, Nigi H. Annual changes of testes size, seminiferous tubules and plasma testosterone concentration of wild Sika deer in Hokkaido. J Vet Med Sci 1992; 54:551–556.
36. Sies H. Oxidative Stress: Oxidants and Antioxidants. Academic, Orlando, FL 1991.
37. Frei B, Stocker R, England L, Ames BN. Ascorbate: the most effective antioxidant in human blood plasma. Adv Exp Med Biol 1990; 264:155–163.
38. Munday R, Winterbourn CC. Reduced glutathione in combination with superoxide dismutase as an important biological antioxidant defense mechanism. Biochem Pharmacol 1989; 38:4349–4352.
39. Ames BN, Cathcart R, Schwiers E, Hochstein P. Uric acid provides an antioxidant defense in humans against oxidant- and radical-caused aging and cancer: a hypothesis. Proc Natl Acad Sci USA 1981; 78:6858–6862.
40. Ingold KU, Webb AC, Witter D, Burton GW, Metcalfe TA, Muller DP. Vitamin E remains the major lipid-soluble, chain-breaking antioxidant in human plasma even in individuals suffering severe vitamin E deficiency. Arch Biochem Biophys 1987; 259:224,225.
41. Packer L. Antioxidant action of carotenoids in vitro and in vivo and protection against oxidation of human low-density lipoproteins. Ann NY Acad Sci 1993; 691:48–60.
42. Frei B, Kim MC, Ames BN. Ubiquinol-10 is an effective lipid-soluble antioxidant at physiological concentrations. Proc Natl Acad Sci USA 1990; 87:4879–4883.
43. Neuzil J, Stocker R. Free and albumin-bound bilirubin are efficient co-antioxidants for alpha-tocopherol, inhibiting plasma and low density lipoprotein lipid peroxidation. J Biol Chem 1994; 269:16,712–16,719.
44. Fraga CG, Motchnik PA, Shigenaga MK, Helbock HJ, Jacob RA, Ames BN. Ascorbic acid protects against endogenous oxidative DNA damage in human sperm. Proc Natl Acad Sci USA 1991; 88:11,003–11,006.
45. Fraga CG, Motchnik PA, Wyrobek AJ, Rempel DM, Ames BN. Smoking and low antioxidant levels increase oxidative damage to sperm DNA. Mutat Res 1996; 351:199–203.
46. Frei B, Stocker R, Ames BN. Antioxidant defenses and lipid peroxidation in human blood plasma. Proc Natl Acad Sci USA 1988; 85:9748–9752.
47. Preston AM. Cigarette smoking-nutritional implications. Prog Food Nutr Sci 1991; 15:183–217.

48. Schectman G, Byrd JC, Hoffmann R. Ascorbic acid requirements for smokers: analysis of a population survey. Am J Clin Nutr 1991; 53:1466–1470.
49. Kallner A, Hartmann D, Hornig D. Steady-state turnover and body pool of ascorbic acid in man. Am J Clin Nutr 1979; 32:530–539.
50. Dawson EB, Harris WA, Teter MC, Powell LC. Effect of ascorbic acid supplementation on the sperm quality of smokers. Fertil Sterile 1992; 58:1034–1039.
51. Luck MR, Jeyaseelan I, Scholes RA. Ascorbic acid and fertility. Biol Reprod 1995; 52:262–266.
52. Dawson EB, Harris WA, Rankin WE, Charpentier LA, McGanity WJ. Effect of ascorbic acid on male fertility. Ann NY Acad Sci 1987; 498:312–323.
53. Harris WA, Harden TE, Dawson EB. Apparent effects of ascorbic acid medication on human semen metal levels. Fertil Sterile 1979; 32:455–459.
54. Ingold KU, Webb AC, Witter D, Burton GW, Metcalfe TA, Muller DP. Vitamin E remains the major lipid-soluble, chain-breaking antioxidant in human plasma even in individuals suffering severe vitamin E deficiency. Arch Biochem Biophys 1987; 259:224,225.
55. Wickramasinghe SN, Fida S. Bone marrow cells from vitamin B12- and folate-deficient patients misincorporate uracil into DNA. Blood 1994; 83:1656–1661.
56. MacGregor JT, Schlegel R, Wehr CM, Alperin P, Ames BN. Cytogenetic damage induced by folate deficiency in mice is enhanced by caffeine. Proc Natl Acad Sci USA 1990; 87:9962–9965.
57. Blount B. Detection of DNA damage caused by folate deficiency and chronic inflammation. Ph.D. thesis 1994; University of California at Berkeley.
58. Naughton CA, Chandler CJ, Duplantier RB, Halsted CH. Folate absorption in alcoholic pigs: in vitro hydrolysis and transport at the intestinal brush border membrane. Am J Clin Nutr 1989; 50:1436–1441.
59. Reisenauer AM, Buffington CA, Villanueva JA, Halsted CH. Folate absorption in alcoholic pigs: in vivo intestinal perfusion studies. Am J Clin Nutr 1989; 50:1429–1435.
60. Anderson MB, Lepak K, Farinas V, Geroge WJ. Protective action of zinc against cobalt-induced testicular damage in the mouse. Reprod Toxicol 1993; 7:49–54.
61. Xu B, Chia SE, Tsakok M, Ong CN. Trace elements in blood and seminal plasma and their relationship to sperm quality. Reprod Toxicol 1993; 7:613–618.
62. Xu B, Chia SE, Ong CH. Concentrations of cadmiun, lead, selenium and zinc in human blood and seminal plasma. Biol Trace Element Res 1994; 40:49–57.
63. Oteiza PI, Olin KL, Fraga CG, Keen CL. Zinc deficiency causes oxidative damage to proteins, lipids and DNA in rat testes. J Nutr 1995; 125:823–829.
64. Kvist U, Kjellberg S, Bjorndahl L, Soufir JC, Arver S. Seminal fluid from men with agenesis of the Wolffian ducts: zinc-binding properties and effects on sperm chromatin stability. Int J Androl 1990; 13:245–252.
65. Bedwal RS, Bahuguna A. Zinc, copper and selenium in reproduction. Experientia 1994; 50:626–640.
66. Block G, Patterson B, Subar A. Fruit, vegetables and cancer prevention: a review of the epidemiologic evidence. Am J Clin Nutr 1991; 18:1–29.
67. Ames BN, Gold LS, Willett WC. The causes and prevention of cancer. Proc Natl Acad Sci USA. 1995; 92:5258–5265.
68. Patterson B, Block G. Food choices and the cancer guidelines. Am J Public Health 1988; 78:282–286.

21   Maternal Nutrition and Preterm Delivery

Theresa O. Scholl and Mary L. Hediger

1. DEFINITION AND IMPORTANCE OF PRETERM DELIVERY

The United States has an infant mortality rate that ranks 20th worldwide. A major cause of this poor rank is an excess of preterm deliveries to US women compared with lower ranking countries, such as Norway *(1)*. Preterm delivery (<37-completed-weeks' gestation) contributes substantially to low birth weight (LBW, <2500 g) but is not synonymous with it. Of all infants weighing <2500 g, 60–70% are born before 37 completed weeks, and the remainder are term infants who were growth-restricted *in utero* (small-for-gestational-age [SGA]) *(2)*. Preterm delivery is held to be the strongest underlying risk factor for infant mortality, accounting for 85% of the early neonatal deaths not because of lethal congenital defects *(3)*. In the United States, it is estimated that nearly three-quarters of all neonatal deaths occur among infants who deliver too early *(4)*.

Although there has been a long-term decline in LBW births in the United States, that decline is attributable primarily to a reduction in the rate of SGA births (i.e., term LBW) *(5)*. In contrast, the rate of preterm birth based on gestation duration has exhibited a secular increase in the United States (9.2% in 1982 to 10.7% in 1992), rising by 14% in a decade *(2,6)*. There has been virtually no change in the incidence of very low birth weight (VLBW, <1500 g)*(7)*, which reflects very preterm delivery (<33-completed-weeks' gestation) in particular.

In addition to increased mortality, infants delivered preterm are at increased short-term risk of complications, including respiratory distress syndrome (RDS), bronchopulmonary dysplasia, intraventricular hemorrhage, and necrotizing enterocolitis. In the longer-term (1–3 yr), such children are at increased risk of seizure disorders, disabilities of the special senses (blindness and deafness), cerebral palsy, and mental retardation. Learning and behavioral deficits persist *(8,9)* and are associated with increased risk of hyperactivity, placement in special education programs, and grade retention among school children who entered life preterm *(10,11)*.

2. NONNUTRITIONAL FACTORS ASSOCIATED WITH PRETERM DELIVERY

One problem hampering the identification of associated risk factors is the heterogeneous nature of preterm delivery. The most common proximate cause is idiopathic preterm labor culminating in a preterm delivery. Another etiology involves premature

From: *Preventive Nutrition: The Comprehensive Guide for Health Professionals*
Edited by A. Bendich and R. J. Deckelbaum Humana Press Inc., Totowa, NJ

rupture of the fetal membranes (PROM) before labor and delivery. In addition, there are numerous complications (e.g., pregnancy-induced hypertension [PIH]) that can, in turn, lead to a medical induction before term and, thus, to an indicated preterm birth *(12)*. Each of the proximate causes may have separate risk factors. Consequently, only a fraction of the factors and exposures that give rise to preterm and very preterm delivery have been identified. These include, most importantly, a history of preterm delivery during a prior pregnancy, as well as young (<17 yr) and older (>35 yr) maternal age, low socioeconomic status, cigarette smoking, substance abuse, black ethnicity, bacteriuria, faulty placentation or vasculopathology, and possibly poor maternal nutritional status (low pregravid weight, anemia early in pregnancy, poor diet, and inadequate weight gain during pregnancy) *(13)* (*see* Chapter 22).

3. FETAL GROWTH AND PRETERM DELIVERY

Whatever the underlying cause, preterm delivery seems to be characterized by suboptimal fetal growth. In a recent study *(14)*, we found for a sample of young, minority mothers (about age 17 yr) that their infants delivering preterm (<37 completed weeks gestation) were already significantly smaller in all fetal growth dimensions by 32 weeks' gestation compared with fetuses at 32 wk of gestation who later delivered at term. The diminished fetal growth was attributable to slower rates of growth from about 16 to 32 weeks' gestation. When stratified by the proximate cause of preterm delivery, infants delivered preterm for medical or obstetric indications (placental abruption, severe pre-eclampsia, nonreassuring heart rate patterns, chorioamnionitis, oligohydramnios) were found to have asymmetric growth patterns, which suggest a growth failure late in pregnancy. On the other hand, infants delivered preterm after PROM or after failed or no tocolytic therapy to halt their spontaneous preterm labor were proportionately smaller in all dimensions, implying an overall slowing of growth that likely originated early in pregnancy and possibly demonstrates a more chronic stress.

In a prior study, Tamura et al. *(15)* evaluated prospectively 148 fetuses of pregnancies at risk for preterm delivery, the majority of which (63%) were measured within 7 d of delivery. They found that an increased percentage (more than three times expected) had abdominal circumferences (AC) and biparietal diameters (BPD) below the 10th percentile of standards. Two studies looked specifically at altered growth with preterm labor. Westgren et al. *(16)* examined the femur length (FL)-AC ratio, which is presumed to be gestational age-independent, in 82 fetuses of gravidas hospitalized for preterm labor; 39 delivered preterm after failed tocolysis, whereas 43 went on to deliver at term. They found that the FL-AC ratio was significantly increased among those with failed tocolysis, implying that the growth of the fetuses delivering preterm was already suboptimal at the time when preterm labor was diagnosed. Similarly, MacGregor et al. *(17)* performed ultrasounds during admission for preterm labor in 78 pregnancies and found that at 31 weeks of gestation significant percentages of nearly all growth measurements (BPD, head circumference [HC], AC, and FL) were suboptimal (below the 25th and 10th percentiles).

Weiner et al. *(18)* used extant charts to estimate fetal weights from ultrasound and compared the estimated fetal weight (EFW) at various gestational ages to published birth weight-for-gestational-age norms. They found that the birth weights of preterm infants were significantly smaller than the EFW of same-aged fetuses who later delivered at term. Secher et al. *(19)* and Ott *(20)* drew the same conclusion based on similarly de-signed studies, comparing EFW derived from ultrasound to birth weights or sonograph-ically-derived standards.

Slowed fetal growth in association with preterm delivery is consistent with findings among both adolescent and adult gravidas that the risk of preterm delivery is increased with low rates of gestational weight gain in the last half of pregnancy *(21–23)*. The low rates of gestational gain may reflect a slowed fetal growth late in pregnancy and thus be a marker for impending preterm birth.

4. MATERNAL NUTRITIONAL STATUS AND PRETERM DELIVERY

4.1. Maternal Pregravid Weight, Height, and Body Mass Index (BMI)

Maternal size (weight, height, and body mass index [BMI]) is often taken to reflect pregravid nutritional status, although these indicators are not very specific. In an at-tempt to disassociate the effects of weight (fatness) from height, the Institute of Medi-cine (IOM) *(24)* has recommended that BMI, defined as weight (kg)-for-height (m)^2, be used to index maternal pregravid status. At a BMI of <19.8 a woman is considered to be underweight, at 19.8–26.0 normal weight, above 26.0–29.0 overweight, and above 29.0 obese. Whereas there is abundant evidence that maternal pregravid BMI has an inde-pendent and positive effect on birth weight, the association between maternal pregravid status and preterm delivery is somewhat less clear.

Only a few studies have shown a relationship specifically between maternal height and preterm delivery. Low maternal height, among women from developing countries, may indicate stunting consequent to long-term nutritional stress. In their study of the risk factors for preterm LBW in India, Mavalankar et al. *(25)* did find that short women (<150 cm) had a better than twofold increased risk of preterm LBW compared with their taller counterparts (155+ cm), but this effect could not be disassociated from that of low maternal weight.

However, in their study of over 13,000 women from Montreal, Kramer et al. *(26)* found a small (odds ratio [OR]=1.17, confidence interval [CI] 95%: 1.05–1.30), but sta-tistically significant, increased risk of preterm delivery (<37 completed weeks) with short stature (≤157.5 cm) independent of pregravid weight. The risk of preterm deliv-ery, however, was confined to those spontaneous deliveries before 37 wk, but not before 34 or 32 wk. Kramer et al. *(26)* speculated that for these women short stature may be a marker for small pelvic size, and thus at increased risk for early onset of labor as a result of pelvic filling.

In several studies underweight has been associated with an increased risk of preterm delivery, especially when gestation duration is estimated using fundal height or ultra-sound criteria *(27–29)*, although the extent to which this represents a size bias in the es-timation of gestation or the extent to which gestational weight gain and diet during pregnancy can overcome the nutritional deficit are not well known.

4.2. Gestational Weight Gain

Most research on gestational weight gain has focused on the relationship between total weight gain and birth weight, and the body of evidence on this topic has been ex-tensively reviewed by the IOM *(24)*. Studies have consistently shown a positive rela-tionship between weight gain and birth weight *(24,30)*. Maternal pregravid weight or

BMI (kg/m^2) and weight gain appear to have independent and additive effects on birth weight outcome. Correlations between weight gain and birth weight range between 0.20 and 0.30. The average magnitude of the effect on birth weight (in women with a normal weight-for-height) is, assuming a base birth weight of about 3000 g, approx 20 g of birth weight for every 1 kg of total gain, and pregravid weight-for-height is a strong effect modifier on birth weight *(31)*. The relationship between gestational weight gain and preterm delivery appears more complex and is still more controversial.

Although cumulative or total weight gain is an important predictor of birth weight, the pattern of weight gain and rates also appear to play significant roles in predicting preterm delivery *(22,32)*. Taking a cue from several earlier studies implicating overall weight gain as a risk factor for preterm delivery *(21,33,34)*, we found that both early and later weight gain during adolescent pregnancy have independent effects on pregnancy outcome. In a multiracial sample of 1790 teenagers from Camden County, NJ, early inadequate weight gain (<4.3 kg by 24 wk of gestation) was associated with an increased risk of SGA infants (below the 10th percentile for standards) *(22,35)*. Preterm delivery (at <37-completed-wk of gestation), on the other hand, appeared unaffected by early inadequate weight gain, but was increased for teenagers with inadequate weight-gain rates (<400 g/wk) late in pregnancy. This occurred even when the total pregnancy weight gain never fell below the targets set in clinical standards (adjusted odds ratio [AOR]=1.69, CI 95%: 1.12–2.55) *(36)*.

Following on our work with teenage mothers, other studies of primarily adult gravidas have also indicated that low rates of weight gain, primarily in the latter half of pregnancy, are associated with preterm delivery *(23,29,37,38)*. Wen et al. *(29)* in their study of over 17,000 low-income black and white gravidas from Alabama found that rates of weight gain of <0.24 kg/wk after 20-wk of gestation increased the risk for preterm delivery (OR=1.52, p<.05) compared with rates between 0.58 and 0.74 kg/wk. Interestingly, Wen et al. *(29)* also noted that women with high or excessive rates of gain (≥0.75 kg/wk) also had an increased risk of preterm delivery (OR=1.71, $p < .05$), although they speculated that this association might be a function of late edema caused by pregnancy-induced hypertension. Confirming the association between low weight gain late in pregnancy and preterm delivery, Siega-Riz et al. *(37)* found for a predominately Hispanic sample (80%) of nearly 5000 women from the West Los Angeles area that inadequate weight gain during the third trimester was predictive of preterm delivery (greater than two times increased risk).

Most recently, Hickey et al. *(38)* studied 1015 nonobese (BMI < 26.0) black and white women from Alabama. In this study, first trimester weight gain averaged 2.48±3.36 kg, second trimester rates of gain averaged 0.49±0.21 kg/wk, and third trimester 0.45±0.28 kg/wk. Whereas low gain or low rates of gain in the first two trimesters were not associated with preterm delivery, a low rate in the third trimester (<0.38 kg/wk with a pregravid BMI <19.8, <0.37 kg/wk with a pregravid BMI 19.8–26.0) was associated with an increased risk of preterm delivery (OR=2.46, CI 95%: 1.53–3.92).

That there is increasing evidence for an association between low rates of maternal weight gain late in pregnancy and preterm delivery does not mean that these low rates are causal. They may reflect maternal nutrition indirectly. For example, early poor nutrition might act by affecting placental development and vascularization, thereby restricting fetal growth, by affecting the integrity of the chorioamniotic membranes (leading to PROM) *(39)*, or by increasing susceptibility to vaginal or urinary tract infection. We have found in previous observational studies of both young and older gravidas that low intakes of iron and zinc are related to an increased risk of preterm delivery *(40,41)*. In the case of zinc, the risk of preterm delivery with low dietary zinc intake was particularly strong (three times increased risk) for those whose rupture of membranes preceded labor *(41)*. On the other hand, the low rates of gestational gain may reflect the slowed fetal growth associated with preterm delivery and be a marker for impending preterm birth.

4.3. Diet and Gestational Weight Gain

One inference arising from the observation that maternal weight gain during pregnancy and infant birth weight and/or gestation duration are positively correlated is that although the maternal diet may influence pregnancy outcome, the influence probably is, at least in part, indirect. That is, during pregnancy maternal diet affects gestational gain, which, in turn, increases the risk of preterm delivery and/or infant LBW when the weight gain is poor. A poor or otherwise inadequate gestational gain thus may reflect an inadequate dietary intake. Although this association appears to be reasonable, a relationship between caloric intake and weight gain during pregnancy has not often been described.

The first report of a positive relationship between diet and weight gain was made by Thomson *(42)*, who found a correlation of 0.30 between caloric intake and weight gain in Scottish primigravidas eating "to appetite." Among Camden gravidas, a significantly lower caloric intake (by about 300 kcal/d) was associated with an inadequate gestational gain *(43)*. After controlling for calories, women with an inadequate gestational weight gain showed little difference in macronutrients (protein, calories) or total grams of food ingested, suggesting that the differences observed were explained for the most part by lower energy intake. This relationship was confirmed subsequently with three 24-hr dietary recalls taken during the course of pregnancy *(41)*. Since intakes were obtained throughout gestation, overall caloric intake was higher (+160 kcal/d) than in the prior study. After control for confounding variables women with inadequate gestational weight gain consumed fewer kcal/d (–173 kcal/d) than did women whose pregnancy weight gain was adequate for gestation.

4.4. Diet and Preterm Delivery

The relationship between poor diet and inadequate gestational weight gain and the observation that slowed fetal growth and low rates of weight gain late in pregnancy were each associated with preterm delivery suggests that a poor maternal diet may increase the risk of preterm delivery. For example, during the Dutch Famine of 1944–1945, third trimester exposure to intense famine shortened gestation by about 4 d, whereas exposure during the first trimester was associated with an excess of preterm birth *(44)*. The famine is better known for its effect on fetal growth and maternal weight. The identification of preterm births presumably was hampered by maternal amenorrhea consequent to the famine, which would have rendered gestational dating insecure for many. Although caloric rationing was implicated as the cause, low energy intake during the famine may have been only a marker for the inadequate consumption of other essential nutrients.

4.4.1. IRON

Iron is an essential element in the production of hemoglobin for the transport of oxygen to tissues and in the synthesis of enzymes that are required to use that oxygen for the production of cellular energy (24). Supplementation with iron is generally recommended during pregnancy to meet the energy demands of both the mother and rapidly growing fetus. Anemia (low hemoglobin levels) and iron-deficiency anemia (IDA) sometimes also serve as indicators of overall poor maternal nutritional status during pregnancy. When overall dietary intake is inadequate, anemia seems to be one of the most obvious symptoms.

When detected early in pregnancy, IDA is associated with lower caloric and iron intake, an inadequate gestational gain over the whole of pregnancy, as well as with a greater than twofold increase in the risk of preterm delivery (40,45). Maternal anemia, when diagnosed before midpregnancy, is also associated with an increased risk of preterm birth (46,47). However, during the third trimester, anemia is a good prognostic sign because it indicates an expansion of the maternal plasma volume and is thus usually associated with a diminution, as opposed to an increased risk of preterm birth (48). On the other hand, high levels of hemoglobin or hematocrit later in pregnancy are associated with an increased risk of preterm delivery. The increased risk with high hemoglobin levels may indicate a failure of plasma-volume expansion and is correlated with an increased risk of PIH.

A number of studies (47–50) have documented this "U-shaped" relationship between low and high maternal hemoglobin and hematocrit levels and preterm delivery (Table 1). Garn et al. (49) noted the relationship in their retrospective analysis of data from over 50,000 white and black women followed as part of the National Collaborative Perinatal Project. Using the lowest recorded pregnancy values of hemoglobin and hematocrit, they demonstrated an increased risk of preterm delivery with hemoglobin levels <100 g/L and with levels >120 g/L. Murphy et al. (50) in a study of nearly 55,000 women from the Cardiff Births Survey found the same "U-shaped" relationship of preterm delivery to hemoglobin levels ascertained at entry to prenatal care (booking). Risk of preterm birth was increased with low hemoglobin levels (<104 g/L) for women entering care before 13 wk of gestation and after 20 wk, whereas for late entrants to care (wk 20–24) risk was also increased when hemoglobin levels were high. Steer et al. (48) in a multiethnic study of over 150,000 women from the North West Thames region of London showed that there was an increased risk of preterm delivery with both low (≤85 g/L) and high (>115 g/L) hemoglobin levels among all ethnic groups. Although African, Afro-Caribbean, and Indo-Pakistani women have higher rates of preterm delivery, their higher rates of anemia did not account for the increased risk of preterm delivery (48).

However, the increased risk of preterm delivery does appear to be specific to iron-deficiency anemia, and not anemia as a result of causes other than iron deficiency. We used data from over 800 women from the Camden Study to examine total anemia, IDA, and anemia as a result of causes other than iron deficiency at entry to prenatal care (16–17 wk of gestation) as risk factors for preterm delivery. At entry to care, the prevalence of anemia (using Centers for Disease Control standards (40) for hemoglobin) was high (27.9%), but the proportion with IDA (anemia with a serum ferritin of <12 µg/L) was lower than anticipated (3.5% of the cohort). Nevertheless, there was a better than twofold increased risk (AOR = 2.66, CI 95%: 1.15–6.17) of preterm delivery with IDA, after control for confounding variables. Anemia from other causes was not associated with preterm delivery. The overall attributable risk for preterm delivery to IDA was only 5.5%, meaning that although there may be direct effects of iron-deficiency on preterm delivery, anemia as a result of other causes may be best viewed as a marker for other pathologic conditions (e.g., bleeding, infection, poor nutritional status) that also increase the risk for preterm delivery.

4.4.2. MICRONUTRIENTS

During pregnancy, low intakes of two micronutrients, zinc *(41)* and folate *(51)*, are associated with lower caloric intake, IDA at entry to care, an inadequate gestational gain during pregnancy, as well as an increased risk of preterm delivery. Zinc is involved either directly in the production of DNA and RNA polymerase or as a catalyst in the synthesis of other enzymes *(52)*. Folic acid functions as a coenzyme in the transfer of single carbon atoms from donors, such as serine and histidine, to intermediates in the synthesis of amino acids, purines, and thymidilic acid *(53)*. Although many other nutrients in addition to these two would be limited in a marginal maternal diet, inadequate intake of either zinc, folate, or both potentially leads to impaired cell division and alterations in protein synthesis. Such alterations are most notable and have the greatest potential to do harm during times of rapid tissue growth, such as pregnancy *(24)* (*see* Chapter 20).

4.4.2.1. ZINC

Using plasma zinc as an indicator of zinc status, Neggers et al. *(54)* found a significant positive correlation between duration of gestation and zinc concentration at entry to prenatal care. Sikorski et al. *(55)* reported a lower zinc index at delivery (composite of zinc in hair, colostrum, and plasma) in women with premature rupture of the membranes at term. With low dietary zinc intake (<40% RDA for pregnancy) in Camden there was a twofold increase in risk of LBW and a threefold increase in risk of preterm delivery *(41)*.

Although observational studies have been suggestive, clinical trials of zinc supplementation have focused on entire groups of low-income women where the mean zinc intake is below the RDA for pregnancy. These trials have yielded equivocal results, perhaps because of an approach that selects a population, as opposed to individuals, at risk. One study demonstrated no effect of supplementation on pregnancy outcome *(56)*. Another trial showed effects that were conditional on maternal weight *(57)*, that is, there was a lower rate of preterm delivery in zinc-supplemented women with normal body weight at delivery. A recent trial *(58)* took a more targeted approach to supplementation and recruited women with plasma zinc levels below the median and randomly assigned them to zinc or placebo. Zinc supplementation was associated with increased gestation duration of approx 0.5 wk ($p = .06$) and an increase in birth weight about half of which was explained by the longer duration of gestation. Consistent with prior results, effects were increased for women with lower pregravid body mass index (BMI < 26.0).

In addition to its effect on protein synthesis, zinc also has antiseptic action *(52)*. In theory, a low zinc intake may be associated with an increased risk of infection during pregnancy leading to fetal membranes that are prone to rupture; conversely, a low plasma zinc level may be an acute phase response to a stressor, such as maternal infection.

Table 1
Maternal Nutrients and Preterm Delivery, Sample Characteristics

Nutrient	Ref.	Study design, size, and setting	Age, yr	SES	Race/Ethnicity	Findings
Iron/anemia	Garn et al. (49)	Observational study of over 50,000 women followed in the National Collaborative Perinatal Project (NCPP), lowest pregnancy values of hemoglobin (Hgb) and hematocrit (Hct).	—	Mixed	Whites and blacks	Maternal Hgb and Hct levels had "U-shaped" relationship to preterm delivery (≤37 wk), with the risk being higher at Hgb <100 g/L and >120 g/L. The increased risk with high Hgb indicated a failure of plasma-volume expansion.
	Murphy et al. (50)	Observational study of nearly 55,000 women in the Cardiff Births Survey, Hgb levels ascertained at entry to prenatal care (booking).	—	Mixed	Welsh	Preterm delivery (<37 completed weeks) showed a "U-shaped" relationship to Hgb levels. At <13 wk, risk was increased about 50% with Hgb <104 g/L; at wk 13–19 risk was not increased; at wk 20–24, risk was increased for low (<104 g/L) and high (>145 g/L) Hgb by over 50%.
	Klebanoff et al. (47)	Case-control study of 1706 (725 preterm, 981 term) deliveries from Kaiser Permanente Births Defects Study, Hct levels measured throughout gestation.	—	—	14% Asian 28% Black 21% Mexican 37% White	Hct values fell during early second trimester and began to increase again at 31–33 wk. Moderate relationship between second trimester anemia (Hct < 10th percentile for ethnicity and gestation) and preterm delivery.

Nutrient	Reference	Study description	Age	SES	Race/ethnicity	Findings
Iron/Iron-deficiency anemia	Scholl et al. (40,45)	Observational study of iron-deficiency anemia (IDA, anemia with serum ferritin < 12 µg/L) among 779 Camden, NJ women	18.4 ± 3.7 (anemia) 18.4 ± 3.9 (no anemia)	78% Medicaid	77% Black (anemia) 56% Black (no anemia)	IDA (found in 12.5% of those with anemia) was found to be associated with lower energy and iron intakes early in pregnancy. The risk of preterm delivery was better than two times with IDA, but was not increased with anemia from other causes.
Iron	Steer et al. (48)	Retrospective analysis of over 150,000 women from the North West Thames region of London, lowest recorded Hgb during pregnancy	—	Mixed	73% White 14% Indo-Pakistani 5% Black 8% Other	Increased risk of preterm delivery (<37 wk completed) with Hgb levels ≤ 85 g/L (AOR = 1.62, CI 95%: 1.35–2.18) and >115 g/L.
Zinc	Cherry et al. (57)	Randomized, controlled trial of zinc supplementation among pregnant New Orleans teenagers assigned to placebo ($N = 556$) or 30 mg zinc supplement ($N = 581$).	17.6 (13.5–19.6)	Low	95% Black	With stratification by maternal weight at delivery, zinc supplementation was related to a lower risk of preterm delivery (<38 wk) among normal weight women (18.3% vs 28%, $p < .05$). Zinc supplemented low weight multiparas had increased gestation duration (+1.2 wk, $p < .008$). There was a tendency ($p < .15$) for weight gain rates to be greater among zinc supplementated women (0.52 kg/wk) compared with placebo (0.42 kg/wk).

(continued)

Table 1 (*Continued*)

Nutrient	Ref.	Study design, size, and setting	Age, yr	SES	Race/Ethnicity	Findings
	Goldenberg et al. (58)	Randomized, controlled trial of zinc supplementation among pregnant Alabama women with plasma zinc below median at entry to prenatal care, assigned to multivitamin tablet with additional 25 mg zinc (N = 294) or placebo (N = 286).	23.9 ± 5.5 (zinc) 22.8 ± 5.4 (placebo)	Low	100% Black	Birth weight increased with zinc supplementation by 126 g (p < .05) and gestation duration by 0.5 wk (p = .06). Women with pregravid BMI <26 had a birth weight increase of 248 g (p < .005) and an increase in gestation of 0.7 wk (p =.08).
	Hunt et al. (56)	Double-blind randomized, controlled trial of multivitamin mineral tablet with 20 mg zinc (N = 106) or placebo (N = 102).	1.0% <17 94.7% 17–34 4.3% ≥35	Low	100% Hispanic (Mexican)	No effect of zinc supplementation on preterm delivery (<37 wk) (5.7% zinc vs 4.4% controls) or low birth weight (4.7% zinc vs 4.4% controls).
	Neggers et al. (54)	Observational study of 476 Alabama women.	21.8 ± 4.9 (12–42)	Low	76.5% Black	Low plasma zinc at entry to prenatal care (7.0–12.2 μmol/L) increased risk of infant LBW eight times compared with women in the highest quartile (15.9–25.4 μmol/L, p < .05). Plasma zinc was linearly related to gestation duration (0.17 wk/μmol/L zinc, p < .05).
	Scholl et al. (41)	Observational study of dietary zinc intake in 818 Camden, NJ pregnant women.	19.2 (≤6 mg zinc/d) 18.7 (>15 mg zinc/d)	Low	60% Black	Low dietary zinc intake associated with twice greater preterm delivery (<37 wk) and infant LBW, 3–4 times greater very early preterm delivery (<33 wk) (p < .05 for each). Risk of preterm delivery with PROM increased 3.5 times with low zinc (p < .05)

Nutrient	Reference	Description	Age	SES	Ethnicity	Results
	Sikorski et al. (55)	Observational study of zinc status in 70 women with term deliveries.	26 ± 4.4	—	Polish	Zinc index compiled from zinc assayed in blood, scalp and pubic hair and colostrum. Zinc index in patients with PROM was lower (4.33 ± 1.18) compared with patients without PROM (5.97 ± 1.39, $p < .05$). Zinc index was inversely correlated with parity ($r = -0.61$).
Folate	Tchernia et al. (65)	Observational study of serum folate in 100 women using iron or iron and vitamin C.	—	—	French	Serum folate lower by 1.1 μg/L in women delivering ≤ 39 wk ($p < .01$).
		Observational study of red cell folate in 100 high-risk women.	—	—	French	Gestation duration reduced by 0.8 wk in women with RBC folate ≤200 μg/L ($p < .025$).
		Supplementation trial (open) of iron vs iron + folate (350 μg/d) in 108 women.	—	—	French	Gestation duration increased by 0.8 wk among iron and folate supplemented women ($p < .001$).
	Blot et al. (64)	Non-randomized, double-blind study of iron and ascorbic acid vs iron, ascorbic acid, and folate (350 μg/d) at six mo gestation in 200 women.	27.5 ± 4.5	34% Low	French	Gestation duration increased by 0.8 wk with folate supplementation, birth weight increased by 158 g, birth length by 1.7 cm ($p < .05$).
	Scholl et al. (51)	Observational study of folate from diet and supplements in Camden, NJ ($N = 832$).	18.8	Medicaid 80%	67% Black	Women with low folate intake (≤240 μg/d) had three times greater preterm delivery and infant LBW ($p < .05$). Risk of preterm delivery without PROM increased 3 times ($p < .05$).

(continued)

397

Table 1 (*Continued*)

Nutrient	Ref.	Study design, size, and setting	Age, yr	SES	Race/Ethnicity	Findings
	Scholl et al. (63)	Observational study of serum and RBC folate in 801 Camden, NJ women.	18.0	Medicaid 80%	67% Black	Odds of preterm delivery decreased by 2.4% per unit increase in serum folate (ng/mL) at wk 28 ($p < .05$).
Calcium	López-Jaramillo et al. (71,72)	Randomized, controlled trial of calcium supplementation among 56 nulliparas at risk for pregnancy-induced hypertension in Quito, Ecuador	19.4 ± 1.8	Low-income clinic patients with overall low calcium intake		Gestation duration longer for 22 supplemented women (2 g calcium/d) vs placebo group ($N = 34$). Gestation 39.2 ± 1.2 wk for calcium supplemented, 37.4 ± 2.3 week for placebo ($p < .01$).
	Villar and Repke (73)	Randomized, controlled trial of calcium supplementation, 190 teenagers in Baltimore, MD.	≤17	Low-income clinic patients	93.7% Black	Gestation duration longer for 94 supplemented teenagers (2 g calcium/d) vs placebo group ($N = 95$). Gestation 39.2 ± 2.7 wk for calcium supplements, 37.9 ± 3.9 wk for placebo ($p < .01$). Lower percentage of preterm delivery (<37 wk) among supplemented (7.4%) vs placebo (21.1%, $p < .01$).
	Belizán et al. (70)	Randomized, controlled trial of calcium supplementation among 1194 gravidas in Rosario, Argentina.	23.7 ± 5.5 (calcium) 23.7 ± 5.7 (placebo)	Mixed		Percent with preterm delivery (<37 wk) among 579 calcium-supplemented women 6.3 vs 6.8% for 588 women receiving placebo.
Fish oils (N-3 fatty acids)	Olsen et al. (76)	Randomized, controlled trial of supplementation with fish oil, 533 women assigned 2/1/1 to fish oil, olive oil, or no oil supplementation, Aarhus, Denmark.	29.4 ± 4.4 (fish oil) 29.7 ± 4.3 (olive oil) 29.1 ± 4.1 (no oil)			Mean gestation duration longer ($p < .006$) for the 266 women receiving fish oil (283.3 ± 11.1 d) compared with olive oil (279.4 ± 13.1 d) or no oil groups (281.7 ± 11.6 d).

4.4.2.2. FOLATE

During gestation marginal maternal folate nutriture has the potential to impair cellular growth and replication in the fetus and/or the placenta which, in turn, could increase the risk of preterm delivery and infant LBW *(24)*. Such adverse outcomes are more prevalent among poor women than those who are better off. Pregnant women living under circumstances where preterm delivery is prevalent have been reported to consume diets with a lower density of vitamins and minerals, including folate *(59,60)*, and to limit consumption of folate-containing dietary supplements *(61,62)*. Our observational data indicate that a low folate intake (<60% RDA for pregnancy) carries approximately a threefold increased risk for preterm delivery, primarily without prior rupture of the fetal membrane (by inference preterm labor), as well as LBW *(51)*. Confirming the relationship of dietary folate and outcome, concentration of serum folate was positively related to folate intake and with preterm delivery and LBW *(63)*. Randomized studies of routine folate supplementation in combination with iron suggested that folate was associated with increased maternal hemoglobin, greater gestational weight gain, as well as an increase in mean gestation duration *(64,65)*. A meta-analysis of existing supplementation studies *(66)* recommended further study of the effect of folate during pregnancy on reducing the rate of preterm delivery and LBW as an "urgent priority" *(66)*. Many of the trials demonstrated a beneficial effect when a folate supplement was used in combination with iron during pregnancy, although these trials were described as methodologically flawed.

4.4.3. OTHER NUTRIENTS

4.4.3.1. CALCIUM

Another element that has received attention for its possible association with preterm delivery is a macromineral, calcium. During pregnancy, there is an increased physiologic demand for calcium. A full-term infant accretes about 30 g of calcium, primarily in the third trimester when the fetal skeleton is actively ossifying, and to meet these needs there is enhanced absorption of calcium from the gut *(67,68)*. Diets low in calcium both in general and especially during pregnancy have been associated with increased blood pressure levels because smooth muscle reactivity is heightened. During pregnancy, this results in an increased risk of PIH, and, thus, hypothetically to preterm delivery. Calcium supplementation trials during pregnancy have been shown to lower blood pressure levels *(69,70)*.

Two calcium supplementation trials among high-risk women (women with very low intakes in Quito, Ecuador and teenagers in Baltimore) showed promising results in decreasing the incidence of preterm delivery. In Ecuador *(71,72)*, length of gestation was increased from 37.4 ± 2.3 wk for the placebo group (N=34) to 39.2 ± 1.2 wk ($p < .01$) for the calcium-supplemented group (N=22). Among teenagers (aged 16 yr) in Baltimore *(73)*, with similar overall dietary calcium intakes, the calcium-supplemented group had a lower incidence of preterm delivery (7.4%) compared with the placebo group (21.1%, $p < .007$). Further, life-table analysis demonstrated an overall shift to a higher gestational age in the calcium-supplemented group.

On the other hand, a large calcium supplementation trial of over 1000 adult women from Argentina showed the expected decrease in the incidence of PIH, but no effect on preterm delivery *(70)*. Thus, the ability of supplemental calcium to decrease the risk of preterm delivery may be confined to high-risk populations in which there is either a severe dietary restriction of calcium intake or, as in the case of adolescents, there is an increased demand for calcium both to meet the needs of the growing fetus and the mother herself.

4.4.3.2. N-3 FATTY ACIDS

Consumption of marine foods rich in n-3 fatty acids is also associated with a longer gestation duration. Ecologic data from the Faroe Islands, where 50% of the diet is derived from marine sources, show that island women bear infants with substantially higher birth weights (about 200 g) and longer gestations than the Danish comparison *(74)*. This difference in gestation was hypothesized to arise from a diminution in prostaglandin $F_{2\alpha}$ and E2 production or an increase in prostacyclin production with high consumption of n-3 fatty acids.

The clinical trial conducted by the People's League of Health *(75)* on 5022 London women between 1938 and 1939 suggested that supplementing the usual British diet, which was, on the average, not markedly deficient, with minerals, vitamins, and halibut oil extended gestation. Fewer infants were born before the 40th wk of gestation to the supplemented women (20% among supplemented born before week 40 vs 24% among the unsupplemented), although there was no difference in mean birth weight.

A recent clinical trial *(76)* of 533 Danish women who received fish oil, olive oil, or no supplement by wk 30 gestation showed that women taking the fish-oil supplement had longer average gestations (4 d) and bore infants with higher average weights (+107 g), which was mostly attributable to the change in gestation. The effect of fish oil was strongest for women with low fish consumption at entry and amounted to an increase of 7.4 d in this group. There was little effect of the supplement on women with high consumption at entry (−1.6 d). Thus, the hypothesized effect of n-3 fatty acids on gestation appears to have a threshold, beyond which there is no effect. Furthermore, in this trial the effect appeared to be specific to the mechanism underlying the initiation of idiopathic preterm labor rather than PROM.

Finally, ecological studies have indicated that the consumption of large quantities of fish during pregnancy is associated with lower blood pressure and thus, in theory, with a lower the incidence of PIH *(77)*. Consistent with this is the reduction in the incidence of pre-eclampsia in the People's League of Health Study *(75)*. However, because of the multiple supplementation regimen, it could not be attributed to the specific use of the fish oil. Thus, use of fish oils during pregnancy may, in some populations, potentially be associated with lower risk of indicated preterm delivery through a reduction in the incidence of PIH.

5. RECOMMENDATIONS

Although the relationship between nutrition and growth, both prenatal and postnatal, is well established, poor maternal nutrition has newly emerged as a risk factor for preterm delivery. As of yet, only a few observational and experimental studies have examined the influence of maternal diet and nutritional status on gestation duration and preterm birth; thus, for greater security the relationship will require further study. In many cases, the influence of maternal diet probably is indirect (e.g., poor diet gives rise to an inadequate gestational weight gain). Poor maternal nutrition may be a surrogate measure for poor fetal growth.

Further studies are required to determine whether poor maternal nutrition is a marker for or a cause of preterm birth. These studies should not focus primarily on macronutrients, since evidence suggests that populations at high-risk of preterm birth appear to have a poor-quality diet. For example, among minority groups from the inner cities of the United States, a high intake of fat (>30% caloric intake from fat) is common, whereas the consumption of fresh fruits and vegetables and whole grains is extremely low *(78)*. Likewise, the lower social class women from London also eat diets that fail to meet ". . . basic maternal needs for a range of nutrients characteristic of whole grain, vegetable and fruit and dairy produce *(59)*." Thus, among the poor of the industrialized world, it is more usual to provide foods high in fat rather than more costly and perishable foodstuffs albeit of higher nutrient density. An alternative nutrient source, vitamin and mineral supplements, are used more frequently among middle-classes than among the poor *(62)*. Thus, as a corollary, for clinical practice it may be prudent to encourage women to eat a healthful diet before and during pregnancy, since a poor diet rarely occurs in isolation. It is also critical to encourage programs that offer early prenatal care; counseling on the adverse effects of cigarettes, alcohol, and drugs, and alternatives for those who cannot comply with this advice.

REFERENCES

1. Wilcox A, Skjaerven R, Buekens P, Kiely J. Birth weight and perinatal mortality. A comparison of the United States and Norway. JAMA 1995; 273:709–711.
2. Ventura SJ, Martin JA, Taffel SM, et al. Advance report of final natality statistics, 1992. National Center for Health Statistics, Hyattsville, MD, 1994; 43:55.
3. Rush RW, Keirse MJN, Howat P, et al. Contribution of preterm delivery to perinatal mortality. Br Med J 1976; 2:965–968.
4. Adams M. The continuing challenge of preterm delivery. JAMA 1995; 273:739–740.
5. Kessel SS, Villar J, Berendes H, Nugent R. The changing pattern of low birth weight in the United States. JAMA 1978; 251:1978–1982.
6. National Center for Health Statistics. Advance report of final natality statistics, 1982. Monthly vital statistics report 33:6(Suppl). US Public Health Service, Hyattsville, MD, 1984: 33:56.
7. National Center for Health Statistics. Health United States 1990. US Public Health Service, Hyattsville, MD, 1991.
8. Aylward G, Pfeiffer S, Wright A, Velhurst S. Outcome studies of low birth weight infants published in the last decade: a meta analysis. J Pediatr 1989; 115:515–518.
9. Saigal S, Rosenbaum P, et al. Intellectual and functional status at school entry of children who weighed 1000 grams or less at birth: a regional perspective of births in the 1980's. J Pediatr 1989; 115:515–520.
10. Astbury J, Orgill A, Bajuk B, et al. Determinants of developmental performance of very low birth weight survivors at one and two years of age. Develop Med Child Neurol 1983; 25:709–711.
11. Blackman J, Lindgren S, Hein H, et al. Long term surveillance of high risk children. Am J Dis Child 1987; 141:1293–1298.
12. Savitz DA, Blackmore CA, Thorp JM. Epidemiologic characteristics of preterm delivery: etiologic heterogeneity. Am J Obstet Gynecol 1991; 164:467–471.
13. Berkowitz GS, Papiernik E. Epidemiology of preterm birth. Epidemiol Rev 1993; 15:414–443.
14. Hediger ML, Scholl TO, Schall JI, Miller LW, Fischer RL. Fetal growth and the etiology of preterm delivery. Obstet Gynecol 1995; 85:60–64.
15. Tamura RK, Sabbagha RE, Depp R, et al. Diminished growth in fetuses born preterm after spontaneous labor or rupture of membranes. Am J Obstet Gynecol 1984; 148:1105–1110.
16. Westgren M, Beall M, Divon M, Platt L. Fetal femur length/abdominal circumference ratio in preterm labor patients with and without successful tocolytic therapy. J Ultrasound Med 1986; 5:243–245.
17. MacGregor SN, Sabbagha RE, Tamura RK, et al. Differing fetal growth patterns in pregnancies complicated by preterm labor. Obstet Gynecol 1988; 72:834–837.

18. Weiner CP, Sabbagha RE, Vaisrub N, Depp R. A hypothetical model suggesting suboptimal intrauterine growth in infants delivered preterm. Obstet Gynecol 1985; 65:323–326.

19. Secher NJ, Kern Hansen P, Thomsen BL, Keiding N. Growth retardation in preterm infants. Br J Obstet Gynaecol 1987; 94:115–120.

20. Ott WJ. Intrauterine growth retardation and preterm delivery. Am J Obstet Gynecol 1993; 168: 1710–1717.

21. Berkowitz GS. Clinical and obstetric risk factors for preterm delivery. Mt Sinai J Med 1985; 52:239–247.

22. Hediger ML, Scholl TO, Belsky DH, Ances IG, Salmon RW. Patterns of weight gain in adolescent pregnancy: effects on birth weight and preterm delivery. Obstet Gynecol 1989; 74:6–12.

23. Abrams B, Newman V, Key T, Parker J. Maternal weight gain and preterm delivery. Obstet Gynecol 1989; 74:577–583.

24. Institute of Medicine, National Academy of Sciences. Nutrition During Pregnancy. Washington, DC: National Academy Press, 1990.

25. Mavalankar DV, Gray RH, Trived CR. Risk factors for preterm and term low birthweight in Ahmedabad, India. Int J Epidemiol 1992; 21;263–272.

26. Kramer MS, McLean FH, Eason EL, Usher RH. Maternal nutrition and spontaneous preterm birth. Am J Epidemiol 1992; 136:574–583.

27. Scholl TO, Hediger ML, Salmon RW, Belsky DH, Ances IG. Influence of prepregnant body mass and weight gain for gestation on spontaneous preterm delivery and duration of gestation during adolescent pregnancy. Am J Hum Biol 1989; 1:657–664.

28. Edwards LE, Alton IR, Barrada MI, Hakanson EY. Pregnancy in the underweight woman: course, outcome, and growth patterns of the infant. Obstet Gynecol 1979; 135:297–302.

29. Wen SW, Goldenberg RL, Cutter GR, et al. Intrauterine growth retardation and preterm delivery: prenatal risk factors in an indigent population. Am J Obstet Gynecol 1990; 162:213–218.

30. Johnston EM. Weight changes during pregnancy and the postpartum period. Prog Food Nutr Sci 1991; 15:117–157.

31. Abrams BF, Laros RK. Prepregnancy weight, weight gain, and birth weight. Am J Obstet Gynecol 1986; 154:503–509.

32. Hediger ML, Scholl TO, Salmon RW. Early weight gain in pregnant adolescents and fetal outcome. Am J Hum Biol 1989; 1:665–672.

33. Papiernik E, Kaminski M. Multifactorial study of the risk of prematurity at 32 weeks of gestation. J Perinat Med 1974; 2:30–36.

34. Berkowitz GS. An epidemiologic study of preterm delivery. Am J Epidemiol 1981; 113:81–92.

35. Brenner WE, Edelman DA, Hendricks CH. A standard of fetal growth for the United States of America. Am J Obstet Gynecol 1976; 126:555–565.

36. Butman M. Prenatal Nutrition: A Clinical Manual. Boston, MA: Massachusetts Department of Health, 1982.

37. Siega-Riz AM, Adair LS, Hobel CJ. Institute of Medicine maternal weight gain recommendations and pregnancy outcome in a predominantly Hispanic population. Obstet Gynecol 1994; 84:565–573.

38. Hickey CA, Cliver SP, McNeal SF, et al. Prenatal weight gain patterns and spontaneous preterm birth among nonobese black and white women. Obstet Gynecol 1995; 85:909–914.

39. Allen SR. Epidemiology of premature rupture of the fetal membranes. Clin Obstet Gynecol 1991; 34:685–693.

40. Scholl TO, Hediger ML, Fischer RL, Shearer JW. Anemia vs iron deficiency: increased risk of preterm delivery in a prospective study. Am J Clin Nutr 1992; 55:985–988.

41. Scholl TO, Hediger ML, Schall JI, Fischer RL, Khoo CS. Low zinc intake during pregnancy: its association with preterm and very preterm delivery. Am J Epidemiol 1993; 137:1115–1124.

42. Thomson AM. Diet in relation to the course and outcome of pregnancy. Br J Nutr 1959; 13:509–523.

43. Scholl TO, Hediger ML, Khoo CS, et al. Maternal weight gain, diet and infant birth weight: correlations during adolescent pregnancy. J Clin Epidemiol 1991; 44:423–428.

44. Stein Z, Susser M, Saenger G, et al. Famine and Human Development: The Dutch Hunger Winter of 1944/45. New York, NY: Oxford University Press, 1975.

45. Scholl TO, Hediger ML. Anemia and iron-deficiency anemia: compilation of data on pregnancy outcome. Am J Clin Nutr 1994; 59 (Suppl):492S–501S.

46. Klebanoff MA, Shiono PH, Berendes HW, Rhoads GG. Facts and artifacts about anemia and preterm delivery. JAMA 1988; 262:511–515.

47. Klebanoff MA, Shiono PH, Selby JV, et al. Anemia and spontaneous preterm birth. Am J Obstet Gynecol 1991; 164:59–63.
48. Steer P, Alam A, Wadsworth J, Welch A. Relation between maternal haemoglobin concentration and birth weight in different ethnic groups. Br Med J 1995; 310:489–491.
49. Garn SM, Ridella SA, Petzold AS, Falkner F. Maternal hematologic levels and pregnancy outcomes. Semin Perinatol 1981; 5:155–162.
50. Murphy JF, O'Riordan J, Newcombe RG, et al. Relation of haemoglobin levels in first and second trimesters to outcome of pregnancy. Lancet 1986; 1:992–995.
51. Scholl TO, Hediger ML, Schall JI, et al. Dietary and serum folate: their influence on the outcome of pregnancy. Am J Clin Nutr 1996; 63:520–525.
52. Pilch SM, Senti FM, eds. Assessment of the zinc nutritional status of the U.S. population based on data collected in the Second National Health and Nutrition Examination Survey, 1976–1980. Bethesda, MD: Life Sciences Research Office, Federation of American Societies for Experimental Biology, 1984.
53. Pilch SM, Senti FM, eds. Assessment of the folate nutritional status of the U.S. population based on data collected in the Second National Health and Nutrition Examination Survey, 1976–1980. Bethesda, MD: Life Sciences Research Office, Federation of American Societies for Experimental Biology, 1984.
54. Neggers YH, Cutter GR, Acton RT, et al. A positive association between maternal serum zinc concentration and birth weight. Am J Clin Nutr 1990; 51:678–684.
55. Sikorski R, Juszkiewicz T, Paszkowski T. Zinc status in women with premature rupture of membranes at term. Obstet Gynecol 1990; 76:675–677.
56. Hunt IF, Murphy NJ, Lleaver AE, et al. Zinc supplementation during pregnancy: effects on selected blood constituents and on progress and outcome of pregnancy in low-income women of Mexican descent. Am J Clin Nutr 1984; 40:508–521.
57. Cherry FF, Sanstead HH, Rojas P, et al. Adolescent pregnancy: association among body weight, zinc nutriture and pregnancy outcome. Am J Clin Nutr 1989; 50:945–954.
58. Goldenberg RL, Tamura T, Neggers Y, et al. The effect of zinc supplementation on pregnancy outcome. JAMA 1995; 274:463–468.
59. Wynn SW, Wynn AM, Doyle W, Crawford MA. The association of maternal social class with maternal diet and the dimensions of babies in a population of London women. Nutr Health 1994; 9:303–315.
60. Johnson DA, Knight EM, Edwards CH, et al. Dietary intake, anthropometric measurements and pregnancy outcome. J Nutr 1994; 124(Suppl):936S–492S.
61. Subar AF, Block G. Use of vitamin and mineral supplements: demographics and amounts of nutrients consumed (The 1987 Health Interview Survey). Am J Epidemiol 1990; 133:1091–1101.
62. Suitor CW, Gardner JD. Supplement use among culturally diverse group of low-income pregnant women. J Am Diet Assn 1990; 90:268–271.
63. Scholl TO, Hediger ML, Schall JI, Khoo CS. Mid-pregnancy circulating folate and poor pregnancy outcome. Paediatr Perinat Epidemiol 1994; 8(4):A4.
64. Blot I, Papiernik E, Kaltwasser JP, et al. Influence of routine administration of folic acid and iron during pregnancy. Gynecol Obstet Invest 1981; 12:294–304.
65. Tcherina G, Blot I, Rey A, et al. Maternal folate status, birthweight and gestational age. Develop Pharmacol Therap 1982; 4(Suppl 1):58–65.
66. Mohammed K. Routine folate supplementation in pregnancy. In: Pregnancy and Childbirth Module (eds, Enkin MW, Keirse MJCN, Renfreq MJ, Nielson JP, eds.) "Cochrane Database of Systematic Reviews" Review No. 03158, April, 1993.
67. Repke JT. Calcium magnesium, and zinc supplementation and perinatal outcome. Clin Obstet Gynecol 1991; 34:262–267.
68. NIH Consensus Development Panel on Optimal Calcium Intake. Optimal calcium intake. JAMA 1994; 272:1942–1948.
69. Repke JT, Villar J. Pregnancy-induced hypertension and low birth weight: the role of calcium. Am J Clin Nutr 1991; 54:237S–241S.
70. Belizán JM, Villar J, Gonzalez L, et al. Calcium supplementation to prevent hypertensive disorders of pregnancy. New Engl J Med 1991; 325:1399–1405.
71. López-Jaramillo P, Narváez M, Weigel RM, Yépez R. Calcium supplementation reduces the risk of pregnancy-induced hypertension in an Andes population. Br J Obstet Gynaecol 1989; 96:648–655.
72. López-Jaramillo P, Narváez M, Felix C, López A. Dietary calcium supplementation and prevention of pregnancy hypertension. Lancet 1990; 335:293.

73. Villar J, Repke JT. Calcium supplementation during pregnancy may reduce preterm delivery in high-risk populations. Am J Obstet Gynecol 1990; 163:1124–1131.
74. Olsen SF, Hansen HS, Sorensen T, et al. Intake of marine fat, rich in (n-3) polyunsaturated fatty acids, may increase birthweight by prolonging gestation. Lancet 1986; 2:367–369.
75. People's League of Health. Nutrition of expectant and nursing mothers. Lancet 1942; 2:10–12.
76. Olsen SF, Sorensen JD, Secher NJ, et al. Randomized controlled trial of effect of fish-oil supplementation on pregnancy duration. Lancet 1992; 339:1003–1007.
77. Popeski D, Ebbeling LR, Brown PB, et al. Blood pressure during pregnancy in Canadian Inuit: community differences related to diet. Can Med Assoc J 1991; 145:445–454.
78. Rogers MA, Simon DG, Zucker LB, et al. Indicators of poor dietary habits in a high risk population. J Am Coll Nutr 1995; 14:159–164.

22 Dietary Polyunsaturated Fatty Acids for Optimal Neurodevelopment

Recommendations for Perinatal Nutrition

Ricardo Uauy-Dagach, Patricia Mena, and Patricio Peirano

1. INTRODUCTION

Multiple studies over the past four decades have addressed the evaluation of the effects of early human malnutrition on central nervous system (CNS) development in experimental animals and humans. From the results of these studies, one can conclude that a reduction in energy and/or essential nutrient supply during the first stages of life have profound effects on somatic growth and organ structural and functional development, especially for the brain. Malnutrition impairs brain development, reducing cell replication cycles and dendritic connections. Different regions of the brain are impacted in specific ways; cell number as measured by DNA content is especially affected by intrauterine malnutrition and early postnatal malnutrition, whereas synaptic connectivity is particularly affected if malnutrition occurs after birth but before the third year of life *(1)*. Beyond the brain's "growth spurt," alterations in dietary precursors may determine, in part, neurotransmitter levels (serotonin, norepinephrine, dopamine, acetylcholine) in specific brain regions, and essential and nonessential lipid supply may affect the structural composition of the brain and of myelin sheaths *(2)*. The functional correlates are also significantly modified by malnutrition; the waking electroencephalographic activity, auditory-evoked potentials, sleep-wake organization, as well as neurovegetative activities during sleep have been demonstrated to be disturbed by early human malnutrition *(2a)*.

The linkage between retarded somatic growth and altered brain development is strong if the nutritional deprivation model is one of early protein energy malnutrition (PEM). This principle has guided many experimental studies and epidemiological evaluations of the nutrition-mental development relationships. Yet, there are multiple instances where somatic growth may proceed unabated whereas brain structure and function are significantly altered. The effect of early anemia on brain function does not affect somatic growth; the impact of taurine deficiency on retinal and brain development on nonhuman primates and on human infants is not dependent on structural proteins since this sulfur amino acid is not incorporated in protein synthesis; the role of n-3 fatty acids as structural components of brain is not associated with effects on growth but rather on modifying membrane function and electric responses. Examples in the

From: *Preventive Nutrition: The Comprehensive Guide for Health Professionals*
Edited by A. Bendich and R. J. Deckelbaum Humana Press Inc., Totowa, NJ

opposite direction, namely of normal mental development and poor growth, are more difficult to find, suggesting that somatic growth is a necessary, but insufficient condition to attain normal mental development. Early malnutrition from pyloric stenosis or cystic fibrosis illustrates the capacity of the brain to recover from malnutrition, but is not by itself sufficient to negate the effect of sustained nutritional deprivation on the developing CNS. An important contribution to the approach of the relationship between nutritional deficiencies and brain development has been the concept that direct effects of PEM on child development seem no longer evident, since PEM coexists with other nutritional deficiencies that can also disrupt child development (3).

The study of the influence of specific nutrients on brain development in preterm neonates is in its infancy. Fetal growth retardation is not an isolated nutritional deprivation, but rather a combination of many restrictions; oxygen, blood supply, overall nutrients, and various growth factors and hormones. It is likely that better nutritional practices in early life contribute significantly not only to improved survival but to better growth and development of very immature infants. Yet this rather obvious conclusion is not well substantiated by objective data. One of the few controlled observations in premature infants revealed that head size at 12 mo was related to the time after birth when very low birth weight (LBW) infants had reached full caloric intake. Since the relationship between head size and later development in preterm infants has been established, this is indirect evidence for an effect of better nutrition on developmental indices in later life. As an example of the complexity of this problem, the increase in protein intake in preterm infants required to optimize somatic growth as studied in the late 1940s was associated with lower IQ scores in later life (4). The classic Harlem Columbia study revealed that higher protein intake fed to pregnant women who where at risk of delivering LBW was in fact associated with increased prevalence of prematurity and lower developmental indices at 12 mo (5) (see Chapter 21).

The research on the effects of energy and caloric intake is reviewed in classic and in recent publications (1,2,3,6). This chapter primarily addresses the role of essential polyunsaturated fatty acids (PUFA) on neural development in the fetus, preterm, and term infants.

2. BACKGROUND ON THE ESSENTIAL PUFAs AND THEIR METABOLISM

2.1. Essentiality of Polyunsaturated Fatty Acids

The concept that specific components of fat may be necessary for the proper growth and development of animals and possibly humans was introduced in 1929 by George and Mildred Burr (7). The essential fatty acids (EFA) were considered of marginal nutritional importance for the human until the 1960s, when clinical signs of EFA deficiency became apparent in infants fed skim milk-based formula and in those given lipid-free parenteral nutrition. Hansen firmly established that linoleic acid (LA) is essential for normal infant nutrition in a clinical and biochemical study of 428 infants fed cow's milk-based formulations with different types of fat (8). Daily LA intake of study infants ranged from 10 mg/kg while fed a fully skimmed milk preparation to 800 mg/kg when a corn/coconut oil-based preparation was fed. He observed dryness, desquamation, and thickening of the skin and growth faltering as frequent manifestations of LA deficiency in young infants (8). More subtle clinical symptoms appear in n-3 EFA deficiency. They include skin changes unresponsive to LA supplementation, abnormal vi-

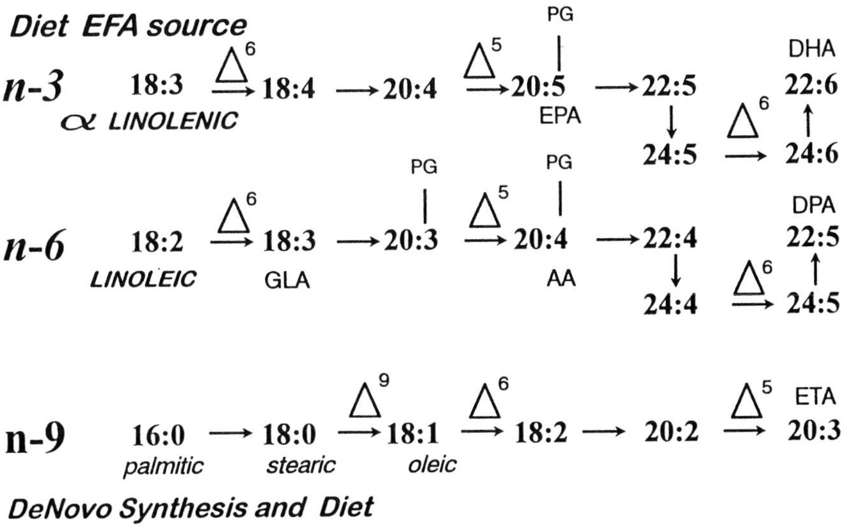

Fig. 1. LCPUFA and EFA metabolism. Parent EFAs are derived from dietary sources for both n-3 (18:3, LNA) and n-6 series (18:2, LA). *De novo* synthesis is able to produce only n-9 LCPUFAs. Elongation occurs two carbons at a time and δ desaturases introduce double bonds at 9,6, and 5 carbons from the carboxylic end of the fatty-acid chain. The final step in the formation of n-3 and n-6 end-products is catalyzed by a peroxisomal β-oxidation. LCPUFAs of interest include 18:3 n-6 (GLA), 20:4 n-6 (AA), 22:5 n-6 (DPA), 20:3 n-9 (ETA), 20:5 n-3 (EPA), and 22:6 n-3 (DHA). EPA, AA, and 20:3 n-6 are immediate precursors of prostaglandins (PG) and other eicosanoids.

sual function, and peripheral neuropathy *(9,10)*. The nervous system manifestations of n-3 deficit are likely caused by an insufficiency of the specific metabolic derivative of α-linolenic acid (LNA), namely docosahexaenoic acid (DHA). Indeed, the high concentrations of DHA in cerebral cortex and retina would suggest its participation in neural and visual function *(11,12)*.

The evidence indicates that in early life C 18 n-3 precursors are not sufficiently converted to DHA to allow for biochemical and functional normalcy. Thus, not only LA and LNA but DHA should be considered essential nutrients for normal eye and brain development in the human. The old practice of administering cod-liver oil to prevent rickets acquires a new dimension based on this new knowledge.

2.2. LCPUFA Metabolic Pathway

The structural role of long-chain polyunsaturated fatty acids (LCPUFA) derived from EFA and the functional correlates of specific fatty acids (FAs) are being increasingly recognized *(13–16)*. The LCPUFAs arachidonic acid, (AA [20:4 n-6]) eicosapentaenoic acid (EPA [20:5 n-3]), and docosahexaenoic acid (DHA [22:6 n-3]) are important membrane components and precursors of potent bioactive oxygenated products. Eicosanoids, such as prostaglandins, leukotrienes, and epoxides, derived from AA and EPA modulate or are required in numerous physiologic processes; a myriad of clinical correlates associated with deficient or excessive EFA intake have been observed *(13–19)*.

Animal tissues, especially the liver, are capable of further elongating and desaturating the parent EFAs, generating a family of compounds for the respective families as shown in Fig. 1. As depicted in the figure, AA can be formed from LA; it becomes essential only if the capacity for elongation and desaturation of LA is limited. This, in fact, occurs in the cat and other felines. Further details on EFA metabolism can be found in referenced reviews *(14,17,19–21)*. The competitive desaturation of the n-3, n-6, and n-9 series by δ-6 desaturase is of major significance since this is the controlling step of the pathway. Sprecher's group has proposed that the last reaction apparently catalyzed by δ-4 desaturation is indeed a three-step path as depicted in Fig. 1. The initial step is an elongation, followed by δ-6 desaturation and then, through a peroxisomal-β-oxidation, the chain is shortened to a 22-carbon PUFA. This latter step has been termed retroconversion *(22)*. The Sprecher pathway has been verified for both DHA and docosapentaenoic acid (DPA [22:5 n-6]) formation. The δ-6 desaturase in the Sprecher pathway is likely different from the enzyme responsible for the initial step of the parent EFA metabolism. If n-3 FAs are absent or deficient in the diet the elongation/desaturation of the n-6 compounds generates a significant elevation of DPA; if both EFAs are lacking eicosatrienoic acid (ETA [20:3 n-9]) accumulates *(13,14)*. The triene/tetraene (ETA/AA) ratio may be used as an index of essential fatty acid deficiency but is not valid as a marker of isolated n-3 deficit *(18)*.

The conversion of parent EFAs to LCPUFA is under active regulation; therefore, the effects of providing AA, EPA, or DHA cannot be reproduced by providing the equivalent amount of LA or LNA *(19,20)*. The uniqueness of the biological effects of feeding human milk on EFA metabolism is based on the direct supply of LCPUFAs bypassing the regulatory step of the δ-6 desaturase. Excess dietary LA associated with some vegetable oils, particularly safflower, sunflower, and corn oils, may decrease the formation of DHA from LNA since the δ-6 desaturase is inhibited by excess substrate. In addition, AA formation is lower when excess LA is provided *(13,14,19,20)*. The inhibitory effect of EPA on δ-5 desaturase activity has been considered responsible for the lower AA observed when marine oil is consumed. Excess LA, as seen in enterally or parenterally fed infants receiving corn oil or safflower oil as the predominant FA supply, will inhibit the elongation/desaturation of the parent EFAs and, thus, lower the LCPUFA supply necessary for membrane synthesis. Marine PUFAs provide minimal preformed AA and substantial amounts of preformed n-3 LCPUFA, such as EPA and DHA *(23)*.

2.3. Effects of PUFAs on Neural Membrane Function

The dry weight of the human brain is predominantly lipid; 22% of the cerebral cortex and 24% of white matter consist of phospholipids. Studies of several animal species and recent evidence from humans have established that brain phospholipids AA and DHA decrease whereas n-9 and n-7 mono- and polyunsaturated fatty acids increase when LA and LNA or only n-3 fatty acids are deficient in the diet *(24–27)*. Typically, n-3 fatty acid-deficient cells have decreased DHA and increased levels of the end product of n-6 metabolism, DPA. Within the subcellular organelles, synaptosomes and mitochondria seem to be more sensitive to a low dietary n-3 supply, as evidenced by the relative abundance of DHA and the changes in composition of these organelles in response to dietary deprivation *(24–27)*.

The functional implications of diet-induced changes in structural lipids have been the subject of much research *(27–29)*. Membrane physiologists have suggested that the fatty acid composition of structural membrane lipids can affect membrane function by modifying membrane fluidity, affecting membrane thickness, changing lipid-phase properties, or specifically interacting with membrane proteins. The changes in neural membranes of greatest potential significance during development are those related to changes in physical properties and to changes that affect membrane excitability. Diet-induced changes in structural lipids affect the functional characteristics of excitable membranes in several animal species and in human neural cell lines *(12,28–31)*.

A deficiency of n-3 fatty acids can change membrane physical properties, including membrane-bound enzymes, receptor activity, antigenic recognition, and signal transduction *(32–36)*. Also, n-3 fatty-acid deficiency affects rotational mobility, as measured by fluorescent diphenylhexatriene probes, less than lateral mobility, as measured by pyrene dimer formation within the lipid bilayer *(37)*. Recently, we found that excited dimer (eximer) pyrene formation in human retinal cells, which occurs when two monomers collide, is increased by DHA supplementation of the culture media *(38)*. Membrane composition changes in human retinoblastoma and neuroblastoma cell lines also affect membrane transport mechanisms. A higher DHA content increases the affinity and transport rates for choline and taurine *(39)*. Furthermore, preliminary studies suggest that the dietary n-3 fatty acid supply may affect nucleotide cyclase activity and ribosylation of guanine nucleotide-binding proteins *(40)*.

The role of membrane lipid composition in determining the electrical properties of cultured neuronal cells exposed to exogenous fatty acids has been investigated *(41,42)*. Both n-3 and n-6 fatty acids induced slower rates of rise, and to a lesser extent a lower amplitude, of Na^+ action potentials. The reverse effects were observed when saturated or *trans*-monoenoic fatty acids were added. It seems likely that these effects were mediated by a change in the number of active Na^+ channels. A change in membrane composition or altered fatty acid availability to the cells could have caused this *(41)*.

N-3 fatty acid supplementation ameliorates the fluidifying effect of ethanol on neural membranes, whereas LA and LNA deficiency potentiates volatile anesthetic action in rats; LA supplementation specifically reverses this effect *(42)*. Changes in eicosanoid and docosanoid production may also explain the effect of PUFA's supplementation on neural function. Phospholipases liberate AA, EPA, and DHA from membrane lipids and make them available to cycloxygenase or lipoxygenase action for production of eicosanoids and docosanoids.

2.4. Sources of Dietary Essential PUFAs

The principal source of PUFA for infants is human milk (HM). The amount of PUFA in HM depends, principally, on the mother's diet during pregnancy and lactation and varies according to postpartum age, preterm or term delivery, and maternal diseases affecting lipid metabolism, such as diabetes, cystic fibrosis, and abetalipoproteinemia. AA is the main n-6 PUFA and DHA is the most important of the n-3 series. The ratio of total n-6 to n-3 is 5–10:1, ranging up to 18:1 if high LA oils are consumed. The ratio of AA to DHA is most commonly 1.5–2:1. The variability in LCPUFA in HM is high and determined mainly by diet. EPA is found in minimal amounts, except in populations consuming high intakes of fish; it is always lower than DHA content *(43,44)*.

Vegetable oils derived from corn, safflower, and sunflower contain predominantly LA; others, such as soy and linseed oils, contain LNA. This latter fatty acid has higher concentrations in chloroplast membranes of green leafy vegetables rather than in oily seeds. Thus, products from animals fed in the wild have different fatty acid composition than grain-fed animals. This is of interest in terms of the higher DHA content of eggs from range-fed chicken. The introduction of egg yolk as a weaning food in some areas

Table 1
Sources of PUFAs for Use in Infant Formula

Source	n-6	n-3
Black current seed oil	GLA	
Borage oil	GLA	
Egg phospholipids	AA	DHA
Evening primrose oil	GLA	
Fish oil		EPA/DHA
Marine oil fractions		DHA
Animal phospholipids	AA	DHA
Single-cell oil	AA	DHA

of the world may represent a useful dietary practice to assure LCPUFA supply in early infancy. In addition, the use of evening primrose oil or black current oil provides 18:3 n-6 linolenic acid (GLA), thus, bypassing the controlling enzyme, δ-6 desaturase, necessary for AA formation. This latter approach has been used by some formula manufacturers to improve AA status in young infants.

Ω-3 polyunsaturated fatty acids of marine origin are formed in the chloroplast of the phytoplankton or microalgae consumed by fish. The main source for the *de novo* synthesis of n-3 fatty acids are marine autotrophic bacteria, microalgae, and protozoa, which constitute the zooplankton and phytoplankton *(45,46)*. Fish, higher in the food chain, incorporate the Ω-3 PUFA and further elongate them to 20 and 22 carbon atom fatty acids containing four, five, and up to six double bonds by the action of specific desaturases. Thus, fish will concentrate EPA and DHA as triglycerides, mainly in the adipose tissue and in the fat of muscle and visceral organs. The higher fat content of fish, the higher its content of n-3 fatty acids. Some marine mammals, such as seals and polar bears, that feed predominantly on fish also accumulate relatively high quantities of n-3 fatty acids in their adipose tissue *(47,48)*. Another important source of LC-PUFA is egg-yolk phospholipids. The concentration of PUFA is different depending on the feed given; the ample use of fish meal in chicken feed has increased egg-yolk DHA *(49,50)*. LCPUFA products for blend in infants' formulas can be successfully produced if chicken feed is carefully monitored and refined lipid extraction procedures are used. This is presently an important LCPUFA source used in European infant formulas.

Bacterial strains and microalgae isolated from the intestinal content of some fish show a remarkably high content of EPA and DHA *(48)*; therefore, efforts have been made to grow these micro-organisms in natural or artificial sea water to obtain EPA and DHA for nutritional or pharmacological use. In addition, selected fungal strains produce concentrated arachidonic acid, which is suitable for human consumption. The industrial production of AA, EPA, and DHA from strains of these single-cell organisms has been successful; however, their expanded use will depend on price and demand for them relative to the concentrates obtained from marine oils. Single-cell oils offer a promising new source of LCPUFAs provided mass production becomes commercially profitable *(45)*. Table 1 summarizes the main sources of LCPUFAs for use in supplementation.

3. PUFA IN HUMAN GROWTH AND DEVELOPMENT

3.1. Significance of PUFAs During Fetal Development

The fetus and the placenta are fully dependent on maternal EFA supply for their growth and development. The diet before pregnancy plays an important role in determining maternal EFA status since these essential nutrients are stored in adipose tissue and can be mobilized over time through lipolysis. The major fat deposition in the human fetus occurs during the third trimester, but key phospholipids in placental vessels and uterine vasculature are dependent on EFA supplied by the mother for eicosanoid formation from the moment of conception *(51)*. Animal studies have demonstrated that preconceptional nutrition determines in part what fats are accreted in the conceptus and placental tissues. In the human, several investigations have shown significant increases in the AA and DHA content of fetal brain tissue during the last trimester of gestation *(52,53)*.

Maternal dietary LA and LNA supply serve as precursors for n-3 and n-6 LCPUFA synthesis by the maternal liver and to a limited degree by the placenta. The placenta selectively transports AA and DHA from the maternal to the fetal compartment; thus, there is an enrichment of these LCPUFAs in circulating lipids in the fetus, especially during the third trimester, when fetal demands for neural and vascular growth are greatest *(50,54,55)*. A total of 600 g of EFAs are transferred from mother to fetus during a full-term gestation; net uptake approximates 2.2 g/d. If conversion is fully efficient, this amount could be supplied by LA and LNA, yet recent studies in the United States by Holman suggest that in fact n-3 LCPUFAs decrease during pregnancy and lactation *(56)*. Similar data have been obtained in Europe *(57)*. A need for LCPUFA supplementation during pregnancy is suggested by these results. This may be particularly important in pregnancy of multiparous women and during multiple pregnancies *(58,59)*.

The use of marine oil supplementation has been proposed in the prevention of pre-eclampsia since maternal blood pressure responses are dependent on AA/EPA balance in the vessel wall. EPA-derived prostanoids oppose the action of AA derivatives, namely EPA has vasodilatory effects and decreases rather than enhances platelet aggregation. Preliminary results from controlled trials support an effect of marine oil in the prevention of severe but not of mild pregnancy-induced hypertension *(60)*. In addition, epidemiological evidence and several randomized controlled studies suggest that marine oil supplementation and fish consumption prolong gestation, reduce the incidence of premature birth, and increase mean birth weight *(61)*. If these results are confirmed, marine oil supplementation during pregnancy would offer a unique way of preventing pregnancy-induced hypertension while providing DHA for neural development. This would represent a clear advantage over the alternative pre-eclampsia preventive strategy using aspirin *(62)*.

3.2. Significance of PUFAs for Preterm Infants

Interest over the past decade has focused on the potential requirements and benefits of dietary n-3 EFAs, LNA, and DHA for optimal growth and development. Studies were designed to investigate in infants the questions posed by the observations of Neuringer and Connor using primate models of n-3 deficiency *(63)*. These investigators developed an animal model of deficiency using safflower oil (LA:LNA = 250:1) as the main source of fat given during pregnancy and postnatally until maturity *(63)*. Similar high ratios are actually still found in powdered infant formulas containing sunflower or safflower oils used in some parts of the world *(64,65)*.

We used the preterm infant fed corn oil-based formula as a model for n-3 deficiency. At the time of our initial studies, 1986, all infants received no DHA; ample LA and virtually no LNA; the ratio of LA to LNA in most infant formula at the time was close to 50:1, thus compromising the endogenous DHA synthesis from LNA. We considered that very-low-birth-weight (VLBW) infants were particularly vulnerable to EFA deficiency given the virtual absence of adipose tissue stores at birth, the possible immaturity of the FA elongation/desaturation pathways, and the inadequate LNA and DHA intake provided by formula. Over the past decade, we and others have conducted studies to evaluate the effect of n-3 FA and VLBW infants examining the effects of LNA or LNA plus DHA supplementation on plasma and tissue lipid composition, retinal electrophysiologic function, the maturation of the visual cortex, and other measures of infant growth and development *(66–69)*.

Infants born at 28–32-wk of gestation and relatively "healthy" were studied. Infants receiving their own mother's fortified human milk served as ex utero controls for the study. We also evaluated some infants who remained in utero and tested them at the equivalent postconceptional age relative to the study infants as in utero controls. If mothers were unable to provide HM their infants were randomly assigned to one of three formula groups varying in EFA. Experimental formula feedings began at d 10 of life and continued until 57 wk postconception (i.e., equivalent to 4 mo postterm). Full details on study subjects, test diets, and experimental protocol can be found in refs. *66–69*.

Composition of red blood cell (RBC) lipids for all diet groups was similar on entry into the study. At 36 and 57 wk postconception, marked differences in DHA content were evident in the RBC lipids of all diet groups. Infants fed the n-3 FA-deficient corn oil-formula had significant reductions in DHA compared to the other formula groups. The marine oil group had DHA concentrations elevated above all other groups. RBC lipids of the HM and marine oil groups showed similar patterns for both total n-3 and n-6 long-chain PUFA. The soy oil group had intermediate DHA values relative to corn and soy/marine oil groups, but differed significantly from the DHA-supplemented soy/marine oil-fed infants *(66,67)*. Retinal function responses demonstrated significantly higher threshold values from rod photoreceptors in the n-3-deficient group (corn oil-fed) at the 36 wk follow-up relative to groups receiving n-3 FAs, as shown in Fig. 2 *(66–67)*. That is, the light intensity required to elicit a 2 μV response (threshold) was greater when plasma DHA levels were low. Higher threshold and lower maximum electroretinogram (ERG) amplitudes in response to high-intensity light were observed when DHA values were low, indicating that the sensitivity and maturity of the rod photoreceptors in n-3 FA-deficient infants were reduced significantly compared to infants fed soy/marine formula or HM. The group of infants born at 35 wk gestational age who acquired EFAs transplacentally and were tested 3–5 d after birth were nearly identical in all rod ERG functional indices to the equivalent conceptional age HM- or soy/marine oil-fed premature infants. The soy oil-fed group had higher threshold values than the soy/marine oil-fed group. At the 57-wk follow-up the corn oil-fed infants consistently had longer implicit times in light-adapted oscillatory potentials; soy oil-fed infants had some peaks differ significantly from the HM-fed infants whereas the

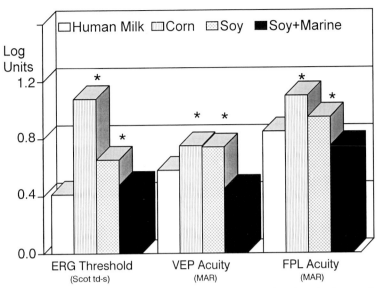

Fig. 2. Rod ERG threshold at 36 wk postconceptional age and visual evoked potential (VEP) and forced-choice preferential looking (FPL) visual acuities of preterm study infants at 57 wk postconceptional age. Rod ERG threshold is the light intensity measured in scotopic troland-seconds (Scot-dt-s) required to induce a b-wave amplitude of 2 μV; higher thresholds are associated with lower photoreceptor sensitivity. Larger log minimum angle of resolution (MAR) visual acuity values are associated with poorer visual acuity. Asterisks within a functional measure indicate significantly different from human milk mean values using ANOVA. For experimental details and data *see* refs. *67,68.*

soy/marine and HM groups were similar in oscillatory potentials. Oscillatory potentials are generated in the inner retina and most likely reflect ganglion cell-amacrine cell interactions *(70).*

The DHA supplemented (soy/marine formula and the HM-fed) groups had lower values for minimal angle of resolution, consistent with better visual acuity, relative to infants fed formulas devoid of DHA at the 57-wk follow-up using either electrophysiologic responses (visual evoked potentials) or behavioral methods (forced choice preferential looking) to assess acuity. A significant positive correlation was found between DHA levels and visual acuity; that is, when DHA levels were high, acuity was better. The group that received soy oil as a source of n-3 FAs had poorer acuity at the 57-wk follow-up relative to the soy/marine oil-fed group, indicating that despite ample LNA, visual function was less mature than in the DHA-supplemented infants. A group of healthy full-term breast-fed infants matched by conceptional age were used as controls. The HM-fed and soy/marine oil-fed groups were virtually identical to the controls, whereas the corn and soy groups had poorer visual acuities, as shown in Fig. 2 *(66).*

These results, in conjunction with those of Carlson, who used behavioral measures of visual acuity and the Bayley scale of psychomotor development, support a need for DHA for optimal neural development in preterm infants *(71–73).* In addition, results from four other groups confirm the need for LCPUFA supplementation of formula to maintain plasma and RBC phospholipid composition at relative concentrations similar to those found in human milk-fed preterm infants *(74–77).*

A possible long-term effect of early feeding on brain development is suggested by results from a controlled trial of preterm infants indicating that feeding HM that contains LCPUFAs by nasogastric tube for 28 d was associated with a +8.3 point IQ difference at 8 yr of age relative to a formula-fed group (devoid of LCPUFAs) after controlling for socioeconomic and other maternal variables *(78)*. These controlled observations in preterm infants indicate that HM may, in fact, offer unique advantages for brain development.

3.3. Significance of PUFAs for Term Infants

Similar questions to those addressed in the previous section on LBW infants have been posed more recently in healthy full-term infants. The finding of lower plasma DHA concentrations in infants fed formula compared to that of breast-fed infants suggests that present formulas provide insufficient LNA or that chain elongation-desaturation enzymes are not sufficiently active during early life to support tissue accretion of DHA. Full-term infants also appear to be dependent on dietary DHA for optimal functional maturation of the retina and visual cortex *(78,80)*. Furthermore, necropsy studies in infants born at term who died from sudden infant death syndrome revealed that brain composition is affected by type of feeding. HM feeding resulted in higher DHA content in the brain cortex as compared to cow's milk-based formula feeding *(81,82)*.

A recently published controlled prospective trial of gamma linoleic acid 18:3 *n*-6 (GLA) and DHA supplementation of full-term infants concluded that there is a need for DHA supplementation in infants who are not breast-fed. Biochemical indices of DHA status and visual acuity maturation of infants receiving only LNA was delayed relative to those receiving formula supplemented with LNA + DHA; these latter infants were similar to the breast-fed control group *(83)*. Infants who receive breast milk for more than 16 wk had better visual evoked potential acuity than those breastfed for shorter times or given formula without LCPUFAs. Additional supportive evidence can be derived from a study of 526 full-term infants born in Groningen, Holland between 1975 and 1979 and followed for 9 yr. There was a significantly lower occurrence of neurological dysfunction in the 135 breast-fed infants (for more than 3 wk) after adjusting for obstetric, perinatal, neonatal neurological, and social differences *(84)*. Other controlled, nonrandomized evaluations have shown a better cognitive development in children fed HM, although there is always the possibility that uncontrolled variables could explain the differences. There appears to be a direct correlation between the duration of breast-feeding and improved performance *(85–87)*.

In addition, several abstracts published during 1995 and 1996 for the most part support the hypothesis that DHA is also required for optimal visual development in term infants. The biochemical data solidly demonstrate that only LCPUFA (DHA or DHA + AA)-supplemented infants have plasma and red cell membrane phospholipid composition similar to the human milk-fed infants. The functional effects of supplementation are in most studies transient; that is, the impact is measurable by 4 mo but not demonstrable at 1 yr of age. Completion of ongoing controlled trials will serve to fully confirm or question these findings.

The possibility of optimizing LNA to DHA conversion by providing sufficient LNA (>0.7% of total energy) and a lower LA: LNA ratio in formula (<10:1) to provide for sufficient DHA has been tested in term infants. Initial results by Ponder et al. indicate that this alternate strategy may be simpler and less expensive than the addition of n-3 LCPUFA to attain biochemical normalcy *(88)*. A study by Innis et al. concluded that the need for DHA supplementation should not be based on the improved visual acuity of breast-fed infants since despite differences in DHA blood content the study revealed no differences in forced choice preferential looking acuity between breast-fed and unsupplemented formula-fed infants *(89)*. The formula used in this study contained 2.1% of total fat as LNA, but no LCPUFAs. On the other hand, the recent publication from Gibson's group in Adelaide indicates that despite providing ample LNA in formula, term infants have compromised visual acuity if only LNA is provided and a normal visual development occurs only if DHA is provided in an amount similar to that found in human milk *(83)*.

3.4. Long-Term Effects of Early Dietary PUFA Supply

The question of reversibility of observed changes in visual function cannot be fully answered from our data on preterm infants since the study was terminated at 57 wk postconception. In the case of the Carlson studies, infants were followed up to 12 mo, demonstrating effects on psychomotor development at that age *(73)*. In our retinal studies most, but not all, the ERG changes at 36 wk were, in fact, reversible based on the 57-wk results.

The possibility of long-term effects cannot be discarded easily considering the results of the 3-yr follow-up of visual acuity maturation in formula vs HM-fed infants. We conducted a 3-yr follow-up of healthy, full-term infants to test if HM feeding, which contains significant amounts of DHA, had an effect on the development of visual function *(79)*. The cohorts were breast-fed from birth to at least 4 mo or fed for 12 mo formula containing ample LA and 0.5% of the total fat as LNA. The breast-fed group was weaned to an oleic acid (18:1)-predominant formula and received egg yolk through 12 mo of age. The breast-fed group maintained higher plasma and RBC membrane phospholipid DHA concentrations throughout the first year of life. At 3 yr of age, stereo acuity, as measured by operant preferential looking (OPL) techniques, was more mature in the breast-fed infants relative to the formula-fed group; 92% of the breast-fed group had mature OPL stereo acuity, whereas 35% of the infants in the formula-fed group met the maturity criteria. Visual recognition in the breast-fed group was also better; whereas only 61% of the formula-fed infants had a perfect score, 93% of the breast-fed group had a perfect score *(79)*. These and the results of a controlled study of LCPUFA supplementation conducted by Makrides et al. *(83)* are suggestive of a DHA effect on visual acuity maturation in term infants.

In addition, the follow-up of phenylketonuric infants, treated with early protein restriction, may also serve to evaluate the effect of LCPUFA deficit. The impact of DHA supplementation on functional development is presently in progress *(90)*. In peroxisomal diseases there is an alteration of the n-3 partial β oxidation necessary to produce DHA. The relevance of DHA supplementation in this condition may be especially relevant if less generalized disease is present *(91)*.

Evidence of potential beneficial long-term effects of DHA supplementation on brain development is suggestive, but proof is lacking. The resolution of this issue should be forthcoming since controlled clinical trials of DHA and DHA+AA supplementation in term infants are now being completed. The follow-up of these infants beyond infancy should help to address the question of long-term effects.

Table 2
Formula with LCPUFAs in Europe

Formula	% Total fatty acids	
Preterm infants		
Aletemil. PreNidal Beba (Nestle)	0.5 GLA	0.1 EPA
	0.1 AA	0.5 DHA
Nutriprem Cow & Gate (Nutricia)	0.6 GLA	0.2 EPA
		0.3 DHA
Prematil (Milupa)	0.2 GLA	
	0.4 AA	0.2 DHA
Humana OF+ (Humana)	0.2 AA	0.2 DHA
Nenatal (Nutricia)	0.6 AA	0.4 DHA
Premilon (Nutricia)	0.45 AA	0.3 DHA
Full-term infants		
Alete PreBeba	0.5 GLA	0.1 EPA
	0.1 AA	0.5 DHA
PreAptamil (Milupa)	0.2 GLA	0.2 DHA
	0.4 AA	
Adapta 90 Inicio (Wander)		0.2 EPA
		0.2 DHA

4. RECOMMENDATION FOR ESSENTIAL PUFAs DURING THE PERINATAL PERIOD

Based on the information reviewed here and other results available to the experts, the European Society for Pediatric Gastroenterology and Nutrition in 1991, the British Nutrition Foundation in 1992, and the recent Food and Agriculture Organization (FAO)/World Health Organization (WHO) consultation on Fats and Oils in Human Nutrition established recommendations for Ω-3 and -6 PUFA intake for mothers and formula-fed infants (92). Over the past few years several infant formula manufacturers have added LCPUFAs to preterm formula and more recently to formulations for term infants. Table 2 summarizes LCPUFA composition of selected formulas in Europe (64,65,93).

4.1. Recommendations for Essential PUFAs During Pregnancy and Lactation

A total of 600 g of EFAs are transferred from mother to fetus during a full-length gestation. Net uptake approximates 2.2 g/d. Thus, the pregnant mother should receive 2–3 g of EFA in addition to her usual intake. This is consistent with the necessary increase in energy during pregnancy as long as the ratio of n-3 to n-6 fatty acids is maintained. During lactation the overall energy supply may be derived from any energy source, but the EFA secreted in HM will be dependent on maternal diet and composition of fat stores. Based on the HM composition of omnivorous women and assuming an output of close to 1 L of milk per day, 3–4 g of EFA are recommended during the first trimester, increasing to 5 g once fat stores are depleted, usually after the fourth month of lactation (94).

4.2. Recommendations for Formula-Fed Infants

Since we recognize not only n-6 but also n-3 as essential nutrients for premature infants, the following provisional recommendations are suggested for the formula-fed infant for the first 6 mo of life:

1. The total EFA requirement (n-6+n-3) for premature infants should be set at 5–6% of total energy, although up to 13% can be provided safely. This represents approx 0.6–0.8 g/kg/d with an upper limit of 1.5 g/kg.
2. The parent n-6 EFA (linoleic acid) supply should be 0.5–0.6 g/kg daily and since desaturase and elongating enzymatic activity may be limited in the premature infant, formulas for these infants should provide 60–100 mg/kg/d as preformed arachidonic acid.
3. The total n-3 FA supply should be 70–150 mg/kg daily. Since desaturase and elongase enzyme activity may be limited in the premature infant, formulas for these infants should provide 35–70 mg n-3 long-chain kg body weight/d as DHA.
4. The total LA supply should not exceed 12% of total energy since excess LA may adversely affect the formation of long-chain PUFAs.
5. The ratio of total n-6:n-3 FA present in the early diet should be maintained within a range of 5:1 to a maximum of 15:1. The ratio of DHA to AA should be from 1:1 to 1:2 since excess DHA may lower conversion of LA to AA.

5. CONCLUSIONS AND RECOMMENDATIONS

Studies presented in this chapter provide clear evidence that dietary n-3 fatty acid deficiency affects eye and brain function of preterm infants as measured by ERG, cortical visual-evoked potentials, and behavioral testing of visual acuity. Preterm infants require DHA in their diet because they are unable to form these in sufficient quantity from LNA provided by soy oil-based formula products. Dietary n-3 and n-6 PUFA supply results in discernible differences in the fatty acid composition of plasma and RBC membrane lipids. Changes in membrane chemical structure are likely responsible for the observed functional effects. Preliminary evidence from term infants suggests that DHA supplementation is also required by this group.

Long-chain PUFAs have demonstrable benefits during development. The effects on neural development are of particular interest. HM is the best and only time-proven source of fat and EFAs in the infant diet. Technological procedures based on chemical and physical separation of the unsaturated fatty acids have permitted the elaboration of concentrated EPA, DHA, and AA for clinical use. The development of single-cell oil sources has allowed the provision of novel forms of LCPUFA delivery. Before the 1990s, low LNA was found in most infant formulas. By now virtually all infant formula in developed countries is supplemented with LNA and several manufacturers in Europe and in Japan have added DHA, DHA, plus AA, or also included GLA in preterm and term formula (93–95). The public health implications of these changes need to be fully evaluated in order to support this practice on a global scale.

REFERENCES

1. Dobbing J, Hopewell JW, Lynch A. Vulnerability of developing brain. VII. Permanent deficit of neurons in cerebral and cerebellar cortex following early mild undernutrition. Exp Neurol 1971; 32:439–447.
2. Levitsky DA, Strupp BJ. Malnutrition and the brain: changing concepts, changing concerns. J Nutr 1995; 125:2212S–2220S.
2a. Pagol I, Peirano P, Bes F, Salzarulo P. Sleep in early human malnutrition. In: Horne JA, ed. Sleep '88. Gustav Fisher Verlag, 1989, pp. 58–62.

3. Pollitt E. A critical view of three decades of research on the effects of chronic energy undernutrition on behavioral development. In: Chronic Energy Deficiency. Schurch B, Scrimshaw N, eds. Laussane, Switzerland: IDECG, 1988.

4. Goldman HI, Goldman JS, Kaufman Y, Lieberman OB. Late effects of early dietary protein intake on low-birth-weight infants. J Pediatr 1974; 85:764–976.

5. Rush D, Stein Z, Susser M. A randomized controlled trial of prenatal, nutritional supplementation in New York City. Pediatrics 1980; 65:683–697.

6. Grantham-McGregor S. A review of studies of the effect of severe malnutrition on mental development. J Nutr 1995; 125:2233S–2238S.

7. Burr GO, Burr MM. A new deficiency disease produced by rigid exclusion of fat from the diet. J Biol Chem 1929; 82:345–367.

8. Hansen AE, Wiese HF, Boelsche AN, Haggard ME, Adam DJD, Davis H. Role of linoleic acid in infant nutrition: clinical and chemical study of 428 infants fed on milk mixtures varying in kind and amount of fat. Pediatrics 1963; 31:171–192.

9. Holman RT, Johnson SB, Hatch TF. A case of human linolenic acid deficiency involving neurological abnormalities. Am J Clin Nutr 1982; 35:617–623.

10. Simopoulos AP. Omega-3 fatty acids in health and disease and in growth and development. Am J Clin Nutr 1991; 54:438–463.

11. Anderson RE, Benolken RM, Dudley PA, Landis DJ, Wheeler TG. Polyunsaturated fatty acids of photoreceptor membranes. Exp Eye Res 1974; 18:205–213.

12. Ballabriga A. Essential fatty acids and human tissue composition. An overview. Acta Paediatr Suppl 1994; 402:63–68.

13. Brenner RR, Peluffo RO. Regulation of unsaturated fatty acid biosynthesis. Biochim Biophys Acta 1969; 176:471–479.

14. Sprecher H. Biochemistry of essential fatty acids. Prog Lipid Res 1981; 20:13–22.

15. Willis AL. Essential fatty acids, prostaglandins, and related eicosanoids. Present Knowledge in Nutrition. Washington, DC: The Nutrition Foundation, Inc., 1984; pp. 90–113.

16. Glomset JA. Fish, fatty acids and human health. New Engl J Med 1985; 312:1253, 1254.

17. Lee AG, East JM, Froud RJ. Are essential fatty acids essential for membrane function? Prog Lipid Res 1986; 25:41–46.

18. Uauy R, Treen M, Hoffman DR. Essential fatty acid metabolism and requirements during development. Sem Perinat 1989; 13:118–130.

19. Uauy R, Hoffman DR. Essential fatty acid requirements for normal eye and brain development. Sem Perinatol 1991; 15:449–455.

20. Innis SM. Essential fatty acids in growth and development. Prog Lipid Res 1991; 30:39–103.

21. Galli C, Simopoulos AP, Tremoli E. Effects of fatty acids and lipids in health and disease. World Rev Nutr Diet 1994; 76:1–149.

22. Voss A, Reinhart M, Shankar S, et al. The metabolism of 7,10,13,16,19-docosapentaenoic acid to 4,7,10,13,16,19-docosahexaenoic acid in the rat liver is independent of a 4-desaturase. J Biol Chem 1991; 266:19,995–20,000.

23. Brockenhorff H, Ackman RG, Hoyle RJ. Specific distribution of fatty acids in marine lipids. Arch Biochem Biophys 1963; 100:93–100.

24. Galli C, Trzeciak HI, Paoletti R. Effects of dietary fatty acids on the fatty acid composition of brain ethanolamine phosphoglyceride: reciprocal replacement of n-6 and n-3 polyunsaturated fatty acids. Biochim Biophys Acta 1971; 248:449–454.

25. Menon NK, Dhopeshwarkar GA. Essential fatty acid deficiency and brain development. Prog Lipid Res 1982; 21:309–326.

26. Bourre JM, Durand G, Pascal G, Youyou A. Brain cell and tissue recovery in rats made deficient in n-3 fatty acids by alteration of dietary fat. J Nutr 1989; 119:15–22.

27. Bourre JM, Francois M, Youyou A. The effects of dietary α-linolenic acid on the composition of nerve membranes, enzymatic activity, amplitude of electrophysiological parameters, resistance to poisons and performance of learning tasks in rats. J Nutr 1989; 119:1880–1892.

28. Wheeler TG, Benolken RM, Anderson RE. Visual membranes: specificity of fatty acid precursors for the electrical response to illumination. Science 1975; 188:1312–1314.

29. Mitchell DC, Litman BJ. A role for phospholipid polyunsaturation in modulating membrane protein function. Proceedings of the 2nd International Congress of the ISSFAL (International Society for the Study of Fatty Acids and Lipids). NIH Bethesda MD USA June 7–16, 1995.

30. Salem N Jr, Shingu T, Kim HY, Hullin F, Bougnoux P, Karanian JW. Specialization in membrane structure and metabolism with respect to polyunsaturated lipids. In: Karnovsky ML, Leaf A, Bollis LC, eds. Biological Membranes: Aberrations in Membrane Structure and Function. New York: Alan R. Liss, Inc., 1988; 319–333.

31. Holh CM, Rosen P. The role of arachidonic acid in rat heart cell metabolism. Biochim Biophys Acta 1987; 921:356–363.

32. Fleisler SJ, Anderson RE. Chemistry and metabolism of lipids in the vertebrate retina. Prog Lipid Res 1983; 22:79–131.

33. Stubbs CD, Smith AD. The modification of mammalian polyunsaturated fatty acid composition in relation to fluidity and function. Biochim Biophys Acta 1984; 779:89–137.

34. Murphy MG. Dietary fatty acids and membrane protein function. J Nutr Biochem 1990; 1: 68–79.

35. Wood JN. Essential fatty acids and their metabolites in signal transduction. Biochem Soc Trans 1990; 18:755–786.

36. Foot M, Cruz TF, Clandinin MT. Effect of dietary lipid on synaptosomal acetylcholinesterase activity. Biochem J 1983; 211:507–509.

37. Lands WEM. Renewed questions about polyunsaturated fatty acids. Nutr Rev 1986; 44:189–195.

38. Treen M, Uauy RD, Jameson DM, et al. Effect of docosahexaenoic acid on membrane fluidity and function in intact cultured Y-79 retinoblastoma cells. Arch Biochem Biophys 1992; 294:564–570.

39. Yorek MA, Bohnker RR, Dudley DT, Spector AA. Comparative utilization of *N*-3 polyunsaturated fatty acids by cultured human Y-79 retinoblastoma cells. Biochim Biophys Acta 1984; 795:277–285.

40. Distel RJ, Robinson GC, Spiergelman BM. Fatty acid regulation of gene expression. Transcriptional and post-transcriptional mechanism. J Biol Biochem 1992; 267:5937–5941.

41. Love JA, Saurn WR, McGee R. The effects of exposure to exogenous fatty acids and membrane fatty acid modification on the electrical properties of NG108-15 cells. Cell Mol Neurobiol 1985; 5:333–352.

42. Evers AS, Elliott WJ, Lefkowith JB, Needleman P. Manipulation of rat brain fatty acid composition alters volatile anesthetic potency. J Clin Invest 1986; 77:1028–1033.

43. Jensen RG, Ferris AM, Lammi-Keefe CJ. Lipids in human milk and infant formulas. Ann Rev Nutr 1992; 12:417–441.

44. Giovannini M, Agostoni C, Riva E. Fat needs of term infants and fat content of milk formulae. Acta Paediatr Suppl 1994; 402:59–62.

45. Iwamoto H, Sato G. Production of EPA by freshwater unicellular algae. J Am Oil Chem Soc 1986; 63:434–438.

46. Cohen Z, Norman HA, Heimer YM. Microalgae as a source of *n*-3 fatty acids. World Rev Nutr Diet Basel: Karger 1995; 77:1–31.

47. Ackman RG. Structural homogeneity in unsaturated fatty acids of marine lipids. A review. J Fish Res Board Canada 1964; 21:247–254.

48. Akimoto M, Ishii T, Yamagaki K, Ohtaguchi K, Koide K, Yazawa K. Production of eicosapentaenoic acid by a bacterium isolated from mackerel intestines. J Am Oil Chem Soc 1990; 67:911–915.

49. Simopoulos AP, Salem N. Egg yolk as a source of long-chain polyunsaturated fatty acids in infant feeding. Am J Clin Nutr 1992; 55:411–414.

50. Sawatzki G, Georgi G, Kohn G. Pitfalls in the design and manufacture of infant formulae. Acta Paediatr Suppl 1994; 402:40–45.

51. Ongari MA, Ritter JM, Orchard MA, et al. Correlation of prostacyclin synthesis by human umbilical artery with status of essential fatty acid. Am J Obstet Gynec 1984; 149:455–460.

52. Clandinin MT, Chappell JE, Leong S, et al. Intrauterine fatty acid accretion rates in human, brain: implication for fatty acid requirements. Early Hum Dev 1980; 4:121–130.

53. Martinez M. Tissue levels of polyunsaturated fatty acids during early human development. J Pediatr 1992; 120:S129–S138.

54. Honstra G, Houwelingen AC, Simonis M, Gerrard JM. Fatty acid composition of umbilical arteries and veins: possible implications for the fetal EFA status. Lipids 1989; 24:511–517.

55. Crawford MA, Costeloe K, Doyle W, Leighfield MJ, Lennon EA, Meadows N. Potential diagnostic value of the umbilical artery as a definition of neural fatty acid status of the fetus during its growth: the umbilical artery as a diagnostic tool. Biochem Soc Tans 1990; 18:761–766.

56. Holman RT, Johnson SB, Ogburn PL. Deficiency of essential fatty acids and membrane fluidity during pregnancy and lactation. Proc Natl Acad Sci USA 1991; 88:4835–4839.

57. Al MDM, Hornstra G, Schouw YT van der, et al. Biochemical EFA status of mothers and their neonates after normal pregnancy. Early Hum Dev 1990; 24:239–248.

58. Houwelingen AC, Zijder EE, Foreman v-Drongelen M, Honstra G. The essential fatty acids status of multi-plets at birth. 2ªInternational Congress of the ISSFAL International Society for the study of fatty acids and lipids. 1995 #67.

59. Al MDM, Houwelingen AC, Honstra G. The effect of pregnancy on the cervonic acid (docosahexaenoic acid) status of mothers and their newborns. 2ªInternational Congress of the ISSFAL International Society for the study of fatty acids and lipids. 1995 #71.

60. Olsen SF, Sorensen JD, Secher NJ, et al. Randomized controlled trial of effect of fish oil supplementation on pregnancy duration. Lancet 1992; 339:1003–1007.

61. Secher NJ, Olsen SF, Sorensen JD. Fish-oil and pre-eclampsia. Br J Obstet Gynaecol 1991; 98:738–740.

62. Sibai BM, Caritis SN, Thom E, et al., and NICHD Maternal Fetal Medicine Units Network. Prevention of pre-eclamsia with low dose-aspirin in healthy nulliparous pregnant women. NEJM 1993; 329:1213–1218.

63. Neuringer M, Connor WE, Van Petten C, et al. Dietary omega-3 fatty acid deficiency and visual loss in infant rhesus monkeys. J Clin Invest 1984; 73:272–276.

64. Hansen J. Appendix: Commercial formulas for preterm infants in Nutritional Needs of Preterm Infants: Scientific Basis and Practical Guidelines, Tsang RC, Lucas A, Uauy R, Zlotkin S, eds. Pawling, New York: Williams and Wilkins by Caduceus Medical Publishers Inc., 1993; 297–301.

65. Koletzko B, Bremer HJ. Fat content and fatty acid composition of infant formulas. Acta Paeditr Scand 1989; 78:513–521.

66. Birch EE, Birch DG, Petrig B, et al. Retinal and cortical function of infants at 36 and 57 weeks postconception. Clin Vision Sci 1990; 5:363–373.

67. Birch EE, Birch DG, Hoffman DR, et al. Dietary essential fatty acid supply and visual acuity development. Invest Ophthal Vis Sci 1992; 33:3242–3253.

68. Uauy RD, Birch DG, Birch EE, et al. Effect of dietary omega-3 fatty acids on retinal function of very-low-birth-weight neonates. Pediatr Res 1990; 28:485–492.

69. Uauy R, Birch E, Birch D, et al. Visual and brain function measurements in studies on n-3 fatty acid requirements of infants. J Pediatr 1990; 120:S168–S180.

70. Sokol S. Visually evoked potentials: theory, techniques, and clinical applications. Surv Ophthalmol 1976; 21:18–44.

71. Carlson SE, Cooke RJ, Rhodes PG, et al. Long-term feeding of formulas high in linolenic acid and marine oil to very low birth weight infants: phospholipid fatty acids. Pediatr Res 1991; 30:404–412.

72. Carlson SE, Werkman SH, Rhodes PG, Tolley EA. Visual-acuity development in healthy preterm infants: effect of marine-oil supplementation. Am J Clin Nutr 1993; 58:35–42.

73. Carlson SE, Werkman SH, Peeples JM, Wilson WM. Growth and development of premature infants in relation to n-3 and n-6 fatty acid status. In: Fatty Acids and Lipids: Biological aspects. Galli C, Simopoulus AP, Tremoli E., eds. World Rev Nutr Diet Karger Basel, Switzerland 1994; 75:63–69.

74. Koletzko B, Schmidt E, Brenner HJ, Haug M, Harzer G. Effects of dietary long chain polyunsaturated fatty acids on the essential fatty acid status of preterm infants. Eur J Pediatr 1989; 148:669–675.

75. Innis SM, Foote KD, MacKinnon MI, King DJ. Plasma and red cell fatty acids of low birth weight infants fed their mothers expressed breast milk or preterm formula. Am J Clin Nutr 1990; 51:994–1000.

76. Clandinin MT, Parrot A, Van Aerde JE, Hervada AR, Lien E. Feeding preterm infants a formula containing C-20 and C-22 fatty acids simulates plasma phospholipid fatty acid composition of infants fed human milk. Early Hum Dev 1992; 31:41–51.

77. Ghebremeskel K, Leightfields M, Leaf A, Costelone K, Crawford M. Fatty acid composition of plasma and red cell phospholipids of preterm babies fed on breast milk and formulae. Eur J Pediatr 1995; 154:46–52.

78. Lucas A, Morley R, Cole TJ. Breastmilk and subsequent intelligence quotient in children born preterm. Lancet 1992; 339:261–264.

79. Birch E, Birch D, Hoffman D, Hale L, Uauy R. Breast-feeding and optimal visual development. J Pediatr Ophthalmol Strabismus 1993; 30:33–38.

80. Makrides M, Simmer K, Goggin M, Gibson RA. Erythrocyte docosahexaenoic acid correlates with the visual response of healthy, term infants. Pediatr Res 1993; 33:425–427.

81. Farquharson J, Cockburn F, Patrick WA, Jamieson EC, Logan RW. Infant cerebral cortex phospholipid fatty-acid composition and diet. Lancet 1992; 340:810–813.

82. Makrides M, Neumann MA, Byard RW, Simmer K, Gibson RA. Fatty acid composition of brain, retina, and erythrocytes in breast- and formula-fed infants. Am J Clin Nutr 1994; 60:189–194.

83. Makrides M, Neumann M, Simmer K, Pater J, Gibson R. Are long-chain polyunsaturated fatty acids essential nutrients in infancy? Lancet 1995; 345:1463–1468.

84. Lanting CI, Fidler V, Huisman M, Touwen BCL, Boersma ER. Neurological differences between 9-year-old children fed breast-milk or formula-milk as babies. Lancet 1994; 344:1319–1322.

85. Rogan JM, Gladen BC. Breast feeding and cognitive development. Early Hum Dev 1993; 31:181–193.
86. Morrow-Tlucak M, Haude RH, Enhart CB. Breastfeeding and cognitive development in the first two years of life. Soc Sci Med 1988; 26:635–639.
87. Taylor B, Wadsworth J. Breast feeding and child development at five years. J Dev Med Child Neurol 1984; 26:73–80.
88. Ponder DL, Innis SM, Benson JD, et al. Docosahexanoic acid status of term infants fed breast milk, or soy oil or corn oil containing infants formula. Pediatr Res 1992; 32:638–688.
89. Innis SM, Nelson CM, Rioux MF, King J. Development of visual acuity in relation to plasma and erythrocyte *n*-6 and *n*-3 fatty acids in healthy term gestation infants. Am J Clin Nutr 1994; 60:347–352.
90. Agostoni C, Riva E, Biasucci G, et al. The effects of *n*-3 and *n*-6 PUFA on plasma lipids and fatty acids of dietary treated phenylketonuric children. 2ᵃInternational Congress of the ISSFAL, International Society for the study of fatty acids and lipids. 1995 #103.
91. Martínez M. Polyunsaturated fatty acids in the developing human brain, red cells and plasma: influence of nutrition and peroxisomal disease. In: Fatty Acids and Lipids: Biological aspects. Galli C, Simopoulus AP, Trenoli E, World Rev Nutr Diet Basel Karger 1994; 75:70–78.
92. European Society of Paediatric Gastroenterology and Nutrition Committee on Nutrition: comment on the content and composition of lipids in infant formulas. Acta Paediatr Scand 1991; 80:887–896.
93. Koletzko B. Long chain polyunsaturated fatty acids in infant formulae in Europe. ISSFAL Newsletter 1995; 2:3–5.
94. FAO/WHO Report of Expert Consultation. The Role of Dietary Fats and Oils in Human Nutrition. FAO Rome 1995; 57:49–55.
95. ISSFAL. Recommendations for the essential fatty acid requirements of infant formula ISSFAL Newsletter 1994;1:4.

PART IV
BENEFITS OF PREVENTIVE NUTRITION IN THE UNITED STATES AND EUROPE

23 Potential Benefits of Preventive Nutrition Strategies

Lessons for the United States

Walter C. Willett

1. INTRODUCTION

For years, the Recommended Dietary Allowances (RDAs) served as nutritional guidelines for individuals and institutions *(1)*. However, these have developed from minimalist criteria primarily aimed at prevention of clinical deficiencies. These guidelines were later supplemented with recommendations to reduce dietary fat and cholesterol. In recent years, attention has focused on specific types of fat and suboptimal intake of dietary factors, even in the absence of recognized clinical deficiency. Dietary factors, including substances not generally considered to be nutrients, now appear involved in the cause or prevention of conditions as diverse as coronary heart disease (CHD), stroke, many cancers, cataracts, and birth defects. The National Research Council (NRC) and the Surgeon General's office *(2,3)* have examined the relationship of diet to health more broadly and issued new recommendations. This brief overview will build on the 1989 NRC report on Diet and Health *(2)* emphasizing subsequent findings.

2. SOURCES OF EVIDENCE

Traditionally, animal experiments and small human metabolic studies formed the basis of dietary recommendations. Inevitably, the study of chronic disease in humans has required epidemiologic approaches. Initially, investigations compared dietary intakes and disease rates among populations in various countries. These analyses highlighted the large differences in disease rates worldwide and provided many hypotheses; however, such studies are limited because many other factors besides diet vary across cultures and the data are inherently aggregated. The next generation of studies were primarily case-control investigations, which mainly examined dietary factors retrospectively in relation to risk of cancer and other diseases. Now, large prospective studies of many thousands of persons are beginning to provide data based on both biochemical indicators of diet and dietary questionnaires that have been rigorously validated *(4)*. Prospective studies are less subject to biases resulting from the retrospective reporting of dietary intakes or the effects of disease on biochemical indicators. Micronutrient supplements can potentially be evaluated in randomized trials; however, trials of dietary interventions may often be unfeasible because of difficulties in maintaining com-

From: *Preventive Nutrition: The Comprehensive Guide for Health Professionals*
Edited by A. Bendich and R. J. Deckelbaum Humana Press Inc., Totowa, NJ

pliance for the necessary long periods, which could be decades. Recent advances in molecular biology have yet to contribute substantially to dietary recommendations, but in the future these approaches may provide useful intermediary endpoints, allow the study of gene–diet interactions, and enhance our understanding of the mechanisms by which dietary factors influence disease. Ultimately, our knowledge is best based on a synthesis of epidemiologic, metabolic, animal, and mechanistic studies.

3. SPECIFIC DIETARY COMPONENTS

3.1. Dietary Fat

Major reviews on diet and health have consistently recommended reducing total fat intake, usually to 30% of energy or less (2,3), to decrease CHD. The classical diet–heart hypothesis has rested heavily on the repeated observation that serum total cholesterol levels predict CHD risk; serum cholesterol has thus functioned as a surrogate marker of risk in hundreds of metabolic studies. These studies, summarized as equations by Keys (5) and Hegsted (6), indicated that, compared with carbohydrates, saturated fats and dietary cholesterol increase and polyunsaturated fat decreases serum cholesterol, whereas monounsaturated fat has no influence. These widely used equations, although valid for total cholesterol, have become less relevant as surrogate variables for CHD risk with the recognition that the high-density lipoprotein cholesterol fraction (HDL) is strongly and inversely related to CHD risk, and that the ratio of total cholesterol to HDL is a better predictor (7–10).

Substitution of carbohydrate for saturated fat (the basis of the American Heart Association diets) tends to reduce HDL as well as total and low-density lipoprotein (LDL) cholesterol; thus, the ratio does not change appreciably (8–10). In contrast, substituting monounsaturated fat for saturated fat reduces LDL without affecting HDL, thus providing an improved ratio (10). In addition, monounsaturated fats, compared with carbohydrate, reduce blood sugar and triglycerides in adult onset diabetics (11). Questions have been raised regarding whether the reductions in HDL resulting from a high carbohydrate diet have the same adverse effect as reductions caused by other factors (12). Although this is difficult to address directly, other factors that influence HDL levels, including alcohol, estrogens, obesity, smoking, exercise, and medications, affect CHD risk in the predicted direction (13,14). The use of the usual cholesterol prediction equations has been further complicated by the recognition that different saturated fats vary in their influence on LDL levels: 18:0, stearic acid (the main fat in chocolate and a major saturated fat in beef fat) has little effect; 16:0, palmitic acid (the main fat in palm oil, also found in beef fat) modestly increases LDL, and 14:0, myristic acid (the main saturated fat in butter and other dairy fats) most strongly increases LDL (10,15).

The optimal amount of polyunsaturated fat intake in the diet remains uncertain. The earlier metabolic studies predicting total serum cholesterol (5,6) suggested that intakes should be maximized, and the American Heart Association recommended intakes of 10% of energy (compared with US averages of about 3% in the 1950s and 6% at present). However, in more recent metabolic studies, the benefits of polyunsaturated fat have been less clear (10) and concerns have arisen from animal studies in which N-6 polyunsaturated fat (typically as corn oil) has promoted tumor growth (16), and the possibility that high intakes of N-6 relative to N-3 fatty acids might promote coronary thrombosis (17,18).

Evidence based on clinical endpoints (as opposed to blood lipid levels) is remarkably sparse. In Keys' pioneering study of diets and CHD in seven countries *(19,20)*, total fat intake had little association with population rates of CHD; indeed, the lowest rate was in Crete, which had the highest fat intake as a result of to the large consumption of olive oil. Saturated fat intake, however, was positively related to CHD in Keys' study. In contrast to international comparisons, little relationship has been seen with saturated fat intake in prospective studies of individuals *(4,21)*, although these studies have not been sufficiently large or rigorous to exclude a modest association. These studies, however, tend to support a modest association between dietary cholesterol and CHD risk *(22)*. An inverse association with polyunsaturated fat was seen in one prospective study conducted at a time when the average intake was low *(21)*, but little relationship has been seen subsequently. Similarly, dietary intervention trials have generally shown little effect on CHD incidence *(23–26)*; in the one trial that clearly reduced CHD mortality *(27)* many components of the diet as well as weight and smoking were changed simultaneously (*see* Chapter 9).

High intake of Ω-3 fatty acids, found primarily in marine fish but also in some vegetable oils and plants, reduces platelet aggregability and prolongs bleeding time *(18)*, slightly reduces blood pressure *(28)*, decreases serum triglycerides, but increases LDL cholesterol *(29)*. Fish consumption was associated with a greatly reduced risk of myocardial infarction in one prospective study *(30)* and in a randomized trial among postinfarction patients *(31)*. However, subsequent data have been less supportive of a major effect of fish consumption on risk of CHD *(32–34)* (*see* Chapter 13).

Trans fatty acids are formed by the partial hydrogenation of liquid vegetable oils in the production of margarine and vegetable shortening and can account for as much as 40% of these products. Intake of partially hydrogenated vegetable fats (which increased from nothing in 1900 to a peak of about 5.5% of total fat in about the 1960s) has closely paralleled the epidemic of CHD during this century, in contrast to intake of animal fat, which has steadily declined over this period *(35)*. *Trans* fatty acids increase LDL and decrease HDL *(35–40)*, as well as raise Lp(a), another lipid fraction implicated in CHD etiology *(39,41)*. Positive associations between intake of *trans* fatty acids and CHD have been seen among regions in the Seven Countries Study *(42)*, in a prospective study of US women *(43)*, a case-control study of men and women *(44)*, and a cross-sectional angiographic study *(45)*. In a multicenter European case-control study, adipose levels of *trans* fatty acids were by far lowest in Spain, also the country with the lowest CHD rates *(46)*. In the same study, the risk of CHD within countries was 40–50% higher among individuals with the highest *trans* fatty acid levels, but this did not quite obtain statistical significance.

Understanding of the interrelationships among dietary fats, blood lipids, and CHD risk has been further complicated by the recognition that antioxidants are likely to play a critical role in preventing atherosclerosis. Experimental evidence suggests that lipid-soluble antioxidants, such as vitamin E, can block the oxidative modification of LDL, an important step in atherogenesis *(47)*. Within Europe, countries with higher blood antioxidant levels have lower rates of CHD *(48)*, and, as described in Section 6., vitamin E supplements have been inversely associated with CHD risk. Because liquid vegetable oils, particularly those that are minimally processed, are the primary source of vitamin E in our diets, reduction of these fats could have adverse effects on CHD risk. Soybean oil may be an exception because it is highly polyunsaturated, yet its primary form of vitamin E, γ-tocopherol, is rapidly excreted and poorly incorporated into tissues and lipoproteins. Thus, diets high in soybean oil, the major fat in the US diet, might result in LDL particularly susceptible to oxidation. In contrast, LDL particles formed on a diet high in monounsaturated fat in the form of olive oil appear to be relatively resistant to oxidation *(49,50)* *(see* Chapter 10).

3.2. Dietary Fat and Cancer

Another major justification for decreasing dietary fat has been anticipated reductions in the risk of cancers of the breast, colon and rectum, and prostate *(2,51)*. The primary evidence has been that countries with low fat intake, also the less affluent areas, have had low rates of these cancers *(51,52)*. These correlations have been primarily with animal fat and meat intake, rather than with vegetable fat consumption.

The hypothesis that fat intake increases breast cancer risk has been supported by animal models *(53,54)*, although no association was seen in a large study that did not use an inducing agent *(55)*. Moreover, much of the effect of dietary fat in the animal studies appears to be because of an increase in total energy intake, and energy restriction profoundly decreases incidence *(16,53,55)*. In most case-control studies, no association between fat intake and breast cancer was observed, although a weak positive association (relative risk = approx 1.07 for 40 vs 30% of energy from fat) was seen in the pooled data from 12 such studies *(56)*. However, these studies are now of diminishing relevance because data from six large prospective studies, including 3400 cases among 280,000 women, have recently been published *(57–62)*. In none of these studies was the risk of breast cancer significantly elevated among those with the highest fat intake, and the summary relative risk for the highest vs lowest category of dietary fat composition is 1.03 *(63)*. In the largest study *(57)*, no reduction in risk was seen even below 25% of energy from fat. Thus, over the range of fat intake consumed by middle-aged women in these studies, which included the present dietary recommendations, dietary fat did not appear to increase breast cancer risk. Effects of much greater fat reductions or influences at early times in life could not be excluded.

The large differences, approximately fivefold, in breast cancer rates among countries are probably the result of many factors. High consumption of soy products, which contain antiestrogenic isoflavonoids *(64)* has been hypothesized to account for the low rates of breast cancer in Japan. Although deserving further research, similarly low rates of breast cancer are uniformly seen in nonindustrialized countries, most of which do not consume soy products. Also, no relation between intake of soy products and breast cancer risk was seen in two recent case-control studies in China *(65)*. Indirect evidence is growing that the powerful effect of energy and growth restriction on mammary cancer incidence in animals also applies to humans. Adult height, in part a marker of early energy balance, is associated with breast cancer rates internationally and in many case-control and cohort studies *(66–68)*. Some of this effect is mediated through delayed ovulation *(69)*; childhood weight gain is the primary determinant of age at menstruation *(70)*, which still averages about 18 yr in China *(71)* *(see* Chapter 6).

Associations between animal fat consumption and colon cancer incidence have been seen more consistently *(72–74)*, although not in all studies *(75)*, whereas little relation has been seen with vegetable fat. Positive associations with animal fat have also been observed for adenomatous polyps, a precursor lesion *(76)*. However, the associations between red meat consumption and colon cancer have been even stronger than the effect of fat in some analyses *(73,74)*, suggesting that relationships with red meat may be because of other components of cooked flesh, such as heat-induced carcinogens *(77)* or the high content of readily available iron *(78)* (*see* Chapter 5).

Like breast and colon cancer, prostate cancer rates are much higher in affluent compared to poor and Eastern countries *(52)*. More detailed epidemiologic studies are few; in subsets of several case-control studies, men with prostate cancer reported higher fat intake than did controls *(79,80)*. In a recent prospective study, a positive association was seen between intake of α-linolenic acid, primarily attributable to consumption of fat from red meat *(81)*.

3.3. Dietary Fat and Body Fatness

Overweight is an important cause of morbidity and mortality (*see* Section 3.3.) and short-term studies have suggested that reducing the fat content of the diet induces weight loss. However, population differences in weight do not appear to be primarily a result of fat intake; in Europe, southern countries with relatively low fat intake have higher rates of obesity than Northern European countries *(82)*. Also, among 65 counties in China, no correlation was seen between body weight and fat intake, which varied from about 6 to 47% of energy *(71)*. Inconsistent associations have been observed in cross-sectional and prospective studies within countries, but such observations are particularly prone to distortion because subjects may alter their diets to modify their weight. In randomized trials of fat reduction, the optimal way to study this relationship, modest weight reductions are typically seen in the short term. However, in three randomized studies lasting a year or longer, reductions in fat to 20–25% of energy had at most a 1.5 kg effect on overall long-term body weight *(83–85)*. In a trial among obese women, a reduction in fat intake to ≈18% of energy reduced weight by only 3.4 kg, and no effect on waist/hip ratio or percent body fat was observed *(86)*. Very low fat intakes, less than 10% of energy, in conjunction with a high volume of bulky food as consumed by some traditional societies, may induce weight loss *(87)*, but long-term studies are needed. However, available evidence suggests that reductions in dietary fat composition over the ranges currently recommended are not likely to have sustained and substantial effects on body fatness.

What can we now say about dietary fat and health? As noted in the executive summary of the NRC report *(2)*, but generally ignored, there is little evidence that dietary fat *per se* is associated with risk of CHD. Metabolic and epidemiological data are presently consistent in suggesting that intake of partially hydrogenated vegetable fats should be minimized. Metabolic data and indirect epidemiologic data support a reduction in saturated fats, particularly from dairy sources, to as low as feasible; because these are not essential nutrients there is no optimal intake. Definitive data are not available on the optimal intake of polyunsaturated and monounsaturated fats, but the metabolic data as well as the experience of Southern European populations suggest that consuming a substantial proportion of energy as monounsaturated fat would be desirable. Available evidence also suggests that fat reduction would have little effect on breast cancer risk, although reducing red meat intake may well decrease the incidence of colon cancer. Browner et al. have estimated that decreasing saturated fat intake so that total fat was reduced from 37 to 30% of energy would reduce mortality in the United States only by 2% *(88)*. This is likely to be an overly optimistic estimate, however, because the calculations did not account for reductions in HDL and assumed major causal association with breast and colon cancer.

3.4. Vegetables and Fruits

Recommendations to eat a generous amount of vegetables and fruits *(2)* are supported by a wealth of epidemiologic data, primarily relating to cancer incidence. In over 200 case-control or cohort studies, persons consuming higher amounts of these foods or having higher levels of carotenoids in their blood experienced reduced risk of various malignancies *(89,90)*. An inverse relation with lung cancer is most strongly supported *(91)*, and has led to the suggestion that β-carotene might be the protective factor *(92)*; this is supported by inverse associations specifically with carrots in multiple studies *(93)*. Intake of fruits and vegetables has also been related to lower risk of stomach cancer in many case-control studies *(89,90,94)*; both the epidemiologic evidence and mechanistic studies *(95)* suggest a possible protective role for vitamin C. Vegetable and fruit consumption has also been inversely related to risk of colon cancer *(96)*, which has been attributed to beneficial effects of dietary fiber, but recent evidence suggests that folic acid might also account for the reduced risk *(74,97)*. Although the numbers of studies are smaller, protective effects have also been seen for cancers of the oral cavity, larynx, pancreas, bladder, and cervix *(89,90,94)*. In a large prospective study, breast cancer incidence was about 25% higher among women with low vegetable intake *(98)*.

Plants contain numerous components, in addition to the micronutrients noted above, that have potential anticancer activity *(90)*; such chemicals could reduce the formation of carcinogens, induce detoxifying enzymes, and block the effects of endogenous estrogens. Although the epidemiologic data on cancer provide solid support for recommendations to consume an abundance of vegetables and fruits, further details about the types and amounts of these foods could permit more precise recommendations.

In the more limited literature on CHD, fiber intake has been related to decreased risk *(4,99,100)*, but the possibility that this association could have been a result of other factors in plants has generally not been explored. Evidence that elevated blood homocysteine is an independent risk factor for CHD and cerebrovascular disease *(101–103)*, and that levels can be reduced by supplements of folic acid and vitamin B-6 *(104,105)* suggest another mechanism. Vegetarians generally have reduced blood pressures, and higher intake of fruits and vegetables has been associated with lower blood pressure even in nonvegetarians *(106)*, but the active factor remains unclear *(see* Chapter 12).

Suboptimal dietary folic acid, which is mainly obtained from fortified breakfast cereals, vegetables, and fruits, definitively increases risk of neural tube defects, the most common severe birth defect *(107,108)*, and may account for more than half of these cases. The effect of low folate intake may be particularly adverse among the approx 10% of the population who are genetically less efficient in utilizing the ingested form of this vitamin *(109)* *(see* Chapter 20).

In both case-control *(110)* and prospective studies *(111)*, intake of dietary antioxidants, including carotenoids and vitamin C has been inversely related to risk of cataracts. Because cataract formation, which is increased by sunlight and cigarette smoking *(112)*, involves the accumulation of oxidized and denatured proteins, this lesion may represent a convenient marker of long-term oxidative damage. High intake of lutein and zeaxanthin in the form of spinach has been associated with a greatly decreased risk of macular degeneration *(113)*. This is particularly notable because lutein and zeaxanthin are the carotenoids specifically concentrated in the macula, where they apparently play a protective role against photo-damage *(114)* (*see* Chapters 14 and 15).

3.5. Starches and Complex Carbohydrates

Because protein varies only modestly across a wide range of human diets, a higher carbohydrate consumption is, in practice, the reciprocal of a low fat diet. For reasons discussed under the topic of fat, a high carbohydrate diet may have adverse metabolic consequences. In particular, such diets are associated with an increase in triglycerides and a reduction in HDL cholesterol *(10)*. These adverse responses may be aggravated in the context of insulin resistance *(115,116)*, which is highly prevalent to some degree in Western populations.

Although direct evidence for benefit in reducing disease risk is limited, several reasons exist to emphasize whole grain and other less refined complex carbohydrates as opposed to the highly refined products and sugar generally consumed in the United States. Adverse consequences of highly refined grains appear to result both from the rapid digestion and absorption of these foods, as well as from the loss of fiber and micronutrients in the milling process. The glycemic response after carbohydrate intake, which has been characterized by the glycemic index, is greater with highly refined foods as compared with less-refined, whole grains *(117)*. The more glycemic response as a result of highly refined carbohydrates is accompanied by increased plasma insulin levels and appears to augment the other adverse metabolic changes as a result of carbohydrate consumption noted above *(117)* to a greater degree than with less refined foods. Diets with a high glycemic index, particularly when associated with low fiber intake, appear to increase the risk of noninsulin-dependent diabetes *(118)*. Anticipated reductions in colon cancer risk by diets high in grain fiber have been difficult to document epidemiologically *(119)* (although inverse associations with vegetables have been seen repeatedly) *(90)*. However, reduced constipation and risk of colonic diverticular disease *(112)* are clear benefits of such diets. The role of soluble fiber, found in oat bran and some other plant foods, in lowering blood lipids has been hotly debated; recent evidence suggests that a small effect may exist with large intakes *(120)*. Risk of myocardial infarction appears to be reduced by higher intake of dietary fiber from grains to a greater degree than can be explained by the effect of fiber on blood lipids alone *(121)*.

The importance of micronutrients in the prevention of many chronic conditions has re-emphasized the problem of "empty calories" associated with diets high in sugar and highly refined carbohydrates. In the standard milling of white flour, as much as 60–90% of vitamins B-6 and E, folate, and other nutrients are lost *(122)*; this may be nutritionally critical for persons with otherwise marginal intakes. Thiamin, riboflavin, and niacin are presently replaced by fortification, but other nutrients remain substantially reduced.

3.6. Protein

Average protein consumption in the United States substantially exceeds requirements *(2)* and adequate intake can be maintained on most reasonable diets, including those without animal products. High intake of animal protein can increase urinary calcium loss *(123)*, contribute to homocysteinemia *(124)*, and has been hypothesized to increase risk of various cancers *(125)*; however, evidence for the latter effect is limited.

3.7. Calcium and Dairy Products

Recommendations to "maintain adequate calcium intake" *(2)*, generally considered to be 800 mg/d for most healthy adults, and to consume dairy products on a daily basis *(126)* derive primarily from the importance of calcium in maintaining bone strength. Although calcium supplements (in conjunction with vitamin D) have reduced fracture incidence in older adults *(127,128)*, uncertainty remains regarding the optimal intake. Intakes as high as 1500 mg/d have been recommended for older women at risk of fractures *(129)*, which are difficult to achieve without supplements. However, some populations have low fracture rates despite minimal dairy product consumption and low overall calcium intake by adults *(130)*. Milk and other dairy products may not be directly equivalent to calcium from supplements, because these foods contain a substantial amount of protein, which can enhance renal calcium losses *(123)*. Few studies have directly addressed the relation of dairy product consumption and fracture incidence; with the exception of one small study *(131)*, higher consumption of calcium or dairy products as an adult has been associated with a higher or no difference in fracture incidence *(132,133)* (*see* Chapter 16).

Inverse associations have been observed between calcium intake and blood pressure in some studies *(134)*, but in a review of trials of supplementation little overall effect was seen *(135)*. Low calcium intake has been associated with risk of colon cancer, but evidence has not been consistent and deserves further examination *(136)*.

Although recommended calcium intakes can be achieved by a high consumption of greens and certain other vegetables, greatly increased intakes would be required for most women to achieve these dietary levels without regular use of milk and other dairy products. However, calcium supplements have been shown to increase bone density and are an inexpensive form of calcium. Thus, dairy product consumption can be considered an optional rather than a necessary dietary component.

3.8. Salt and Processed Meats

Reduction of salt (sodium chloride) intake from an average of approx 8–10 to < 6 g/d will, on average, decrease blood pressure to a small degree. In a recent review Law et al. *(137)* concluded that a 3 g/d reduction would reduce the incidence of stroke by 22% and of CHD by 16%. Although the decrease in risk of cardiovascular disease achieved by reducing salt consumption is small for most individuals, the overall number of deaths potentially avoided is large, supporting policies to reduce the salt consumption, particularly in processed foods and by institutions. In a number of case-control studies, the consumption of salty and pickled foods has been associated with stomach cancer *(138)*. However, since this cancer is relatively rare in the United States, further benefit from reducing salt intake would be small.

4. BODY WEIGHT

Although the NRC made the recommendation to "balance food intake and physical activity to maintain appropriate body weight" *(2)* without any specific weight recommendations, the document was cited as the justification for the revised 1990 US guidelines for weight. These guidelines included substantial increases after age 35 to much heavier weights than the earlier and widely used Metropolitan Life recommendations *(139)*. Unfortunately, the new guidelines appear to have been based on unpublished data that did not account for confounding influences of such factors as smoking (which is a strong cause of premature death and is also associated with low body weight) or the fact that many individuals, particularly at older ages, have low body weights because of chronic illness (140). More detailed analyses indicate that middle-aged persons of even average weight have a high prevalence of abnormalities of blood glucose and lipids as well as blood pressure (141), and experience substantial increases in myocardial infarction (142,143), diabetes (144), hypertension (145), and gallstones (146), as well as total mortality rates (147,148) compared to their leaner counterparts. Thus, the older, leaner weight guidelines are probably closer to optimal, and the best health experience is achieved by avoiding increases in weight during adulthood. As noted earlier, dietary fat composition over a wide range appears to have little relationship with weight maintenance; in contrast, regular exercise and avoidance of extreme inactivity, such as excessive television watching, is crucial (149).

5. ALCOHOL

Many adverse influences of heavy alcohol consumption are well recognized, but moderate consumption has both beneficial and harmful effects, greatly complicating decisions for individuals. Overwhelming epidemiologic data indicate that moderate consumption reduces risk of myocardial infarction (150,151), two drinks a day decrease risk by about 30–50%. Although it has been suggested that this effect may be because of antioxidants in red wine (152), similar protective effects for equivalent amounts of alcohol have been seen for all types of alcoholic beverages (153). On the other hand, modest positive associations with risk of breast cancer incidence have been observed in approx 30 studies (154,155) for similar levels of alcohol intake, possibly because alcohol appears to increase endogenous estrogen levels (156,157). The overall effect of alcohol, as represented by total mortality, appears beneficial up to about two drinks per day in men (158). Overall, a similar relation with total mortality is seen among women, but no net benefit was observed among those at low risk of CHD because of their age or lack of coronary risk factors (159). Furthermore, the risk of transition from moderate alcohol consumption to addiction and uncontrolled drinking has not been well quantified.

6. VITAMIN SUPPLEMENTS

Because populations can be identified with very low rates of almost every major disease, vitamin supplements may not further enhance health among populations consuming ideal diets. Only recently are data emerging that address the effects of vitamin supplements against the background of actual diets in the United States, which appear far from ideal (94).

The most firmly established benefit, based on case-control, cohort, and randomized studies, is that folic acid supplements in the amounts contained in multivitamins can reduce the risks of neural tube defects by approx 70% (107,160). This is probably only a sentinel indicator of suboptimal folate intakes, because associations have also been seen with colonic neoplasias and low folate intake, along with suboptimal vitamin B-6, is likely to contribute to elevated blood homocysteine levels and risk of cardiovascular disease (102,103).

As noted above, vitamin E supplements well beyond the dietary range have been associated with decreased risk of CHD. In two recent prospective studies, men and women who consumed the highest amounts of vitamin E (mostly from supplements)

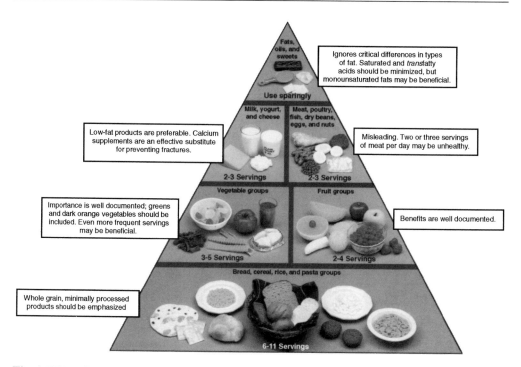

Fig. 1. USDA food pyramid, Annotated. Optimal food intakes for children and pregnant or lactating women may need further consideration. (Modified figure reproduced with permission of Nasco Nutrition Teaching Aids.)

had an approx 40% lower risk of myocardial infarction compared with those having low vitamin E intakes *(161,162)*. The maximum reduction in risk appeared to be at levels of 100 or more IU/d, well above intakes achievable by diet alone. In one case-control study, use of vitamin E supplements was associated with a 50% reduced risk of oral cancer *(163)*. Vitamin C supplementation was associated with lower risk of CHD in one national study *(164)*, but the data available did not distinguish vitamin C from other supplements. No protective effect of vitamin C was observed in another prospective study *(162)*. Apart from a possible reduction in risk of cataracts *(112)*, there is little evidence at present that high doses of vitamin C have substantial benefits. Although no overall benefit of supplemental vitamin A was seen in a large prospective study of breast cancer, an inverse relation with risk was seen among women with below-average vitamin A intakes *(98)* (*see* Chapter 14).

The effects of vitamin supplementation on risk of chronic diseases have been examined in only a few randomized trials. In a randomized trial conducted in a region of China with low consumption of fruits and vegetables, a supplement containing β-carotene, vitamin E, and selenium reduced incidence of stomach cancer *(165)*. Benefits from additional micronutrients may not be limited to those in extreme poverty; in a Canadian trial a multivitamin/mineral supplement reduced risks of infections by 50% among older persons *(166)*, possibly a result of an enhancement of immune status (*see* Chapter 18).

Current evidence, although far from complete, suggests that supplements of folate and possibly other vitamins, at the US RDI level, which for folate is twice the current RDA level, contained in most nonprescription multivitamin preparations may have substantial benefits for at least an important but unidentified subgroup of the US population, perhaps characterized by increased requirements as well as by suboptimal diets. Because intakes of folate as well as other micronutrients appear marginal for many Americans *(89,94)*, the risks of using multivitamins appear nonexistent, and the cost of supplements is low (especially compared with that of fresh fruits and vegetables), the use of a daily or several-times-a-week multivitamin appears rational for the majority of Americans, given current knowledge. A similar argument can be made for vitamin E supplements at levels above the RDA (15 IU), although further data are highly desirable. For other vitamins and minerals there is presently limited evidence of benefit of supplements over the RDA levels. Intake of vitamins A and D at levels substantially above the RDA can potentially be harmful *(2)*; in a recent study, intake of supplements containing more than 10,000 IU/d of preformed vitamin A was associated with risk of specific birth defects *(167)*. Thus, women planning pregnancy should be counseled to take multiple vitamins with folic acid that do not contain vitamin A at more than the RDA level of 8000 IU/day *(168)*.

7. RECOMMENDATIONS

Any set of dietary recommendations must be made with the clear qualification that information is currently incomplete and conclusions are subject to change with new data. Most of the major causes of morbidity and mortality in the United States develop over many decades and large-scale nutritional epidemiologic studies have only begun in the last 10–15 yr; a full picture of the relation between diet and disease will require additional decades of careful investigation. Nevertheless, combining metabolic, clinical, and epidemiologic evidence, several general recommendations that are unlikely to change substantially can be made to those who are interested in consuming a healthy diet.

1. Stay lean and active throughout life. For most individuals, body weight should not increase by more than 5–10 pounds after age 21. Because most of us work at sedentary jobs, weight control will usually require conscious regular daily exercise as well as some effort to avoid overconsumption of calories.
2. Vegetables and fruits should be consumed in abundance (five servings per day is minimal) and include green leafy and orange vegetables daily.
3. Grains should be consumed primarily in a minimally refined form, and intake of simple sugars should be low.
4. Red meat should be consumed only occasionally and in low amounts if at all; nuts and legumes as well as poultry and fish in moderation are healthy alternatives.
5. Animal fats and *trans* fatty acids from partially hydrogenated vegetable oils should be avoided as much as possible. On the other hand, olive oil and possibly other primarily monounsaturated fats appear to be healthy alternatives. Highly polyunsaturated fats, such as corn and soybean oil, may also be healthy alternatives, but theoretical concerns exist regarding high consumption of these oils. Unless explicitly stated otherwise, it is safest to assume that deep-fried fast foods and most commercially prepared foods contain *trans* fatty acids.

6. The optimal consumption of dairy products and calcium intake is not known, but high consumption of milk is not likely to be necessary or beneficial for middle-aged and older adults. Adequate calcium intake may be particularly important for growing children, adolescents, and lactating women; supplements should be considered if dietary sources are low.

7. Unless one is extremely careful about a healthy food selection at every meal, consuming a daily RDI-level (DV) multivitamin containing folic acid provides a sensible nutritional safety net. Definitive evidence exists that use of a folic acid-containing multivitamin supplement during the early weeks of pregnancy can prevent a large fraction of neural tube defects and the Public Health Service recommends that women who are potentially child-bearing consume 400 µg of folic acid daily, the level found in most multivitamin supplements *(169)*. For most people, this intake is difficult and unreliable to achieve by diet alone. As noted above, benefits of folic acid supplementation may extend to prevention of myocardial infarction, stroke, and colon cancer, although this is not proven. Because menstrual losses of iron may not be adequately replaced by iron intake on the low-energy diets of women in a sedentary society, it may make sense for most premenopausal women to use a multivitamin that also contains iron.

Pending further data, the use of a vitamin E supplement at 400–800 IU/d is reasonable for most middle-aged and older persons as substantial evidence suggests that this will reduce risk of myocardial infarction. Although not proven, substantial evidence also suggests that use of vitamin C supplements at the level of 500 mg/d can reduce risk of cataract, which may be sufficient reason for some individuals to consider using this. Although there is no documented harm from these supplements at the levels of intake suggested, long-term effects need to be examined in further studies. Also, personal physicians should be made aware of any nutritional supplements that are being consumed in the event of possible interactions with medications or diagnostic tests. Further, use of supplements should not be considered as an alternative to eating a healthy diet because foods contain a wide variety of additional factors that are likely to contribute to good health.

8. Finally, be adventuresome in eating! Unfortunately, most of us in the United States are heirs to the rather monotonous Northern European dietary tradition centered on the consumption of meat and dairy products. Contemporary food processing has added to the deleterious effects of this diet by the removal of dietary fiber and micronutrients through overrefining of foods, and has profoundly and adversely altered the biological effects of vegetable oils through the process of partial hydrogenation. To further aggravate matters, the worst aspects of diet tend to be the most heavily marketed and promoted. Fortunately, healthy diets do not have to be invented or discovered through new technological advances. Existing foods together with the lessons of various cultural models of eating based primarily around minimally processed foods from plant sources provide a means of achieving a diet that is both healthy as well as interesting and enjoyable.

REFERENCES

1. Food and Nutrition Board. Recommended Dietary Allowances, 10th rev. ed. Washington, DC: National Academy Sciences, 1989.
2. National Research Council—Committee on Diet and Health. Diet and Health: Implications for Reducing Chronic Disease Risk, Washington, DC: National Academy Press, 1989.
3. Department of Health and Human Services. The Surgeon General's Report on Nutrition and Health, Washington, DC: Government Printing Office, (DHHS publication [PHS] 50210), 1988.
4. Willett WC. Nutritional Epidemiology. New York: Oxford University Press, 1990.

5. Keys A. Serum-cholesterol response to dietary cholesterol. Am J Clin Nutr 1984; 40:351–359.

6. Hegsted DM. Serum-cholesterol response to dietary cholesterol: a re-evaluation. Am J Clin Nutr 1986; 44:299–305.

7. Castelli WP, Abbott RD, McNamara PM. Summary estimation of cholesterol used to predict coronary heart disease. Circulation 1983; 67:730–734.

8. Ginsberg HN, Barr SL, Gilbert A. Reduction of plasma cholesterol levels in normal men on an American Heart Association step 1 diet or a step 1 diet with added monounsaturated fat. New Engl J Med 1990; 322:574–579.

9. Mensink RP, Katan MB. Effect of monounsaturated fatty acids versus complex carbohydrates on high-density lipoprotein in healthy men and women. Lancet 1987; 1:122–125.

10. Mensink RP, Katan MB. Effect of dietary fatty acids on serum lipids and lipoproteins: a meta-analysis of 27 trials. Arteriosclerosis Thromb 1992; 12:911–919.

11. Garg A, Grundy SM, Koffler M. Effect of high carbohydrate intake on hyperglycemia, islet cell function, and plasma lipoproteins in NIDDM. Diabetes Care 1992; 15:1572–1580.

12. Brinton EA, Eisenberg S, Breslow JL. Increased apo A-I and apo A-II fractional catabolic rate in patients with low high density lipoprotein-cholesterol levels with or without hypertriglyceridemia. J Clin Invest 1991; 87:536–544.

13. Sacks FM, Willett WC. More on chewing the fat: the good fat and the good cholesterol. New Engl J Med 1991; 325:1740–1742.

14. Mannitari M, Huttunen JK, Koskinen P, et al. Lipoproteins and coronary heart disease in the Helsinki Heart Study. Eur Heart J 1990; 11:26h–31h.

15. Denke MA, Grundy SM. Effects of fats high in stearic acid on lipid and lipoprotein concentrations in men. Am J Clin Nutr 1991; 54:1036–1040.

16. Welsch CW. Relationship between dietary fat and experimental mammary tumorigenesis: a review and critique. Cancer Res 1992; 52(Suppl 7):2040S–2048S.

17. Renaud S, Kuba K, Goulet C, Lemire Y, Allard C. Relationship between fatty-acid composition of platelets and platelet aggregation in rat and man. Relation to thrombosis. Circ Res 1970; 26:553–564.

18. Leaf A, Weber PC. Cardiovascular effects of n-3 fatty acids. New Engl J Med 1988; 318:549–557.

19. Keys A. Seven Countries: a multivariate analysis of death and coronary heart disease. Cambridge, MA: Harvard University Press, 1980.

20. Verschuren WM, Jacobs DR, Bloemberg BP, et al. Serum total cholesterol and long-term coronary heart disease mortality in different cultures. Twenty-five-year follow-up of the Seven Countries Study. JAMA 1995; 274:131–136.

21. Shekelle RB, Shryock AM, Paul O, et al. Diet, serum cholesterol, and death from coronary heart disease: the Western Electric Study. New Engl J Med 1981; 304:65–70.

22. Shekelle RB, Stamler J. Dietary cholesterol and ischemic heart disease. Lancet 1989; 1:1177–1179.

23. Multiple Risk Factor Intervention Trial Research Group. Multiple Risk Factor Intervention Trial: risk factor changes and mortality results. JAMA 1982; 248:1465–1477.

24. Stamler J, Wentworth D, Neaton JD. Is the relationship between serum cholesterol and risk of premature death from coronary heart disease continuous and graded? Findings in 356,222 primary screenees of the Multiple Risk Factor Intervention Trial (MRFIT). JAMA 1986; 256:2823–2828.

25. Frantz ID, Dawson EA, Ashman PL. Test of effect of lipid lowering by diet on cardiovascular risk. The Minnesota coronary survey. Arteriosclerosis 1989; 9:129–135.

26. Sacks F. Dietary fats and coronary heart disease. Overview. J Cardiovasc Risk 1994; 1:3–8.

27. Hjermann I, Holme I, Leren P. Oslo Study Diet and Antismoking Trial; results after 102 months. Am J Med 1986; 80:7–11.

28. Bonaa KH, Bzerve KS, Staume B, Gram IT, Thelle D. Effect of eicosapentaenoic and docosahexaenoic acids on blood pressure in hypertension: a population-based intervention trial from the Tromso study. New Engl J Med 1990; 322:795–801.

29. Kestin M, Clifton P, Belling GB, Nestel PJ. N-3 fatty acids of marine origin lower systolic blood pressure and triglycerides but raise LDL cholesterol compared with N-3 and N-6 fatty acids from plants. Am J Clin Nutr 1990; 51:1028–1034.

30. Kromhout D, Bosscheiter EB, de Lezenne Coulander C. The inverse relation between fish consumption and 20-year mortality from coronary heart disease. New Engl J Med 1985; 312:1205–1209.

31. Burr ML, Fehily AM, Gilbert JF. Effects of changes in fat, fish, and fibre intakes on death and myocardial reinfarction. Lancet 1989; ii:757–761.

32. Vollset SE, Heuch I, Bjelke E. Fish consumption and mortality from coronary heart disease (letter). New Engl J Med 1985; 313:820,821.

33. Ascherio A, Rimm EB, Stampfer MJ, Giovannucci E, Willett WC. Dietary intake of marine n-3 fatty acids, fish intake and the risk of coronary disease among men. New Engl J Med 1995; 332:977–982.

34. Morris MC, Manson JE, Rosner B, Buring JE, Willett WC, Hennekens CH. Fish consumption and cardiovascular disease in the Physicians' Health Study: a prospective study. Am J Epidemiol 1995; 142:166–175.

35. Booyens J, Louwrens CC. The Eskimo diet. Prophylactic effects ascribed to the balanced presence of natural *cis* unsaturated fatty acids and to the absence of unnatural *trans* and *cis* isomers of unsaturated fatty acids. Med Hypothesis 1986; 21:387–408.

36. Mensink RPM, Katan MB. Effect of dietary *trans* fatty acids on high-density and low-density lipoprotein cholesterol levels in healthy subjects. New Engl J Med 1990; 323:439–445.

37. Zock PL, Katan MB. Hydrogenation alternatives: effects of trans fatty acids and stearic acid versus linoleic acid on serum lipids and lipoproteins in humans. J Lipid Res 1992; 33:399–410.

38. Judd JT, Clevidence BA, Muesing RA, Wittes J, Sunkin ME, Podczasy JJ. Dietary trans fatty acids: effects of plasma lipids and lipoproteins of healthy men and women. Am J Clin Nutr 1994; 59:861–868.

39. Nestel P, Noakes M, Belling B. Plasma lipoprotein and Lp[a] changes with substitution of elaidic acid for oleic acid in the diet. J Lipid Res 1992; 33:1029–1036.

40. Sundram K, Anisah I, Hayes KC, Jeyamalar R, Pathmanathan R. *Trans*-18:1 raises cholesterol more than *cis*-mono or saturated fats in humans. FASEB 1995; 9:2549 (abstract).

41. Mensink RP, Zock PL, Katan MG, Hornstra G. Effect of dietary cis and trans fatty acids on serum lipoprotein [a] levels in humans. J Lipid Res 1992; 33:1493–1501.

42. Kromhout D, et al. Dietary saturated and *trans* fatty acids, cholesterol and 15-year mortality from coronary heart disease. The Seven Countries Study. Prev Med 1995; 24:308–315.

43. Willett WC, Stampfer MJ, Manson JE, et al. Trans-fatty acid intake in relation to risk of coronary heart disease among women. Lancet 1993; 341:581–585.

44. Ascherio A, Hennekens CH, Buring JE, Master C, Stampfer MJ, Willett WC. Trans fatty acids intake and risk of myocardial infarction. Circulation 1994; 89:94–101.

45. Siguel EN, Lerman RH. Trans fatty acid patterns in patients with angiographically documented coronary artery disease. Am J Cardiol 1993; 71:916–920.

46. Aro A, Kardinaal AFM, Salminen I, et al. Adipose tissue isomeric trans fatty acids and risk of myocardial infarction in nine countries: the EURAMIC study. Lancet 1995; 345:273–278.

47. Steinberg D, Witztum JL. Lipoproteins and atherogenesis: current concepts. JAMA 1990; 264: 3047–3052.

48. Gey KF, Brubacher GB, Stahelin HB. Plasma levels of antioxidant vitamins in relation to ischemic heart disease and cancer. Am J Clin Nutr 1987; 45(s):1368–1377.

49. Reaven P, Parthasaranthy S, Grasse BJ, Miller E, Steinberg D, Witztum JL. Effects of oleate-rich and linoleate-rich diets on the susceptibility of low density lipoprotein to oxidative modification in mildly hypercholesterolemic subjects. J Clin Invest 1993; 91:668–676.

50. Berry EM, Eisenberg S, Friedlander Y, et al. Effects of diets rich in monounsaturated fatty acids on plasma lipoproteins: the Jerusalem Nutrition Study. Nutr Metab Card Dis 1995; 5:55–62.

51. Prentice RL, Sheppard L. Dietary fat and cancer. Consistency of the epidemiology data, and disease prevention that may follow from a practical reduction in fat consumption. Cancer Causes Control 1990; 1:81–97.

52. Armstrong B, Doll R. Environmental factors and cancer incidence and mortality in different countries, with special reference to dietary practices. Int J Cancer 1975; 15:617–631.

53. Ip C. Quantitative assessment of fat and calorie as risk factors in mammary carcinogenesis in an experimental model in: Recent Progress on Nutrition and Cancer. New York: Wiley-Liss, 1990,107–117.

54. Freedman LS, Clifford C, Messina M. Analysis of dietary fat, calories, body weight, and the development of mammary tumors in rats and mice: a review. Cancer Res 1990; 50:5710–5719.

55. Appleton BS, Landers RE. Oil gavage effects on tumor incidence in the national toxicology program's 2-year carcinogenesis bioassay. In: Poirier LA, Newberne PM, Pariza MW, eds. Adv Exp Med Biol 1985;99–104.

56. Howe GR, Hirohata T, Hislop TG, et al. Dietary factors and risk of breast cancer: combined analysis of 12 case-control studies. J Natl Cancer Inst 1990; 82:561–569.

57. Willett WC, Hunter DJ, Stampfer MJ, et al. Dietary fat and fiber in relation to risk of breast cancer: an eight year follow-up. JAMA 1992; 268:2037–2044.

58. Mills PK, Beeson WL, Phillips RL, Fraser GE. Dietary habits and breast cancer incidence among Seventh-day Adventists. Cancer 1989; 64:582–590.

59. Kushi LH, Sellers TA, Potter JD, et al. Dietary fat and postmenopausal breast cancer. J Natl Cancer Inst 1992; 84:1092–1099.

60. Howe GR, Friedenreich CM, Jain M, Miller AB. A cohort study of fat intake and risk of breast cancer. J Natl Cancer Inst 1991; 83:336–340.
61. Graham S, Zielezny M, Marshall J, et al. Diet in the epidemiology of postmenopausal breast cancer in a New York State cohort. Am J Epidemiol 1992; 136:1327.
62. Van den Brandt PA, Van't Veer P, Goldbohm RA, et al. A prospective cohort study on dietary fat and the risk of postmenopausal breast cancer. Cancer Res 1993; 53:75–82.
63. Hunter DJ, Willett W. Diet, body size, and breast cancer. Epidemiol Rev 1993; 15:110–132.
64. Adlercreutz H. Western diet and western diseases: some hormonal and biochemical mechanisms and associations. Scand J Clin Lab Invest 1990; 50 (Suppl 201):3–23.
65. Yuan JM, Wang QS, Ross RK, Henderson BE, Yu MC. Diet and breast cancer in Shanghai and Tianjin, China. Br J Cancer 1995; 71:1353–1358.
66. Micozzi MS. Nutrition, body size, and breast cancer. Yearbook Phys Anthropol 1985; 28:175–206.
67. Vatten LJ, Kvinnsland S. Body height and risk of breast cancer. A prospective study of 23,831 Norwegian women. Br J Cancer 1990; 61:881–885.
68. Swanson CA, Jones DY, Schatzkin A, Brinton LA, Ziegler RG. Breast cancer risk assessed by anthropometry in the NHANES I epidemiological follow-up study. Cancer Res 1988; 48:5363–5367.
69. Henderson BE, Ross RK, Pike MC. Toward the primary prevention of cancer. Science 1991; 254:1131–1138.
70. Meyer F, Moisan J, Marcoux D, Bouchard C. Dietary and physical determinants of menarche. Epidemiol 1990; 1:377–381.
71. Chen J, Campbell TC, Junyao L, Peto R. The Diet, Lifestyles, and Mortality Characteristics of 65 Rural Populations in the People's Republic of China. Oxford: Oxford University Press, 1987.
72. Whittemore AS, Wu-Williams AH, Lee M, et al. Diet, physical activity and colorectal cancer among Chinese in North America and China. J Natl Cancer Inst 1990; 82:915–926.
73. Willett WC, Stampfer MJ, Colditz GA, Rosner BA, Speizer FE. Relation of meat, fat, and fiber intake to the risk of colon cancer in a prospective study among women. New Engl J Med 1990; 323:1664–1672.
74. Giovannucci E, Rimm EB, Ascherio A, Stampfer MJ, Colditz GA, Willett WC. Alcohol, low-methionine-low-folate diets, and risk of colon cancer in men. J Natl Cancer Inst 1995; 87:265–273.
75. Phillips RL, Snowdon DA. Association of meat and coffee use with cancers of the large bowel, breast, and prostate among Seventh-Day Adventists: preliminary results. Cancer Res 1983; 43:2403–2408.
76. Giovannucci E, Stampfer MJ, Colditz GA, Rimm EB, Speizer FE, Willett WC. Relationship of diet to risk of colorectal adenoma in men. J Natl Cancer Inst 1992; 84:91–98.
77. Gerhardsson de Verdier M, Hagman U, Peters RK, Steineck G. Meat, cooking methods and colorectal cancer: a case-referent study in Stockholm. Int J Cancer 1991; 49:520–525.
78. Babbs CF. Free radicals and the etiology of colon cancer. Free Med Biol Med 1990; 8:191–200.
79. Kolonel LN, Yoshizawa CN, Hankin JH. Diet and prostatic cancer: a case-control study in Hawaii. Am J Epidemiol 1988; 127:999–1012.
80. Graham S, Haughey B, Marshall J, et al. Diet in the epidemiology of carcinoma of the prostate gland. J Natl Cancer Inst 1983; 70:687–692.
81. Giovannucci E, Rimm EB, Stampfer MJ, Colditz GA, Ascherio A, Willett WC. Intake of fat, meat, and fiber in relation to risk of colon cancer in men. Cancer Res 1994; 54:2390–2397.
82. Seidell JC, Derenberg I. Obesity in Europe—scaling an epidemic. Int J Obesity 1995; 19 (Suppl 3):51–54.
83. National Diet-Heart Study Research Group. The National Diet-Heart Study Final Report. Circulation 1968; 18(s):1–154.
84. Sheppard L, Kristal AR, Kushi LH. Weight loss in women participating in a randomized trial of low-fat diets. Am J Clin Nutr 1991; 54:821–828.
85. Lee-Han H, Cousins M, Beaton M. Compliance in a randomized clinical trial of dietary fat reduction in patients with breast dysplasia. Am J Clin Nutr 1988; 48:575–586.
86. Kasim SE, Martino S, Kim PN, et al. Dietary and anthropometric determinants of plasma lipoproteins during a long-term low-fat diet in healthy women. Am J Clin Nutr 1993; 57:146–153.
87. Shintani TT, Hughes CK, Beckman S, O'Connor HK. Obesity and cardiovascular risk intervention through the ad libitum feeding of a traditional Hawaiian diet. Am J Clin Nutr 1991; 6:1647s–1651s.
88. Browner WS, Westerhouse J, Tice JA. What if Americans ate less fat? A quantitative estimate of the effect on mortality. JAMA 1991; 265:3285–3291.
89. Block G, Patterson B, Subar A. Fruit, vegetables, and cancer prevention: a review of the epidemiologic evidence. Nutr Cancer 1992; 18:1–29.
90. Steinmetz KA, Potter JD. Vegetables, fruit and cancer. I. Epidemiology. Cancer Causes Control 1991; 2:325–357.

91. Willett WC. Vitamin A and lung cancer. Nutr Rev 1990; 48:201–211.
92. Peto R, Doll R, Buckley JD, Sporn MB. Can dietary beta-carotene materially reduce human cancer rates? Nature 1981; 290:201–208.
93. Fontham ET. Protective dietary factors and lung cancer. Intl J Epidemiol 1990; 19 (Suppl 1):32–42.
94. Block G, Abrams B. Vitamin and mineral status of women of childbearing potential. Ann NY Acad Sci 1993; 678:244–254.
95. Correa P, Haenszel W, Cuello C, Tannenbaum S, Archer M. A model for gastric cancer epidemiology. Lancet 1975; 2:58–60.
96. Trock B, Lanza E, Greenwald P. Dietary fiber, vegetables, and colon cancer: critical review and meta-analyses of the epidemiologic evidence. J Natl Cancer Inst 1990; 82:650–661.
97. Giovannucci E, Stampfer MJ, Colditz GA, et al. Folate, methionine and alcohol intake and risk of colorectal adenoma. J Natl Cancer Inst 1993; 85:875–884.
98. Hunter DJ, Manson JE, Colditz GA, et al. A prospective study of intake of vitamins C, E and A and risk of breast cancer. New Engl J Med 1993; 329:234–240.
99. Morris JN, Marr JW, Clayton DG. Diet and heart: a postscript. Br Med J 1977; 2:1307–1314.
100. Khaw KT, Barrett-Connor E. Dietary fiber and reduced ischemic heart disease mortality rates in men and women: a 12-year prospective study. Am J Epidemiol 1987; 126:1093–1102.
101. Stampfer MJ, Malinow MR, Willett WC, et al. A prospective study of plasma homocyste(e)ine and risk of myocardial infarction. JAMA 1992; 268:877–881.
102. Kang SS, Wong PWK, Norusis M. Homocysteinemia due to folate deficiency. Metabolism 1987; 36:458–462.
103. Selhub J, Jacques PF, Bostom AG, et al. Association between plasma homocysteine concentrations and extracranial carotid-artery stenosis. New Engl J Med 1995; 332:286–291.
104. Kang SS, Wong PWK, Cook HY, Norusis M, Messer JV. Protein bound homocyst(e)ine—a possible risk factor for coronary artery disease. J Clin Invest 1986; 77:1482–1486.
105. Wilcken DEL, Dudman NPB, Tyrrell PA. Homocystinuria due to cystathionine B-synthase deficiency—the effects of betaine treatment in pyridoxine-responsive patients. Metabolism 1985; 34:1115–1121.
106. Ascherio A, Stampfer MJ, Colditz GA, Rimm EB, Litin L, Willett WC. Correlations of vitamin A and E intake with the plasma concentrations of carotenoids and tocopherols among US men and women. J Nutr 1992; 122:1792–1801.
107. MRC Vitamin Study Research Group. Prevention of neural tube defects: results of the Medical Research Council Vitamin Study. Lancet 1991; 338:131–137.
108. Werler MM, Shapiro S, Mitchell AA. Periconceptional folic acid exposure and risk of occurrent neural tube defects. JAMA 1993; 269:1257–1261.
109. van den Put NMJ, Steegers-Theunissen RPM, Frosst P, et al. Mutated methylenetetrahydrofolate reductase as a risk factor for spina bifida. Lancet 1995; 346:1070,1071.
110. Jacques PF, Hartz SC, Chylack LT, McGandy RB, Sadowski JA. Nutritional status in persons with and without senile cataract: blood vitamin and mineral levels. Am J Clin Nutr 1988; 48:152–158.
111. Hankinson SE, Stampfer MJ, Seddon JM, et al. Nutrient intake and cataract extraction in women: a prospective study. Br Med J 1992; 305:335–339.
112. Hankinson SE, Willett WC, Colditz GA, et al. A prospective study of smoking and risk of cataract surgery in women. JAMA 1992; 268:994–998.
113. Seddon JM, Ajani UA, Sperduto RD, et al. Dietary carotenoids, vitamins A, C, and E, and advanced age-related macular degeneration. JAMA 1994; 272:1413–1420.
114. Schalch W. Carotenoids in the retina: a review of their possible role in preventing or limiting damage caused by light and oxygen. In: Free Radicals and Aging, Emerit I, Chance B, eds. Basel, Switzerland: Birkhauser Verlag 1992:280–298.
115. Jeppesen J, Hollenbeck CB, Zhou MY, et al. Relation between insulin resistance, hyperinsulemia, post-heparin plasma lipoprotein lipase activity, and postprandial lipemia. Arteriosclerosis Thromb Vasc Biol 1995; 15:320–324.
116. Jeppesen J, Chen YDI, Zhou MY, Schaaf P, Coulston A, Reaven GM. Postprandial triglyceride and retinyl ester responses to oral fats effects of fructose. Am J Clin Nutr 1995; 61:787–791.
117. Jenkins DJ, Wolever TM, Taylor RH, et al. Glycemic index of foods: a physiological basis for carbohydrate exchange. Am J Clin Nutr 1981; 34:362–366.
118. Salmeron J, Ascherio A, Rimm E, Colditz G, Spiegelman D, Stampfer M. Carbohydrate quality and risk of non-insulin-dependent diabetes in women. Am J Epidemiol 1995; 141:S67 (abstract).
119. Willett W. The search for the causes of breast and colon cancer. Nature 1989; 338:389–394.

120. Jenkins DJ, Wolever TM, Rao AV. Effect of blood lipids of very high intakes of fiber in diets low in saturated fat and cholesterol. New Engl J Med 1993; 329:21–26.
121. Rimm EB, Ascherio A, Giovannucci E, Spiegelman D, Stampfer MJ, Willett WC. Vegetable, fruit and cereal fiber intake and risk of coronary heart disease among men. JAMA 1996; 275:447–451.
122. Schroeder HA. Losses of vitamins and trace minerals resulting from processing and preservation of foods. Am J Clin Nutr 1971; 24:562–573.
123. Lutz J, Linkswiler HM. Calcium metabolism in postmenopausal women and osteoporotic women consuming two levels of dietary protein. Am J Clin Nutr 1981; 34:2178–2186.
124. Gruberg ER, Raymond SA. Beyond Cholesterol. New York: St. Martin's, 1981.
125. Youngman LD, Campbell TC. The sustained development of preneoplastic lesions depends on high protein intake. Nutr Cancer 1992; 18:131–142.
126. Welsh S, Davis C, Shaw A. Development of the food guide pyramid. Nutr Today 1992; 27:12–23.
127. Chapuy MC, Arlof ME, Duboeuf F, et al. Vitamin D3 and calcium to prevent hip fractures in elderly women. New Engl J Med 1992; 327:1637–1642.
128. Heaney RP. Thinking straight about calcium. New Engl J Med 1993; 328:503–504.
129. Office of Medical Applications of Research: National Institutes of Health. Osteoporosis. JAMA 1984; 252:799.
130. Nordin BEC. International patterns of osteoporosis. Clin Orthop 1966; 45:17–20.
131. Holbrook TL, Barrett-Conner E, Wingard DL. Dietary calcium and risk of hip fracture: 14-year prospective population study. Lancet 1988; 2:1046–1049.
132. Wickham CAC, Walsh K, Cooper C, et al. Dietary calcium, physical activity, and risk of hip fracture: a prospective study. Br Med J 1989; 299:889–892.
133. Michaelsson K, Holmberg L, Mallmin H, et al. Diet and hip fracture risk: a case-control study. Intl J Epidemiol 1995; 24:771–782.
134. McCarron DA, Morris CD, Henry HJ, Stanton JL. Blood pressure and nutrient intake in the United States. Science 1984; 224:1392–1398.
135. The Trials of Hypertension Prevention Collaborative Research Group. The effects of nonpharmacologic interventions on blood pressure of persons with high normal levels. JAMA 1992; 267:1213–1220.
136. Bostick RM, Potter JD, Sellers TA, McKenszie DR, Kushi H, Folsom AR. Relation of calcium, vitamin D, and dairy food intake to incidence of colon cancer in older women. Am J Epidemiol 1993; 137:1302–1317.
137. Law MR, Frost CD, Wald NJ. By how much does dietary salt reduction lower blood pressure? III—Analysis of data from trials of salt reduction. Br Med J 1991; 302:819–824.
138. Correa P, Fonthorn E, Pickle LW, Chen J, Lin Y, Haenszel W. Dietary determinants of gastric cancer in South Louisiana inhabitants. J Natl Cancer Inst 1985; 75:645–653.
139. U. S. Department of Agriculture: U. S. Department of Health and Human Services. Nutrition and your health. Dietary guidelines for Americans, 3rd ed. Washington, DC: U.S. Government Printing Office, 1990.
140. Manson JE, Stampfer MJ, Hennekens CH, Willett WC. Body weight and longevity. A reassessment. JAMA 1987; 257:353–358.
141. Garrison RJ, Kannel WB. A new approach for estimating healthy body weights. Int J Obesity 1993; 17:417–423.
142. Lew EA, Garfinkel L. Variations in mortality by weight among 750,000 men and women. J Chronic Dis 1979; 32:563–576.
143. Willett WC, Manson JE, Stampfer MJ, et al. Weight, weight change, and coronary heart disease in women: risk within the 'normal' weight range. JAMA 1995; 273:461–465.
144. Colditz GA, Willett WC, Stampfer MJ, et al. Relative weight and increased risk of diabetes in a cohort of US women. Am J Epidemiol 1987; 126:750,751 (abstract).
145. Witteman JC, Willett WC, Stampfer MJ, et al. Relation of moderate alcohol consumption and risk of systemic hypertension in women. Am J Cardiol 1990; 65:633–637.
146. Maclure KM, Hayes KC, Colditz GA, Stampfer MJ, Speizer FE, Willett WC. Weight, diet and risk of symptomatic gallstones in middle-aged women. New Engl J Med 1989; 321:563–569.
147. Lindsted K, Tonstad S, Kuzma J. Body mass index and patterns of mortality among Seventh-day Adventists. Int J Obesity 1991; 15:397—406.
148. Manson JE, Willett WC, Stampfer MJ, et al. A prospective study of body weight and mortality in women. New Engl J Med 1995; 333:677–685.
149. Gortmaker SL, Dietz WH, Cheung LW. Inactivity, diet, and the fattening of America. J Am Diet Assoc 1990; 90:1247–1252.

150. Klatsky AL, Armstrong MA, Friedman GD. Risk of cardiovascular mortality in alcohol drinkers, ex-drinkers, and nondrinkers. Am J Cardiol 1990; 66:1237–1242.

151. Rimm EB, Giovannucci EL, Willett WC, et al. A prospective study of alcohol consumption and the risk of coronary disease in men. Lancet 1991; 338:464–468.

152. Renaud S, de Lorgeril M. Wine, alcohol, platelets, and the French paradox for coronary disease. Lancet 1992; 339:1523–1526.

153. Maclure M. A demonstration of deductive meta-analysis: ethanol intake and risk of myocardial infarction. Epidemiol Rev 1994; 15:328–351.

154. Longnecker MP. Alcoholic beverage consumption in relation to risk of breast cancer: meta-analysis and review. Cancer Causes Control 1994; 5:73–82.

155. Longnecker MP, Newcomb PA, Mittendorf R, et al. Risk of breast cancer in relation to lifetime alcohol consumption. J Natl Cancer Inst 1995; 87:923–929.

156. Reichman ME, Judd JT, Longcope C, et al. Effects of alcohol consumption on plasma and urinary hormone concentration in premenopausal women. J Natl Cancer Inst 1993; 85:722–727.

157. Hankinson SE, Willett WC, Manson JE, et al. Alcohol, height, and adiposity in relation to estrogen and prolactin levels in postmenopausal women. J Natl Cancer Inst 1995; 87:1297–1302.

158. Boffetta P, Garfinkel L. Alcohol drinking and mortality among men enrolled in a American Cancer Society prospective study. Epidemiology 1990; 1:342–348.

159. Fuchs CS, Stampfer MJ, Colditz GA, et al. Alcohol consumption and mortality among women. New Engl J Med 1995; 332:1245–1250.

160. Willett WC. Folic acid and neural tube defect: Can't we come to closure? Am J Public Health 1992; 82:666–668.

161. Stampfer MJ, Hennekens CH, Manson JE, Colditz GA, Rosner B, Willett WC. A prospective study of vitamin E consumption and risk of coronary disease in women. New Engl J Med 1993; 328:1444–1449.

162. Rimm EB, Stampfer MJ, Ascherio A, Giovannucci E, Colditz GA, Willett WC. Vitamin E consumption and the risk of coronary heart disease in men. New Engl J Med 1993; 328:1450–1456.

163. Gridley G, McLaughlin JK, Block G, Blot WJ, Gluch M, Frauneril JF. Vitamin supplement use and reduced risks of oral and pharyngeal cancer. Am J Epidemiol 1992; 135:1083–1092.

164. Enstrom JE, Kanim LE, Klein MA. Vitamin C intake and mortality among a sample of the United States population. Epidemiology 1992; 3:194–202.

165. Blot WJ, Li JY, Taylor PR, et al. Nutrition intervention trials in Linxian, China: supplementation with specific vitamin/mineral combinations, cancer incidence, and disease-specific mortality in the general population. J Natl Cancer Inst 1993; 85:1483–1492.

166. Chandra RK. Effect of vitamin and trace-element supplementation on immune responses and infection in elderly subjects. Lancet 1992; 2:1124–1127.

167. Rothman KJ, Moore LL, Singer MR, et al. Teratogenicity of high vitamin A intake. New Engl J Med 1995; 333:1369–1373.

168. Oakley GP, Erickson JD. Vitamin A and birth defects. New Engl J Med 1995; 333:1414–1415.

169. Anonymous. Recommendations for the use of folic acid to reduce the number of cases of spina bifida and other neural tube defects (review). Morbidity/Mortality Weekly Report (MMWR) 1992; 41(RR-14):1–7.

24 Nutrient Addition to Foods

The Public Health Impact in Countries with Rapidly Westernizing Diets

Paul A. Lachance

1. INTRODUCTION

In January 1943, President Franklin Delano Roosevelt signed "War Food Administration Order No. 1" mandating the enrichment of commercial white bread and flour, corn flour, and rice with thiamine, riboflavin, niacin, and iron. Thus began the first recognition in any country, even a developed country, that the human person is a social being with no inborn or instructive urges to prevent the occurrence of malnutrition. The human population is in an ever-changing world and thus faces a continuing evolution in lifestyle and technology. Food choices are increasingly diverse, yet the need for nutrients must be met despite the fact that the need for daily energy (kilocalories) has been diminished to a minimum by automated sophistications in technology. The technology for the addition of nutrients to food, spanning simple restoration, public health enrichment, fortification, and the addition of a balanced array of nutrients, namely, nutrification, has been applied in varying degrees to each of the major food groups (cereal grains, dairy, fruit and vegetable, and protein foods) and, therefore, the technology provides nutrient additions that are practically unavoidable in the daily consumption of food. In modern food processing, an increasingly wider array of nutrients are either removed or incorporated into food products and thus there follows an impact on the public health. Initially, nutrient addition technology provided a safe and significant approach to thwarting outright nutrient deficiencies. Today the need is to provide for the routine practice of the restoration of nutrients as food processing and preparation practices change; and to practice inherently balanced (to protein content) nutrification of foods that serve as meal alternatives. These interventions are needed in order to realize the public health benefits that such practices would contribute to thwarting the pathogenesis of the chronic killer diseases in modern developed countries. The practice of nutrient addition would optimize the daily intake of nutrients and other health promoting factors that occur in food, while concurrently diminishing or eliminating those food chemical factors that may promote disease processes. This must be accomplished without compromising the food attributes of color, flavor, and texture that make food and eating psychologically as well as physiologically satisfying.

From: *Preventive Nutrition: The Comprehensive Guide for Health Professionals*
Edited by A. Bendich and R. J. Deckelbaum Humana Press Inc., Totowa, NJ

2. NUTRIENTS ARE INVISIBLE

The human has no inborn physiological or instructive urges to keep him/her on the safe side of malnutrition. We have food tastes (1), and food fashions (2,3), but these cannot be relied on as a sound guide to realizing nutrition, least of all in technically sophisticated communities, such as in the Western world. We must recognize that the human person is a social being with both instincts and habits, who in the Western world is evolving in an increasingly sophisticated and systematized technological culture controlled to a significant degree by economics.

Food processing technology has often preceded the scientific principles underlying the technology. The pharmacist Nicholas Appert in 1809 demonstrated the value of the heat processing of food in glass. His work was prompted by a prize offered by Napoleon for foods with extended shelf life to meet military situations with unpredictable and lengthy supply lines. Commercial canning began in 1812 in Britain and 1817 in the United States. It was nearly 50 yr later that Louis Pasteur explained that food spoilage was caused by micro-organisms that could be inactivated by heat. By the end of the 19th century, canned meat, fruits and vegetables, condensed milk, and condensed soup were readily available. A revolution in agricultural research and its rapid relay to farmers began in the United States with the signing by Abraham Lincoln of the Morrill Act, which established the "land grant universities" that became the agricultural and mechanical (A & M) or state universities of the United States. Other Western countries have adapted, with varying success, the land grant strategy of identifying and conducting directly applicable research that is actively transferred to farmers and consumers via the creation of "technology" universities and institutes.

At the turn of the 20th century, vitamins were unknown and macronutrients were the basis of nutrition. Work was manual and energy requirements were substantial. The most amply consumed daily foods were cereal grain products (4), especially bread; whereas fruits and most vegetables were seasonal. Meat and potatoes were important, but without refrigeration, meat processing was a "Jungle." In the United States, the Upton Sinclair book (5) by that title led in 1906 to the Pure Food and Drug Act and the Meat Inspection Act. Food regulations date back to the Roman Empire, but specific codification was slow to emerge. Today, most Western countries have food regulations, and the European community has led in the standardization among countries of such regulations by creating and evolving the Codex Alimentarius. Codification, however, serves to constrain innovation, and, therefore, must have openings to permit the rapid introduction of innovative changes—a need that evades current codification philosophies.

3. FOOD TECHNOLOGY

In our generation, no less than 90% of the food consumed in our Western technological society has benefited (e.g., shelf-life has been extended) in some manner from food technology before the food is purchased by the ultimate consumer. The effect of science and technology on dietary customs is proving a potent force in the change of food habits, even where older cultures are well established, e.g., Chinese food in America; fast food chains in Japan, China, and Russia. The modern technologist can alter the methods of food processing and food distribution (6) as though the nutrient composition of the daily diet was of no greater biochemical importance than clothing style or choice of automobile.

4. NUTRIENT BALANCE FROM FOOD COMBINATIONS

There is no conventional food that is perfect or a nutrition panacea. The goal is to make food combinations that accord a balanced array of nutrients from foods; that are desirable and convenient at the lowest cost and at caloric intake levels that do not promote obesity *(7)*, yet allow for some "fun" foods each day. Malnutrition both of deficiency and excess can and does exist in highly technological societies *(8)*. Assuring adequate nutrition on the basis of a balanced intake of commodity foods is impractical because a substantial percentage of the American, and an increasing number of Western diets, are derived from preprepared convenience foods with varying nutritive value. This is complicated by lifestyles that are hectic and no longer dictated by a farming environment in which meals had to revolve around the need to meet the schedule for milking animals and agronomic duties. Today's consumers often skip meals and have intermittent periods of no food (dictated by commuting and flight schedules) on the one hand; and then periods of frequent food contacts dictated by business events, or leisure-time (live or remote sports events) snacking. Further, there is a health conscience that during at-home cooking often calls for "restraint" *(9)* in the composition of the foods selected, but "disinhibition" occurs on occasions of away-from-home eating, be it the selection of fast-foods on the way home or the selection of foods at a restaurant chosen for celebrating accomplishments. The choices of ready-to-eat foods number in the thousands, with few designed to be inherently balanced in nutrient content. Food nutritive value, and, therefore, the benefits to the diet, would require that a conscious recognition of nutritive value had to be in place from product concept through development and market place distribution.

5. A BRIEF HISTORY OF NUTRIENT ADDITION TO FOOD

An early nutrient addition attempt *(10)* occurred in 4000 BC when the Persian physician Melampus, medical advisor to Jason and the Argonauts, prescribed sweet wine laced with iron filings to strengthen the sailors' resistance to spears and arrows. Boussingault, a French physician, recommended *(11)* in 1833 the addition of iodine to table salt to prevent the development of goiter. However, realistic large-scale nutrient additions to food could not take place until the 20th century, when both biochemical and physiological knowledge and the availability of economical and chemically defined forms of the nutrients were on hand and could be incorporated into food products in a meaningful and controlled manner. Between the end of World War I and the end of World War II, iodine added to salt became a routine practice, with dramatic reductions in the incidence of goiter. Later, vitamins A and D were added to margarine, vitamin D to milk, and thiamine, riboflavin, niacin, and iron to flour and bread. There has been a reluctant appreciation of the role of nutrient restoration, public health enrichment, and fortification or nutrification of food as an essential prerequisite to optimal health and consequent reduction in health care costs.

6. CHANGES IN LIFESTYLE

There is a new style of living *(12)* with more mobility, job changing, divorces, and one-parent homes. Food consumption in the Untied States and Western countries has shifted from traditional to varying patterns. A majority of women are in the work force at least part-time. There are more two income households and more male and female single homemakers, all with less time for meal preparation. Skipped meals are more commonplace (13). There are fewer occasions where household members eat together. Snacking is a common practice regardless of age, providing about 20% of kilocalories. The share of the food dollar spent to eat away from home was 47% in 1994 at food costs two and one-half-times greater than that prepared at home. Much of this money goes to fast-food purchases. The nutrient density of food eaten away from home is slightly lower than at home. If the practice continues, individuals will be putting themselves at greater risk of certain nutrient inadequacies (calcium, magnesium, vitamin A, vitamin B6, folic acid, and ascorbic acid) (14). Very few at-home meals are prepared from basic food commodity ingredients. Many foods eaten in food service establishments are in fact prefrozen and are then further cooked and/or reheated on-site. In major institutions (e.g., schools, prisons) entire meals may be preplated prefrozen at an origin miles away. The associated microwaves needed to prepare such ready-to-reheat food has resulted in a booming business in the United States, Japan, Korea, and the United Kingdom (15).

7. CHANGES IN TECHNOLOGY

The food supply can be divided into "intact" and "partitioned" (6,16). An intact food is recognizable as a commodity product of agriculture. An intact food may be either "garden" fresh, i.e., just harvested, or the food may be "market fresh" and has been specially stored and/or transported for days or months. One pea or a dice of carrot in a soup or stew is discernible as intact. Partitioned grains, such as wheat flour or corn oil, are the result of milling, which partitioned the grain into bran, germ (for oil), and flour. The practice of partitioning predates modern technology since it served to extend the useful shelf life of the commodity and to provide ingredients for increased food variety. With the same technology, one can partition commodities usually considered nonedible, such as cotton into lint and seed, and cottonseed into edible oil and flour. Given a series of partitioned ingredients, one may "formulate" or "fabricate" other foods. Formulated foods include baked goods, in particular bread, and delicacies, such as ice cream. Formulated foods follow a recipe and can be prepared at home. Foods that are processed from ingredients into products that emulate more a classic item are said to be "fabricated." Margarine is intended to look and taste like butter. "Cool Whip" looks like and functions longer than whipped cream. Some fabricated products can be incorporated (hidden) within an intact food or recipe, such as "Hamburger Helper" (soy protein) ingredients, which extend ground meat and even macaroni and cheese entrees. A fabricated tomato sauce look-alike derived from starch and spices can extend pizza sauce. Fabricated foods follow a specification and require specialized processing equipment to manufacture.

A food chemist requires that ingredients be defined and predictable. A number of ingredients, such as sucrose and most oils, are refined. In the process of partitioning and/or refining, micronutrient vitamins and minerals can be either lost and ignored or specifically removed as chemicals interfering with a desirable color, flavor, or texture attribute. On the other hand, a desirable nutrient (e.g., vitamin E) or ingredient (natural flavor) can be stripped from an oil or other food fraction.

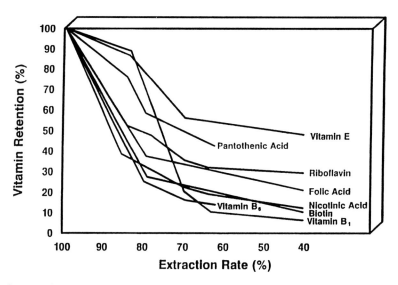

Fig. 1. The milling of wheat to flour entails several separation steps. The overall extraction of flour endosperm from the bran, aleurone, and germ is 70–75%. The resultant flour has considerably poorer nutritive value as compared to whole wheat. Patent flour has a longer shelf life than whole wheat flour. Only thiamine, riboflavin and niacin are restored in "enriched" flour. Enrichment began unofficially in 1938 and became temporarily compulsory during World War II.

8. NUTRIENT LOSSES WITH FOOD PROCESSING AND PREPARATION

There is no question that milling cereal grains has a dramatic negative effect on nutritive value, and the loss can be correlated to the "extraction rate" (amount of milling) and "patent" (blending percentage). The nutrient-rich aleurone layer is just below the bran, so the more bran is removed, the more aleurone remains with the bran. The effects of the milling process used to obtain flour on the vitamin micronutrients of wheat are well known (Fig. 1) *(17,18)*. Minerals undergo a similar pattern of loss. A generalization can be made that a similar pattern of results is to be expected with the milling of all cereal grains, in particular wheat, corn, and rice, the three most significant grains in the world supply of food. The technological reality is that with fortification/nutrification one can provide both the fashion of white bread or corn muffins and the nutrients and health benefits of whole wheat or corn products *(19)*. We can do the same for other cereal products as well *(20,21)*. This experience reinforced the basis for the 1974 NAS/NRC proposal *(22)* on the fortification of cereal-grain products, which recommended the restoration of eight vitamins and four minerals rather than the existing 1942 practice of restoring three vitamins and one mineral. Since the ingredients permitted for the production of many cereal grain products (e.g., breads, pastas) are fixed and governed by federal Standard of Identity or EEC Codex Alimentarius regulations, changes to such formulations require a cumbersome change in the regulations. In the United States, the 1974 NAS recommendations for the updated restoration of regulated cereal products were never implemented because of bureaucratic inertia. Since ready-to-eat (RTE) breakfast cereals are *not* controlled by a Standard of Identity regulation, they invariably provide a profile of 25–35% US Recommended Dietary Allowances (RDA) or

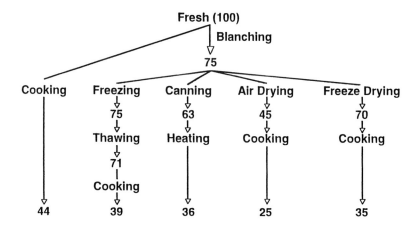

Fig. 2. The nutrients labile to heat, oxygen, UV light, or pH are the vitamins. Minerals are lost primarily through leaching. The greatest loss of nutrients occurs at final preparation (cooking at home or food service establishment). The choice of food processing preservation method enhances retention with freezing > canning > air drying. Numbers represent percent of nutrients remaining after processing.

Recommended Daily Intakes) (RDI) of eight or more key nutrients that complement the milk nutrients. Milk is associated with over 90% of RTE cereal use. This latter experience points to the responsible approaches the industry has taken in absence of specific regulations.

Some developed countries with certain cultural food traditions were slow to permit the fortification of RTE breakfast cereals. However, their extensive use was eventually recognized and countries have adopted reference RDI standards.

Principles (Fig. 2) *(6,23,24)* based on substantial reviews of the literature can be made concerning vitamin losses with the processing and preparation of raw foods (mineral losses are for the most part attributable to leaching, which varies with the recovery process, if any, e.g., discarded product water, cooking water, meat drippings, and so forth). The nutrient content of raw foods of plant origin vary with genetic strain, stage of maturity, soil, climate, fertilizer, and other growing conditions. The highest nutritive value is often just under the peel of fruits and vegetables, yet peelings are often discarded, or if retained, ironically also retain the highest concentrations of naturally occurring toxicants as well as possible agricultural residues. Most commodity (intact) foods are not necessarily feasible for fortification but their products are. For example, instant potato products can be restored with vitamin C. Jams and jellies are regulated by federal Standards of Identity and since nutrients were not recognized as approved ingredients in the late 1930's, micronutrients are not restored. Fruit-flavored drinks are not regulated and are often fortified with vitamin C, yet most fruits contain several other nutrients (e.g., carotenoids, folic acid, potassium) that are not restored. Only one fruit juice product (orange) is fortified with calcium. Other major food groups have some foods that are fortified. In many Western countries, vitamins A and D are added to margarine to emulate butter *(25)*. Vitamins A and D are added to dry and liquid skim milk and vitamin A to some dairy products as a restoration in the case of vitamin A, and as a public health enrichment in the case of vitamin D *(26)*. Currently, there is an ongoing international program to enhance the intakes of vitamin A, iron, and iodine in third world communities by fortification and other technologies *(27)*.

9. NUTRITION AND NUTRIFICATION

Recent NHANES III evidence *(28)* indicates that obesity now affects 34% of the US population. However, the average per capita caloric intake has decreased over the years, and is invariably below expectations in adolescent and career-age women. An intake average of 1500 kcal or even slightly more makes it difficult to obtain a full array of the RDA nutrients. The most limiting nutrients appear to be vitamin B-6, folic acid, magnesium, and zinc *(12)*. When consuming <1200 kilocalories daily, there is an evident need for the selection of high nutrient density foods or the use of micronutrient supplements *(29)*. In 1993, The Food and Nutrition Board of NAS/NRC Institute of Medicine posed a series of questions to the scientific community relevant to future RDAs. One question was, "Should concepts of chronic disease prevention be included in the development of allowances? For which nutrients and other food components?" The concept of prevention was actually stated in the first edition in 1943 of the RDAs "to insure good nutrition and the protection of all body tissues." Since that time, considerable data have emerged. In 1991, John Weisburger *(30)* called for new approaches to improved, balanced nutrition for health promotion and disease prevention. In 1993, in anticipation of Food and Nutrition Board Hearings on future RDAs, a workshop of leading clinical and basic nutritionists and other scientists agreed that a change in the RDAs to reflect health promotion would benefit the public health. Block and Langseth *(31)* have, for example, reviewed numerous reports on the role of antioxidants in the disease prevention. Lachance and Langseth *(32)* provided highlights of the Rutgers Workshop and have pointed to emerging data that higher than current RDAs can benefit the unborn fetus (e.g., preventing neural tube defects *[33,34]*) and the elderly (e.g., cataract formation and the aging process *[35]*).

There are questions regarding levels to recommend and the relationship of these levels to the levels associated with possible toxicity of some nutrients. Lachance *(36)* has proposed that the floor for more optimal nutrient intakes minimally can be those levels provided by ideal diets (actual food combination menus spanning weeks). On these grounds (Table 1), the antioxidant nutrient RDAs for C, E, and β-carotene equivalents would be approximately three times greater than that arrived at for the 1989 (10th edition) RDAs and the value for folacin would double and return to the 1980 RDA. As a public health intervention, the practice of the full restoration of wheat, corn, and rice cereal grain products with B6, folic acid, magnesium, and zinc to the nutrient levels of the whole grain would foster the public health, and in fact, was recommended by a subcommittee of the Food and Nutrition Board in 1974 but refused publication for comment (changes to the Standards of Identity regulations) by the Food and Drug Administration. In fact, a proposal (docket # 92P-0064/CP1) by several American clinical nutritionists to make mandatory the 1942 optional "enrichment" of cereal grain products (e.g., bread, rolls, and pasta) with calcium and vitamin D has been before the FDA since February 1992, and has not been acted on to date.

There is also a need to recognize the positive health effects of the Ω-3 fatty acids and nonnutrients, such as soluble and insoluble dietary fiber and possibly an array of protective chemical factors in certain foods rich in phytochemicals (e.g., catechins, nonvita-

Table 1
Health Factors of USDA/NCI Recommended Diets[a,b]

Dietary health factor	USDA[c]	HHS (NCI)[d]	RDA (1989) Adult
Calories	1695	1604	>1520
Protein, g	84 ± 8	84 ± 5	50–63
Total fat, g	59 ± 6	52 ± 6	Not specified
Percentage of calories from fat	31	30	30
Polyunsaturated fat, g	15 ± 4	12 ± 4	Not specified
Percentage of calories from PUFA	8	6.7	Not specified
Saturated fat, g	19 ± 4	17 ± 4	Not specified
Percentage of calories from saturated fat	10	9.5	<10
P/S ratio	0.8	0.8	Not specified
Cholesterol, mg	238 ± 97	188 ± 33	<300 mg
Total carbohydrate, g	216 ± 15	212 ± 12	>200 g
Dietary fiber	28 ± 3.4	30 ± 3.0	Not specified
Total vitamin A activity	9689	11183	800–1000 RE, μg
Preformed vitamin A, IU	919	1018	Not specified
Provitamin A (carotene), mg	5.2	6.0	Not specified
Percentage of provitamin A (carotene)	90.5	90.9	Not specified
Vitamin E, total	27	23	8–10
Vitamin C, mg	225	217	60
Thiamin (B$_1$), mg	1.7	1.6	1.1–1.5
Riboflavin (B$_2$), mg	1.9	1.8	1.3–1.7
Niacin (B$_3$), mg	24	24	15–19
Vitain B$_6$, mg	1.4	1.3	1.6–2.0
Vitamin B$_{12}$, mg	3.2	2.9	2.0
Folic acid, mg	353	381	180–200
Calcium, mg	1004	1017	800
Phosphorus, mg	1371	1420	800
Sodium, mg	1887	1955	>500
Potassium, mg	3464	3480	>2000
Magnesium, mg	362	388	280–350
Iron, mg	14	14	10–15
Zinc, mg	13	13	12–15

[a]Calculations of the recommended daily dietary food menus suggested to thwart heart disease (Dietary Guidelines) or to thwart cancer (Five-a-Day program) reveal a remarkable similarity in nutrient compositions, as compared to the RDA (1989), with substantially lower recommendations for antioxidants and folic acid.

[b]Copyright Food and Nutrition Press, Trumbull, CT.

[c]US Dept. of Agriculture.

[d]US Dept. of Health and Human Services, Natl. Cancer Inst., National Inst. of Health.

min A precursor carotenoids, diallyl sulfides, flavonoids, polyphenols, and so forth). The benefits to public health would include increases in the quality of life (e.g., the forestalling of cataracts and other morbidities) and substantial decreases in health care costs for high tech rescue medicine and an optimized health promotion cost effectiveness by replacing high cost but low benefit environmental interventions with low cost but high benefit metabolic optimization and healthy life-style practices (37).

The technology of fortification during the past 50 yr includes the in-process point for addition of micronutrients, the mode of addition, and the market forms of the fortifi-

Table 2
Percent Nutrient Contribution of Enrichment and Fortification
to Foods in the United States[a,b]

	1970[c]	1985[d]
Vitamin A	10	13
Vitamin C	10	8
Thiamine (B_1)	40	24
Riboflavin (B_2)	15	20
Niacin (B_3)	20	18
Vitamin B_6	4	6
Folic acid	—	6
Vitamin B_{12}	2	4
Iron	25	24

[a]The contribution of the enrichment and fortification of foods to average nutrient intakes, as estimated from national food consumption survey data, reveals the importance of nutrient addition rationales for public health.
[b]Copyright from The Institute of Food Technologists.
[c]Friend, B. (1970) National Food Situation 142:29.
[d]Lachance PA, Fisher MC, Stanton JL, (1988). Unpublished and Calculated from USDA Continuing Survey of Food Intakes of Individuals 1985.

cants. These technological decisions are dependent on such factors as knowledge concerning stability, bioavailability, sensory problems, safety, cost, production practicality, and reliability (38).

Estimates have been made of the contribution to the dietary intake of the average American consumer from fortificant nutrients (Table 2) (39,40). One could argue that the absence of the existing public health intervention of nutrient additions to food would have resulted in some classic nutrient deficiency diseases occurring in the US population. As changes in society and technology continue, the promise is that the nutrient restoration of food can further augment the public health. A case in point: folic acid restoration of flour to thwart neural tube defects and to enhance the other benefits of a more optimal folic acid intakes. FDA has recently acted on repeated petitions for such action.

The nutrient contribution of 2 oz. (slices) of white bread as currently "enriched" vs fully restored is demonstrated in Fig. 2A, B (41). When one recognizes that the largest single purveyor of hamburger rolls in the United States and in most developed Western countries is a single leading fast food company; considers the nutritive profile of the most frequently purchased fast food meal combinations; and realizes that the NLEA food labeling requirements are **optional** for food service meals in the United States (such labeling varies from minimal to none in other Western countries), the public health import of the restoration of cereal-grain products, such as recommended by the 1974 NAS report, becomes common sense. The per capita consumption of wheat flour in the United States is 138 lb/yr. The restoration of folic acid at a level of 0.4 mg/lb would provide the average adult consumer (including women of child-bearing age) a 100 µg/d folic acid average *additional* intake (Fig. 3) (42), and thus a 50% increase from the current mean intake of 210 µg/d for women 19–50 yr of age (42,43). Folic

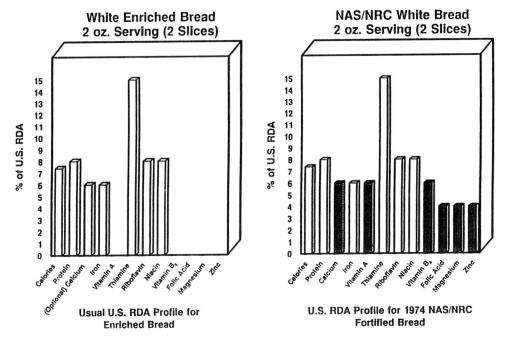

Fig. 3. The percent US RDI nutrient contribution of two slices of enriched bread compared to nutritive values if the 1974 Food and Nutrition Board recommendations had been adopted. Concern for the incidence of neural tube defect incidence has led to the policy recommendation that folic acid be added to wheat and corn products as part of the Standard of Identity in 1998. Restoration of nutrients should not require any justification.

acid is nontoxic. Intake in excess of 1 mg/d has been suggested, but not demonstrated, to possibly mask B-12 deficiency symptoms. This problem, if it exists, might be minimized by adopting a wider fortification policy for vitamin B-12! Even if a consumer were to ingest a multivitamin tablet daily containing 400 µg folic acid, the probability of exceeding 1 mg/d intake is low.

The first comprehensive overview of the science and technology of nutrient additions to food and the delivery of nutrients though formulated and fabricated food systems was published in 1991 *(44)*. Although the science of nutrition has many gaps in its knowledge, as does food science, the technology of nutrition and food technology has evolved because of the need for practical solutions in spite of the gaps in basic science. With small steps in science, technology is able to take giant leaps because science-based ideas become plausible inventions and advances. A major argument opposing food nutrification has been that insufficient science is available to justify the practice. Imagine where the world would be if we applied such an argument in all fields of technical endeavor.

Food delivery systems of various types were established and evolved long before food as a nutrient delivery system was discovered. Currently, fabricated food systems have evolved both, with nutrient delivery (e.g., infant formula, medical foods) and without nutrient delivery (spun vegetable protein meat replacers, surimi seafood products) being a consideration. The most sophisticated practice of nutrification (a balanced array of nutrient additions to a food to assure complete sustenance) has occurred with the advances in infant formulas and medical foods. Chemically defined diet research led to enteral and parenteral preparations to meet specific metabolic diseases and situations of impaired gastrointestinal physiology and are also vital to rehabilitating nutritionally debilitated patients *(45)*.

10. NUTRIENT ADDITION TECHNOLOGY IS A MAJOR CONTRIBUTOR TO PREVENTIVE MEDICINE

The most common practice of nutrient additions to food has occurred with public health enrichment, restoration, and fortification practices. These practices were initially motivated by the presence of deficiency diseases and the need for intervention on a broad scale. The practice of improving the nutritional and health status of the population is collectively one of the greatest accomplishments in nutrition and preventive medicine and ranks among the milestones in the history of public health. Some form of public health nutrification is found in practically all countries, either as a matter of policy or as a component of military feeding and/or child nutrition programs. In these applications, nutrient addition is not tied to deficiency diseases and medical pathologies but to public health and performance considerations. Nutrient addition to food is an emerging technology in the issues of the nutrition needs of the elderly, the role of food in the quality of lifestyles, the role of "designer" (nutraceutical) foods *(46)* in cancer and other chronic disease prevention, and possibly the role of nutrients and other food ingredients in psychosocial and behavioral phenomena *(47)*.

11. THE FUTURE OF NUTRIENT ADDITION TECHNOLOGY

Nutrient addition food technology has its limitations and is not a panacea for all malnutrition situations. The future of the technology will depend on:

1. the continued ingenuity of food technologists in food fabrication;
2. the improved understanding of the interactions in nutrition among nutrients, other food ingredients, and drugs that alter human performance;
3. the continued open debate on the role and benefits of nutrification vis à vis education, safety, and alternative interventions;
4. continued dietary, biochemical, and clinical research; and
5. new advances in basic nutrition, particularly at the molecular level

12. SUMMARY/RECOMMENDATIONS

In summary, the question is not one of the benefits that can be derived from the practice of restoration, and if necessary, public health enrichment, nor the capability to process or manufacture such foods, but of determining which foods should benefit from nutrient addition, with which nutrients, and at what level. The public health goal must be to assure a balanced, and if possible, optimal nutrient intake without compromising the choice of foods and without fear of creating a nutrient safety problem because of indiscriminate use or inferior process control. Two concurrent nutrient addition rationales appear to be fully justified: The public health and product development policy of restoring nutrient levels in products to those nature has provided is a self-evident and safe practice to adopt and practice. We have more than 50 yr of very successful experience and benefit. Furthermore, all products that serve to meet the alternative of partial or full

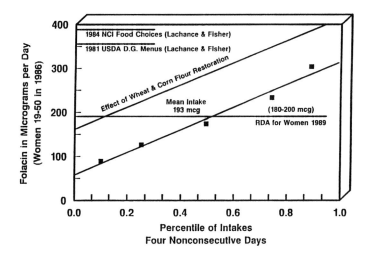

Fig. 4. The restoration of folic acid to wheat and corn cereal grain products would conservatively enhance the current intake of women 19–50-years of age by 100 μg/d. The mean intake would rise to approx 300 μg/d. Promotion of foods such as citrus and leafy green vegetables could also stimulate intakes of naturally occurring folates. Daily users of multivitamin supplements would gain an additional 400 μg/d. Folic acid is nontoxic. Vitamin B12 deficiency has not been demonstrated to be masked by folate intakes below 2 mg/d.

meal replacement should be nutrified with a balanced array of micronutrients complementing the protein contribution to the daily RDA/RDI. The minimal reference standard to assure the eradication of deficiency diseases and the thwarting of chronic degenerative diseases should be possible based on ideal dietary pattern of nominal foods.

REFERENCES

1. Clark FL. Human food habits as determining the basic patterns of economic and social life. In: Proceedings of the 7th international Congress of Nutrition, Vol. 4. Hamburg, 1966; pp. 18–24.
2. Jerome NW. American culture and food habits: communicating through food in the USA. In: Dimensions of Nutrition. Dupont J, ed. Boulder, CO: Associated University Press, 1970; 223–234.
3. Leininger M. Some cross-cultural universal and non-universal functions, beliefs and practices of food. In: Dimensions of Nutrition. Dupont J, ed. Boulder, CO: Associated University Press, 1970; 153–172.
4. Lachance PA. The role of cereal-grain products in the U.S. diet. Food Technology 1981; 35:49–58.
5. Sinclair U, The Jungle. 1906.
6. Lachance PA. Food production, processing, distribution and consumption. In: Nutrition Policy in Public Health. Bronner F, ed. New York: Springer Publishing Co. (in press).
7. Lachance PA. Human obesity—IFT Scientific Status Summary. Food Tech 1994; 48:127–138.
8. Christakis G. Nutrient influence on optimal health. In: Nutrient Additions to Food: Nutritional, Technological and Regulatory Aspects. Bauernfeind JC, Lachance PA, eds. Trumbull, CT: Food and Nutrition Press, 1991; 495–518.
9. Klesges RC, Isbell TR, Klesges LM. Relationship between dietary restraint, energy intake, physical activity, and body weight; a prospective analysis. J Abnorm Psychol 1992; 98:499–503.
10. Richardson D. Iron fortification of foods and drinks. Chem Industry 1983; 13:498–501.
11. Boussingault M. Memoir sur des salines iodiferes des Andes. Ann Chem Physique 1833; 54:163–177.
12. Lachance PA, Bauernfeind JC. Concepts and practices of nutrifying foods. In: Nutrient Additions to food: Nutritional, Technological and Regulatory Aspects. Bauernfeind JC, Lachance PA, eds. Trumbull, CT: Food and Nutrition Press, 1991; 19–86.

13. Fisher MC, Lachance PA. Nutrition evaluation of published weight-reducing diets. J Am Diet Assoc 1985; 85:450–454.
14. Ries CP, Kline K, Weaver SO. Impact of commercial eating on nutrient adequacy. J Am Diet Assoc 1987; 87:463–468.
15. Anonymous, Ready-to-eat foods usage tied to microwave ovens. Food Engineering International 1989; 14(8):23.
16. Lachance PA. Sorting out the confusion in the nutrition revolution era. Food Prod Dev 1974; 8(5): 63–69.
17. Moran R. Nutritional significance of recent work on wheat flour and bread. Nutr Abstracts Rev 1959; 29:1–10.
18. Anonymous. Wheat in human nutrition. Rome: Food and Agricultural Organization, 1970.
19. Cort WM, Borenstein B, Harley JH, et al. Nutrient stability of fortified cereal products. Food Technol 1976; 30:52–60.
20. Rubin SH, Emodi A, Scialpi L. Micronutrient addition—cereal grain products. Cereal Chem 1977; 54:895–904.
21. Emodi A, Scialpi L. Quality of bread fortified with ten micronutrients. Cereal Chem 1980; 57:1–3.
22. Food and Nutrition Board. Proposed fortification for cereal-grain products. Washington: National Academy of Sciences, 1974.
23. Mapson LW. The effects of processing on the vitamin content of foods. Brit Med Bull 1956; 12:73–77.
24. Adams CE, Erdman JW Jr. Effects of home preparation practices on nutrient content of foods. In: Nutritional Evaluation of Food Processing. New York: Karmas E, Harris RS, eds., Van Nostrand Reinhold, 1987; 557–605.
25. Bauernfeind JC. Foods considered for nutrient addition: fats and oils. In: Nutrient Addition to Foods: Nutritional, Technological and Regulatory Aspects. Bauernfeind JC, Lachance PA, eds. Trumbull, CT: Food and Nutrition Press, 1991; pp. 265–280.
26. DeRitter E. Foods considered for nutrient addition: dairy products. In: Nutrient Addition to Foods: Nutritional, Technological and Regulatory Aspects. Bauernfeind JC, Lachance PA, eds. Trumbull: Food and Nutrition Press, 1991; 367–394.
27. Anonymous. Enriching lives: overcoming vitamin and mineral malnutrition in developing countries. World Bank Publications, Philadelphia, PA, 1995; 88 pp.
28. Johnson C. Phase one of NHANES III. Obes Health 1993; 7:10 (abstract).
29. Food and Nutrition Board. Dietary supplements in Diet and Health: Implications for reducing chronic disease risk. Washington, DC: National Academy Press, 1989; 509–525.
30. Weisburger JH. Nutritional approach to cancer prevention with emphasis on vitamins, antioxidants, and carotenoids. Am J Clin Nutr 1991; 53S:226–237.
31. Block G, Langseth L. Antioxidant vitamins and disease prevention. Food Tech 1994; 48(7):80–84.
32. Lachance PA, Langseth L. The RDA concept: time for a change? Nutr Revs 1994; 52:266–270.
33. Bendich A. Folic acid prevention of neural tube defects: critical assessment of FDA proposals to increase folic acid intakes. J Nutr Ed 1994; 26:294–299.
34. Willett WC. Folic acid and neural tube defect: can't we come to closure? Am J Public Health 1992; 82:666–668.
35. Russell RM, Suter PM. Vitamin requirements of elderly people: an update. Am J Clin Nutr 1993; 51:358–361.
36. Lachance PA. Diet-health relationship. In: Food Safety Assessment. ACS Symposium Series # 484. Finely JW, Robinson SF, Armstrong DJ, eds. Washington, DC; American Chemical Society, 1992; 278–296.
37. Doll R. The lessons of life: keynote address to the nutrition and cancer conference. Cancer Res 1992; 52(Suppl 7): 2024–2029.
38. Borenstein B. Gordon HT. Addition of vitamins, minerals and amino acids to foods. In: Nutritional Evaluation of Food Processing. Karmas E, Harris RS, eds. New York: Van Nostrand Reinhold, 1987; 609–626.
39. Lachance PA. Nutritional responsibilities of food companies in the next century. Food Technol 1989; 43(4): 144–150.
40. Cook DA, Welsh SO. The effect of enriched and fortified grain products on nutrient intake. Cereal Foods World 1987; 23:191–196.
41. Bauernfeind JC, DeRitter E. Foods considered for nutrient addition: cereal grain products. In: Nutrition Addition to Foods: Nutritional, Technological and Regulatory Aspects. Bauernfeind JC, Lachance PA, eds. Trumbull: Food and Nutrition Press, 1991; pp. 143–210.
42. Lachance PA. Diet and health. In: Food Safety Assessment. Finley JW, Robinson SF, Armstrong DC, eds. Washington, DC: American Chemical Society, 1992; 484:278–296.

43. Block G, Subar A. Estimates of food intake from a food frequency questionnaire: the 1987 national health interview survey. J Am Dietetic Assoc 1992; 92:969–977.
44. Bauernfeind JC, Lachance PA, eds. Nutrient Addition to Foods: Nutritional, Technological and Regulatory Aspects. Trumbull, CT: Food and Nutrition Press, 1991; 622 pp.
45. Hagen RE, Thomas MR, Bushnell JJ. Foods considered for nutrient addition: formulated special purpose foods, In: Bauernfeind JC, Lachance PA, eds. Nutrient addition to foods: nutritional, technological and regulatory aspects. Trumbull, CT: Food and Nutrition Press, 1991; 395–432.
46. Ramarathnam N, Osawa T, Ochi H, Kawakishi S. The contribution of plant food antioxidants to human health. Trends Food Sci Tech 1995; 6:75–82.
47. Lachance PA. Recommended dietary allowances for growth, development and performance. Asia Pacific J Clin Nutr 1995; 4 (Suppl 1):7–12.

25 Nutrition and Food Policy in Norway

Effects on Reduction of Coronary Heart Disease

Kaare R. Norum, Lars Johansson,
Grete Botten, Gunn-Elin Aa. Bjørneboe,
and Arne Oshaug

1. THE EARLY HISTORY OF THE NORWEGIAN NUTRITION AND FOOD POLICY

Nutrition and food policy has a relatively long history in Norway. It started around 1930 when an official school breakfast was introduced for all children in primary schools [1]. At the same time the Norwegian Medical Association took the initiative to study the interrelation among income, nutrition, and health [2]. This issue created an intense debate in the society and both medical doctors and leading economists took part in the discussion. It is interesting that prominent economists, two of whom [3] later received Nobel Prizes, published papers on diet, nutrition, and income [3,4]. At the same time, the League of Nations raised the issue that it should be a collective duty of a society to take on the responsibility for a nutrition and food policy. In Norway, the General Director of Health, Karl Evang, strongly subscribed to that idea, arguing that the question of the citizen's diet was a national responsibility, demanding solutions through appropriate measures in many sectors in the society. The idea of prevention and health promotion as intersectorial work has since gradually gained support in our country and is now a platform in the newly formed health promotion policy. The establishment of a National Nutrition Council (NNC) in Norway in 1937 was closely related to development in the League of Nations. A specific task of the NNC was to create a nutrition and food policy that the government and Parliament could adopt.

The nutritional problems in Norway at that time were caused by poverty, and the measures in the nutrition policy were closely linked to stimulate economic growth and equal distribution. Nutritional information was also considered very important.

In 1939, a major initiative was taken in Norway to improve the nutritional status of the population, with the participation of the Ministries of Health, Agriculture, Fishery, and Trade. This initiative was mainly taken as means to prepare the population for difficulties if Norway were to be involved in the war in Europe.

During World War II, 1940–1945, when the national food supplies were scarce, few negative nutritional effects were observed in the adult population. On the contrary, mortality from coronary heart disease (CHD) decreased [5].

From: *Preventive Nutrition: The Comprehensive Guide for Health Professionals*
Edited by A. Bendich and R. J. Deckelbaum Humana Press Inc., Totowa, NJ

The idea behind the establishment of the Food and Agricultural Organization of the United Nations (FAO) after World War II in 1945 was a "marriage" between food production and health promotion through better nutrition. FAO requested each of its member nations to establish a nutrition council that should prepare and coordinate implementation of an intersectorial food and nutrition policy. Karl Evang played an important role in the planning of FAO, and when he was back in Norway after the war, he organized in 1946 a reestablishment and strengthening of the NNC, within the Ministry of Health and Social Affairs. In other FAO member countries similar councils were organized within the Ministries of Agriculture, and the link to health promotion was less obvious.

The NNC has, since it was reorganized in 1946, always had a task to give advice to the government concerning nutrition and dietary issues; i.e., formulate recommended dietary allowances and guidelines on fortification of food with vitamins and other micronutrients. The fortification policy has been very restrictive. The main fortification has been adding vitamins A and D to margarine (in recent years also to butter), iodine to salt, and iron to brown cheese and some infant food. Flour and milk are not fortified. However, production of flour for bread is regulated so that the extraction rate has to be higher than 78% in white flour.

Until around 1950 the main challenges for the Norwegian nutrition and food policy were to ensure enough food for all people. After 1950, however, the dietary problems changed in character. The country's economy became much better, and the market flourished with foods. People could now eat the formerly recommended energy-rich food in abundance, and no one expected that this could create health problems. After years of food rationing, plentiful food came on the market. Problems connected with overnutrition and unbalanced diet became more prevalent. There was a substantial increase in mortality from CHD (6), an increase that was associated with changes in food habits and lifestyle. The responsibility for the society to address this problem became more obvious. The General Director of Health set down an expert committee to give him advice. This resulted in an official Norwegian report on the relationship between dietary fat and cardiovascular disease. The experts recommended a decrease in the fat content of the national diet to 30% of dietary energy, mainly by reducing the intake of saturated fat (7). The report formed a basis for subsequent work, with the formulation of an official integrated Norwegian nutrition and food policy. However, it took quite some time before this new nutritional challenge became an important target in an official nutrition and food policy.

2. THE STRUGGLE FOR INTRODUCING NEW RECOMMENDATIONS IN GOVERNMENT POLICIES

As the suggested relationship between diet and CHD gradually gained acceptance, the NNC made several attempts to influence government policy goals in line with the new knowledge. The major effort was a suggestion to the Directorate of Health in 1964 to prepare a white paper on nutrition policy. The proposal gained no political support.

Toward the end of the 1960s, the NNC redefined its approach to a more politically oriented strategy, seeking support among Parliamentary members. By lobbying, the NNC members persuaded members of the Parliament to make use of their opportunities to question ministers (Cabinet members) directly in the Parliament about diet and health. Also, consumer interests and concern with food and health were growing. This brought nutritional issues to the attention not only of the Parliamentary members and ministers, but also of the media and the general public.

In 1970, NNC launched an expert seminar that resulted in a report discussing the various aspects of an integrated approach to health and agriculture. The seminar was followed up in 1971 by a nutrition policy conference, sponsored by the agricultural organizations and the food industry. Selected Parliamentary members and Cabinet ministers were invited, along with nutritional experts, the press, and representatives and experts selected by the sponsoring institutions.

These efforts brought considerable attention to the issues of nutrition, health, and agriculture. Yet, they were not sufficient in creating actual changes at a policy level. Until 1973, the main actors responsible for the nutrition policy, the Ministry of Social Affairs and the Directorate of Health, still were rather passive, and made no explicit effort to bring about policy changes. Parallel to the increased attention on nutritional issues, a concern about agricultural policy was growing both at the political and popular level. There was a fear that the support for the most peripheral rural areas would decrease as a result of the economic cost of having agricultural production in remote areas.

3. THE FIRST WHITE PAPER ON NUTRITION AND FOOD POLICY

At the FAO/WHO World Food Conference in Rome in 1974, it was again stated that each nation should have a nutrition and food policy. The Norwegian delegation at the conference was headed by the Minister of Agriculture, Torstein Treholt. He stated in his main address to the conference that the industrialized countries should also formulate a nutrition policy. When he returned to Norway, he took the initiative to formulate a Norwegian nutrition and food policy. A white paper was presented to the Parliament through Report No. 32 (1975–1976) "On Norwegian nutrition and food policy" from the Ministry of Agriculture *(8)*. The goals and considerations that this policy should coordinate may be summed up in the following four major objectives:

1. Healthy dietary habits should be encouraged.
2. A nutrition and food policy should be formulated in accordance with the recommendations of the World Food Conference.
3. For reasons connected with the question of supply, the policy should aim at increased production and consumption of domestic food and at strengthening the ability to increase rapidly the degree of self-sufficiency in the food supply.
4. For regional policy reasons the highest priority should be placed on utilizing the food production resources in the economically weaker areas.

Furthermore, it was stated that a primary task of the nutrition and food policy was considered to be an *active coordination* of these four major goals.

3.1. Objective 1

The Government said in 1975 that:

The relationship between diet and health, for instance between diet and cardiovascular diseases, is not yet entirely understood. However, there is sufficient knowledge of this relationship to recommend alterations in the diet which are desirable from the point of view of preventing these diseases.

The aforementioned unfavorable health tendencies, particularly in respect of cardiovascular diseases, as well as the gradual understanding that is being gained of the connection between nutrition and health, make it necessary for the Government to base itself on expert recommendations, issued by the National Nutrition Council, when planning Norwegian nutrition and food policy.

The Government will prepare a policy which will contribute to the following:

- *The beneficial aspects of the diet are to be preserved. Conditions will be arranged so that the diet is better adapted to nutritional requirements, while general demands for taste, variety and diversity are stressed. The different nutritional requirements of special groups such as children and young people, pregnant and breastfeeding mothers, the elderly, etc. must also be taken into consideration.*
- *In order to obtain a better adaptation of the diet to nutritional requirements it is especially important to curtail the proportion of fat in the energy supply. An objective should be to reduce the proportion of fat to 35% of the energy supply through a gradual alteration of the diet.*
- *The decrease in the supply of fat should be replaced by foods containing starch—primarily cereals and potatoes. There should be an attempt to limit the proportion of sugar in the energy supply.*
- *The proportion of polyunsaturated fatty acids in the total fat intake should be increased.*

It should be noted that the goal for the average fat consumption in the Policy Document was 35% energy, whereas the NNC had advocated for 30%. The official goal was a compromise between the NNC and the agricultural lobby who feared that a lower fat target would lead to a reduced consumption of meat and dairy products.

In this first white paper it was pointed out that the central question was which **means** were to be taken to influence the production and consumption of food products in accordance with the objectives of the policy. Emphasis was put on collaboration among the public sector; the organizations, enterprises, and employees in the relevant economic sectors; the voluntary organizations; and the various categories of households. In particular, the information/education/training measures were emphasized, aiming at motivating people to adopt better dietary habits, securing a broad general knowledge of the main principles of a nutritionally healthy diet, and providing the possibility to acquiring the necessary skills (8).

The means used have thus addressed a wide range of areas, such as public and professional education and information (at universities, for teachers, adult education, mass media, consumer organization media, conferences, and meetings with primary schools and professional groups); setting of consumer and producer price and income subsidies jointly in nutritionally justifiable ways; the adjustment of absolute and relative consumer food price subsidies; the ensurance of low prices for food grain, skimmed and low fat milk, vegetables, and potatoes; the avoidance of low prices for sugar, butter, and margarine; the marking of regulations to promote provision of healthy foods by retail stores, street vendors, and institutions; and the regulation of food processing and labeling.

The NNC was and still is responsible for the follow-up of national nutrition and food policy. It did not have any decentralized organization to instruct, and funds and staff were limited. In implementing activities, cooperation with other sectors and organizations was important. NNC took responsibility for contact with the school system, the health sector, the local food control authority, the consumer organizations, NGOs/voluntary organizations, the food industry, food retailers and wholesalers, and mass media.

The NNC had regular meetings with major companies in the food industry, organizations dealing with restaurants and institutional catering, politicians, and the mass media. The NNC focused on providing such services as distributing printed material, giving lectures, arranging seminars, and stimulating activities by providing funds for information and public education campaigns and new methods for health promotion at the municipal level.

One of the successes of the Norwegian food and nutrition policy was the information and public education done by the NNC, especially by the use of programs on the national public television, and nationwide, long-lasting nutrition campaigns.

Higher training or education at the university level was also important. The Nordic School of Nutrition, University of Oslo, has trained nutritionists since 1965, and by 1990 almost 500 nutritionists from the Nordic countries had graduated. More than two-thirds are Norwegian, of whom about 20% specialized in clinical nutrition (9). They form a cadre of professionals who are working in many different organizations and at different levels, being key in the implementation of many nutrition-related activities.

The development in the Medical Faculty, University of Oslo, where in the early 1970s nutrition education was virtually nonexistent, has also been important. Nutrition as a subject developed first as an elective, then later as a compulsory course, where students were exposed to nutrition as an area of applied biochemistry and physiology with some lectures including diet, clinical nutrition, and nutrition policy. In 1990, the teachers running the course also produced a tailor-made textbook for nutrition in medical training (10). The wide contact the medical doctors have with the public, their role in preventive and curative health work, and the status they have in peoples' minds make them important nutrition communicators.

Two other projects in the health sector were of great importance for implementation of the nutrition policy. First, the "Oslo Study," a randomized prospective study, showed that a change in diet reduced CHD in middle aged men with initially high blood cholesterol levels (11). The men in the treatment group reduced their saturated fat intake, which led to a 10% reduction in their blood cholesterol level, whereas the control group did not get any dietary advice, and their blood cholesterol level remained unchanged. After 5 yr the coronary incidence in the treatment group was only half of that in the control group. The results of the "Oslo Study" convinced both the population and the politicians of the importance of changing to a more lean diet. Second, the National Health Screening Service has been and still is conducting health surveys in all parts of Norway (12). All inhabitants 40 yr of age are offered a health examination, including measurement of blood lipids, blood pressure, and chest X-ray. Persons with high-risk factors for CHD are referred to the local health authorities for follow-up. The health surveys are done with 2–3 yr interval and have given valuable information on CHD risk factors, body mass index, and other health parameters in different parts of Norway, and have documented changes in these parameters during the period the country has had an active nutrition policy (13).

3.2. Objective 2

In 1975 the Government said:

Taking the recommendations from the World Food Conference as a starting point, it would be right to view the nutrition and food policy in relation to the global situation as regards production and supplies. As part of solving the world's food problems, the developed countries were recommended to increase their food production and to implement measures for improving their own pattern of consumption. Such measures must, however, make allowances for the developing countries' trade interests as promoted through international organizations.

The means used to achieve this include earmarking emergency grain in Norway, provision of aid and support to poor countries, support to UN agencies by contributing to the World Food Program, and increased trade with poor countries. In 1991, about the equivalent of 32 million US dollars was granted for multilateral food aid, in addition to humanitarian food assistance channeled through NGOs *(9)*.

3.3. Objectives 3 and 4

The Norwegian government encouraged farmers to increase production of food grain, potatoes, vegetables, and low-fat milk. Measures were introduced to stabilize milk and meat production to avoid overproduction. In collaboration with farmer's organizations it was tried to produce more grass-fed than grain-fed beef. Furthermore, the pork produced was less fatty than before. A new system to market potatoes and improve their quality has been established.

Furthermore, there has been an integration of support, such as support to fisheries and to fodder production for dairy cattle in northern mountain areas and in remote regions; encouragement of wheat production and discouragement of dairy production in the southern part of the country, provision of transport and other subsidies to retailers in outlying regions; and an integration of agriculture and food policy with other economic planning initiatives.

The link between the food policy and district policy is a reflection of an official policy in Norway for the last 50 yr: support to remote areas of the country in order to diminish migration to centers and cities. This district policy has also been part of the Norwegian defense policy.

In 1982 the government presented a follow-up white paper; Report No. 11 (1981–1982) "On the Follow-Up of Norwegian Nutrition Policy" *(14)*. This time the Ministry of Health and Social Affairs was responsible for the report. Note that the word "Food" was taken out of the title. This was a sign that the policy regarded health as a more important issue compared to agriculture. In 1993, the Nutrition and Food Policy was integrated in Report No. 37 (1992–1993) "Challenges in Health Promotion and Prevention Strategies" *(15)*, which brought nutrition even closer to health, and now with an emphasis on nutrition's role in health promotion. These three white papers define the nutritional goals to be achieved for Norway and the measures that the government intends to employ to improve the Norwegian diet. In all three reports it is underlined that dietary changes should be voluntary. Although it will remain entirely an individual decision what to eat, it is a public and community responsibility to ensure that the circumstances are as good as possible to enable the person to choose a nutritionally favorable diet.

4. RESISTANCE AGAINST THE NUTRITION AND FOOD POLICY

The progress in implementing the nutrition policy was low the first years after its approval by the Parliament in 1976. Two main reasons were that the dairy and meat industries were against the policy, and that the Nutrition Council had little power and political influence.

The dairy industry tried to counteract the policy by inviting foreign experts who claimed that milk, butter, and other dairy products had no influence on risk factors for CHD, and that, therefore, the Norwegian nutrition policy was built on false premises. This led to a survey among leading scientists in the field of atherosclerosis and lipid metabolism *(16)*. The survey clearly showed that the Norwegian nutrition policy was built on a solid scientific basis. (Interestingly, this survey came to play an important role in the US Congressional hearings March 23, 1977 on McGovern's document on dietary goals for the United States.)

The NNC tried to get the dairy industry to produce a low-fat milk for the Norwegian market, but the dairy industry resisted. However, after NNC had organized a successful consumer-based campaign for consumption of skimmed milk instead of whole milk, the dairy industry gave in, and in collaboration with NNC a low-fat milk was introduced in 1984. Since then there has mainly been good collaboration between NNC and the dairy industry, which has gradually produced several low-fat dairy products.

The Norwegian nutrition and food policy also has internal conflicts. Thus, the objective to increase local food production led to more Norwegian wheat for human consumption. However, Norwegian grain was more expensive than wheat on the international market, and simultaneously with an official campaign to eat more cereals, the bread got more expensive!

The first white paper on nutrition and food policy gave two official agencies the task to coordinate the implementation of the nutrition policy: the NNC and the Inter-Ministerial Coordinating Committee on Nutrition (IMC). The latter was formed in order to coordinate all political sectors involved in the nutrition and food policy. The IMC was supposed to be chaired by the Deputy Minister of Health and Social Affairs and to consist of leading civil servants from nine ministries. However, IMC never worked as planned, probably because of competing priorities among the different ministries. The inactivity of IMC at first also deactivated the NNC, rendering it a body with a lot of good intentions but with little power and political influence. Later, however, because the inactivity of IMC, the NNC itself took direct political contact with the Government and members of the Parliament. Thus, gradually NNC gained both power and political influence.

5. SOME RESULTS OF THE NORWEGIAN NUTRITION AND FOOD POLICY

Public surveys have revealed that the knowledge of food, diet, nutrition, and health has increased in the Norwegian population in the last 15 yr. Furthermore, these surveys have shown that the attitudes concerning healthy dietary habits have been more positive in the last 15 yr. These changes in knowledge and attitude are reflected in a change in the diet of the population (*see* Tables 1 and 2).

Dietary data are obtained from the annual reports of the NNC presenting food consumption data based on wholesale figures, and from the household consumption sur-

Table 1
Food Consumption at Wholesale Level. Kg/Person/Yr

Food	1970	1975	1980	1985	1990	1993
Cereals	71	75	80	75	79	81
Potatoes, unrefined[a]	79	71	60	63	51	48
Potatoes, refined[b]	7	8	12	17	19	23
Vegetables	40	37	51	47	55	58
Fruits	67	74	75	85	72	81
Meat	43	52	55	54	54	59
Egg	10	10	11	13	11	11
Fish, approximate[c]	30	35	—	—	40	40
Whole milk, 3.8%	172	169	164	124	56	50
Low-fat milk, 1.5%	—	—	—	28	84	85
Skimmed milk, 0.1%	14	26	28	30	31	29
Cheese	9	10	12	13	13	14
Cream	6.7	6.7	7.1	6.7	6.8	6.7
Butter	5.4	4.7	5.6	4.8	3.3	3.1
Margarine, total	19	18	16	14	13	14
Low fat margarine	0	0	0	0.2	2.4	2.7
Oil and other fats[d]	4.4	4.2	4.7	4.1	4.0	3.9
Sugar, syrup, honey, and so forth	42	32	43	42	41	43

[a]Potatoes not for industrial uses.
[b]Potatoes used to produce potato products.
[c]Figures for fish consumption are only approximate.
[d]Includes cooking oils, cooking fats, and fat used in food manufacturing for mayonnaise, salads, chocolate, biscuits, and so forth.
Source: Norwegian Nutrition Council

veys published by the Norwegian National Bureau of Statistics, which provide figures concerning food entering the household. Although figures are somewhat uncertain for some food groups i.e., fish, they nevertheless provide a basis on which to draw certain conclusions regarding development in food consumption during the last 20 yr (Table 1).

The consumption of cereal products showed a positive trend up to the beginning of the 1980s. After a decrease for some years the consumption has again increased in the last few years. The consumption of wholemeal flour has risen in recent years, and now comprises about 21% of total sales compared to 17% in 1975. The proportion of cereals of Norwegian origin have risen considerably, flour milled from Norwegian cereals comprising approx 30% of total flour consumption, whereas in 1975 not a single grain produced in Norway was consumed by humans, only by domestic animals.

The total milk consumption has decreased. From 1970 to 1985, the consumption of skimmed milk rose, and the use of whole milk decreased. After an initiative from the NNC, the Norwegian Dairies introduced a partially skimmed milk (low-fat milk) with a fat content of 1.5% into the Norwegian market in 1984. This milk now has a considerable share of the market compared with whole milk and skimmed milk. The consumption of cream has remained at a stable level, but the consumption of cheese has increased. Milk and other dairy products are still the major sources of saturated fat in the Norwegian diet. NNC advocated that partially skimmed milk should replace whole

Table 2
Dietary Energy and Energy-Providing Nutrients at Wholesale Level/Person/D

Nutrient	1970	1975	1980	1985	1990	1993
Energy, kcal	2860	2900	3170	3020	2910	2980
Protein, g	85	86	94	94	94	96
Fat, g	126	129	135	122	111	112
Carbohydrate total, g	352	345	390	378	377	392
Starch, g	185	174	185	174	177	185
Sugar, g	115	91	120	118	118	122
Dietary fiber, g		21	23	24	22	23
Percentage distribution of energy						
Protein	12	12	12	13	13	13
Fat	39	40	38	35	35	34
Carbohydrate[a]	49(16)	48(13)	50(15)	51(16)	52(16)	53(17)

[a]Values in parentheses are % energy from sugar.
Source: Norwegian Nutrition Council

milk in school milk programs. In 1984 most of the school milk was whole milk, but in 1993 most of it was replaced by low-fat milk and skimmed milk.

Consumption of fruit and vegetables has increased over a long period. Norwegian-produced vegetables make up 70% of total consumption of vegetables, whereas import comprises about 70% of the total amount of fruit consumed. The consumption of potatoes has decreased, but the share of processed potato products is increasing. Potatoes as raw materials for further processing now comprise about 30% of all potato sales, compared to 10% in 1975. In particular, the sale of potato chips has increased.

Meat consumption has increased considerably. However, the meat produced contains less fat than before. The basis for estimation of fish consumption is uncertain, but is estimated to about 40 kg/person/yr.

The consumption of edible fat has dropped steadily over several years. The decrease has been a result of reduced consumption of margarine and butter. The proportion of soft margarine (i.e., with a relatively large content of vegetable oils) has increased and now makes up 56% of total margarine consumption compared to 42% in 1979. The consumption of low-fat margarine has increased.

Calculations based on wholesale figures and consumer consumption surveys show that the energy of fat in the diet increased from about 20% in 1900 to 40% in 1975 (17). Now it has decreased to 34% of energy of fat (Table 2).

The dietary fatty acid pattern has changed the last 20 yr, with less saturated and trans-fatty acids and relatively more unsaturated fatty acids (17). The dietary content of cholesterol/1000 kcal increased from below 100 mg in the beginning of the century up to 180 mg at 1950, and later decreased to approx 150 mg/1000 kcal (17).

The main changes in Norwegian nutrition from 1975–1993 have been a reduction of fat, mainly because of a reduction in saturated fat, and an increase in consumption of vegetables, fruits, and cereals. Concomitantly with these changes the surveys done by the National Health Screening Service have shown that blood cholesterol has decreased by about 10% in the Norwegian population (13). These changes are reflected in a large reduction in the mortality as a result of CHD among middle-aged men and women (Fig. 1).

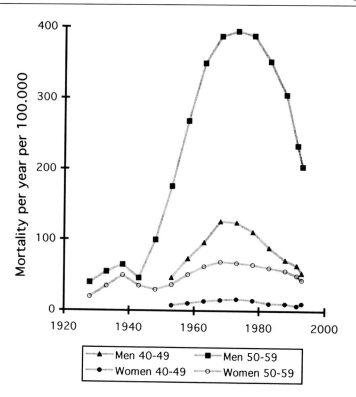

Fig. 1. Mortality from CHD in Norway. The data are compiled from the Norwegian National Bureau of Statistics.

The nutrition policy in Norway from 1975–1990 was to a large extent aimed at a reduction in premature CHD. This goal has to some extent been obtained, and the nutrition policy of today has, therefore, been somewhat changed compared to what was formulated in 1975.

6. THE NUTRITION AND FOOD POLICY IN NORWAY OF TODAY

In Report No. 37 to the Storting (1992–1993) "Challenges in Health Promotion and Prevention Strategies" *(15)*, the Nutrition and Food Policy is integrated into the Health policy. The Policy is based on the experiences gained during the follow-up of the preceding Parliamentary white papers. The current Norwegian Nutrition and Food Policy has the following four main goals:

1. To reduce the prevalence of dietary-related diseases and damage to health in the population. To ensure such a reduction the government intends to implement a policy that will support the following main objectives:

   - A national diet in line with the recommendations of the NNC.
   - Breast-feeding of babies continuing at a high level.
   - Reducing the nutrition-related differences in health status in the population,
   - Integrating dietary treatment in primary and secondary prevention of diet-related diseases within the health services.

The goals deal with both the national diet, including that of infants, the present inequality in health, especially cardiovascular diseases, and ways to change approaches within the health services. Special emphasis should be placed on changes in food consumption so it fulfills the following nutritional goals, which are in line with the present recommendations given by the NNC:

- Reducing the proportion of energy in the diet from fat to 30% by lowering the proportion of saturated fat.
- Increasing the fiber content of the diet to 25 g/person/d by increasing the consumption of cereals, potatoes, vegetables, and fruit.
- Having sugar contribute no more than 10% of the energy.
- Reducing salt intake to 5 g/person/day.
- Increasing consumption of fish.
- Promoting dairy products, meat, and meat products with lower fat content.
- Reducing consumption of butter, hard margarine, high fat potato products, and snacks.
- Avoiding frequent intake of grilled, fried, smoked, or salted foods.

2. To ensure food safety. The policy shall facilitate the following objectives:

- That foods are free of infectious agents and do not contain approved food additives in quantities that are a risk to health.
- That consumer demands for food quality, safety, and security are met. Special emphasis should be placed on improving the mapping, monitoring, and warning systems for food-borne diseases. Included in this part of the policy is ensuring that the water supply satisfies the quality requirements laid down by the Norwegian authorities.

3. To strengthen consumers' influence on the Nutrition and Food Policy, the government will ensure that consumers have a real possibility of providing themselves with a health-promoting diet. In order to maintain this, a consumer policy that stimulates a health-promoting diet through differential prices, food availability, food labeling/claims, and information and marketing will be implemented.

4. To contribute to safe production, distribution, and marketing of food products and to safe consumption patterns in terms of health, the environment, and appropriate use of resources. Food production shall satisfy society's requirements for safe and ethical acceptable norms and allow for protection of animals and plants, genetic resources, and environmental resources. This aspect of the nutrition and food policy is an adjustment to sustainable development, meaning that production should be ecologically sustainable on a long-term basis. This links the modern nutrition and food policy to international work for environmental protection and human rights for food and health. In this respect, it is appropriate to quote the following recommendations regarding food production from The Brundtland Commission: "The industrialized countries must reduce overproduction of agricultural products, so that world market prices will reflect the real production costs. In the short-term this implies higher costs for food importing from developing countries. But it will mean a real stimulus to increase production in developing countries" *(18)*.

Traditionally, the Norwegian nutrition and food policy has been linked to the world food situation. This is also the case today. At the International Nutrition Conference held in Rome, December 1992, a declaration and a plan of action were approved *(19)*.

The primary objectives are to eliminate famine and to reduce, as much as possible, the prevalence of disease and suffering caused by hunger and malnutrition. At the national level, it was expected that each country should prepare a plan of action by the end of 1994. Based on the objectives in the plan of action, the Ministry of Health and Social Affairs emphasized the need to strengthen cooperation between ministries and subordinate bodies as well as between local and central levels, the private sector, and other relevant agencies *(15)*.

7. GOVERNMENTAL IMPLEMENTATION BODIES

At the ministerial level two official bodies are given the responsibility to coordinate the implementation of the Nutrition and Food Policy: The National Food Control Authority and The National Nutrition Council. The Inter-Ministerial Coordinating Committee on Nutrition mentioned earlier did not fulfill its intentions and has been abandoned from the current nutrition policy.

The National Food Control Authority was established in 1988 in order to administer legislation related to food. It is responsible for coordinating and guiding the executive control system, which consists of 82 local food control authorities covering all municipalities in Norway. These local food control offices are responsible for inspecting production, import, storage, and transport of food. During the last few years the work of some local food control authorities has been strengthened and involved itself in broader nutritional work in collaboration with the local health services.

The National Nutrition Council was established in 1937 and reorganized in 1946. The Council is today an expert body consisting of 23 members and 10 employees. Competence in nutritional biology, clinical nutrition, epidemiology, agricultural economy, community nutrition, and nutrition policy is represented in the expert body, which cooperates closely with research institutions. The mandate for the Nutrition Council is:

- Be an advisory body to Ministries and others in matters concerning food supply and nutrition.
- Describe and evaluate the nutritional situation in Norway.
- Propose new strategies and measures in order to reach nutritional goals.
- Give assistance and proposals to research councils and research institutions.
- Contribute in promoting and coordinating professional work on diet and nutrition, nationally and internationally.
- Be actively engaged in nutrition education and ensure that public information on nutrition is according to recommendations.

One important task for the Council is the formulation of the Norwegian dietary guidelines. Such guidelines were first published in 1954, have been the theoretical basis for nutrition-related health promotion, and incorporated as the scientific basis in the Nutrition and Food Policy. The latest revised guidelines (from 1989) have been prepared in cooperation with the other Nordic countries *(20)*.

During the last few years the administration of the Council has been strengthened from being a small secretariat to an efficient administrative body with broad nutritional knowledge, operating in close contact both with the Ministry of Health and with the Council and its members. This has been very important in order to enable the NNC to implement and coordinate nutrition-related activities in many different sectors of the society. An intersectorial approach is one of the most important elements in the Norwegian nutrition and food policy.

8. IMPORTANT CHARACTERISTICS OF THE NUTRITION AND FOOD POLICY AND ITS IMPLEMENTATION

A basis for the policy is an agreement on the idea that many factors affect the diet and the prevalence of diet-related health problems. Of major importance for the implementation of the Norwegian nutrition and food policy is the consensus achieved about the goals and the strategies of the policy. This has been achieved by forming the goals of the policy on a scientific basis and by stimulating scientists to participate in the implementation of the policy. As a consequence, the message given to the public has been consistent, whether voluntary organizations or public agencies have submitted the message. The Norwegian experience has shown that the content of a strategy intended to influence the diet in a desired direction should define:

1. The Goal. The strategic effort must be expressed generally and in terms of principle. Thematically, the objective can be linked to reduced risk of disease, better growth and development, more optimal supply of nutrients, or a healthier diet in general. The target groups should be identified.
2. The Measures. These may be implemented in a number of arenas. Often, several arenas will be used simultaneously in a total effort to achieve the goals. Where to invest the efforts depends on knowledge of nutrition problems in the population. Epidemiological surveys are required to provide information on relevant conditions. It is particularly important to identify groups that may be more susceptible than the population in general. The monitoring of the Norwegian nutrition and food situation has been strengthened considerably through several nation-wide nutrition surveys and screening programs.

It is important to encourage the sale of healthy food. The NNC has worked to influence consumers' choices by information and advice through various communication channels. The goal has been to influence what consumers purchase by, e.g., adequate labeling, marketing, and by changing the relative prices and the availability of different foods. Cooperation with manufacturers and merchants has been important during this process.

The strategies for disease prevention and health promotion are often grouped into mass strategies, target group strategies and high-risk group strategies. The mass strategy involves the whole population. Several long-lasting nation-wide campaigns have been important elements of the mass strategy initiated by the NNC. In these campaigns the public radio and television have been frequently used to give information about how to prepare and consume a healthy and low-fat diet. In target group strategies the focus has been directed at various groups of the population e.g., school children, infants, and immigrants. The national high-risk strategies have been based on screening of large groups of the adult population to identify persons at high-risk for nutrition-related disorders, and then introducing measures directly specifically toward the identified individuals (12,13).

The choice of strategy includes identifying the arena for intervention. Relevant arenas include public services, especially the health and social welfare services, including the curative and preventive health services. Organizations, such as governmental organizations, employer's and employee's organizations, and the various nongovernmental organizations, have been major contributors in the work to promote health through a better nutrition. The food industry has also been of major importance, and the retailers are relevant arenas for strategic nutritional work.

9. CONCLUDING REMARKS

In our opinion the official nutrition and food policy white papers *(8,14,15)* have been very useful strategic documents in the efforts to improve public health in Norway the last 20 yr, as documented above. The NNC has played an important role in the implementation by formulating a consistent and scientific basis for the policy. The council has often been consulted in connection with widespread efforts in various sectors, the health sector included, and has formed premises for various political decisions.

We have learned a lot about forming and carrying out a nutrition and food policy:

- It takes time to get politicians interested in the issue. In order to get a comprehensive policy, the government needs to develop a policy that has broad political support and is not subject to changes linked to specific governments in power.
- A nutrition and food policy must address both problems related to inequality and lack of food (malnutrition), as well as cardiovascular diseases and other health problems related to too much food and changes in lifestyle (overnutrition).
- The nutrition message to the public must be scientifically based, consistent, credible, and relevant for the target groups of the population. It must be practical and easy to understand.
- An effective administrative body (e.g., a nutrition council) and a strong secretariat are needed so that it is clear who has the daily responsibility to implement the policy.
- The Nutrition Council must report to the Ministry in charge and the Parliament at regular intervals.
- The members of the Nutrition Council should be independent experts in nutrition, diet, and health with broad experience.
- Cooperation between the Nutrition Council, NGO's, food industry, and other key actors is important.

Today, we can see several changes in Norwegian eating habits. The consumption of cereals, vegetables, fruit, and low-fat milk has increased. Furthermore, there has been a reduction in the intake of margarine, butter, and whole milk. This has led to a reduction of total fat from 40 to 34% of the food energy, mainly by a reduction of saturated fat. Concomitantly with the changes in the diet, there has been a reduction in the level of plasma cholesterol in the population, and a reduction in death from CHD. This reduction is nearly 50% in men aged 40–49 yr, and also substantial in other age groups and among women. It is most probable that the Norwegian nutrition and food policy has played an important role in changing dietary habits and, thus, contributed to the decline in heart disease.

REFERENCES

1. Natvig H. Textbook in Hygiene. Fabritius, Oslo. 1958; pp. 496–498.
2. Hertzberg G. Ernæring, helse, miljø (Nutrition, health and environment). Garnæs's Boktrykkeri, Bergen, 1934.
3. Frisch R, Haavelmo T. Etterspørslen etter melk i Norge (Demand for milk in Norway). Statsøkonomisk Tidsskr, 1938; pp. 1–62.

4. Wold KG. Kosthold og levestandard. En økonomisk undersøkelse (Nutrition and the Standard of living. An Economic Investigation). Fabritius, Oslo, 1941.
5. Strøm A, Jensen RA. Mortality from Circulatory Diseases in Norway 1940–45. Lancet 1950; I:126–129.
6. Central Bureau of Statistics. Health Statistics 1987. Central Bureau of Statistics, Oslo, 1987.
7. Nicolaysen, R, Eeg-Larsen N, Jervell A, Owren PA, Hjort PR, Eggen Øgrim M, Gran FC. Betenkning om forholdet mellom fett og hjerte-kar-sykdommer (Fat and coronary heart disease). Nasjonalforeningen for folkehelsen/Det Norske råd for hjerte- og karsykdommer, Oslo, 1963.
8. Ministry of Agriculture. Report No. 32 to the Storting (1975–76). On Norwegian nutrition and food policy. Royal Norwegian Ministry of Agriculture, Oslo, 1975.
9. Oshaug A. Nutrition Security in Norway? A Situation Analysis. Scand J Nutr 1994; 38:1S–68S.
10. Bjørneboe GE, Drevon CA, Norum KR, eds. Mat og medisin. Generell og klinisk ernæring (Food and medicine. General and clinical nutrition). Universitetsforlaget, Oslo, 1994; pp. 1–391.
11. Hjermann I, Holme I, Velve Byre K, Leren P. Effect of diet and smoking intervention on the incidence of coronary heart disease. Report from the Oslo Study Group of a randomized trial in healthy men. Lancet 1981; II:1303–1310.
12. Bjartveit K, Foss OP, Gjervig T, Lund-Larsen P. The cardiovascular disease study in Norwegian counties. Background and organization. Acta Med Scand 1979; 634:1–38.
13. Bjartveit K, Stensvold I, Lund-Larsen PG, Gjervig T, Krüger Ø, Urdal P. Hjerte- og karundersøkelser i norske fylker. Bakgrunn og gjennomføring. Status 1986–90 for risikomønster blant 40–42 åringer i 14 fylker (Coronary Heart Disease Surveys in Norwegian Counties). Tidsskr Nor Lægeforen 1991; 111:2063–2072.
14. Ministry of Health and Social Affairs. Report No. 11 to the Storting (1981–82). On the follow-up of Norwegian Nutrition Policy. Royal Norwegian Ministry of Health and Social Affairs, Oslo, 1981.
15. Ministry of Health and Social affairs. Utfordringer i helsefremmende og forebyggende arbeid (Challenges in health promoting and preventive work). Report No. 37 to the Storting (1992–93). Royal Norwegian Ministry of Health and Social Affairs, Oslo, 1993.
16. Norum KR. Some present concepts concerning diet and prevention of coronary heart disease. Nutr Metabol 1978; 22:1–7.
17. Johansson L, Drevon CA, Bjørneboe GE. The Norwegian diet during the last hundred years in relation to coronary heart disease. Eur J Clin Nutr 1996; 50:277–283.
18. World Commission on Environment and Development (The Brundtland Commission): Our Common Future. Palais Wilson, 52 Rue des Paquis, Geneve, 1987.
19. International Conference on Nutrition. World declaration and plan of action for nutrition. FAO and WHO, Rome, 1992.
20. Standing Nordic Committee on Food. Nordic Nutrition Recommendations. National Food Administration, Uppsala, Sweden, 1989.

26 Prevention of Pediatric Obesity

Examining the Issues and Forecasting Research Directions

Myles S. Faith, Angelo Pietrobelli, David B. Allison, and Steven B. Heymsfield

1. INTRODUCTION

The obesity community appears to be taking a strong stance on the prevention of childhood obesity. Unlike other issues for which there is less consensus, obesity and other health researchers appear to have placed obesity prevention at the top of the research agenda. Given the increasing prevalence of pediatric obesity in the United States and its pervasive health and economic costs *(1,2)*, various health organizations have clearly prioritized research to better understand the causes of obesity and to promote the development of innovate prevention strategies *(3,4)*. This interest is fortified by the health status objectives of Healthy People 2000 *(5)*, which calls for the prevalence of overweight among adolescents in the year 2000 not to exceed the 1976–1980 rate of 15% *(5)*.

Perhaps the loudest call to action has come from the National Institute of Diabetes and Digestive and Kidney Diseases' National Task Force on Prevention and Treatment of Obesity. In a recent position paper, this organization outlined five long-term goals, one of which was "the prevention of obesity" *(3)*. Furthermore, designating the prevention of obesity and its comorbidities "the most compelling new research need in the obesity field today" *(6)*, this organization called for the formation of an "Obesity Prevention Initiative" *(6)*. Other prominent organizations have also called for more research into the prevention of obesity, including the Institute of Medicine at the National Academy of Sciences *(4)*.

This chapter examines issues in the prevention of childhood obesity rather than adult obesity. Thus, prevention efforts, such as worksite programs or large-scale community efforts, except as they relate to the prevention of childhood obesity, are not included. Detailed discussions on these programs are available elsewhere *(7–9)*. The chapter is broadly divided into four sections. The first section discusses why the prevention of childhood obesity is a high priority. The second section reviews causal mechanisms of childhood obesity. The role of genetic and environmental factors is described, as well as their implications for the design and implementation of prevention programs. In the third section, existent programs for the prevention of childhood obesity and their clini-

From: *Preventive Nutrition: The Comprehensive Guide for Health Professionals*
Edited by A. Bendich and R. J. Deckelbaum Humana Press Inc., Totowa, NJ

cal efficacy are reviewed. Finally, more fundamental theoretical issues for future prevention research with children and adolescents are examined.

2. PRIORITIZING THE PREVENTION OF CHILDHOOD OBESITY

2.1. Increasing Prevalence of Childhood Obesity

Broadly speaking, obesity can be defined as an excess of adiposity. Although adipose tissue cannot be directly measured in living humans, various indirect measures are available for use among children and adolescents (10,11). These measures include the body mass index (BMI: weight in kg/height in m^2) and weight-for-stature indexes (12); skinfold measures (13); electrical bioimpedance analysis (13); and, recently, more sophisticated body composition techniques, such as dual-energy X-ray absorptiometry (13–15). More detailed descriptions of the advantages and limitations of these methodologies are provided elsewhere (10,11).

The most recent data on the prevalence of childhood obesity comes from the third National Health and Nutrition Examination Survey (NHANES-III), a nationally representative survey of the United States civilian noninstitutionalized population. Overweight was defined as any BMI score exceeding the 85th age- and sex-specific percentile, using 1960's scores as the reference comparison group (16,17). Using this definition, 22% of all children and adolescents measured between 1988 and 1991 were classified overweight. When defined as any BMI score exceeding the 95th percentile, 10.9% of the child and adolescent population was classified as overweight (18). Examining trends in the prevalence of overweight among children and adolescents during five time periods spanning from 1963–1991, these authors noted a substantial increase in the prevalence over this 17-yr period, with the greatest increases from the 1976–1980 period onward. For example, the age-adjusted prevalence of overweight among 6–11-yr-old girls was 15.8% between 1976 and 1980 (using the 85th percentile on BMI as the criterion), but 22.7% between 1988 and 1991 (18). Comparable rates for boys in this age range were 19.9 and 22.3%, respectively. Additional data are provided elsewhere (19).

Studies that have used skinfold measures to assess subcutaneous body fat have also documented an increased prevalence of childhood and adolescent obesity over the past several decades (20–22). Kuczmarski (21) traced changes in the median value of triceps skinfold thickness between 1963–1965 and 1976–1980. He noted a substantial increase in the median triceps skinfold measurement over time, particularly among males age 6–11 and females age 12–17. Changes were less notable for children younger than 6 yr old. Also noteworthy was the increasing skinfold thickness corresponding to the 95th percentile of the population. This increase was greatest for males age 6–11 yr.

Studies comparing prevalences of obesity among children from different ethnic groups were reviewed by Kumanyika (23). Several differences between ethnic groups have been detected and deserve consideration. For example, the greater prevalence of pediatric obesity among American Indians compared to other groups is of concern (24,25). Also noteworthy is the finding that the prevalence of obesity is increasing at a faster rate among Black than White 9–10-yr-old girls (26). Such findings might indicate subgroups of individuals in greater need of effective prevention programs.

3. COMORBIDITIES IN CHILDHOOD

The growing interest in prevention is also fueled by the mounting number of studies documenting the health risks of pediatric obesity. These risks include elevated blood pressure, glucose intolerance, hyperinsulinimia, and dyslipidemias, among others *(27)*.

3.1. Blood Pressure

Several studies have documented an association between adiposity and elevated blood pressure among pediatric and adult samples *(28–31)*. For example, the Muscatine Study of adolescents and young adults found that hypertension was twice as prevalent among overweight than normal weight subjects *(30)*. Another study examined data from over 3000 5–18-yr-old males and females *(31)* and found that fatness in excess of 25% in males and 30% in females was associated with increased risk for hypertension. Similar findings have also been noted among 5- and 6-yr old Hispanic children *(32)*. A recent study also found that, compared to nonobese adolescents, obese adolescents had greater cardiac mass and increased isovolumic relaxation time, indicative of increased heart work *(33)*.

3.2. Hyperinsulinemia and Glucose Intolerance

Body fatness is a reliable correlate of hyperinsulinemia and glucose intolerance among adolescent males and females *(34–38)*. It has been proposed that hyperinsulinemia may underlie the association of obesity, hypertension, and glucose intolerance *(39)*. Although most studies have used adult subjects, there are supportive data from pediatric samples *(37,40)*. To the extent that the model is accurate, possible mechanisms include increased sodium retention, stimulation of the central nervous system, and abnormal vascular regulation *(33)*.

3.3. Lipids and Lipoproteins

Pediatric obesity is associated with elevated levels of total cholesterol, low-density lipoprotein (LDL) cholesterol, and triglycerdes, and decreased levels of high-density lipoprotein (HDL) cholesterol *(41–44)*. Furthermore, there appears to be an association between central adiposity and adverse lipid profiles that is independent of total body fat *(45)*. This association is more pronounced among individuals who have already begun sexual development and have moderate to high levels of total body fat *(45)*. Other studies measuring body composition have obtained comparable findings regarding children's lipid profiles *(46,47)*.

3.4. Respiratory Abnormalities

In nonobese individuals, there is usually little fat deposition in the neck and in peripharynx regions. However, among adult obese subjects, increased neck adiposity has been associated with respiratory abnormalities, such as hyperventilation and obstructive apnea *(48)*. Similarly, increased neck adiposity is associated with respiratory abnormalities during sleep among pediatric samples. Examples of conditions that interfere with sleep include subclinical nocturnal desaturation, or decreased oxygen saturation (<90%) in red blood cells *(49)*, and adenoidal tonsillar hypertrophy *(50)*.

Subcutaneous adiposity at the chest and mediastinal levels limits activity of the thoracic cage, and when also associated with abdominal fat, can interfere with diaphragmic breathing *(50)*. Among adults, thoracic adiposity is associated with breathing difficulties during sleep *(51)*. These findings have been documented among pediatric subjects as well, and may partially explain why their respiratory performance is lower during rest and more pronounced during exercise *(50)*.

3.5. Pseudogynecomastia

Pseudogynecomastia is excessive deposition of fat in the chest and is particularly prevalent during adolescence. Although of minimal health risk, our clinical experience suggests that pseudogynecomastia has negative effects on body image among obese male adolescents. This issue is an important one in light of evidence that obesity is associated with body image dissatisfaction *(52,53)*.

3.6. Mortality

Finally, several longitudinal studies have assessed the long-term impact of childhood obesity on mortality and morbidity *(54–57)*. For example, Must and colleagues *(55)* used 55-yr follow-up data to evaluate the relative risks of mortality given obesity during adolescence. Among males, the relative risks for all-cause mortality and atherosclerostic cerebrovascular disease were 1.8 and 13.2, respectively. The effect of BMI during adolescence on all-cause mortality among males appeared to independent of adulthood BMI. Among females, however, the association between childhood obesity and adult mortality was not significant even after controlling for adult BMI. Such findings suggest that among males the health effects of childhood obesity may not be short-term and may persist into later life.

4. MECHANISMS OF CHILDHOOD OBESITY

4.1. Genetic Influences

It is said that the acorns do not fall far from the oak tree, implying that children grow up to be quite similar to their parents. Similarly, it is well-established that individuals within families tend to be similar with regard to their obtained degree of fatness. This within family similarity could be a result of either genetic influences or a shared common environment. Among animal breeders, it has long been known that selective breeding for fatness and leanness is possible, indicating a strong genetic influence on adiposity in domestic animals *(58)*. Among humans, there is also now substantial evidence that genetic factors exert a strong influence on adiposity *(59–61)*.

One of the earliest investigators to provide data in support of this assertion was Clark *(62)*, who evaluated a small sample of twins and showed that adiposity was correlated more strongly among monozygotic twins (identical; MZ) than dyzygotic twins (fraternal; DZ). However, it was not until the 1980s that genetic influences on human obesity became widely recognized. Probably the greatest influence on the developing interest on this topic was the work by Dr. Albert J. Stunkard and colleagues. Through a series of twin and adoption studies *(63–66)*, Stunkard and colleagues demonstrated that a substantial proportion of the variance in BMI was because of genetic variation. Since then, numerous other twin, family, and adoption studies have been conducted *(60)*. Collectively, these studies strongly suggest that at least 50% of the variation in BMI is a result of within-population genetic variation *(61)*. For reasons outlined elsewhere *(67)*, it is the opinion of the authors that approx 70% of the within population variation in BMI in 20th century developed countries is as result of genetic variation.

It is interesting to note the differences in heritability across the age span. Heritability is defined as the proportion of within-population phenotypic variance that results from within-population genotypic variance. The degree of heritability is relatively stable throughout the lifespan after age 4. However, prior to age 4, the heritability of BMI is somewhat lower *(68)*.

4.2. Environmental Influences

Understanding the genotypic influences on adiposity is important for numerous reasons. In the present context, it increases our understanding of the nature of environmental influences on obesity. It has been noted that BMI "tracks" throughout the lifespan *(69–71)*. In other words, people who tend to be fatter at one point in life tend to be fatter at another point in life. Similarly, people who tend to be thinner than average at one point in life tend to be thinner at another point in life. Put differently, it has been noted that obese children often grow up to be obese adults. This being the case, it has been suggested that if we could prevent childhood obesity then we will likely reduce the prevalence of adult obesity even if we exert no direct influence on the adult population. However, such an analysis assumes that the environmental influences on obesity at one point during the lifespan carry over to other points in the lifespan. This is an empirical question. Recently, several studies have addressed this issue *(68,72,73)*. These studies have generally found that although environmental influences are important, they are also transitory. In other words, the environment may have great influence on an individual's degree of adiposity at each point during the lifespan. However, these environmental effects do not persist with time. Thus, all of the tracking that is observed appears to be a result of the genotype, which exerts a constant influence on degree of adiposity throughout the lifespan. This being the case, it is doubtful that effective environmental interventions that promote childhood weight loss will persist into adulthood without sustained environmental change.

In regard to the effect of environmental influences on childhood obesity onset and maintenance, behavioral geneticists typically distinguish between shared (or common) and nonshared (or unique) environmental effects. Shared environmental effects include those aspects of the environment that are common to individuals raised in the same household, whereas nonshared environmental effects refer to those unique experiences that influence one family member but not another. Contrary to popular belief, numerous twin and adoption studies have documented that shared environmental effects have no significant effect on BMI or obesity *(61)*. On the other hand, nonshared environmental influences do have a significant effect on BMI and obesity and, according to most estimates, explain approx 30% of the total variance in BMI. Of course, the challenge for researchers is to identify these nonshared environmental effects and to explore their implications for prevention programs. However, because the effects of nonshared environmental influences do not seem to persist over time *(68)*, short-term environmental manipulations should have minimal effect on long-term weight loss.

Finally, it should be noted that several studies have identified some environmental correlates of pediatric obesity. First, there may be a small but positive association between socioeconomic status and obesity among children living in industrialized societies *(74)*. However, this trend may change during adolescence. There is some evidence that girls from low-income families become heavier after adolescence, whereas girls from high-income families become leaner after adolescence *(75)*. Indeed, among adult females there is a negative association between socioeconomic status and adiposity *(74)*. Second, there is correlational evidence that family discord is associated with increased BMI among children and adolescents *(76,77)*. Along these lines, a European study recently completed a 10-yr follow-up of children who were either apparently neglected or not neglected by their parents *(78)*. Neglected children were 9.8 times more likely to become obese adolescents than nonneglected children, thus suggesting that environmental stressors might contribute to obesity development.

Third, there is strong evidence that television viewing is associated with obesity among children *(79–81)*. This is probably because of the incompatibility of television viewing and physical activity *(82)*, although other explanations are possible *(83)*. Indeed, one noteworthy study compared the frequency of sports participation among children living in three towns with differential exposure to television. Compared to children living in towns with television, those living in a town without it participated in more sports *(84)*.

Finally, the prevalence of childhood obesity varies across geographic regions within the United States and during seasons *(85,86)*. The prevalence of obesity, measured by anthropometry, was greater in the Northeast and Midwest than in the West and was also greater during the fall and winter than during the summer. These various findings regarding environmental correlates of childhood obesity might be useful in the design and/or application of prevention efforts. However, as we discuss below, few of these findings have been incorporated into the design and/or implementation of prevention trials.

5. PREVENTION OF CHILDHOOD OBESITY

Public health researchers have traditionally described three types of prevention: primary prevention, secondary prevention, and tertiary prevention *(4)*. Primary prevention is the closest concept to true prevention, in which a medical condition is prevented through early and aggressive intervention. Ideally, intervention completely preempts or interrupts the emergence of the condition even before its early stages. Thus, the primary prevention of pediatric obesity would require early-life detection of excessive adiposity or the identification of genetic markers to target individuals who would probably become obese if left untreated. Once identified, primary preventive services would be aggressively introduced to circumvent the emergence of obesity.

Secondary prevention refers to early intervention soon after signs of a condition emerge, although not as immediately as primary prevention. For example, the secondary prevention of pediatric obesity entails prompt intervention services soon after a child is assessed as obese. Some believe that elementary school personnel could be effective and practical agents of secondary prevention services *(87)*. However, as discussed below, existent data are not universally consistent with this hypothesis.

Finally, tertiary prevention refers to intervention after a condition has manifested itself for a period of time. For example, intervention with a 15-yr-old obese teen who has been overweight his whole life is an example of tertiary prevention. The encouraging outcomes of several prominent behavioral interventions for pediatric obesity are examples of tertiary intervention *(88,89)*. Ironically, the phrase "tertiary prevention" may be a misnomer since the goal is not actually to prevent but rather to treat an existent disease *(4)*. Furthermore, the distinction between secondary and tertiary obesity prevention is somewhat arbitrary, with the determining variable being how long the child has been obese.

There has been surprisingly little research on the prevention of pediatric obesity despite its increasing prevalence and associated health risks. Still, there have been attempts to prevent pediatric obesity at the primary, secondary, and tertiary levels *(90–93)*.

5.1. Primary Prevention Studies

To our knowledge, there is only one controlled primary prevention study in the literature in which weight changes were reported *(94)*. In this study, the researchers used nutrition education with the parents of 80 neonates. These parents received a nutritional guide, "The Prudent Diet," to guide food preparation for the children once they reached an age of 3 mo and a weight of 13 lb. This guide gave very specific recommendations for food selections, portion sizes, and calorie content. The parents of 50 control infants received instructions on a "conventional" diet for their infants. At 3-yr follow-up, the data clearly indicated the effectiveness of the intervention. Among female subjects measured after 3 yr, 16.7% of the control infants were overweight in comparison to none of the experimental group. Among male subjects, 34.8% of the control group was overweight in comparison to 2.56% of the experimental group.

Recently, Fitzgibbon and colleagues *(95)* described an obesity prevention pilot program for African-American mothers and their preadolescent daughters. This report described a 6-wk controlled intervention study, with treated families receiving what was described as an education and skills-based approach for managing health behaviors. Compared to control subjects, there was a nonsignificant tendency for mothers and daughters in the experimental group to report decreased daily fat intake. Mothers and daughters in the experimental groups also reported increased nutritional knowledge compared to control subjects. Unfortunately, changes in BMI or other indexes of fatness were not reported.

5.2. Secondary and Tertiary Prevention Studies

5.2.1. SCHOOL-BASED INTERVENTIONS

Most secondary and tertiary prevention programs have been conducted within school settings. There have been a variety of school-based programs, some of which were school-wide, targeting both obese and nonobese children *(96–98)*, whereas others specifically targeted obese children *(99–101)*. These programs tend to be multifaceted, including nutrition education and school-based exercise components.

Stimulus-control techniques, self-monitoring, and problem-solving were components of these programs.

Resnicow *(87)* reviewed six controlled interventions that specifically targeted overweight children. With interventions lasting from 12 wk to 18 mo, children in the treatment groups gained significantly less weight over time than control subjects in five out of the six studies. Despite these findings, a number of issues restrict enthusiasm. As Resnicow points out, subjects were not always randomly assigned to groups. Second, moderators of treatment outcome have not been systematically addressed across studies. Finally, there are few long-term follow-up data on children undergoing such programs and the available data are not encouraging *(100)*.

Especially noteworthy are the recent findings from one of the largest and most comprehensive school-based health interventions to date *(102)*. This controlled intervention studied over 5000 ethnically diverse children from 96 schools in California, Louisiana, Minnesota, and Texas. Despite the magnitude of this program, the Child and Adolescent Trial for Cardiovascular Health, 3-yr health outcomes on a variety of measures, including BMI and skinfolds, were unimpressive. Significant changes were primarily noted on self-reported measures of food intake and exercise.

Finally, evidence for the limitations of school-based interventions comes from a recent meta-analytic review by Haddock et al. *(103)* that, in part, compared the effectiveness of school-based vs nonschool-based treatments for pediatric obesity. Compared to nonschool-based programs, school-based programs were significantly less effective at reducing percentage overweight among obese children receiving treatment as opposed to those receiving no treatment. That is, treatments were more effective when conducted outside of the school setting. This finding suggests that school-based interventions must also target the home or other after-school environments if they are to successfully promote sustained weight loss.

5.2.2. Behavioral Weight-Loss Interventions

In contrast to the discouraging results for adults *(104)*, comprehensive behavioral interventions do promote long-term weight loss in obese children *(88,89,105,106)*. These promising findings primarily come from Leonard Epstein's research program, which includes diet modification and lifestyle exercise promotion. This program has resulted in sustained weight loss even at 10-yr follow-up *(89)*.

Although not primary prevention, these findings provide important insights into variables that might moderate the efficacy of primary prevention programs. For example, the greatest reductions in percentage overweight at 10-yr follow-up were found in treatments incorporating parental involvement in treatment, and activity-promoting lifestyle changes or aerobic exercise rather than calisthenics *(89)*. In another study, the greatest reductions in percentage overweight and percentage body fat were associated with treatments targeting the reduction of sedentary behavior rather than exercise promotion or a combination of the two *(107)*.

Taken together, these findings suggest that the efficacy of prevention programs might be enhanced by enlisting consistent parental input, perhaps necessary for tight regulation of the child's environment. Furthermore, the promotion of lifestyle activities might also be beneficial. However, as mentioned previously, any environmental manipulations would need to be maintained in order to promote sustained long-term weight-loss *(73)*.

6. APPROACHES TO PREVENTION: THEORETICAL PERSPECTIVES

There are different strategies for approaching the prevention of pediatric obesity. Four dimensions of prevention effort research include: targeting, philosophy, punitiveness, and timing.

6.1. Target of Prevention Efforts: "Shotgun" vs "Rifle" Approaches

One fundamental consideration for prevention research is the target of intervention. That is, prevention efforts can target entire populations or specific individuals within the population (i.e., high-risk individuals). The former, a "shotgun" approach, strives to hit most people with modest impact, whereas the latter, a "rifle" approach, strives to aggressively intervene with some at-risk subgroup. The shotgun approach might utilize psychoeducational approaches, including information dissemination via mass media and community activism, to reach most individuals within a community. Such strategies have traditionally been used in community prevention efforts with adults as well as many school-based programs with children.

In the "rifle" approach, aggressive prevention services would depend on prescreening children for obesity or markers of future obesity. For example, given the high heritability of obesity, prevention efforts might target children whose parents and other family members are obese. Recently, an expert panel proposed a two-level screening protocol for determining which adolescents might be most appropriate for prevention services *(108)*. The first level of these guidelines is a BMI exceeding the 95th percentile for a given age and sex, or a BMI >30, whichever is smaller. The second level assesses the following four criteria: elevated blood pressure, total cholesterol, large increments in BMI, and concern by the adolescent about his/her weight. Any adolescent who meets the first level criterion and any one of the second level criteria would be considered appropriate for preventive services.

There are advantages and limitations to both the shotgun and rifle approaches. The shotgun approach has the appealing goal of addressing a mounting public health problem by targeting the majority of children in the population rather than a select, albeit high-risk, subsample. Despite this ambitious goal, the disappointing outcomes from community intervention trials with adults and school-based programs with children are quite sobering and do reveal a poor track record. Such data suggest that modifications to previous shotgun efforts might be necessary if such approaches are to have even a modest impact on pediatric obesity.

As noted above, however, previous shotgun approaches have primarily relied on psychoeducational information dissemination and community activism to promote weight change. More aggressive forms of environmental manipulation, including legislative changes, seem not to have been attempted on a population level. Changes of this magnitude might include, for example, raising taxes on high-fat breakfast foods to discourage their consumption. In other words, the success of the shotgun approach to preventing obesity might rest on the implementation of bolder and broader environmental changes than have been previously attempted.

Regarding the rifle approach, there is clearly room for more prevention studies in this area. It should be noted, however, that all interventions using this approach share the common challenge of identifying the most appropriate children or adolescents for intervention. This challenge is not a simple one given that not all obese children become obese adults, particularly if obese at younger ages *(69–71)*. Thus, researchers run the risk of intervening with young children who might otherwise "outgrow" their obesity if left untreated, although the probability of this decreases as children remain obese into the teenage years. Ultimately, advances in the molecular genetics of obesity might help to better identify obese children who are the best candidates for prevention services. Until that time, much might be learned from aggressive prevention trials that target children based on the best markers currently available.

6.2. Philosophy of Prevention Methods (Inoculation vs Environmental Manipulations)

Prevention strategies can be fundamentally geared toward changing the child ("inoculation") or changing the environment ("environmental manipulation"). Inoculation approaches emphasize teaching children skills to avoid overeating, to select low-fat foods, and to devote more time to physical exercise despite an increasingly sedentary environment. This philosophy has guided most school-based interventions.

Environmental manipulations, on the other hand, include such prevention strategies as the taxation of fattening foods *(109)*, installing signs in public settings to promote activity over sedentary behaviors *(110)*, prompts in supermarkets to guide food selection *(111)*, changing the marketing of certain food products to subgroups *(112)*, the development and implementation of fat substitutes and other advances in food science *(113)*, involving parents in intervention to better control their children's environment *(89)*, and the direct provision of nutritionally sound meals to obese individuals in lieu of their own supermarket shopping *(114)*.

In terms of the relative efficacy of inoculation vs environmental manipulations for promoting weight loss, there appears to be no controlled studies comparing prevention programs differing on this dimension. However, the disappointing results from community prevention trials with adults and the limited success of school-based programs suggest that inoculation methods might have limited effectiveness for reducing pediatric obesity. Furthermore, as previously mentioned, environmental influences on body weight are transient *(68)*. More aggressive and sustained inoculation strategies might be necessary before effects on obesity status can be detected.

6.3. Punitiveness of Prevention Efforts (Punitive vs Nonpunitive Approaches)

Prevention programs can include punitive or nonpunitive strategies. The taxation of fattening foods is an example of a punitive strategy that has already been used to target alcohol and cigaret sales *(115,116)*. Examples of non-punitive strategies include subsidizing gymnasium membership fees, price reductions for low- or fat-free foods in restaurants and supermarkets, and perhaps tax rebates for weight loss.

There are no data comparing the relative efficacy of punitive vs nonpunitive approaches. Given this absence of data, non-punitive strategies may be more desirable than punitive strategies strictly on humanitarian grounds.

6.4. Timing of Prevention Efforts: Rifle Approach

Interventions targeting high-risk children must decide the optimal time to begin intervention. One position is that there may be critical periods during the lifespan that are pivotal for the development of obesity and might be ideal for prevention services. For example, Dietz *(117)* suggested three possible critical periods: the first and second trimesters of pregnancy, the period of "adiposity rebound" between 5 and 7 yr of age, and adolescence.

It has also been suggested that the earliest possible intervention might be the most efficacious ones *(104)*. Unlike interventions with older children, efforts targeting younger children might not have to challenge eating patterns that have been practiced over many years. Early interventions that provide overexposure to lower fat and lower total calorie, as opposed to higher fat and higher calorie foods, might promote a greater liking for these foods *(118–120)*.

Despite these arguments, data to support the critical periods hypothesis are somewhat limited. For example, Allison and colleagues *(72)* concluded that the intrauterine period was a critical period for the development of adulthood height, but not BMI. Other behavioral genetics studies have also demonstrated that environmental influences on BMI are transient *(68)*. Such findings are inconsistent with the critical periods hypothesis and suggest that the duration of the intervention may be more important than the age at which it is initiated.

7. FUTURE DIRECTIONS: INTEGRATING BASIC RESEARCH INTO PREVENTION TRIALS

There is much concern about the increasing prevalence of childhood obesity and its associated health risks. However, there is rejuvenated interest among obesity researchers for the development of new and innovative prevention programs. Specifically, the obesity field has witnessed in recent years tremendous advances in its basic understanding about the onset and nature of obesity. Much of these data come from basic research in behavioral and molecular genetics, body composition measurement, and physiology. The information derived from such research is of enormous value and will ultimately help researchers to develop more effective prevention programs for children. For example, basic research might help to identify which children are the most appropriate candidates for obesity prevention services and which specific environmental variables should be targeted for manipulation. Indeed, it might be unrealistic to expect that strides in prevention research will occur without a serious appreciation of more basic processes. As new findings into the onset, nature, and maintenance of pediatric obesity continue to accumulate, such data should be used to guide the next generation of prevention studies.

8. RECOMMENDATIONS

Given the literature reviewed in this chapter, the following general clinical suggestions are offered regarding pediatric obesity prevention/treatment. More detailed discussions can be found in the references.

1. Increase and sustain the child's overall activity level. General lifestyle changes are associated with long-term weight loss in obese children and appear to be essential for obesity prevention. Thus, for example, the environment should be structured such that obese children select stairs over elevators, walking over being driven, and outdoor play vs indoor television viewing. More formal exercise regimens should be carefully structured since adherence tends to fail when prescribed intensity levels are too high *(121)* or if the situation permits teasing from peers *(122)*.

2. Parental involvement in treatment is highly desirable. Longitudinal research has documented the efficacy of behavioral interventions that involve parents compared to those that do not *(89)*. Even when obese parents regain their own lost weight, their children are often able to maintain weight loss if adhering to a regimen *(123)*.

3. Environmental changes must be sustained. Because the effects of environmental influences on body mass appear to be transient *(68)*, weight loss will probably be regained unless changes to the environment are sustained. Once a caregiver has identified the most effective environmental changes for a given child, every effort should be made to preserve these modifications.

4. Consult a health professional when considering more substantial dietary modification. Although behavioral interventions do not interfere with growth when properly implemented *(105)*, it is important that dietary modification not be too restrictive and that nutritional demands be met.

In sum, until more data become available from controlled prevention studies, the best recommendation may be a multifaceted approach *(124)* that incorporates increased activity, dietary modification, and family involvement, especially among higher risk families, such as those with a history of obesity and associated health-risk factors.

ACKNOWLEDGMENTS

This work was supported in part by NIH grants DK26687 to the Obesity Research Center, R29DK47256-01A1 awarded to Dr. Allison, training grant T32DK37352 to support Dr. Faith, and a scholarship awarded to Dr. Pietrobelli from the University of Milan, H San Raffaele, Italy.

REFERENCES

1. Colditz GA. Economic costs of obesity. Am J Clin Nutr 1992; 55:503S–507S.
2. Seidell JC. The impact of obesity on health status: some implications for health care costs. Int J Obes 1995; 19:S13–S16.
3. The National Task Force on Prevention and Treatment of Obesity. Towards prevention of obesity: research directions. Obes Res 1994; 2:571–584.
4. Weighing the Options: Criteria for Evaluating Weight-Management Programs. Washington, D.C.; National Institute of Medicine Academy Press, 1995.
5. Healthy People 2000. Washington, D.C.: US Dept. of Health & Human Services, 1990.
6. Hirsch J. Obesity prevention initiative. Obes Res 1994; 2:569,570.
7. Jeffery RW. Community programs for obesity prevention: The Minnesota Heart Health Program. Obes Res 1995; 3:283S–288S.
8. Taylor CB, Stunkard AJ. Public health approaches to weight control. In: Stunkard AJ, Wadden T, eds. Obesity: Theory and Therapy. New York: Raven Ltd, 1993: 335–353.
9. Jeffery RW. Public health approaches to the management of obesity. In: Eating Disorders and Obesity.A Comprehensive Handbook. Brownell KD, Fairburn CG, eds. New York, London: Guilford; 1995; pp. 558–563.
10. Goran M. Obesity in children: recent advances in energy metabolism and body composition. Obes Res 1995; 3:277–289.
11. Heymsfield SB, Allison DB, Heshka S, Pierson RN Jr. Assessment of human body composition. In: Handbook of Assessment Methods for Eating Behaviors and Weight-Related Problems. Allison DB, ed. Thousand Oaks, CA: Sage;1995; 515–560.
12. Hamill PV, Drizd TA, Johnson CL, Reed RB, Roche AF, Moore WM. Physical growth: National Center for Health Statistics percentiles. Am J Clin Nutr 1979; 32:607–629.
13. Goran MI, Driscoll P, Johnson R, Nagy TR, Hunter G. Cross-calibration of body composition techniques against dual X-ray absorptiometry in young children. Am J Clin Nutr 1996; 63:299–305.

14. Gutin B, Cucuzzo N, Islam S, Smith C, Moffatt R, Pargman D. Physical training improves body composition of black obese 7- to 11-year-old girls. Obes Res 1995; 305–312.
15. Pietrobelli A, Faith MS, Allison DB, Gallagher D, Chiumello G, Heymsfield SB. Body mass index as a measure of adiposity among children and adolescents. Manuscript in preparation.
16. National Center for Health Statistics. Plan, operation, and response results of a program of children's examinations. *Vital Health Stat* 1967; N:5.
17. National Center for Health Statistics. Plan and operation of a Health Examination Survey of U.S. youths 12-17 years of age. Vital Health Stat 1969; N:8.
18. Troiano RP, Flegal KM, Kuczmarski RJ, Campbell SM, Johnson CL. Overweight prevalence and trends for children and adolescents. Arch Pediatr Adolesc Med 1995; 149:1085–1091.
19. CDC. Prevalence of overweight among adolescents—United States, 1988–1991. MMWR 1994; 43:818–821.
20. Dietz WH, Gortmaker SL, Sobol AM, Wehler CA. Trends in the prevalence of childhood and adolescents obesity in the United States. Pediatr Res1984; 19:198S.
21. Kuczmarski RJ. Trends in body composition for infants and children in U.S. Clin Rev Food Sci Nutr 1993; 33:375–387.
22. Gortmaker SL, Dietz WH, Sobol AM, Wehler CA. Increasing pediatric obesity in the United States. Am J Dis Child 1987; 141:535.
23. Kumanyika S. Ethnicity and obesity development in children. In: Prevention and Treatment of Childhood Obesity. Williams CL, Kimm SYS, eds. The New York Academy of Sciences, 1993; 81–92.
24. Hauck FR, Gallagher MM, Yang-Oshida M, Serdula MK. Trends in anthropometric measurements among Mescalero Apache Indian preschool children. Am J Dis Child 1992; 146:1194–1198.
25. Sugurman JR, White LL, Gilbert TJ. Evidence for a secular change in obesity, height, and weight among Navajo Indian school children. Am J Clin Nutr1990; 52:960–966.
26. Campaigne BN, Morrison JA, Schumann BC, Falkner F, Lakatos E, Sprecher D, Schreiber GB. Indexes of obesity and comparisons with previous national survey data in 9- and 10-year-old black and white girls: the National Heart, Lung, and Blood Institute Growth and Health Study. J Pediatr 1994; 124:675–680.
27. Johnston FE. Health implications of childhood obesity. Ann Inter Med 1985; 103:1068–1072.
28. Allison DB, Heshka S, Heymsfield SB. Evidence for a major gene with pleiotropic effects for a Cardiovascular Disease Risk Syndrome in children under 14. Am J Disabilities Child 1993; 147:1298–1302.
29. Falkner B, Kushner H, Onesti G, Angelakos ET. Cardiovascular characteristic in adolescents who develop essential hypertension. Hypertension 1981; 3:521–527.
30. Lauer RM, Connor WE, Leaverton PE, Reiter MA, Clarke WR. Coronary heart disease risk factors in school children: the Muscatine Study. J Pediatr 1975; 86:697–708.
31. Williams DP, Going SB, Lohman TG, Harsha DW, Srinivasan SR, Webber LS, Berenson GS. Body fatness and risk for elevated blood pressure, total cholesterol, and serum lipoprotein ratios in children and adolescents. Am J Public Health 1992; 82:358–362.
32. Gutin B, Basch C, Shea S, Contento I, DeLozier M, Rips J, Irigoyen M, Zybert P. Blood pressure, fitness, and fatness in 5- and 6-year-old children. JAMA 1990; 264:1123–1127.
33. Rocchini AP. Hemodynamic and cardiac consequences of childhood obesity. In: Prevention and Treatment of Childhood obesity. (Williams CL, Kimm SYS, eds.), The New York Academy of Sciences, 1993, 46–56.
34. Bandini LG, Schoeller DA. Total body fat distribution and glucose tolerance in adolescents. Am J Clin Nutr 1986; 43:696.
35. Freedman DS, Srinivasan SR, Burke GL, et al. Relation of body fat distribution to hyperinsulinemia in children and adolescents: the Bogalusa Heart Study. Am J Clin Nutr 1987; 46:403–410.
36. Jacot JP, Zuppinger KA, Joss EE, Donatin A. Evidence for two types of juvenile obesity on the basis of body composition and insulin release following small doses of glucose. Klin Wochenschr 1973; 51:1109–1114.
37. Jiang X, Sathanur R, Weihang Bao, Berenson GS. Association of fasting insulin with blood pressure in young individuals. Arch Intern Med 1993; 153:323–328.
38. Voors AW, Harsha DW, Webber LS, Radhakrishnamurthy B, Srinivasan SR, Berenson GS. Clustering of anthropometric parameters, glucose tolerance, and serum lipids in children with high and low b and pre-b-lipoproteins: Bogalusa Heart study. Arteriosclerosis 1982; 2:346–355.
39. Modan M, Halkin H, Almog S, et al. Hyperinsulinemia: a link between hypertension, obesity and glucose intolerance. J Clin Invest 1985; 75:809–817.
40. Rocchini AP, Katch V, Kveselis D, Moorehead C, Martin M, Lampman R, Gregory M. Insulin and renal retention in obese adolescents. Hypertension 1989; 14:367–374.
41. Baumgartner RN, Siervogel RM, Chumlea WC, Roche AF. Association between plasma lipoprotein cholesterols, adiposity and adipose tissue distribution during adolescence. Int J Obes 1989; 13:31–41.

42. Frerichs RR, Webber LS, Srinivasan SR et al. Relation of serum lipids and lipoproteins to obesity and sexual maturity in white and black children. Am J Epidemiol 1978; 108:486–496.

43. Fripp RR, Hodgson JL, Kwiterovich PO, Wernwr JC, Sculsler HG, Whitman V. Aerobic capacity, obesity, and arteriosclerotic risk factors in male adolescents. Pediatrics 1985; 75:813–818.

44. Smoak CG, Burke GL, Webber LS, et al. Relation of obesity to clustering of cardiovascular disease risk factors in children and young adults: the Bogalusa Heart Study. Am J Epidemiol 1987; 125:364–372.

45. Freedman DS, Srinivasan SR, Harsha DW, Webber LS, Berenson GS. Relation of body fat patterning to lipid and lipoprotein concentrations in children and adolescents: the Bogalusa Heart Study. Am J Clin Nutr 1989; 50:930–939.

46. Bellu' R, Ortisi MT, Scaglioni S, Agostoni C, Saitta Salanitri V, Riva E, Giovannini M. Lipid and apoprotein A-I and B levels in obese school-age children: results of a study in the Milan area. J Pediatr Gastroenterol Nutr 1993; 16:446–450.

47. Durant RH, Baranowski T, Rhodes T, Gutin B, Thompson WO, Carroll R, Puhl J, Greaves KA. Association among serum lipids and lipoprotein concentration and physical activity, physical fitness, and body composition in young children. J Pediatr 1993; 123:185–192.

48. Horner RL, Mohiaddin RH, Lowell DG, et al. Sites and sizes of fat deposits around the pharynx in obese patients with obstructive sleep apnea and weight matched controls. Eur Respir J 1989; 2:613–622.

49. Silvestri JM, Weese-Mayer DE, Bass MT, et al. Polysomnography in obese children with a history of sleep-associated breathing disorders. Pediatr Pulmonol 1993; 16:124–129.

50. Chiumello G, Brambilla P, Manzoni P, Beccaria L, Pietrobelli A. Obesita' distrettuale e complicanze in eta' pediatrica ed adolescenziale. Abstract Book UICO 1994. Naples.

51. Kopelmann PG. Sleep apnea and hypoventilation in obesity. Int J Obes 1992; 16:S37–S42.

52. Friedman MA, Brownell KD. Psychological correlates of obesity: moving to the next research generation. Psychol Bull 1995; 117:3–20.

53. Mendelson BK, White DR. Relationship between body-esteem and self-esteem among of obese and normal children. Percept Mot Skills 1982; 54:899–905.

54. DiPietro L, Mossberg HO, Stunkard AJ. A 40 year history of overweight children in Stokholm: life-time overweight, morbidity, and mortality. Int J Obes 1994; 18:585–590.

55. Must A, Jacques PF, Dallal GE, Bajema CJ, Dietz WH. Long-term morbidity and mortality of overweight adolescents. New Engl J Med 1992; 327:1350–1355.

56. Nieto FJ, Szklo M, Comstock GW. Childhood weight and growth rate as predictors of adult mortality. Am J Epidemiol 1992; 136:201–213.

57. Hoffmans MDAF, Kromhout D, deLezenne Coulander C. The impact of body mass index on 78,612 18-year old Dutch men on 32-year mortality from all causes. J Clin Epidemiol 1988; 41:749–756.

58. Abplanalp H, Tai C, Vapolitano D. Differences in body fat of six inbred lines of white leghorns derived from a common base population. Poultry Sci 1984; 63:418–424.

59. Allison DB, Heshka S, Neale MC, Lykken DT, Heymsfied SB. A genetic analysis of weight residualized for height among 4020 twin pairs with an emphasis on sex specific effects. Health Psychol 1994; 13:362–365.

60. Bouchard C. The Genetics of Obesity. Boca Raton, FL: CRC, 1994.

61. Grilo CM, Pogue-Geile MF. The nature of environmental influences on weight and obesity: a behavior genetic analysis. Psychol Bull 1991; 110:520–537.

62. Clark PJ. The heritability of certain anthropometric characters as ascertained from measurements of twins. Am J Hum Genet 1956; 8:49–54.

63. MacDonald A, Stunkard AJ. Body-mass index of British separated twins. New Engl J Med 1990; 332:1530.

64. Stunkard AJ, Harris JR, Pedersen NL, McClearn GE. The body-mass-index of twins who have been reared apart. New Engl J Med 1990; 21:1483–1487.

65. Sorensen TIA, Holst C, Stunkard AJ, Skovgaard LT. Correlations of body mass index of adult adoptees and their biological and adoptive relatives. Int J Obes 1992; 16:227–236.

66. Sorenen TIA, Price RA, Stunkard AJ, Schulsinger F. Genetics of obesity in adult adoptees and their biological siblings. Br Med J 1989; 298:87–90.

67. Allison DB, Kaprio J, Korkeila M, Koskenvuo M, Neale MC, Hayakawa K. The heritability of BMI among an international sample of monozygotic twins reared apart. Manuscript under review.

68. Cardon LR. Genetic influences on body mass index in early childhood. In: Turner JR, Cardon LR, Hewitt JK, eds. Behavior Genetic Approaches in Behavioral Medicine. New York: Plenum, 1995; 133–143.

69. Charney E, Goodman HC, McBride M, Lyon B, Pratt R. Childhood antecedents of adult obesity. Do chubby infants become obese adults? New Engl J Med 1976; 295:6–9.

70. Guo S, Roche AF, Chumlea WC, Siervogel RM, Gardner JD. The predictive value of childhood body mass index values for adult overweight. Am J Clin Nutr 1994; 159:810–819.

71. Serdula MK, Ivery D, Coates RJ, Freedman DS, Williamson DF, Byers T. Do obese children become obese adults? A review of the literature. Prev Med 1993; 22:167–177.

72. Allison DB, Paultre F, Heymsfield SB, Pi-Sunyer FX. Is the intra-uterine period *really* a critical period for the development of adiposity? Int J Obes 1995; 19:397–402.

73. Fabsitz RR, Carmelli D, Hewitt JK. Evidence for the independent genetic influences on obesity in middle age. Int J Obes 1992; 16:657–666.

74. Sobal J, Stunkard AJ. Socioeconomic status and obesity: a review of the literature. Psychol Bull 1989; 105:260–275.

75. Garn SM, Clark DC. Trends in fatness and the origins of obesity: Ad Hoc Committee to Review the Ten-State Nutrition Survey. Pediatrics 1976; 57:443–456.

76. Mendelson BK, White DR, Schliecker E. Adolescents' weight, sex, and family functioning. Int J Eating Disord. 1995; 17:73–79.

77. Kinston W, Loader P, Miller L. Emotional health of families and their members where a child is obese. J Psychosom Res 1987; 31:583–599.

78. Lissau I, Sorensen TIA. Parental neglect during childhood and increased risk of obesity in young adulthood. Lancet 1994; 343:324–327.

79. Dietz WH, Gortmaker SL. Do we fatten our children at the television set? Obesity and television viewing in children and adolescents. Pediatrics 1985; 75:807–812.

80. Loncard E, Mamelle N, Billette A, Miginiac M, Munoz F, Rey S. Risk factors for obesity in a five year old population. Parental *versus* environmental effects. Int J Obes 1992; 16:721–729.

81. Satoshi S, Yamada F, Masuda K, Tada M. TV game play and obesity in Japanese school children. Percept Mot Skills 1993; 76:1121–1122.

82. Vara LS, Epstein LH. Laboratory assessment of choice between exercise or sedentary behavior. Res Q Exerc Sport 1993; 64:356–360.

83. Klesges RC, Shelton ML, Klesges LM. Effects of television on metabolic rate: potential implications for childhood obesity. Pediatrics 1993; 91:281–286.

84. Murray JP, Kippax S. Children's social behavior in three towns with differing television experience. J Commun 1978; 18:19–29.

85. Dietz Jr WH, Gortmaker SL. Factors within the physical environment associated with childhood obesity. Am J Clin Nutr 1984; 39:619–624.

86. Price RA, Cadoret RJ, Sunkard AJ. Genetic contributions to human fatness: an adoption study. Am J Psychiatr 1987; 144:1003–1008.

87. Resnicow K. School-based obesity prevention. In: Prevention and Treatment of Childhood Obesity. Williams CL, Kimm SYS, eds. The New York Academy of Sciences, 1993; 154–166.

88. Epstein LH, Valoski A, Wing RR, McCurley J. Ten-year follow up of behavioral, family-based treatment for obese children. JAMA 1990; 264:2519–2523.

89. Epstein LH, Valoski A, Wing RR, McCurley J. Ten-year outcomes of behavioral family-based treatment of childhood obesity. Health Psychol 1994; 13:373–383.

90. Dietz WH. Prevention of childhood obesity. Pediatr Clin North Am 1986; 33:823–833.

91. Allison DB, Engle C. Prevention of obesity. In: Proceedings of the Seventh International Congress of Obesity. John Libbey & Co., 1996; pp. 607–612.

92. Kanders BS. Pediatric obesity. In: Weighing the Options: Criteria for Evaluating Weight-Management Programs. Washington, DC: National Academy Press, 1995; 210–233.

93. Williams SK, Kimm SYS. Prevention and Treatment of Childhood Obesity. New York: Annals of the New York Academy of Sciences, 1993.

94. Pisacano JC, Lichter H, Ritter J, Siegal AP. An attempt at prevention of obesity in infancy. Pediatrics 1978; 61:360–364.

95. Fitzgibbon ML, Stolley MR, Kirschenbaum DS. An obesity pilot program for African-American mothers and daughters. J Nutr Ed 1995; 27:93–99.

96. Killen JD, Robinson TN, Telch MJ. The standard adolescent heart health program. Health Educ Q 1989; 16(2):263–283.

97. Resnicow K, Cohn J, Reinhardt J, et al. A three year evaluation of the Know Your Body program in minority school children. Health Educ Q 1992; 19:463–480.

98. Walter HJ, Hofman A, Vaughan RD, Wynder EL. Modification of risk factors for coronary heart disease. New Engl J Med 1988; 318:1093–1100.

99. Brownell KD, Kaye FS. A school-based behavior modification, nutrition education, and physical activity program for obese children. Am J Clin Nutr 1982; 35:277–283.

100. Foster GD, Wadden TA, Brownell KD. Peer-led program for the treatment and prevention of obesity in the schools. J Consult Clin Psychol 1985; 53:538–540.

101. Lansky D, Vance MA. School-based intervention for adolescent obesity: Analysis of treatment, randomly selected control, and self selected control subjects. J Consult Clin Psychol 1983; 51:147–148.

102. Luepker RV, Perry CL, McKinlay SM, Nader PR, Parcel GS, Stone EJ, et al. Outcomes of a field trial to improve children's dietary patterns and physical activity. The Child and Adolescent Trial for Cardiovascular Health (CATCH). JAMA 1996; 275:768–776.

103. Haddock CK, Shadish WR, Klesges RC, Stein RJ. Treatments for childhood and adolescent obesity. Ann Behav Med 1994; 16:235–244.

104. Wilson GT. Behavioral treatment of obesity: thirty years and counting. Adv Behav Res Ther 1994; 16:31–75.

105. Epstein LH, Wing RR. Behavioral treatment of childhood obesity. Psychol Bull 1987; 101:331–342.

106. Epstein LH. Methodological issues and ten-year outcomes for obese children. In: Prevention and Treatment of Childhood Obesity. Williams CL, Kimm SYS, eds. The New York Academy of Sciences, 1993; 237–249.

107. Epstein LH, Valoski AM, Vara LS, McCurley J, Wisniewski L, Kalarchian MA, Klein KR, Shrager LR. Effects of decreasing sedentary behavior and increasing activity on weight change in obese children. Health Psychol 1995; 14:109–115.

108. Himes JH, Dietz WH. Guidelines for overweight in adolescent preventive services: recommendations from an expert committee. Am J Clin Nutr 1994; 59:307–316.

109. Jeffery RW. Population perspectives on the prevention and treatment of obesity in minority populations. Am J Clin Nutr 1991; 53:1621S–1624S.

110. Brownell KD, Stunkard AJ, Albaum JM. Evaluation and modification of exercise patterns in the natural environment. Am J Psychiatry 1980; 137:1540–1545.

111. Winett RA, King AC, Altman DG eds. Health Psychology and Public Health. An Integrative Approach. Pergamon, New York; 1989.

112. Williams JD, Achterberg C, Sylvester GP. Target marketing of food products to ethnic minority youth. In: Prevention and Treatment of Childhood Obesity. Williams CL, Kimm SYS, eds. New York: The New York Academy of Sciences, 1993; 107–114.

113. Jackson MY, Proulx JM, Pelican S. Obesity prevention. Am J Clin Nutr 1991; 53:1625S–1630S.

114. Jeffery RW, Wing RR. Long-term effects of interventions for weight loss using food provision and monetary incentives. J Consult Clin Psychol 1995; 63:793–796.

115. Warner K. Smoking and health implications of a change in the federal cigarette excise tax. JAMA 1986; 255:1028–1032.

116. Levy D, Sheflin N. New evidence on controlling alcohol use through price. J Stud Alcohol 1983; 44:929–937.

117. Dietz WH. Critical periods in childhood for the development of obesity. Am J Clin Nutr 1994; 59:955–959.

118. Johnson SL, Birch LL. Parents' and children's' adiposity and eating style. Pediatrics 1994; 94:653–661.

119. Fisher JO, Birch LL. 3-5 year-old children's fat preferences and fat consumption are related to parental adiposity. Am Diet Assoc 1995; 95:759–764.

120. Marinho H. Social-influence in the formation of enduring preferences. J Abnorm Soc Psychol 1942; 37:448–468.

121. Epstein LH, Koeske R, Wing RR. Adherence to exercise in obese children. J Cardiac Rehab 1984; 4:185–195.

122. Wilfley DE, Brownell KD. Physical activity and diet in weight loss. In: Advances in Exercise Adherence. Dishman RK, ed. Champaigne, IL: Human Kinetics, 1994; 361–393.

123. Epstein LH, Valoski AM, Kalarchian MA, McCurley J. Do children lose and maintain weight loss easier than adults: A comparison of child and parent weight changes from six months to ten years. Obes Res 1995; 3:411–418.

124. Epstein LH. Family-based behavioral intervention for obese children. Int J Obesity 1996; 20 (Suppl. 1):S14–S21.

PART V
IMPLICATIONS OF PREVENTIVE NUTRITION
FOR THE FAR EAST, SOUTH AMERICA,
AND DEVELOPING AREAS

27 Effect of Westernization of Nutritional Habits on Obesity in Latin America

Recommendations for the Region

S. Jaime Rozowski and Manuel Moreno

1. INTRODUCTION

Latin American countries have a rather heterogeneous situation in demography, culture, and socioeconomic status leading to a wide range of health profiles in their population. Migration of the population from rural to urban areas has led to the growth of large cities, generally without an adequately organized urbanization. The number of cities in Latin America with more than two million inhabitants has increased from four in 1950 to 14 in 1985. Those with more than 100,000 inhabitants have increased from 55 to 216 in the same period of time (1). In industrialized countries this urbanization usually brings along progress in technology and social organization. However, in developing countries the benefits of urban growth tend to be only in the upper socioeconomic levels. In the lower socioeconomic groups, urbanization usually leads to a relative decrease in income that (from the nutritional point of view) shifts consumption toward high-calorie foods with a reduced nutrient density, with a trend toward incorporating eating habits of the more industrialized nations. In fact, this trend is shown by the majority of people in what could be called "nutritional westernization," characterized by an increase in the consumption of the so-called fast foods coupled with a tendency toward decreased physical activity.

The incorporation of these new trends has led the Latin American region as a whole and every country in particular to change morbidity and mortality profiles where rates as a result of chronic diseases have increased above that of infectious diseases, the usual killers of the past. Currently, chronic diseases are the main cause of death in most of the Latin American countries (1).

An example is the case of Chile, where the infant mortality rate in 1955 was approx 120/1000 live births, mainly as a result of malnutrition and the infectious diseases. At that time, cancer and cardiovascular diseases accounted for 25.8% of all deaths in the country (2). Now the infant mortality rate is estimated to be 12/1000 live births, with cancer and cardiovascular diseases accounting for 50% of all deaths (*see* Chapter 28).

The Panamerican Health Organization (PAHO) has classified Latin American countries into four groups according to their demographic characteristics: Group 1, coun-

From: *Preventive Nutrition: The Comprehensive Guide for Health Professionals*
Edited by A. Bendich and R. J. Deckelbaum Humana Press Inc., Totowa, NJ

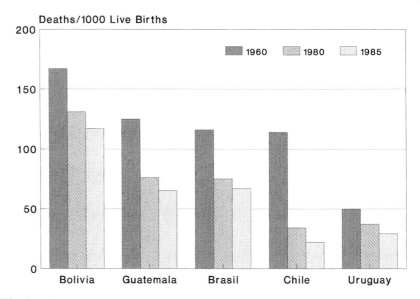

Fig. 1. Infant mortality rate in selected countries in Latin America (data from ref. *1*).

tries with high mortality and high birth rates, belonging to the first stages of demo-graphic transition, e.g., Bolivia and Haiti; Group 2, countries that have a high birth rate and moderate mortality rates, e.g., El Salvador, Guatemala, Honduras, Nicaragua, Paraguay, and Peru; Group 3, countries that have moderate birth and growth rates, and a low mortality rate, including Brazil, Colombia, Chile, Costa Rica, Dominican Republic, Ecuador, Mexico, and Venezuela; and Group 4, countries that have the most advanced demographic transition in the region, with low birth rates and moderate mortality rates, e.g., Argentina, Cuba, Puerto Rico, and Uruguay *(1)*.

Figure 1 shows the infant mortality rates from 1960 to 1985 in five countries that rep-resent the demographic groups cited above. Although all of these countries show a re-duction in this indicator, this decline has been variable, with Chile showing the largest relative decrease between 1960 and 1980. These data are also reflected in the proportion of individuals older than 65-yr of age as shown in Fig. 2, where the data from 1950 and 1990 are shown and projected to the year 2000. The proportion of the older than 65-yr group has increased 66% in Brazil and 50% in Chile and Uruguay in comparison with the year 1950 *(3)*. In countries with slower development, such as Bolivia and Guatemala, the increase in this segment of the population has been minimal or nonexis-tent. These data point to the aging of the population, which, when coupled with a de-cline in early deaths, necessarily forecasts an increase in the prevalence of chronic dis-eases of the aged.

The increase in adult population causes a growing demand on health services, to not only take care of the nutritional needs of the mother and child (malnutrition and micronutrient deficits), but also provide for the treatment of nontransmissible chronic diseases (NTCD) and its associated risk factors. Thus, it seems urgent to decrease the nutrition-related risk factors involved in NTCD, such as overweight and high intake

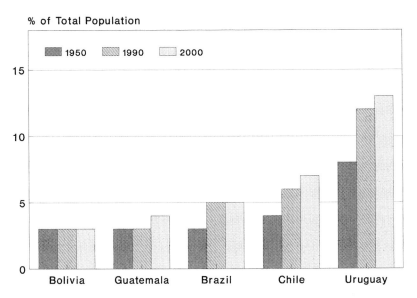

Fig. 2. Proportion of individuals older than 65-yr of age in selected countries in Latin America (data from ref. *3*).

of saturated fats; one mechanism is through health promotion via healthy lifestyle programs (*see* Chapter 26).

2. SOCIOECONOMIC CHANGES

A thorough discussion of socioeconomic changes in the region is beyond the scope of this chapter. However, it is important to discuss some aspects that are relevant from the nutritional point of view. The gross national product (GNP) of the different countries in Latin America has shown substantial increases in the last decades. Nevertheless, this increase has not always been accompanied by an improvement in the health situation. For instance, Brazil, which in 1990 had one of the largest GNP per capita in all of Latin America, still had an infant mortality rate of 57.5/1000 live births that year, higher than those of countries with lower GNP, such as Chile and Uruguay *(4)*.

The increase in GNP and in the general well-being of many countries has produced in many cases an influx of foreign fast-food enterprises with a wide range of food items at very low cost and, therefore, at the reach of people from all socioeconomic levels. For instance, a chain of fast-food restaurants had a recent offer in Santiago, Chile in which hamburgers were advertised for the equivalent of US$ 0.60. At this price, practically everyone can take advantage of this offer.

A different situation arises when the availability of nutritionally balanced foods is examined. As an example, in the case of Costa Rica, the proportion of income necessary to purchase the basic food basket in 1987–1988 was such that 20% of the population needed far more than the average income to purchase the basket *(5)*. Another 40% of the population needed between 40 and 60% of their income for the same purchase indicating that for a large proportion of the population it takes a major effort to feed themselves properly (Fig. 3).

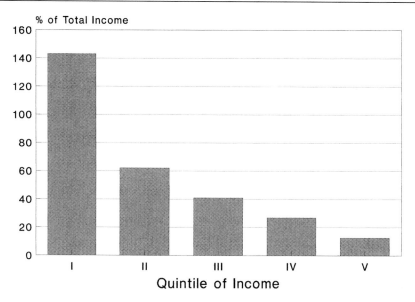

Fig. 3. Income necessary to purchase the basic food basket (as proportion of total income). Costa Rica 1987–1988. Quintiles of income are I (lowest) to V (highest) (adapted from ref. *13*).

3. FOOD HABITS

A thorough analysis of food habits in Latin America is hampered by the lack of national food consumption surveys. Except for a few countries, most information available is from small surveys that are often not representative of the population. In addition, most of these surveys are published in local journals that are not always widely available.

There is a great diversity of national nutritional habits in Latin America. In the southern cone countries (Chile, Argentina, and Uruguay), wheat represents the main component of the national diets, with the addition of meat and dairy products in Argentina and Uruguay. Corn is the main staple in Mexico and Central America (with the exception of Costa Rica). The rest of the countries have a rather diverse diet, combining the three main cereals (wheat, corn, and rice). In the Andean countries (Peru, Bolivia, Ecuador) and Paraguay, potatoes represent an important contributor to the national diets. In many countries, sugar has become an important contributor of calories, representing about 10% of caloric intake as an average. However, in some groups it can provide as much as 20% of dietary calories *(6)*.

Socioeconomic level is a major determinant of food intake. The structure of national diets has shown a tendency to change in most of the countries when income per capita has increased. Lipid calories increase because of a higher supply of fat (butter, margarine, and different types of oils), with a high proportion from animal fat. Calories from complex carbohydrates tend to decrease and the ones from sugar tend to increase. Protein calories tend to remain stable or to increase slowly but with a rapid rise in the intake of proteins from animal origin. These changes can also be observed in the different socioeconomic groups within a particular country. One example of this is shown in Fig. 4, which shows the type of foods consumed in three groups of Brazilians. As the aver-

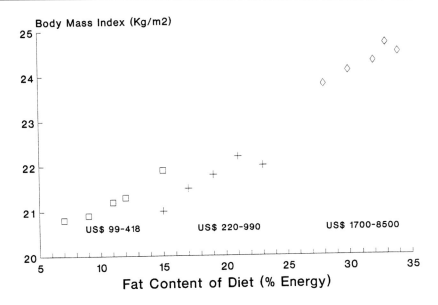

Fig. 4. Household diet and body mass index in Brazilian men, according to dietary staples. US-dollars figures indicate ranges of annual income in each of the groups/Dietary staples are: □ cassava, rice, beans; + rice, beans, lard; ◇ wheat, rice, oil, meat, milk (adapted from ref. 7).

age income increases we observe an increase in the intake of calories with a concomitant change in the basic food items consumed and the nature of the fats in the diet. In this way, the group with the higher income consumes a diet richer in saturated fats when compared with the groups of less income (7). In addition, increases in body mass index (BMI) parallel increases in income and dietary fat content.

In general, family income and urbanism are important determinants of the differences in food regimens among families within the same country. Urban families from low socioeconomic levels have an intake that is about 40% greater in cereal calories than high socioeconomic level families. People in the upper socioeconomic level have an intake of animal proteins that is 80% greater than the poorer ones (6). In general, countries tend to adopt the industrialized food model that is characterized by a high intake of energy and animal proteins and fats, with a tendency to replace simple and traditional foods by industrialized and widely distributed products.

3.1. Food Consumption in Chile According to Socioeconomic Level

The problems described above regarding an analysis of food consumption can also be applied to Chile. The last food consumption survey at the national level was done in 1974 (8). The survey divided the country in regions, and included an assessment of socioeconomic level in the population. Important differences were found in the consumption of protein according to income. Although only 5% of the population in the highest income quintile was consuming less than the requirement of protein (0.75 g/kg body weight), 51% of the poorest quintile consumed less protein than the requirements (8).

More recent data can be found in the surveys of the National Institute of Statistics (INE), which conducts family budget surveys based on amount of money actually spent

Table 1
Daily Calorie and Protein Intake Per Person[a,b], Chile, 1969–1988[c]

Quintile of income	Calorie intake			Protein intake, g		
	1969	1978	1988	1969	1978	1988
I	1925	1626	1425	54	47	39
II	2113	1875	1805	62	51	47
III	2422	2176	2112	68	64	57
IV	2830	2504	2259	84	77	60
V	3160	3186	2805	100	106	81
All	2587	2328	2133	74	71	58

[a]Values for 1969 cover the entire country. Those for 1978 and 1988 cover the Greater Santiago region.
[b]The values for 1978 and 1988 include food distributed by government programs.
[c]Source: ref. 12.

on different items. Surveys have been performed in 1969, 1978, and 1988 (9–11). Recently Cabezas (12) analyzed food consumption based on the three INE surveys (Table 1). Calorie intake fell since 1969 for all groups studied, the decrease being most pronounced in the first quintile. The author attributes the drop in calorie intake in the high-income groups to concerns about excessive intake of saturated fats and cholesterol (12). The average drop in calorie consumption from 1969 to 1988 was 17.5%. It is striking to notice that, according to this study, the lowest income quintile consumes, on the average, half the calories of the highest income group.

The direct, positive relationship between income and food intake is observed in many other smaller studies published and it also involves protein and most vitamins. The patterns of fat consumption are a little more confusing. Although it is estimated that the current intake of fat is 20%–25% of total calories, these data do not take into account the influence of foods high in fats from fast-food outlets.

The principal foods consumed by the rich and poor in Chile are, qualitatively, essentially the same. Over time and socioeconomic sectors, the dominant contributor to total calories in the diet have been bread and other cereals. Although bread consumption in Chile has decreased by about 25% in the last two decades, it was estimated at a level of 90 kg/person/yr in 1987 (13). The consumption of specific items in the low-income populations can be determined as much by their availability as it is by price. The choices of food available in poor areas tend to be more limited than in the high-income neighborhoods, where the presence of large competing supermarkets allows for a much wider availability of different types of food.

Based on the recommendations to lower the risk of chronic diseases, the average Chilean diet could be considered a relatively healthy one. However, the differences in consumption trends and nutrient intake between the different socioeconomic groups are substantial. The wealthier 60% of the population consumes a diet quantitatively different from the poorer 40%. In addition, the prevalence of obesity in poor groups (see Section 4.) suggests a pattern of consumption or intra-household distribution of food that is not reflected in the average values given in the different studies. Nutritional studies that concentrate on these populations that can accurately determine within-family variations are necessary to clarify the risks for these populations.

3.2. Fast-Food Outlets: A Growing Presence in Latin America

Fast-food restaurants have shown a striking increase in some Latin American countries, like Chile, Argentina, Brazil, and Uruguay, where most of these traditionally American restaurants have had explosive growth. These type of restaurants are attractive for the population because of the low cost, easy accessibility, and good taste of saturated fat. They are particularly attractive for the low-income population because they provide a clean place where they can eat a tasty meal. The food is also within their financial means. Aware of their success, many middle-income local food service stores have turned into fast-food outlets with mass produced items. As a result, items like hamburgers and french fries are more frequently consumed compared to years ago, when their intake was only sporadic.

An example of fast foods sold at a relatively low price is an offer by a fast-food chicken outlet in Santiago, Chile that consisted of a deep-fried chicken drumstick, three small fried cheese turnovers (empanadas), a portion of french fries, and a glass of soda. The cost was equivalent to $2.15. The estimated nutritional content was 1000 calories, with 40–45% of the calories coming from fat.

4. OBESITY

The last decades have witnessed a dramatic increase in the prevalence of obesity in developed countries. The importance of this condition has also grown substantially in some developing countries, such as Brazil *(14)* and Chile *(15)*.

It is well accepted that obesity is a major risk factor for mortality, particularly from cardiovascular disease *(16,17)*. An association has been found between obesity and hypertension, diabetes, lipid disorders, and ischemic heart disease. The condition is also related to other chronic diseases like cholecystitis, certain types of cancer, osteoarthritis, and pulmonary disease *(18)*. This makes obesity a major public health concern that, if prevented, would have a multiplying effect on the improvement of adult health *(19)*.

Obesity can be described as a nutritional disease with serious consequences. Its prevalence increases with age and although the increase in weight with age has been accepted as inevitable, recent data show that this weight gain augments the risk of mortality in women *(17)*. The treatment of obesity is difficult and usually unsatisfactory, therefore making its prevention very important.

There are few studies that allow a comparison of the prevalence of obesity in different countries in Latin America. The Food and Nutrition Surveillance System (SISVAN) of FAO reviewed the prevalence of obesity in adults in Latin America utilizing information provided by member countries *(20)*. The cut-off point utilized was a BMI of 25 kg/m². The results are shown in Fig. 5. The prevalence of obesity was high, reaching as high as 50% in some countries. Unfortunately, in some cases the information provided by the different countries was outdated, which makes comparisons difficult. For instance, the information from Chile was from 1975 whereas that from Uruguay was from 1991. The latter showed the highest prevalence for both sexes, with half of the population with a BMI >25kg/m². The prevalence of obesity was higher in women than in men and showed a tendency to increase with age, reaching a maximum around the sixth decade.

The highest prevalence of obesity at an early age (20–30 yr old) has been found in Costa Rica, Cuba, Chile, and Peru *(20)*. When comparing the prevalence of overweight

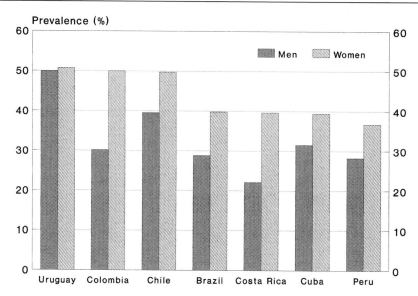

Fig. 5. Prevalence of obesity (BMI > 25 kg/m²) in Latin-American countries. Only countries with samples that had a degree of representation were taken from the original data (adapted from ref. *20*).

and obesity in Latin America with that in the Hispanic population in the United States *(21)*, there is a similar prevalence in women, with an even higher prevalence in women from some Latin American countries.

A national survey was carried out in 1989 in Brazil using a representative sample of 14,455 households and compared with a previous survey of 55,000 households performed in 1974–1975 *(14)*. The results of prevalence are shown in Table 2.

An increase in prevalence was observed in both overweight and obesity in the period of time between the two surveys. Women were 2.5 times as likely as men to be obese, but the highest relative increase was seen in men, where prevalence almost doubled in 15 yr. In men the prevalence was much higher in urban areas than in rural areas and showed a direct relationship with income. In both sexes the more developed regions were associated with a higher prevalence of overweight/obesity *(14)*.

The prevalence of obesity is particularly high in Chile. In 1987 Berrios et al. studied the prevalence of risk factors, including obesity, in 475 males and 728 females above 15 yr of age from Santiago *(15)*. Using cut-off points of 27.3 kg/m² for women and 27.8 kg/m² for men, the authors showed an overall prevalence of 13 and 20% in men and women, respectively. Prevalence increased with age, was higher in women than in men up to 55 yr of age, and showed an inverse relationship with socioeconomic level in women (Fig. 6). The marked decrease in prevalence seen in men above 65 yr of age could be a result of sampling problems and/or a selective mortality. The same authors have recently reported preliminary data from a follow-up study in 1992 showing a prevalence of 20 and 37% in men and women, respectively (Berrios X, Jadue L, personal communication). The prevalence of obesity in poor women was as high as 50% in the follow-up study.

The profile of obesity found by Berrios et al. in terms of its relationship to socioeconomic level is interesting. The inverse relationship seen in women is similar to that usually seen in more developed countries *(20,21)*. On the other hand, the higher prevalence

Table 2
Prevalance (%) of Overweight/Obesity Among Brazilian Adults in Two National Surveys[a]

	1989		1974/1975	
	Men (n = 16,783)	*Women* (n = 17,168)	*Men* (n = 63,138)	*Women* (n = 65,169)
Overweight (BMI 25–29)	22.5	26.4	14.4	18.9
Obese (BMI > 30)	4.8	11.7	2.5	6.9
Overweight/obese (BMI > 25)	27.3	38.1	16.9	25.8

[a]Source: ref. *14*.

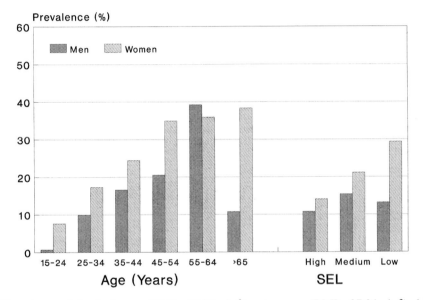

Fig. 6. Prevalence of obesity in men (BMI > 27.8 kg/m^2) and women (BMI > 27.3 kg/m^2) older than 15-yr of age in Santiago, Chile. SEL: Socioeconomic level (adapted from ref. *15*).

in women compared to men is not often seen in developed countries *(22)*. Men in Santiago showed no relationship between socioeconomic level and obesity, opposite to the results of the Brazilian study, in which a direct relationship was seen *(14)*. This is a pattern more in agreement with developed countries *(23)*. Although it is hard to define the reasons for these profiles of obesity, the differences could be because of lifestyle factors and the stage of transition from a diet high in complex carbohydrates and low in fat to one with a higher content of animal fats and proteins.

If we extrapolate a prevalence found by Berrios in Santiago to the whole country, in absolute terms the number of obese people increased by one million in a period of 5 yr. The problem of obesity in Chile is not only confined to adults and adolescents, but it is also present in increasing numbers in children. Preschool children have a prevalence of obesity (weight/height index >2 SD) of 10.7%, the highest of that age group in Latin-America *(7)*.

4.1. Prevalence of Conditions Related to Obesity in Chile

4.1.1. DIABETES

There are only a few studies on the prevalence of diabetes in Chile. These are usually restricted to relatively small samples that may not be representative of the general population. A study of 16,306 individuals published in 1960 showed a prevalence of diabetes of 1.26%. This study also showed that 10% of those did not know their condition *(24)*. A study performed a few years later in 3136 public workers > 30-yr old found a prevalence of diabetes of 3%. Prevalence of obese, normal weight, and thin individuals were 4.5, 2.1, and 0.3%, respectively *(25)*.

In what is probably the best study of prevalence, Mella et al. in 1979 found a prevalence of diabetes in 1100 adult individuals in Santiago of 5.3% *(26)*. The diagnosis was done according to the World Health Organization DATA Group *(27)*. Of the identified diabetics, 43.7% did not know their condition. The prevalence was similar in men and women, although in most age groups men had a higher prevalence, and there was no difference according to socioeconomic level. Overweight people (>120% Metropolitan Life) showed a higher prevalence than normal individuals *(26)*.

As a cause of death diabetes has increased from 1.5% of all deaths to 2.0% (a 33% increase) between 1969 and 1989 *(28)*, although it is difficult to assess the accuracy of reporting since diabetes is usually not reported as the primary cause of death.

These data suggest that there has been an increase in the prevalence of diabetes in Chile. However, because of the reduced sample utilized in the studies cited above, it is difficult to make a definite conclusion.

4.1.2. LIPID DISORDERS

Since 1969 cardiovascular diseases constitute the first cause of death in Chile, representing 30% of all deaths. The well-known association between altered lipid levels and cardiovascular disease and the association between obesity and lipid disorders makes it important to examine the lipid profile of Chileans.

In 1961–1963 Arteaga et al. studied 467 blue-collar workers 15–64 yr old *(29)* and found average serum cholesterol levels of 188.4 mg/dL. The same group in the early 1970s compared 100 subjects with coronary heart disease (CHD) with 123 apparently healthy individuals and found average levels of serum cholesterol of 211 and 278 mg/dL for the healthy and the CHD individuals, respectively *(30)*. Triglycerides levels were 52.9 and 92.3 mg/dL, respectively.

In 1983 Chamorro et al. studied 828 professional males (middle- to high-income level) without history of CHD *(31)*. They observed a marked increase in cholesterol and triglyceride levels with age showing values that seemed to be higher than those of previous studies *(32)*. In the population studied, 52% of the subjects older than 41 yr of age had serum cholesterol levels above 220 mg/dL.

A study of 1164 blue-collar workers at the national electricity company in 1987 showed average values of serum cholesterol of 206 and 200 mg/dL for men and women, respectively *(33)*. HDL cholesterol levels were 53.6 and 46.8 mg/dL and triglyceride levels were 110.2 and 160.2 mg/dL, respectively.

An interesting finding was reported in 1988 by Albala et al. *(34)* who compared obese women (height/weight index >120%) of high and low socioeconomic level (SEL). Serum cholesterol levels were much higher in women from high SEL compared

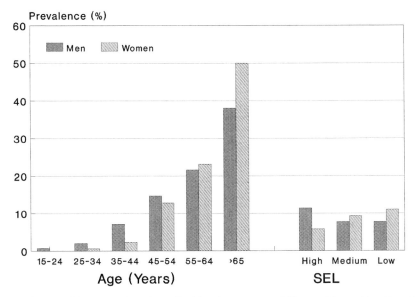

Fig. 7. Prevalence of hypertension (systolic blood pressure ≥160 mm Hg and/or diastolic blood pressure ≥95 mm Hg) in men and women older than 15-yr of age in Santiago, Chile. SEL: Socioeconomic level (adapted from ref. *15*).

with those in low SEL (227 and 179 mg/dL, respectively). Triglyceride levels were also significantly higher in the high SEL group (150 mg/dL) when compared with the low SEL group (107 mg/dL). Calorie intake was similar in both groups. The authors attribute the low cholesterol levels in the obese women of low SEL to the level of fat in the diet coming mainly from lard in this group as opposed to dairy products in the diet of women of high SEL. One could also speculate that a diet high in bread and cereals can also conduce to obesity.

Berrios et al. in the study cited previously measured serum cholesterol in a subsample of approx 600 men and women in 1987 *(35)* and again in 1992 (Berrios X, Jadue L, personal communication). They found in the first study that 33.8% of women and 40% of men had cholesterol levels above 200 mg/dL. In the 1992 study they found that 42.5% of men and 46% of women had serum cholesterol levels above 200 mg/dL.

The studies cited above suggest that the average levels of blood cholesterol have increased in the population of Santiago. However, it is doubtful that we can extrapolate these results to the whole country. To reach a definite conclusion it is necessary to perform a national survey which can assess the changes in serum lipids in the face of the changes in food intake that have occurred in the last decade.

4.1.3. HYPERTENSION

Although no national survey on the prevalence of hypertension or on salt consumption have been performed recently, epidemiological data show that about one-sixth of the Chilean population have high blood pressure levels *(36)*. The information that is currently used comes mainly from two publications. In a pediatric population, Lagomarsino et al. *(37)* found a prevalence of hypertension of 1%. In the survey of adults in Santiago, Berrios et al. found an overall prevalence of hypertension (systolic blood pressure ≥ 160 mm Hg and/or diastolic blood pressure ≥ 95 mm Hg) of 8.6% in men and 9.1% in women *(15)*. Prevalence increased with age and in women it decreased with higher socioeconomic level (Fig. 7), in a trend similar to the one seen in obesity in the same population, where an inverse relation was found between obesity and socioeconomic level.

Hospitalizations because of hypertension increased progressively in the country from 35/100,000 inhabitants in 1950 to 75/100,000 inhabitants in 1982 *(38)*. However, the rates decreased to 58/100,000 inhabitants in 1989, most probably a result of the use of new antihypertensive drugs that greatly reduced the need for hospitalizations as a result of the disease.

Preventive activities in hypertension in Chile have included the identification of people carrying the disease by screening and the normalization of blood pressure levels *(39,40)*. However, the coverage has been low and mainly confined to the major cities. It is estimated that coverage of the program has covered only 20% of the people.

5. RECOMMENDATIONS FOR THE REGION

It is particularly difficult to propose general recommendations to an area as diverse as Latin America, where nutritional problems range from severe malnutrition to high prevalence of obesity. However, as economic development progresses the region will be faced with a range of problems in adults that will seriously burden the health system. Coherent prevention programs must be implemented to reduce the impact of diseases of "nutritional excess" on the health system, and to improve the quality of life of the population as it ages *(7,41)*. An additional concern is that the chronic, prolonged illness of an adult has an effect on the health and well-being of other members of the household *(42)*.

The reality is that the influence of foreign food companies in Latin American countries will increase in the future. Consumption of prepared foods, either from large supermarkets or from fastfood outlets, will be more prevalent, either by convenience, by price, or both. This consumption will increase the intake of fats, refined carbohydrates, and salt in the diet. The way to counteract this trend is to improve the nutrition education of the population. It would be expected that the industry will respond to public demands, so it is expected that an educated consumer will force industry to develop foods with a low-fat content, rich in complex carbohydrates, and low in salt.

The programs proposed below are directed to the prevention of chronic diseases and concentrate mainly on nutritional aspects. They were originally developed for Chile *(19)*. This country is in an ideal position to implement health promotion and disease prevention (HP/DP) programs. The country has an efficient health infrastructure, a high level of awareness in the medical and paramedical professions, very good professional training with a high proportion of foreign-trained professionals, and a wide reach of the mass media. It is estimated that there are currently in the country more than 4,500,000 radios and 2,500,000 television sets. In addition, newspapers reach a large proportion of the population, which is more than 90% literate.

Other countries in the region show very different characteristics compared with Chile, so a generalization of recommendations might not be applicable. Nevertheless, these recommendations can be adjusted to the needs of each particular country.

Because of the limited resources available, an effective program of HP/DP should be "multiple disease" focused and have as a general goal the creation of a level of awareness that will guide the individuals in the food choices they make in daily living. It should involve all levels of education (including elementary schools, both public and private) as well as local health facilities and community groups. The program should also stimulate and welcome the participation of the food industry to improve labeling (for which, as far as we know, regulations do not exist in the majority of countries in the region) and to diminish the use of food items known to have an undesirable effect on health.

The HP/DP program has to be part of a coherent health and nutrition policy with clear targets for promoting the concept of healthy nutrition *(41,43)*. The general framework of a prevention program can be defined by the following components:

1. To develop a general awareness of the problem.
2. To identify in the public those groups at risk.
3. To remove or add those factors that affect the development of the disease (for instance, to instruct people on the consumption of saturated fats [remove], to promote physical activity [add]).
4. To treat those individuals where the disease is already present.

The goals of a particular program, once the diagnosis has been made, should be clearly defined and attainable, taking into account the different socioeconomic groups in the population and the realities of daily living.

The goals and objectives outlined below concentrate in three major areas: nutrition education, the control and prevention of obesity, and the promotion of exercise. In terms of cost/benefit these areas are probably the most advantageous in developing countries.

The following describes the programs for nutrition education and for control and prevention of obesity. The discussion of a program for the promotion of exercise is beyond the scope of this Chapter. Several programs and recommendations were used to formulate the goals and specific objectives outlined below. These include the North Karelia Program in Finland *(44,45)*, the MRFIT program in the United States *(46,47)*, the Honolulu Heart Program in Hawaii *(48,49)*, the recommendations of the National Academy of Sciences *(50)*, and others *(7,51–54)*. The goals and objectives were adapted from the Model Standards of Healthy Communities 2000 *(53)*, although the objective years have been adapted to the reality of Chile according to the authors.

5.1. Nutrition Education

The nutrition literacy of Chileans is low. An education program directed to the general population can create an awareness directed to the proper food choices. The vehicles for the program should include:

1. Posters disseminated in public places like health clinics and hospital waiting rooms, government offices, schools, banks, pharmacies, public transportation, and other places where people have the opportunity to read announcements;
2. Nutrition education leaflets with specific messages for distribution through health services, voluntary organizations, and schools;
3. Articles in newspapers;

4. Radio announcements of short duration (1–2 min) dedicated to a particular subject (e.g., high caloric foods);
5. School programs to provide nutrition instruction and to transfer the message to the family (e.g., in the North Karelia project schoolchildren gave their fathers a Father's Day card with a health message); and
6. Television "shorts" with specific messages and development of specific television programs.

Although the cost of some of these components can be very high, it can be diminished by enlisting governmental and nongovernmental organizations (e.g., government-owned or university owned radio and television stations).

The goals of this program should be:

1. To increase awareness of the relationship between diet and heart disease, high blood pressure, diabetes, certain cancers, and other conditions.
2. To increase awareness of the ideal range of body weight and provide information on sound weight control strategies.
3. To provide information and education on healthy food choices at the point of purchase, at home, the workplace, and school.
4. To provide information on selection and preparation of healthy diets.
5. To stimulate the food industry to make available to the public a wide choice of low-fat, low-sodium processed foods, and to develop clear labels for these products. This aspect also involves the establishment of government policy in terms of food labeling.

The specific objectives for the year 2005 should be:

1. That the proportion of the population that can identify the principal dietary factors related to chronic diseases should be at least 60%.
2. That 75% of the nation's schools should provide sound nutrition education as part of a health curriculum in the Basic and Middle cycles.
3. That 60% of adults should be able to identify foods that are low in sodium, low in saturated fat content, high in calories, and good sources of fiber.
4. That 75% of adults should understand the concept of losing weight by reducing caloric intake or by increasing physical activity, or both.
5. That 75% of adults should be able to use food labels to make nutritious food selections.
6. To maintain fat consumption in the diet to 25% or less of calories and saturated fat intake to 10% or less of calories. This level of fat consumption is being advocated as an optimal diet to prevent CHD and certain types of cancer (55). Although a substantial proportion of the population seems to be at these levels already, there is a trend in some groups to increase fat consumption.
7. To decrease salt consumption so that at least 50% of home food preparers do not add salt during preparation and at least 60% of people do not add salt at the table.
8. That 60% of adults have a basic knowledge of the food groups and make an effort to increase (or maintain) consumption of complex carbohydrates and fiber-containing foods.

5.2. The Control and Prevention of Obesity

The prevalence of obesity in Chile is high. A program to prevent overweight and obesity can be implemented within the general context of the Nutrition Education Program outlined above. In addition, certain measures need to be more specific. The vehicles for this program would be similar to the ones specified above.

The goals of this program should be:

1. To increase awareness that physical inactivity is associated with an increased risk of developing obesity and its disease correlates, and of the beneficial effect of exercise in relation to CHD, hypertension, and obesity.
2. To increase awareness of the ideal range of body weight and provide information on sound weight control strategies (same as goal #2 of nutrition education).
3. To disseminate information on appropriate exercise regimens to reduce the risk of CHD in adults.

The specific objectives of the program for the year 2005 should be:

1. To reduce the prevalence of overweight in adults aged 20 and above to no more than 20% in adult females and 10% in adult males. Note: Special objectives will have to be defined to groups where the prevalence is particularly high, for instance, poor women.
2. To increase the proportion of people 15 and older that engage in moderate exercise to 30% or more.
3. To increase to 50% the proportion of overweight people that are engaged in some form of physical activity combined with appropriate dietary practices to achieve ideal body weight.
4. To increase to 50% the proportion of people 20 and older aware that regular exercise reduces the risk of heart disease, helps maintain appropriate body weight, retards the development of osteoporosis, and enhances self-esteem.

6. CONCLUSION

The social and economic changes that are occurring in Latin American countries are having a strong influence in the eating habits of the population. Although the lack of reliable information precludes a thorough analysis, there has been a rise in the prevalence of nontransmittable chronic diseases and its risk factors, with obesity becoming a more prevalent disease in a population where this pathology used to be considered a disease of the rich. In Chile, the prevalence of obesity shows levels comparable to the industrialized countries. The need to counteract the changes in lifestyle and nutrition should be of utmost importance to the governments, who should aim to create a level of nutrition literacy and a "consciousness" in the population toward appropriate food choices and in this way promote a healthy pattern of eating. It is highly desirable to find an optimal national diet that, in conjunction with economic development, will maximize health benefits and minimize health hazards.

REFERENCES

1. Pan American Health Organization. Health Conditions in the Americas. 1990 Edition. Washington, DC: Pan American Health Organization, 1990.
2. Ministerio de Salud Pública. Situación y Atención de la Salud en Chile. Santiago, Chile, 1993.
3. CELADE (Economic Commission of Latin America and the Caribean). Anuario Estadistico, 1990.
4. The World Bank. World Tables 1992. Johns Hopkins University, Baltimore, MD, 1992.
5. Costa Rica. Informe Conferencia Internacional de Nutrición, 1992.
6. FAO/PAHO. Situación Alimentaria y Nutricional de América Latina. Santiago, Chile: Food and Organization of the United Nations and Pan-American Health Organization, 1993.
7. WHO Study Group Diet, nutrition, and the prevention of chronic diseases. Technical Report Series Nr. 797. Geneva: World Health Organization, 1990.
8. Ministerio de Salud. Encuesta Continuada Sobre el Estado Nutricional de la Poblacion Chilena (ECEN). July 1974–June 1975.

9. Instituto Nacional de Estadistica. II Encuesta Nacional de Presupuestos Familiares 1968–1969. Santiago de Chile, 1969.
10. Instituto Nacional de Estadistica. III Encuesta Nacional de Presupuestos Familiares December 1977–November 1978. Santiago de Chile, 1979.
11. Instituto Nacional de Estadistica. IV Encuesta Nacional de Presupuestos Familiares December 1987–November 1988. Santiago de Chile, 1989.
12. Cabezas KM. Cambios en la estructura de consumo alimenticio en Chile 1969–1988. Documento de Trabajo PET No. 82, Santiago, Chile, February 1991.
13. Round Table. Tendencia en el consumo de pan en Chile. Rev Chil Nutr 1987; 15:46–48.
14. Sichieri R, Coitinho DC, Leao MM, et al. High temporal, geographic and income variation in body mass index among adults in Brazil. Am J Public Health 1994; 84:793–798.
15. Berrios X, Jadue L, Zenteno J. Prevalencia de factores de riesgo de enfermedades crónicas. Estudio en población general de la región metropolitana 1986–1987. Rev Méd Chile 1990; 118:597–604.
16. Pi-Sunyer X. Health implications of obesity. Am J Clin Nutr 1991; 53:1595S–630S.
17. Manson JA, Willet WC, Stampfer MJ, et al. Body weight and mortality among women. New Engl J Med 1995; 333:677–685.
18. Garrow JS. Obesity and Related Diseases. London: Churchill Livingston, 1988.
19. Rozowski SJ, Albala C. Adult Nutrition in Chile. Monograph prepared for the World Bank, 1992.
20. FAO/SISVAN. Informe final de la IV Mesa Redonda sobre sistemas de vigilancia alimentaria y nutricional de América Latina y el Caribe. Quito, September 30–October 2, 1991.
21. Pawson IG, Martorell L, Mendoza FE. Prevalence of overweight and obesity in US Hispanic populations. Am J Clin Nutr 1991; 53:1522S–1528S.
22. Flegal KR, Harlan WR, Landis JR. Secular trends in body mass index and skinfold thickness with socioeconomic factors in young adult women. Am J Clin Nutr 1988; 45:535–543.
23. Sobal J, Stunkard AJ. Socioeconomic status and obesity. Psychol Bull 1989; 105:260–275.
24. Canessa L, Valiente S, Jaramillo I, et al. Encuesta de morbilidad diabética en Chile. Rev. Méd Chile 1960; 88:22–28.
25. Valiente S, Arteaga A. Problemas nutricionales colectivos de Chile. Bol Of Sanit Panam 1965; 58:405–411.
26. Mella I, García de los Rios, Parker M, et al. Prevalencia de la diabetes en el Gran Santiago, Chile Rev Méd Chile 1981; 109:869–75.
27. WHO Study Group. Expert Committee of Diabetes Mellitus. Technical Report Series Nr. 646, 1980.
28. Ministerio de Salud. Anuario Estadístico. Santiago de Chile, 1990.
29. Arteaga A, Valiente S, Taucher E. Relación entre colesterol y acidos grasos de la dieta. Rev Méd Chile 1963; 91:888–894.
30. Arteaga A, Soto S, Valdivieso J, et al. Estudio nutricional y metabólico en la enfermedad coronaria. Rev Méd Chile 1973; 101:519–523.
31. Chamorro G, Costa E, Valenzuela G, et al. Riesgo cardiovascular en dos poblaciones laborales chilenas. Rev Med Chile 1980; 108:697–699.
32. Chamorro G, Arteaga A, Casanegra P, et al. Factores de riesgo de enfermedad cardiovascular aterioesclerótica y prueba de esfuerzo en hombres de nivel profesional en Santiago. Rev Méd Chile 1983; 111:1009–1017.
33. Kauffman R, Hidalgo C, Roesller E, et al. Examen médico preventivo en trabajadores asintomáticos: Diseño y resulñtados iniciales de un programa institucional. Rev Méd Chile 1991; 119:617–625.
34. Albala C, Villaroel P, Olivares S, et al. Mujeres obesas de alto y bajo nivel socioeconómico: Composición de la dieta y niveles séricos de lipoproteínas. Rev Méd Chile 1989; 117:3–9.
35. Berrios X, Jadue L. Factores de riesgo de enfermedad ateroesclerótica en Chile. Bol Escuela Med U Católica 1991; 20:76–79.
36. Medina E, Kaempfer AM, Martinez L, et al. Estudio de morbilidad en la población de 12 ciudades chilenas. Rev Méd Chile 1988; 116:476–483.
37. Lagomarsino E, González E, y cols: "Hipertensión Arterial en Pediatria." Rev Chil Pediatría 1990; 61:2S–7S.
38. Ministerio de Salud. Anuario de egresos hospitalarios. Chile, 1989.
39. Medina E. Una politica de prevención de enfermedades cardiovasculares. Bol Hosp San Juan de Dios 1986; 33:36–44.
40. Escobar MC. Enfermedades cardiovasculares: experiencia chilena en el manejo de la hipertensión arterial. Corporación de Promoció Universitaria. Documento de Trabajo No. 39/90, 1990.

41. Kane RL, Radosevich DM, Vaupel JW. Compression of morbidity: issues and irrelevancies. In: Improving the Health of Older People. Kane RL, Evans JG, Macfayden, eds. New York: Oxford University Press on behalf of The World Health Organization, 1990; 30–49.
42. Over M, Ellis RP, Huber JH, Solon O. The consequences of adult health. In: Health of Adults in the Developing World. Feachem RGA, Kjellstrom T, Murray CJL, Over M, and Prillips MA, eds. Washington, DC: The World Bank, 1991.
43. Glasunov IS, Grabauskas V, Holland WW, Epstein FH. An integrated programme for the prevention and control of noncommunicable diseases. A Kaunas report. J Chron Dis 1983; 36:419–436.
44. Kottke TE, Nissinen A, Puska P, et al. Message dissemination for a community-based cardiovascular disease prevention programme (the North Karelia Project). Scand J Prim Health Care 1984; 2:99–104.
45. Pietinen P, Vartiainen E, Korhonen HJ, et al. Nutrition as a component in community control of cardiovascular disease (the North Karelia Project). Am J Clin Nutr 1989; 49:1017–1024.
46. Benfari RC. (for the MRFIT). The Multiple Risk Factor Intervention Trial (MRFIT). III. The Model for intervention. Prev Med 1981; 10:426–442.
47. Multiple Risk Factor Intervention Trial Research Group. Mortality after 10 1/2 years for hypertensive participants in the Multiple Risk Factor Intervention Trial. Circulation 1990; 82:1616–1628.
48. Worth RM, Kagan A. Ascertainment of men of Japanese ancestry in Hawaii through World War II selective service registration. J Chronic Dis 1970; 23:389–397.
49. Curb JD, Marcus EB. Body fat, coronary heart disease, and stroke in Japanese men. Am J Clin Nutr 1991; 53:1612S–1615S.
50. Committee on Diet and Health, National Research Council. Diet and Health: Implications for Reducing Chronic Disease Risk. Washington, DC: National Academy Press, 1989.
51. Department of Health and Human Services (USDHHS). Healthy People 2000. National Health Promotion and Disease Prevention Objectives. Washington, DC: Public Health Service, 1990.
52. Department of Health and Human Welfare. Promoting Health/Preventing Disease. Objectives for the Nation. Washington, DC: US Government Printing Office, 1980.
53. American Public Health Association. Healthy Communities 2000: Model Standards. APHA, Washington, DC, 1991.
54. Bengoa JM, Torun B, Behar M, Scrimshaw N, eds. Guias de Alimentacion. Bases para su Desarrollo en America Latina. Caracas: United Nations University and Fundacion Cavendes, 1988.
55. Wynder EL, Weisburger JH, Ng SK. Nutrition: the need to define "optimal" intake as a basis for public policy decisions. Am J Public Health 1992; 82:346–350.

28   Prevention of Malnutrition in Chile

Fernando Mönckeberg

1. INTRODUCTION

During the last thirty years, a progressive and continuous improvement in the health and nutrition of infants and preschool children has taken place in Chile. Biomedical indicators show that Chile has reached one of the highest levels in the region, although during this period per capita gross national product (GNP) has not changed substantially. Also during this same period, economic policies have changed drastically, ranging from a planned, centralized economy, to an open, liberal economy from 1976 until the present. In the last thirty years the country has confronted many severe economic and political crises. A socialist government was overthrown by a military coup in 1973. Two severe economic crises occurred in 1975 and 1982, associated with high unemployment rates that, in the latter period, reached 20% of the total labor force. Despite these numerous changes and crises, malnutrition and infant and preschool child mortality have continued to decrease.

The situation was quite different prior to the early 1960s *(1)*. Chile had one of the highest infant mortality rates in Latin America (120 per thousand). This decreased to 11 per thousand in 1994, the lowest rate in the region (Fig. 1). This decline in the infant death rate resulted from a remarkable decrease in infant mortality caused by respiratory and diarrheal disease in children <1-yr old (Table 1). A similar trend has been observed in preschool child mortality, which has declined from 14 per thousand in 1960 to 0.6 per thousand in 1994.

At the same time, the percentage of children with malnutrition has also been reduced dramatically, from 37% in 1960 to 5.9% in 1994. Second and third-degree malnutrition similarly decreased from 5.9% to 0.2% (Table 2). Maternal nutrition has improved if we consider that the percentage of newborns with low birth weight (below 2.5 kg) has diminished from 11.6% to 5.0% from 1975 to 1988.

2. GENERAL CONSIDERATIONS

It is self-evident that malnutrition is the result of poverty and underdevelopment. Many authors have demonstrated that in any given country there is a close relationship between the level of underdevelopment and the percentage of children suffering from malnutrition. In Chile, however, this correlation does not exist. The nutritional condition of children up to 5 yr of age is much better than the socioeconomic realities of the country would predict (Fig. 2) *(2)*.

From: *Preventive Nutrition: The Comprehensive Guide for Health Professionals*
Edited by A. Bendich and R. J. Deckelbaum Humana Press Inc., Totowa, NJ

Table 1
Chile: Infant Motality (0–1 yr of Age) as a Result
of Respiratory and/or Diarrheal Disease, 1962–1994
(per 100,000 Live Births)[a]

Year	Respiratory disease	Diarrheal disease
1962	4.118	1.350
1963	4.107	1.239
1964	3.715	1.541
1965	3.601	1.444
1966	3.683	1.614
1967	3.432	1.520
1968	3.060	1.391
1969	2.955	1.280
1970	2.793	1.476
1971	2.404	1.198
1972	2.186	1.087
1973	1.825	972
1974	1.757	888
1975	1.331	718
1976	1.277	637
1977	784	571
1978	704	386
1979	661	292
1980	502	210
1981	440	139
1982	220	110
1983	250	110
1984	240	90
1985	247	70
1986	242	70
1987	238	68
1988	206	62
1989	170	41
1990	161	36
1991	158	30
1992	141	24
1993	139	19
1994	133	14

[a]Source: Informe Anual, 1994 (Santiago, Chile: Ministry of Health).
Note: The figures for infant mortality reflect the deaths of children from
0–12 mo old.

Table 2
Percentage of Malnourished Children (0–6 y) in Chile 1960–1994[a]

Year	Total	Mild	Moderate	Severe
1960	37.0	31.1	4.1	1.8
1970	19.3	15.8	2.5	1.0
1980	11.5	10.0	1.4	0.2
1990	8.0	7.7	0.2	0.1
1994	5.9	5.8	0.1	0.1

[a]Source: Informe Anual, 1994 (Santiago: Ministry of Health), p. 18.

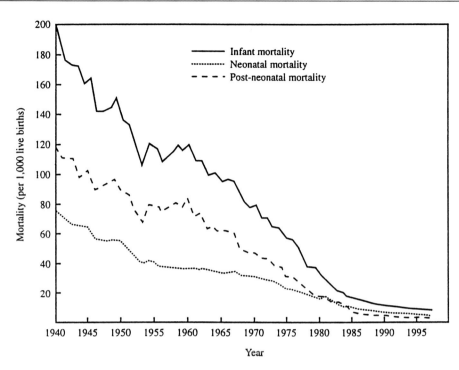

Fig. 1. Decline in infant mortality in chile from 1940 to 1988. Source: Ministry of Health, Chile.

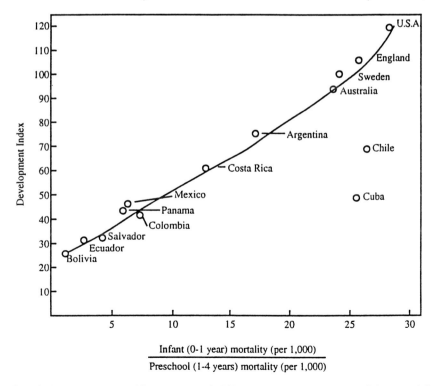

Fig. 2. Correlation between nutritional status of children below 6 yr of age and degree of development in selected countries. Note: Degree of development has been calculated using an indicator developed by the Institute of Social Development of the United Nations, based on 80 different items. Lower numbers indicate less development. The infant and preschool mortality rates have been selected as indicators of nutritional status. Source: ref. 2.

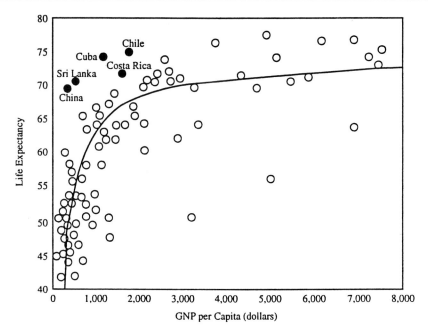

Fig. 3. Life expectancy in relation to GNP. Note: Line of central tendency is a freehand curve. Source: UNICEF Commission on Health Research Development, Health Research: Essential Link to Equity in Development. New York: Oxford University Press; 1990, p. 10.

Similarly, studies have shown a close relationship between life expectancy and per capita GNP. Again, this relationship is not observed in the case of Chile, where the life expectancy is much higher than what would be expected from the per capita GNP (Fig. 3) *(3)*.

This anomaly calls for close analysis because it demonstrates that under certain conditions it is possible to improve health and nutrition even when there is no substantial economic development. These facts, as observed in Chile, contradict the claims of many economists who believe that progress in health and nutrition only can be achieved through a substantial degree of sustained economic development. In this view, economic growth creates new resources that permeate the different strata of the society, ultimately improving living conditions even among the lowest socioeconomic groups.

From our point of view, however, this economic analysis is not plausible. Development itself cannot be achieved if a high percentage of the population is already damaged as a consequence of poverty and malnutrition and barely able to survive because of poor health conditions. Malnutrition, poverty, and underdevelopment constitute a truly vicious cycle that works to hinder economic growth.

Considering these two different points of view and given an environment of limited resources, two different strategies arise for preventing malnutrition and improving health conditions: focusing the effort on achieving large-scale economic growth and development; and focusing efforts on targeted health, nutrition, and education interventions to improve the well-being of the population, especially the most deprived groups.

With respect to the first strategy, one might conclude that if a society were to devote all efforts to economic development and to generating expanded economic resources, then increased wealth would benefit greater numbers of individuals overtime, eventually reaching the entire population. However, two questions arise from this approach. The first is how long would it take under the best circumstances for this wholesale improvement to occur, taking into account the realities existing in poor countries? Poor countries, for the most part, lack adequate technologies and the capability either for generating or for acquiring these technologies. These countries tend to have inefficient infrastructure, lack trained workers, and have a low savings capacity and little investment capital. Also, they are burdened by a large foreign debt. The logical answer, then, is that on average, economic development would take a long time, probably many generations, to accomplish. The second question is whether it is possible to have significant and continuous development in countries in which 30–60% of their population has been physically and psychologically damaged over generations as a result of poverty and malnutrition. The answer, again, is negative.

If we seek to achieve socioeconomic development, which is the ultimate objective, the essential point is to break out of the vicious cycle created by underdevelopment, malnutrition, and poor health conditions. Human resources are one of the most important, albeit insufficiently recognized, factors for social development. Modern society has become very complex, and the demands on the knowledge and skills of its members grow constantly. Incorporating individuals as useful members of the community is unlikely if the environment deprives them of well-being and impedes full expression of their genetic potentialities.

Under these conditions, even if some economic improvement occurs, it is not likely to reach the lowest socioeconomic strata, where malnutrition and disease is most prevalent. This assertion is confirmed by many observations. During the decade of 1970–1980, for example, economic progress was observed in Latin America, but this only led to a widening gap in economic circumstances among different groups. Thus, although the poorest 20% of the population did not increase its per capita income, the richest 10% increased its income by about $400 on average *(4)*.

Protecting the human resources of a country is a difficult, long-term task. At least four areas have to be considered: health, nutrition, sanitation, and education. A strategy has to be adopted to develop the human resources in each of these four areas, and to coordinate programs among the sectors. Individuals must be protected from the moment they are born, or even before, by adequate nutrition, sanitation, health care, education, and housing. These components must be well coordinated because they are interrelated and interdependent.

It is obvious that all nations would benefit from a nutrition and health policy. Yet a universal health and nutrition policy would require considerable resources, and the ultimate decision rests at the political level. In a situation of underdevelopment, governments have many urgent priorities to confront, and often political decisions on health and nutrition take a back seat and are postponed. Unfortunately, those who suffer from extreme poverty and malnutrition are not well organized and lack the means to exert political pressure. Furthermore, results take a long time to become visible, and policy makers frequently need to have immediate results.

In my experience, political decisions supportive of a national health and nutrition policy do not happen spontaneously. Rather, they must be induced. In the case of Chile, the University (Universidad de Chile), especially our Institute (Instituto de Nutrición y Technología de los Alimentos, INTA) has played a very significant role. Pragmatically, whereas the first priority of a politician is to achieve power, the first priority of a government is to remain in power. On the basis of this assumption, support for a desired political decision will be obtained only when the decision will bring benefits to political supporters. In other words, to provoke a favorable political decision, malnutrition and health problems have to become visible political issues.

For many years we have developed a defined communications strategy to create awareness of nutritional and health problems in the community. With this purpose in mind, we have utilized for years the mass media, including the training of journalists, in an attempt to create awareness about the adverse effects of malnutrition and poor health on individuals and the whole society.

Only when this communications stage has been reached will politicians become disposed to incorporate health and nutrition programs or interventions into their political platforms. Although their actions sometimes are employed for propaganda purposes, substantive policy and technical criteria have slowly gained ground in this way. Thus, a stage is reached when practically all the candidates for public office have programs aimed at eradicating malnutrition and improving health conditions. In this sense, election periods are especially important.

As a general rule, to be successful as a planner, it is necessary to calculate not only the nutritional or the health cost/benefit relationship of a given program, but also the political costs and benefits. Only those professionals who have calculated the nutritional cost/benefit ratio of a given program will then be able to translate that data into a political equation, having proven to be successful in getting their ideas implemented.

Another notable consideration is to implement nutritional and health policies that last over time, beyond the tenure of the current government. Very frequently in Latin America new governments have a tendency to change what the previous ones have done. The success observed in Chile is because, in great part, programs have been maintained and perfected over time. In this respect, our institute has played a crucial additional role (5). Every political system or government has its supporters and enemies. Programs, with their successes and failures, necessarily will come to be identified with the government in power. Professional planners responsible for these programs will, therefore, also come to be identified with a particular government.

The crucial point for the professional is to reach an acceptable balance between political involvement and independence. This is perhaps the key point: to keep the programs running beyond the term of the government in power. In this sense, we have been in an exceptional position because our interventions have been carried out in a university setting and from the vantage point of a highly respected institution. It is essential to gain the confidence of the government in power and also of the community. The whole team of experts participating in a health and nutrition program have to be cautious not to get involved with contingent, changing, and short-lived issues. This is extremely difficult, especially in Latin American universities, because they can easily become instruments promoting a particular political point of view despite the essential need to remain outside of the power struggle. Therefore, it is important for professionals to win support from all sides and to remain aloof from partisan political battles.

Finally, a nutritional and health policy has to be flexible in the sense that it has to be adaptable to the socioeconomic strategy of the government. Planners try many times to do exactly the opposite, that is, to adapt government socioeconomic policies to the needs of a nutrition and health policy. Lack of flexibility is unrealistic and underlies many failures. Policy has to be developed in such a way that it is compatible with different political philosophies and political realities, ranging from a socialist economic system to a liberal, market economy. This has been the case in Chile, where nutritional and health policies have survived shifts from one extreme to the other. During the last thirty years, in spite of different governments and economic strategies, the basic principles behind health and nutrition have been maintained, and program efficiency and coverage have been improved. In addition, new interventions were implemented regardless of changing circumstances. This means that health and nutrition policies have to be flexible and were not linked to any particular political group or ideology.

3. PRIMARY HEALTH CARE

In a underdeveloped country, a high percentage of people are born into extremely impoverished conditions and are subject to high risk. They also are totally marginalized, living outside the socioeconomic structures of society. Because of this, it is difficult to reach them with the basic services provided by the government. For most families, this poverty has persisted for many generations. Furthermore, they do not anticipate any change in their lot, nor do they perceive the benefits they could obtain from the services provided by the government. People living in extreme poverty frequently lack the capacity to become organized, and they do not and cannot exert political pressure to obtain favorable legislation. Many governments have organized health systems for groups that can exert pressure, such as blue- or white-collar workers, the military, and the middle class, but ignore or pay little heed to marginal rural and urban groups.

From our point of view, the first step in a sound nutrition and health policy is to organize a national health infrastructure. This would cover the entire population, especially the lower socioeconomic groups, and offer free services for those who cannot afford them. This policy has taken effect in Chile: In 1952, several organizations that provided health care were merged and transformed into the National Health Service. Since then, preventive medicine has been provided free of charge to the entire population.

In the beginning, only a small percentage of the population was covered, but coverage has extended to the whole country, excluding only those who can afford private medical care. At present, the National Health Service has 35,000 hospital beds and 1480 health clinics and health centers throughout the country. The National Health Service employs 58,000 persons, including 4520 physicians, 1365 dentists, 2090 registered nurses, 1690 midwives, 768 social workers, 710 nutritionists, and 24,480 nurses aides.

In the thirty years that the service has been in operation, coverge has been not only extended but made more effective. The personnel has developed an attitude of service and commitment to the community, whose respect they have gained. In turn, the population has become aware of its rights and responsibilities in relation to health care. Thus, for example, examinations during pregnancy have increased considerably, 98% of births now take place in hospitals, and an estimated 95% of all children are regu-

Table 3
Amounts of Food Distributed Monthly by National Health Service to Children
and Mothers[a]

| | | | Composition, per 100 g | |
Group	Product	Amount, kg/mo	Calories	Protein, g
Children				
0–5 mo	Milk, 26% fat	3	496	27
6–23 mo	Milk, 26% fat	2	496	27
2–5 yr	Weaning food	1.5	420	20
Women				
Pregnant	Milk, 12% fat	2	410	31.6
Nursing	Milk, 26% fat	3	496	27

[a]Source: ref. 2. Note: In each instance, "milk" means powdered milk.

larly given immunizations. As a consequence, the incidence of such diseases as measles and whooping cough has declined considerably, and poliomyelitis and tetanus neonatorum have been eradicated. Regular check-ups of children have become routine and provide weight-for-age data for over 90% of the preschool children, who are evaluated every 3 mo.

Family planning has been included among health activities since 1966 and has resulted in a considerable decrease in fertility. Currently, a large percentage of women are using contraceptives, which has contributed to the decline in population growth from an annual rate of 2.9% to the present rate of 1.48%. The decrease has taken place mainly in the low socioeconomic groups. Because of this, a significant decrease in infant mortality and malnutrition has been observed. From 1962–1981, the crude birth rate decreased from 38 to 23 per thousand, in particular among families with four or more children, where the greatest incidence of malnutrition is usually found. There also have been fewer births to women 35 years of age or older, a situation that has contributed to the decline in neonatal mortality. The decrease in the birth rate is responsible for 20% of the reduction in the infant mortality rate (6).

From the beginning, a program of nutritional intervention was implemented throughout the National Health Service. It includes free distribution of powdered milk for every child up to two, and weaning foods for children between two and five. The program also includes powdered milk distribution to lactating and pregnant mothers (Table 3).

The food is distributed through the primary health care centers and acts as a motivation for undertaking other health care activities. Food distribution has been extremely important not only from the nutritional point of view, but as a mechanism to attract mothers to the health care centers as well. To achieve these goals, the products distributed and their packaging and display have been of excellent quality. Special care has been taken to avoid the feeling that these programs are designed for poor people. The same products and services compete successfully in the open market.

The food distribution program started in 1951. In the beginning, the amount of milk dispensed was limited, but increased gradually as the National Health Service devel-

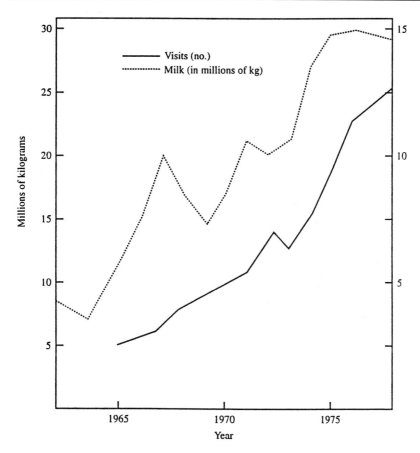

Fig. 4. Prenatal visit and amount of food distributed. Note: As food distribution increases, so does the number of visits of pregnant women. Source: ref. *12*.

oped. Figures 4 and 5 show that a close relationship exists between the amount of food distributed and the number of visits to a primary health care facility. The linkage between attendance at health care centers and food distribution means that in the public mind both programs are interrelated and complementary.

In short, an efficient health care infrastructure and rational nutritional programs have been two basic factors that explain the dramatic decline in malnutrition and infant and preschool mortality in Chile between 1960 and 1974. The improvements during this period served as a foundation for progress later on. The implementation of the health system with its broad coverage has led not only to effective nutritional programs oriented at target groups, but also to other interventions, such as family planning, health controls, immunizations, health and nutrition education, and the promotion of breast-feeding. The fact that the community has developed a true "culture of health" and has awakened to the need to preserve it through the health service is of paramount importance.

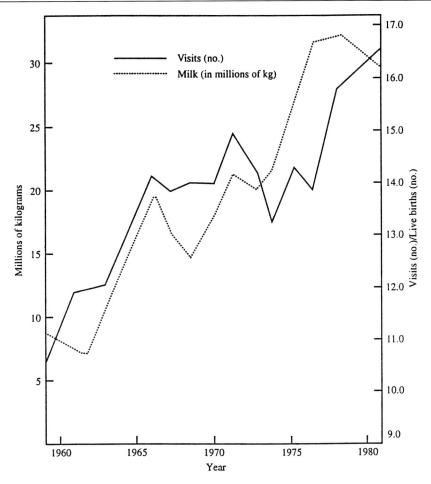

Fig. 5. Children attended by the National Health Service and amount of milk distributed. Note: As milk distribution increases, utilization of medical services. Source: ref. *12*.

4. OUR EXPERIENCE IN NUTRITIONAL POLICY

Despite all of these advances, in 1974 malnutrition in Chile still affected 16% of the preschool children, and infant and preschool mortality was 64 per thousand. A new strategy was, therefore, required and for this purpose the government created the Council for Food and Nutrition (Consejo Nacional para la Alimentación y Nutrición; CONPAN) in 1974. This was an autonomous, interministerial agency entrusted with the preparation and coordination of a nutritional policy for the country. The agency had a council composed of the ministers of health, economy, education, agriculture, work, social welfare, and planning. CONPAN had an executive coordinator to supervise the technical and administrative coordination of the agency's activities, a position I had the privilege of undertaking.

CONPAN resulted in a new nutrition policy with the aim of ensuring the best possible nutritional situation for the entire population within the limits of the country's resources. Special emphasis was placed on protecting the most vulnerable groups. The new policy encompassed the entire food chain and the concerns for food security, food production, imports, food marketing, income, quality control, nutrition education, micronutrient disorders, nutritional diseases, and sanitation *(7)*.

We soon realized that these concepts were absolutely theoretical. To articulate a nutrition policy is one thing; to try to implement it is a completely different issue. Numerous obstacles became apparent. Resources were limited; bureaucratic resistance surfaced; vested interests emerged; finally, rivalries among different ministers arose, reflecting the fact that few would accept interference in their own areas of responsibility. We learned the hard way than an ideal nutrition policy may be an impossible dream and that, perhaps, after all, it may be unnecessary. Therefore, we concentrated our efforts on specific interventions aimed at improving the nutritional condition of specific target groups.

CONPAN had a short life and was disbanded by a government decree. After that, we changed the strategy to establish direct relationships with particular ministers and with key people in the different sectors. This approach proved to be much more effective. Our conclusion was that one should not pretend to have a comprehensive nutrition policy or an official body to coordinate the interventions of the different sectors. Coordination and evaluation are extremely difficult tasks in any government. The essential points are to exert leadership, to have credibility based on scientific and technical authority, and to exhibit flexibility and, most of all, persistence and patience. Again, it should be noted that this has been the critical role played by the university and, more specifically, by INTA.

In retrospect, I think the rather brief existence of CONPAN was necessary. Methodologies for solving significant problems were developed and many of the interventions that were designed have been successfully implemented afterward. Above all, the government became aware of the need for scientifically based programs that seek to help groups that have been excluded from the economic and political structures of the country. After describing this experience, I have to say that in the end, considerable progress has been achieved during this last period, which I will attempt to summarize by sectors—health and nutrition, education, and agriculture.

4.1. Health and Nutrition Sector

A data collection system was developed specifically targeted to the nutritional condition of children up to 6 yr of age. Every child under the care of the National Heath Service (an estimated 1.35 million children) is measured every 3 mo and his or her weight for age is calculated. Basic information is gathered about families to examine socioeconomic conditions and related health risk factors. Information about weight at birth is collected regularly for all the deliveries in the hospitals of the country.

4.1.1. FOOD AND NUTRITION INTERVENTIONS

Targeted food interventions for families in extreme poverty have been developed. For these groups, a food distribution program, including staples, such as rice, wheat flour, and oil, was established through the primary health care centers. The objective of this program is to improve the nutrition of both the children and their families. Selected for this program are families with children of low birth weight (2.5 kg), children whose weight increase has been inadequate for 2 mo, and children born to mothers under 20 yr of age. Also participating are families with five or more children and those with severe socioeconomic problems.

Table 4
Clinical Progress of Marasmic Infants During 4 Mo of Treatment[a]

Statistic	at admission	at 50 d	at 100 d	at 150 d
Weight deficit for age, g				
Group A	56 ± 8	54 ± 13	48 ± 12	40 ± 13
Group B	55 ± 5	35 ± 8	21 ± 6	16 ± 3
		$p < 0.001$	$p < 0.001$	$p < 0.001$
Height deficit for age, cm				
Group A	76 ± 10	70 ± 17	65 ± 14	65 ± 14
Group B	82 ± 13	50 ± 14	32 ± 6	21 ± 7
		$p < 0.001$	$p < 0.001$	$p < 0.001$
Psychomotor development quotient				
Group A	56 ± 8	60 ± 11	64 ± 14	65 ± 12
Group B	55 ± 5	71 ± 10	80 ± 8	85 ± 1
		$p < 0.01$	$p < 0.001$	$p < 0.001$

[a]Source: Monckeberg F. Nutrition in the 1980s. Liss, 1980, p. 141. Notes: Group A consisted of 80 infants treated in a conventional pediatric hospital. Group B consisted of 80 infants treated in a CONIN center.

4.1.2. TREATMENT OF MALNOURISHED CHILDREN

Children suffering from severe malnutrition now have access to treatment. This program has had a direct influence on infant mortality. A 1974 study showed that approx 8200 children a year, on average, became severely malnourished. A follow-up study confirmed that infants with severe malnutrition prior to 6 mo of age had an 85% chance of dying before they were 1 yr old. Analysis of cases of severe malnutrition showed that almost all occurred in children under 2 yr of age, and 80% of the affected children were 6 mo of age.

A pilot project was started in 1975 to tackle this program, with the aim of rehabilitating infants with severe malnutrition. For this purpose a specialized Nutritional Recovery Center was set up with 40 beds for infants. Each malnourished infant remained an inpatient until fully recovered; he or she was given appropriate food and underwent a program of cognitive, affective, and motor stimulation. The mother was involved in the treatment and received education and training. The results of this pilot study were impressive. No deaths occurred among the children in treatment, although inpatient mortality previously had been about 25%, and very satisfactory rehabilitation was attained in both nutritional and psychomotor status (Table 4 and Fig. 6).

In view of the successes of the pilot project, INTA set up a private foundation, called the Chilean Nutrition Foundation (Corporación para la Nutrición Infantil; CONIN) to extend the pilot program throughout the country. Within three years, with funds amounting to US $9 million provided by the community, 33 centers were built, equipped, and put into operation in different cities of the country. The installed capacity covers all needs. With 1500 beds, it is possible annually to treat 34,000 severely malnourished children, thus bringing them to full recovery.

Each center has 40–60 beds, full medical facilities, a kitchen with milk distribution, and a laundry. The staff encompasses a full-time manager and six health professionals,

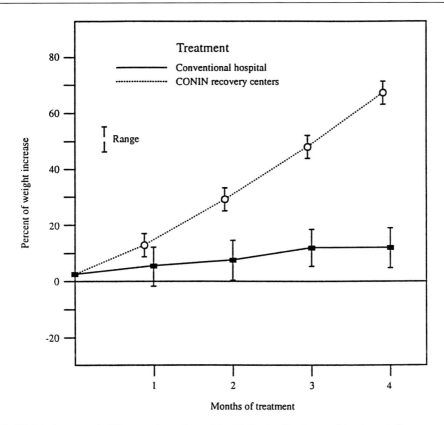

Fig. 6. Weight increase in 70 severely malnourished infants after 4 mo of treatment. Source: ref. *8*.

including a pediatrician, nutritionist, registered nurse, nursery teacher, and a social worker. Forty nurses' aides work in three shifts, and 80 volunteers work on individual stimulation programs and follow-up visits at home. Operational costs are financed under an agreement with the National Health Service (which covers 80% of the costs) and partly by CONIN-raised funds *(8)*. The cost per day is $6.50/child and the total cost of rehabilitating one severely malnourished infant is $600. CONIN has a staff of 1400 along with 2300 voluntary workers.

The program has had a notable impact in reducing the number of children suffering from severe malnutrition and in reducing the incidence of infant malnutrition. It is estimated that CONIN helps prevent almost 2000 deaths annually among infants under 12 mo of age. In terms of overall infant mortality, this means that the program is responsible for over 20% of the reduction in infant mortality. During the years in which the program has been operational, over 55,000 infants have been rehabilitated with an average mortality rate of 2%. Follow-up studies show that 98% of the children who have recovered continue to have satisfactory weight gain at home, and only 1.8% have required readmission in a center.

CONIN now has embarked on a new program that rehabilitates low-birth-weight babies before returning them to their mothers. Studies have shown that this is a high-risk group that contributes significantly to mortality during the first 2 mo of life. Affected infants remain in a center for 30 d, during which time the mothers receive instruction on child care *(9)*.

4.1.3. BREAST-FEEDING

Because a large share (85%) of Chile's population lives in urban areas, and perhaps as a result of the system of free milk distribution, there has been an abrupt decline in the practice of breast-feeding. In 1940, 85% of the infants were breast-fed up to the age of 6 mo. By 1967 this proportion had decreased to 25% and by 1974 to 19% *(10)*. This decline undoubtedly contributed to the increase in early, severe malnutrition. Consequently, an extensive program was introduced to promote breast-feeding, using both the mass media (e.g., radio, television, magazines) and formal education. In particular, a firm stand was taken on this issue in the professional medical community and in the schools that train child health care workers, such as midwives, nurses, and health educators. Professional and auxiliary personnel have received instruction provided by the National Health Service. Printed materials illustrating the importance of breast-feeding and how to advance it have been prepared and distributed.

As a consequence, there has been a noticeable change of attitude in the population and among health care personnel. Breast-feeding has increased significantly. More than 70% of mothers now breast-feed their children during the first 90 d, representing an 88% increase in breast-feeding during the first 3 mo of life *(11)*.

4.1.4. NUTRITION EDUCATION

A nutrition education program was created by CONPAN and included nutrition training at both the elementary and intermediate school levels. Textbooks have been prepared, although they have not been put in use. However, in the health sector, there has been considerable progress with a nutrition training. It has been possible to staff each national health service clinic with a nutritionist who is responsible for implementing the nutrition education program. Nutritionists, who are required to undergo five years of university courses, have been carrying out important work in both the prevention and the treatment of malnutrition.

4.1.5. RURAL HEALTH CARE

Because 85% of Chile's population is urban, the National Health Service has adequate coverage in urban areas, but it has been more difficult to provide coverage in rural areas, especially in the most isolated regions. Medical and nutritional care for rural communities is provided by health posts, each of which has a full-time health worker whose activities are complemented by regular visits of health teams. These health posts also provide nutrition programs.

To increase health care availability for pregnant rural women and provide adequate access to the nearest maternity facility, a program known as Hostels for Rural Mothers was implemented. The idea was to build these accommodations near maternity hospitals and to allow pregnant women from rural areas to stay there during the 15 d prior to, and up to 10 d after, the delivery. The women also receive instruction from hospital staff concerning nutrition, breast-feeding, and child care. Sixty-four of these hostels have been set up in conjunction with maternity hospitals in primary health care areas. Along with other measures they have significantly decreased neonatal mortality by reducing the risks inherent in delivery.

4.2. Educational Sector

4.2.1. PRIMARY EDUCATION

During the past thirty years a considerable improvement has occurred in elementary education. In 1960, more than 30% of the population was illiterate; the rate now stands at <49%. Only 10% of the children in 1960 had completed elementary education. Today, 85% of the children complete eight years of elementary education.

It is particularly important to draw attention to the emphasis that has been placed on education for mothers because this has a strong bearing on malnutrition and infant mortality. The latter is five times higher among mothers who have not completed elementary education than among those who have *(12)*. Progress in the educational field is particularly noticeable among women who were illiterate during their child-bearing years. This figure fell to 6% by 1982. In the period 1969–1982, there was a noticeable decrease in the number of births to women with a low level of education (i.e., either without education or with only elementary-level education).

4.2.2. SCHOOL FOOD PROGRAMS

The school feeding program, although technically not a nutritional intervention program since it only can provide limited daily calories and protein, has had a very important effect in reducing school desertion. CONPAN reviewed the program, reaching the conclusion that its implementation should be transferred to private agencies that could provide the complete service and leaving to the Ministry of Education the role of evaluation and control. This reorganization improved the quality of the service, and accomplished the goal of combating school desertion. At present, the program during 180 d of the school year supplies 1,230,000 breakfasts and 620,000 lunches daily to 4000 schools across the country.

4.2.3. PRESCHOOL FOOD PROGRAMS

The largest proportion of malnourished children in Chile live in deprived urban areas as a consequence of the massive migration to the cities that took place during the last decade. Almost every city has a belt of shantytowns surrounding it. Experience shows that it is difficult to prevent malnutrition in children from population groups with a low socioeconomic and educational level, even when free food is provided. Moreover, a number of studies indicate that extreme poverty causes damage to the physical and intellectual capabilities of individuals. This damage is the result not only of malnutrition, but of other factors inherent in chronic poverty.

Against this background, CONPAN supported the development of a day care center program for preschool children living in extreme urban poverty. Children attending the centers during the day have all their food provided and also undergo psychomotor and affective stimulation. During the last 10 yr 1300 such centers have been built and equipped, covering 180,000 preschool children between the ages of two and six. According to earlier estimates by CONPAN, the program will eventually cover 210,000 children, which is the number believed to be at risk of malnutrition and living in extreme poverty in urban areas *(13)*.

4.2.4. HOMELESS CHILDREN

A program for homeless and troubled children is designed to provide care in live-in centers for children from 2–12 yr of age. These children include orphans, abandoned

Table 5
Urban Coverage of Potable Water and Sewage Services,
1970–1994

Year	Potable water, %	Sewage, %
1970	72.3	41.2
1980	92.5	65.3
1990	97.3	78.1
1994	98.9	88.7

children, and children who display maladjusted behavior. The aim is to restore the child to a normal behavioral situation, to combat child vagrancy, and to improve the conditions of life. The program has been extended and improved through the building of new centers and now covers 52,000 children.

4.3. Sanitation Sector

Overcrowding and inadequate sanitation in urban areas are common to all Latin American countries. The situation has become worse in the past few decades as a result of the explosive growth of the population and increased migration to the cities. In 1974, a high percentage of the population in Chile lived in extremely impoverished areas that lacked sanitation facilities. Inadequate sanitation adversely affects child nutrition and gives rise to gastrointestinal and other infectious diseases. Diluted, contaminated infant formulas are one of the main contributors to the shift in the incidence of malnutrition to the early months of life and this, in turn, is associated with high risk of death.

For these reasons, CONPAN developed a program that emphasized the importance of sanitation in preventing early malnutrition. During the initial stage of this program, a brick-and-timber sanitary unit was built on the plots of 300 families living in a slum area. Each unit had a kitchen, a bathroom, and an outdoor sink for washing clothes. The kitchen was equipped with shelves and a sink; the bathroom had a lavratory, a flush toilet, and a shower. Hot water also was supplied. The unit was connected to the general sewage system (14).

The results demonstrated a significant causal link between environmental sanitation and improvements in both nutrition and the quality of life. Perhaps the most significant result was the striking change in the attitudes of the families. The pessimistic and fatalistic approach to life, hopelessness, and acceptance of the miserable life prevailing in the community before the sanitary unit was installed changed into a sincere and deeply felt desire for improvement in their living conditions. This resulted in increased individual efforts and in motivation to meet the challenge of improving the quality of life.

The results led to the development of a nationwide sanitation program to improve the sanitary situation of the urban population. In the past 10 yr 220,000 sanitary units have been built in different cities of the country. In 1960, only 40% of the population had drinking water in their homes, and only 35% had an adequate sewage system. At present, 99% of the population have drinking water at home, and 88% live in housing connected to a sewage system (Table 5). There is no doubt that improved sanitary conditions also have been important factors in the decrease in malnutrition and in the improvements in health conditions.

4.4. Agriculture Sector

Agriculture and food production are fundamental elements in any nation's development process and a precondition to raising the state of health and nutrition among people. As I have emphasized earlier, the economic development of Chile as expressed in per capita GNP, for the most part, has not been very considerable during the last 40 yr. From the beginning of the present century, the Chilean economy was based primarily on the export of raw materials: first nitrates, and later copper. Industrial development started only after World War II, but this development was based on import substitution, with a high degree of protectionism. Agricultural development was retarded because of artificially fixed prices, the high cost of imported commodities, and the lack of incentives. As a consequence, agricultural production increased less than population growth, and the failure of agricultural production to keep pace resulted in the ever-increasing importation of food.

In 1970, a socialist government was elected and an agrarian reform was implemented. This reform resulted in the expropriation of more than 60% of the total land under cultivation in the country. Agricultural production came almost totally under government control. A year later, agricultural production had nearly collapsed. Enormous amounts of food, equivalent to 70% of all the requirements, had to be imported *(14)*.

Three years later, in 1973, a military defeated the socialist government, and a free and open market economy was created. In 1974, CONPAN and the Ministry of Agriculture established a new agricultural policy based on the following principles:

1. Transfer of state-owned land to peasants and farmers;
2. Free-market prices for every agricultural product and elimination of all state subsidies;
3. Guaranteed prices for basic products;
4. Technology transfer to farmers;
5. Construction of an irrigation infrastructure; and
6. A new credit policy.

As a result of these changes, a rapid increase in agricultural production was achieved with an annual growth rate of 7% during the last 10 yr. The value of food imports fell from 700 million in 1973 to 200 million annually at present. In the last 11 yr a remarkably strong agricultural sector, consisting of fruit and vegetable production and agroindustrial development, has been established. Today, this has become one of the most dynamic economic sectors, which in 1995 accounted for 2300 million/yr in exports. The success of Chile's agricultural sector has led not only to a sharp decline in costly food imports, but also to a substantial increase in rural employment and income and, correspondingly, to a marked improvement in health and nutrition.

5. SUMMARY

The Chilean experience demonstrates that it is possible to implement targeted interventions in health, sanitation, education, and food production that lead to substantial improvements in the population's health and nutrition status despite the persistence of poverty and underdevelopment. This result is important because it shows that it was possible to prevent to a large extent the physical and psychological injury of large numbers of Chile's infants and children. By hindering the full expression of the genetic potential of the population, negative societal and environmental factors impede development. We maintain that the capabilities of the population constitute the most precious asset of any country. If we want to reach satisfactory levels of development, this resource must be carefully protected and nurtured. Our experience may be useful to other countries with whom we share similar problems. Of course, the successful utilization of our experience requires an analysis of local realities and the adaptation of the programs to these realities.

It is important to stress that the process described in this chapter took place over several decades. Its success resulted mainly from the persistence and continuity of programs over time and continued improvements in their implementation. In the future, periodic adaptation of programs to the prevailing circumstances, along with sound economic strategies to improve the situation of the poorer groups, will have to be implemented to consolidate the advances already made. If these conditions are not met, these gains may be lost because they already exceed the economic limits of the country; that is, what might be expected given the limited economic growth and limited income that are evident in many parts of the country.

REFERENCES

1. Mönckeberg FS, Valiente S, Mardones F. infant and preschool nutrition: economical development versus intervention strategies, the case of chile. Nutr Res 1987; 7:327.
2. Mönckeberg F. The Possibilities for nutrition intervention in Latin America. Food Tech 1981; 35:115–121.
3. Commissions on Health Research Development. *Health Research: Essential Link to Equity in Development*. Oxford University Press, 1990; pp. 10.
4. Terra JP. Situación de la Infancia en Latinoamérica y el Caribe Remarks at the Annual Meeting of UNICEF, Mexico City, May 16–18, 1979.
5. Mönckeberg F. Socioeconomic development and nutritional status: efficiency of intervention programs. In Nutrition Intervention Strategies in National Development. Underwood, ed. New York: Academic Press, 1983; 31.
6. Taucher E. Effects of Declining Fertility on Infant Mortality Levels. New York: Rockefeller Foundation, 1986. unpublished report.
7. Mönckeberg F, Valiente S, eds. *Food and Nutrition Policy in Chile* Santiago: Instituto de Nutrición y Technológea de los Alimentos, 1976.
8. Möncherberg F, Riumallo J. Nutrition recovery centers: the Chilean Experience, in: Nutrition Intervention Strategies in National Development Underwood BA, ed., New York: Academic 1983, p. 31–42.
9. Mönckeberg F. Treatment of severe malnutrition during the first year of life. In: Nutrition in the 1980s: Constraints on Our Knowledge. New York: 1981; 141.
10. Gonzalez N, et al. Evaluación preliminar del programa de pomento a la lactancia materna. Rev Chilean Pediatr 1982; 54:360.
11. Valiente S, et al. Evolución de la mortalidad infantil y otros indicadores Conexos en Chile, entre 1962 y 1981. Unpublished Report.
12. Gonzalez N, Infante A, Schlesinger L, Mönckeberg F. Effectiveness of suplementary feeding programs in Chile. In: Nutrition Intervention Strategies in National Development. (Underwood B ed), New York, Academic Press, 1983; pp. 101–109.
13. Schlesinger L, et al. Environmental sanitation: a nutrition intervention. In: *Nutrition Intervention Strategies in National Development*. Underwood Academy: 1983; p. 241.
14. Mönckeberg F. Crear para competir y Competir para Seguir Creando. Santiago: Editorial Andrés Bello, 1980.

29 Effects of Western Diet on Risk Factors of Chronic Diseases in Asia

Kaichi Kida, Takuo Ito, Sei Won Yang, and Vichai Tanphaichitr

1. INTRODUCTION

Infectious diseases and malnutrition were the major medical problems in most Asian countries before the World War II and are still so today in some parts of Asia. The structure of diseases has been dramatically changed in many Asian countries after World War II, in parallel with a rapid development of the economy followed by Westernization of lifestyles. The GNP has been increased by 20 times in Japan, 43 times in Korea, and 17 times in Thailand in the past 25 yr and lifestyles in housing, clothing, and eating have been westernized in these countries. Westernization of diets is seen in an increase of protein and fat consumption at meals and the prevalence of American style fast foods, such as hamburgers and fried chicken. In Japan, Korea, and Thailand, the three leading causes of death today are neoplasms, heart disease, and cerebrovascular disease, as they are in Europe and North America. The cost for cardiovascular disease in Japan in 1992 was US$44 billion, accounting for 6% of the national budget. Chronic diseases resulting from atherosclerosis are not only a medical, but also a growing economic problem in Asian as well as Western countries. Thus, more attention is required aimed at prevention of risk factors for these chronic diseases by nutritional intervention. In this chapter, the relationship between Westernization of diets and chronic diseases based on atherosclerosis or their risk factors in Asian countries is reviewed. Nutritional recommendations are described in reference to prevention of risk factors for chronic diseases based on atherosclerosis.

2. EPIDEMIOLOGY OF CHRONIC DISEASES AND THEIR RISK FACTORS

2.1. Chronic Diseases

Heart disease, which develops from atherosclerosis and/or hypertension, has been linearly increasing year by year and has recently become one of the major causes of death in Japan, Korea, and Thailand *(1)*. Although the death rate from ischemic heart disease has increased several-fold in Japan and Korea in the last 20–50 yr, it is still substantially lower than in Europe and North America; 9.9/100,000 in 1950 to 41.4/100,000 in 1992 in Japan *(2)*, and 2.2/100,000 in 1983 to 12.5/100,000 in 1992 in Korea *(3)* (Fig. 1). In Thailand, the death rate from heart disease increased from

From: *Preventive Nutrition: The Comprehensive Guide for Health Professionals*
Edited by A. Bendich and R. J. Deckelbaum Humana Press Inc., Totowa, NJ

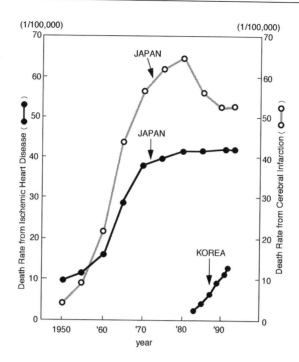

Fig. 1. Yearly change in death rates from ischemic heart disease and cerebral infarction in Japan and Korea.

40.3/100,000 in 1987 to 56.0/100,000 in 1992, a period of only 5 yr. The prevalence of ischemic heart disease in one Thai community serially studied increased from 7/1000 in 1976 to 17/1000 in 1983 *(4)*.

Cerebrovascular diseases are also emerging as a leading cause of death in Japan and other Asian countries *(1)* (Fig. 1). Although the death rate from total cerebrovascular diseases in Japan has gradually decreased during the past 25 yr, the death rate from cerebral infarction and its contribution to total cerebrovascular diseases have greatly increased over 40 yr; from 4.0/100,000 in 1950 to 52.4/100,000 in 1993 *(2)* (Fig. 1). In Korea, the death rate from cerebrovascular diseases increased from 65.4/100,000 in 1983 to 80.4/100,000 in 1992 *(3)*. In Thailand, the death rate from hypertension and cerebrovasular diseases increased from 12.8/100,000 in 1987 to 16.9/100,000 in 1992 and the prevalence of hemiplegia as a result of cerebrovascular diaseases in one town increased from 1.5/1000 in 1976 to 6.6/1000 in 1983 *(4)*.

2.2. Risk Factors

Both hypercholesterolemia and hypertension are now proved to be major risk factors for ischemic heart disease and cerebrovascular diseases among Japanese, similar to Caucasian populations *(5,6)*. Nationwide surveys demonstrate that serum total cholesterol levels have increased by 20–30 mg/dL between 1960 and 1990 in both adults and children in Japan *(7–11)* (Table 1). The average total cholesterol levels of Japanese adults today are still lower than those of American adults, but those of Japanese children are now similar or even slightly higher than those of American children. All school children 9–12 yr old (approx 10,000 school children) have been screened for serum choles-

Table 1
Yearly Change in Serum Total Cholesterol Levels in Japan

	1960 (7)	1970 (8)	1980 (9)	1990 (10)	1993 (11)
Males					
30–39 yr	167 ($n = 676$)	188 ± 33 ($n = 239$)	192 ± 38 ($n = 897$)	196 ± 35 ($n = 620$)	203 ± 39 ($n = 475$)
40–49 yr	175 ($n = 1043$)	194 ± 45 ($n = 1043$)	197 ± 38 ($n = 1533$)	204 ± 37 ($n = 788$)	208 ± 39 ($n = 558$)
50–59 yr	175 ($n = 878$)	181 ± 45 ($n = 623$)	199 ± 39 ($n = 1081$)	200 ± 37 ($n = 758$)	206 ± 37 ($n = 583$)
60–69 yr	179 ($n = 428$)	169 ± 43 ($n = 334$)	193 ± 40 ($n = 594$)	197 ± 38 ($n = 674$)	200 ± 38 ($n = 574$)
Females					
30–39 yr	187 ($n = 396$)	184 ± 42 ($n = 184$)	178 ± 34 ($n = 591$)	186 ± 32 ($n = 992$)	190 ± 32 ($n = 780$)
40–49 yr	192 ($n = 325$)	179 ± 36 ($n = 377$)	191 ± 39 ($n = 705$)	200 ± 35 ($n = 1124$)	205 ± 35 ($n = 867$)
50–59 yr	207 ($n = 216$)	194 ± 44 ($n = 273$)	211 ± 41 ($n = 735$)	218 ± 37 ($n = 995$)	225 ± 38 ($n = 852$)
60–69 yr	194 ($n = 104$)	189 ± 44 ($n = 142$)	214 ± 39 ($n = 597$)	223 ± 38 ($n = 870$)	223 ± 37 ($n = 751$)

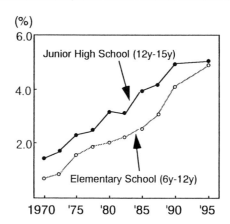

Fig. 2. Yearly change in obesity among school children (Rohrer Index ≥ 160) in Matsuyama, Japan. The number of children in elementary schools and junior high schools are approx 30,000 and 15,000 in a year.

terol, blood pressure, and obesity every year in the town of Matsuyama since 1989. Their serum total cholesterol levels have increased by 5 mg/dL for these 7 yr. The prevalence of hypercholesterolemia (≥200 mg/dL) is 15.7% (780/4972) in school children of 9–10 yr and 8.3% (418/5024) in those of 12–13 yr in Matsuyama; their average total cholesterol levels are 172.4 ± 25.3 at the age of 9–10 yr (n = 4972) and 165.7 ± 24.7 at the age of 13 yr (n = 5024) (Kida K, Matsuyama Study 1995). The prevalence of hypertensive diseases (hypertension and diseases from hypertension) in Japan has increased from 8.0/1000 in 1965 to 15.6/1000 in 1975, and 30.7/1000 in 1985 *(12)*. The prevalence of hypertension among adults 30 yr old or more in 1990 was 29.7% in men and 26.2% in women *(10)*. That among school children is 13/1000 in boys and 16/1000 in girls of 9–10 yr and 14/1000 in boys and 21/1000 in girls of 12–13 yr (Kida K, Matsuyama Study 1995). It is well established that obesity is associated with hyperlipidemia and hypertension among Japanese *(13,14)*. The average BMI (weight/height^2) among Japanese adults has been increasing during the past 40 yr and estimated prevalence of adulthood obesity (BMI ≥ 30) in Japan today is 2.1% in men and 3.3% in women, which is still lower than those in Western countries *(15)*. Nevertheless, the prevalence of obesity (160 or more of Rohrer Index, weight/height^3) among Japanese school children has remarkably increased by 3–5 times during the past 30 yr (Kida K, Matsuyama Study 1995) (Fig. 2). School children with hypercholesterolemia or obesity in Matsuyama are provided with health education, including diet and excercise recommendations, by school dietitians and school nurses. Improvement of serum total cholesterol or obesity is achieved in more than 50% of children after this instruction (Kida K, Matsuyama Study) (Fig. 3, Table 2).

In Korea, the average total cholesterol levels of children are comparable with those of Japanese or American children and the prevalence of hypercholesterolemia (≥200 mg/dL) among school children is reported to be 5–23% *(16)*. The prevalence of obesity has increased by 70% in boys and by 35% in girls over only 4 yr, from 1984 to 1988; these rates are now 12.4% among boys and 11.6% among girls in Seoul and Cheju *(17,18)*. In Thailand, a survey of coronary risk factors and nutritional conditions among

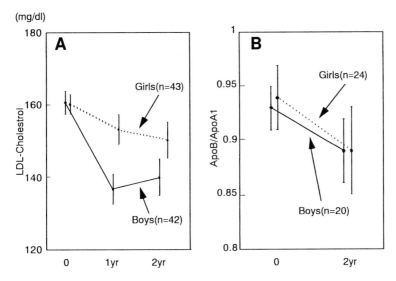

Fig. 3. Effect of intervention on LDL-cholesterol levels and ratio of ApoB/ApoA1. Children with 140 mg/dL or more of serum LDL-cholesterol and those with 0.8 or more of ApoB/ApoA1 ratio were given nutritional education by school dietitians and followed up for 2 yr.

Table 2
Effect of Intervention on Obesity Among School Children in Matsuyama (Longitudinal Study)

	Percent overweight	
	9–10 yr	*12–13 yr*
Intervention group		
Boys (*n* = 339)	33.0 ± 0.6 →	30.1 ± 0.9[a]
Girls (*n* = 261)	31.0 ± 0.7 →	23.4 ± 1.0[b]
Nonintervention group		
Boys (*n* = 82)	31.1 ± 1.3 →	33.9 ± 1.6
Girls (*n* = 111)	31.2 ± 1.0 →	30.0 ± 1.6

[a]$p < 0.05$, mean ± SE.
[b]$p < 0.001$, mean ± SE.

3495 workers was done in 1985 and reported that the prevalence of hypercholesterolemia (≥ 200mg/dL), hypertension ($\geq 141/91$) and obesity (BMI ≥ 25) was respectively 71.3, 9.6, and 25.5% in men and 65.4, 4.3, and 21.4% in women. In 1991, the later survey was done among 519 hospital staff people, who were expected to be more motivated for health. This study demonstrated that the prevalence of hypercholesterolemia, hypertension, and obesity was 33.4, 4.6, and 18.2% in men and 40.2, 1.8, and 27.0% in women, lower than those in the former survey but still high *(4,19)*. This suggests that motivation and education play an important role in reducing these risk factors. Thus, risk factors for chronic disease, including hypercholesterolemia, hypertension, and obesity, have increased over only a few decades in Asian countries, and are now compatible or even exceed those in Western countries.

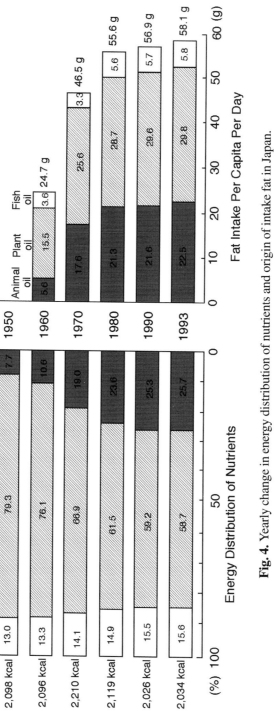

Fig. 4. Yearly change in energy distribution of nutrients and origin of intake fat in Japan.

Table 3
Yearly Change in Intake of Nutrients per Capita per Day in Korea

Nutrients	1971	1976	1981	1986	1991	1992
Energy, kcal	2072	1926	2052	1930	1930	1875
Carbohydrate, g	422	380	394	343	325	313
% Energy	81.5	78.9	76.8	71.0	67.4	66.8
Fat, g	13.1	20.0	21.8	28.1	35.6	34.5
% Energy	5.7	9.3	9.6	13.1	16.6	16.6
Protein, g	67.0	60.4	67.2	74.2	73.0	74.2
% Animal origin	11.6	20.2	32.2	41.2	42.7	46.6

3. NUTRITIONAL STATES

In Japan, the total energy intake per capita per day has not significantly changed for the past 40 yr; 2098 kcal in 1950, 2184 kcal in 1965, 2119 kcal in 1980, and 2034 Kcal in 1993 *(11)* (Fig. 4). On the other hand, the percent energy intake from fat has increased 3.3 times during these 40 yr; 7.7% in 1950, 14.8% in 1965, 23.6% in 1980, and 25.7% in 1993. Intake of fat of animal, plant, and fish origin has been increased respectively by 4, 1.9, and only 1.6 times during these 30 yr, and the ratio of fat from animal, plant, and fish is now 4:5:1 in Japan *(11)* (Fig. 4). The percent energy intake from saturated fatty acids (S), monounsaturated fatty acids (M), and polyunsaturated fatty acids (P) in Japan was 2, 3, and 4%, respectively in 1955, but it became 8, 9, and 9%, respectively, in 1985, which indicates that fat intake, particularly fat of animal origin, greatly increased in these 30 yr *(20)*. The ratio of n-6 polyunsaturated fatty acids/n-3 polyunsaturated fatty acids increased from 2.8 in 1955 to 3.8 in 1985 *(20)* and 4.1 in 1990 *(21)*. The increase in the ratio of n-6/n-3 polyunsaturated fatty acids might be attributed to a relative decrease in intake of fat of fish origin and an increase in intake of plant oils containing a large amount of linoleic acid. In fact, the energy intake from linoleic acid was increased 2.5 times, from 2.6% in 1955 to 6.4% in 1985 in Japan *(20,22)*. The protein intake per capita per day has not changed in the past 30 yr in Japan, but protein of animal origin increased 1.7 times and protein of plant origin decreased by 34% in this period *(11)*. The change in the quantity and quality of nutrients might reflect Westernization of diets of Japanese people. Furthermore, occasions to eat meals outside at restaurants or even at American-style fast-foods bars, where fat-rich foods, such as hamburgers and fried chicken, are served, have remarkably increased in Japan during the past 30 yr; 11.3% in 1965, 16.1% in 1980, and 19.6% in 1993 *(11)*. The eating habits of Japanese have, thus, been Westernized in quantity, quality, and manner.

A similar pattern is seen in Korea *(23)* (Table 3). Eating habits have been greatly Westernized during the past 20 yr. The total energy intake per capita per day has slightly decreased, whereas the percent energy from fat has been increased by three times; 5.7% in 1971, 9.6% in 1981, and 16.6% in 1992 *(23)*. The ratio of fat from animal, plant, and fish was 19:69:12 in 1971 and was 25:62:13 in 1990. The ratio of S:M:P is reported to be 2:2.8:1 and that of n-6/n-3 to be 4.9 in 1990 *(23)*. The protein intake per capita per day was increased only by 1.1 times, whereas protein of animal origin increased 4.4 times from 1981–1992 *(23)*. The expense for fast foods and instant foods increased from 7.7% in 1973 to 12.9% in 1983 and occasions to eat meals outside the home also increased, from 2.8% in 1977 to 8.9% in 1986 *(23)*. In Thailand as well, Westernization

Table 4
Cohort Study on Eating of Fish and Sex-, Age-Adjusted Death Rate (Relative Risk)
from Chronic Diseases in Japan, 1966–1982

	Eating of fish					
Cause of death	Every day	Sometimes	Rarely	Never	χ^2	P
Total death	1.0	1.07	1.12	1.32	9.13	<0.0001
Cerebrovascular diseases	1.0	1.08	1.10	1.10	4.54	<0.0001
Heart diseases	1.0	1.09	1.13	1.24	3.92	<0.0001
Hypertension	1.0	1.55	1.89	1.79	4.14	<0.0001
Liver cirrhosis	1.0	1.21	1.30	1.74	3.77	<0.0001
Stomach cancer	1.0	1.04	1.04	1.44	2.14	<0.05
Liver cancer	1.0	1.03	1.16	2.62	2.11	<0.05
Uterus cervix cancer	1.0	1.28	1.71	2.37	4.14	<0.0001
observed person • year	1,412,740	2,186,368	203,945	28,943		

of diets can be seen in increased fat intake by people in Bangkok. Fat currently accounts for 30% of total energy intake (19).

4. ATHEROSCLEROSIS AND NUTRITION

It is well established that the origin of dietary fat and its composition of fatty acids are related to the risk of cardiovascular diseases resulting from atherosclerosis. The epidemiological study with Eskimos in Greenland and many other studies demonstrate that fish oils or n-3 polyunsaturated fatty acids could play a role in preventing cardiovascular diseases (see Chapter 12) (24–28). Epidemiological studies with Japanese have shown similar results. The death rates from ischemic heart disease and cerebral infarction were lower by 2.6 and 9.2 times, respectively, in the town of Higashi-Izu, where people eat more fish than in Tokyo (29). More recently, a large scale epidemiological investigation was done to look at the effect of eating fish on the risk of chronic diseases among adults in Japan. The 55,523 deaths out of 265,118 cohort from 1966–1982 were analyzed in reference to their intake of fish. The study revealed that the total death rate and the death rate from cerebrovascular disease, heart disease, hypertension, and cancer were significantly lower in people who ate fish every day compared to those who did so sometimes, rarely, or never (30) (Table 4). Looking at the degree of development of atherosclerosis in living subjects by measuring pulse-wave velocity of the aorta, it was 7.0 ± 1.1 m/s in a fishermen's village where 90% of people eat fish every day, and death from ischemic heart disease is low. The pulse-wave velocity was significantly slower (less sclerotic) than the value of 7.7 ± 1.3 m/s in a farmer's village where only 11% of people eat fish every day, and death from ischemic heart disease is high (31). Furthermore, renarrowing of coronary arteries after percutaneous transluminal coronary angioplasty (PTCA) for ischemic heart disease was significantly decreased, from 37% in controls ($n = 43$) to 20% in subjects who were orally given 1.6 g/d of eicosapentenoic acid (EPA) for 3–4 mo ($n = 30$) (32), as confirmed by a large-scale double-blind investigation (33). A multi-center study in Japan demonstrated that EPA was effective in arteriosclerosis obliterans (ASO) as assessed by the diameter of ulcers on the skin; 7.4 ± 1.87 mm in controls ($n = 25$) vs 6.0 ± 1.59 mm in subjects treated with 1.8 g/d of EPA for 6 wk ($n = 18$) (34).

Table 5
Nutritional Recommendations in Japan, Korea, and Thailand

	Japan (37)	Japan (Matsuyama)	Korea (41)	Thailand (42)
Fat intake (% total energy)	20–25 (≥18 yr) 25–30 (1–17 yr)	20–25 (≥1 yr)	20	<30
Fat intake from animal:plant:fish	4:5:1[a]	3:4:2		
Fish meat, g/animal meat, g		1.0–1.5		
S:M:P	1:1.5:1.0[a]	1:1.5:1.5	1:1~1.5:1	1:1:1
n-6/n-3	4[a]	3–(2)		

[a]Reasonable at present.

These data indicate that oils of fish orgin or n-3 polyunsaturated fatty acids could be beneficial in preventing atherosclerosis and related chronic diseases.

Another characteristic of the Japanese diet is a high intake of salt (NaCl), which likely plays an essential role in hypertension as an important risk factor for atherosclerosis. The salt intake per capita per day in Japan today is 12.8 g, i.e., 6.4 g/1000 kcal, which has not changed in the past 30 yr (11). About 50% of total salt is from soy sauce, soy bean paste and salted vegetables (11). People in the eastern part of Japan consume 1.3 times more salt than those in the Kinki district, including Osaka and Kyoto (11). Public education in a community for 8 wk successfully reduced salt intake of the residents by 3.8 g/d and lowered the systolic blood pressure by 4.7 mm Hg and diastolic blood pressure by 3.9 mm Hg (35).

5. NUTRITIONAL RECOMMENDATIONS

Taking the rapid increase in chronic diseases based on atherosclerosis and Westernization of diets into consideration, much attention is paid to reduction of chronic diseases by establishing a nutritionally appropriate lifestyle in Japan. The most recent recommendations appear in the fifth edition of Recommended Dietary Allowance for Japanese issued by the Ministry of Health and Welfare of Japan in 1994 (36) (Table 5). The recommended energy intake was calculated by the formula; $E = (1 + A) \times B \times 10/9$, where E is the recommended energy intake (kcal/d), B is the basal metabolic rate (kcal/d) estimated from body surface, and A is the coefficient for intensity of daily activities. The energy intake from fat is recommended to be 25–30% of total energy intake for young people of 1–17 yr and 20–25% of total energy intake for adults of 18 yr or more. These recommendations are in contrast to the previous recommendations, which was 25–30% of total energy for all people (37). The ratio of S:M:P among fatty acids is recommended to be 1:1.5:1 and the ratio of n-6/n-3 of polyunsaturated fatty acids to be 4.0 according to the results of analyses of the present nutritional conditions of Japanese people. The intake of salt (NaCl) is recommended now at 10 g/d or less and should be reduced to 7–8 g/d if possible.

There are a few arguments relating to these recommendations. There are no apparent reasons to elevate the upper limit of fat intake to 30% of the total energy for young people from 25% for adults. In fact, hypercholesterolemia is found in 8.3–15.7% of school children (Kida K, Matsuyama Study, 1995). Furthermore, pathological studies in Japan as well as in the United States have revealed that atheroscrelosis takes place with high

Table 6
Menus of Typical Japanese and Korean Meals and Their Composition of Nutrients

	Japan			Korea		
	Breakfast	*Lunch*	*Dinner*	*Breakfast*	*Lunch*	*Dinner*
	Steamed rice	Steamed rice	Steamed rice	Steamed rice	Steamed rice with barley	Steamed rice
	Soybean soup	Beef and vegetable in sukiyaki style	Grilled mackerel pike	Seaweed soup	Beanpaste pot stew	Kimuchi pot stew
	Grilled salmon	Salad	Stewed radish	Soybean curd	Baked fish (a hair-tail)	Beel boiled in soy sauce
	Pickled radish	Fruit	Grilled salmon	Fried food	Soybean boiled with soy sauce	Soybean sprout
	Stewed vegetable	Low-fat milk	Grated yam	Cucumber salad	Spinach	Anchovy boiled in soy sauce
	Fruit		Spinach with egg in soup	Laver	Kimchi	Kimchi
				Kimchi		Apple
				Milk		
Total energy		1967 kcal			1890 kcal	
% energy (carbohydrate/fat/protein)		63/20/17			63/20/17	
S:M:P		1:1.2:1.1			1:1.3:0.6	
n-6/n-3		2.1			5	
Salt		7.7 g			18.5 g	

532

frequency even in young people and is related to their blood cholesterol levels *(38–40)*. Our study group of Matsuyama, therefore, recommends that fat intake should not exceed 25% of the total energy in school children and adolescents of 6–17 yr. Even infants, except babies and young infants, should not be exposed to fat-rich diets since the period of infancy is critical toward setting eating habits in later life (Table 5). Although no definite consensus on the ideal composition of fat and fatty acids is established, it is obvious from animal experiments and epidemiological studies that fat of animal origin should be reduced and the ratio of n-6 to n-3 of polyunsaturated fatty acids should be lowered as much as possible. The authors do not think it is rational to set the recommended values for the composition of fat and fatty acids from the results of analyses of the average diets in Japan today that are unfavorably Westernized in terms of fat. It might be feasible for Japanese to take more fat of fish orgin and less of animal origin and at the same time to reduce linoleic acid (n-6 polyunsaturated fatty acid) intake by avoiding oil or food fortified with linoleic acid, so that the ratio of n-6/n-3 of polyunsaturated fatty acids may be lowered to the level of 2.8, which was the ratio in 1955. Our study group of Matsuyama, accordingly, recommends the ratios of S:M:P among fatty acids and of n-6/n-3 of polyunsaturated fatty acids be 1:1.5:1.5 and 3.0–(2.0), respectively (Table 5). Regarding salt intake, the recommended intake of salt, 10.0 g/d, is still high compared with those in many other parts of the world. Our study group of Matsuyama also recommends intake of salt to be 8.0 g/d. The recommended salt intake of 8.0 g/d is not far below the 10.8 g/d level found in the Kinki district, one of the most traditional, and at the same time, most modernized places in Japan.

In Korea, the recommended fat intake is 20% of total energy intake and recommended ratios of S:M:P and n-6/n-3 are 1.0:1.0–1.5:1.0 and 4–10, respectively *(41)*. In Thailand, it is recommended that the fat intake should not exceed 30% of total energy intake with equal distribution of S, M, and P among fatty acids *(42)*.

Table 6 presents a typical sample of menus of Japanese and Korean meals for a breakfast, lunch, and dinner. The Japanese menu fits the recommendation of our study group of Matsuyama. The menus of meals are neither too Westernized nor too traditional or "old fashioned" so that all generations of people may accept it as part of daily life today. Efforts are needed to educate the community, governmental organizations, and nongovernmental organizations, including food industries and mass medias, to understand the role of nutrition and usefulness of Asian traditional diets in prevention of chronic diseases based on atherosclerosis and their risk factors.

REFERENCES

1. WHO: World Health Statistics Annual, 1993.
2. Statistics and Information Department, Minister's Secretariat, Ministry of Health and Welfare of Japan. Vital Statistics of Japan, 1993.
3. National Statistics Office, Republic of Korea. Annual Report on Case of Death Statistics, 1994.
4. Leelagul P, Tanphaichitr V. Current status on diet-related chronic diseases in Thailand. Intern Med 1995; 11:28–33.
5. Tarui S. Distribution of phenotypes of hyperlipidemia and relationship between serum lipid levels and development of cardiovascular complications in Japan. Report of Study Group on Primary Hyperlipidemia, Ministry of Health and Welfare of Japan 1987; pp. 17–26.
6. Ueda K, Omae T, Hasuo Y, Kiyohara Y, Fujii I, Wada J, Kato I, Kawano H, Shinkawa A, Omura T, Fujishima M. Progress and outcome of elderly hypertensives in a Japanese comminity: results from a long-term prospective study. J Hyperten 1988; 6:991–997.

7. Research Committee on Atherosclerosis in Japan, Ministry of Education and Culture of Japan.Total serum cholesterol levels in normal subjects in Japan. Jpn Circ J 1965; 29:505–510.

8. Research Committee on Hyperlipidemia in Japan, Ministry of Education and Culture of Japan. Total serum cholesterol and triglyceride levels in normal subjects in Japan. J Jpn Atherosclerosis Soc 1973; 1:101–108.

9. Research Committee on Familial Hyperlipidemia in Japan, Ministry of Education and Culture of Japan. Changes of serum total cholesterol and triglyceride levels in normal subjects in Japan in the past twenty years Jpn Circ J 1983; 47:1351–1358.

10. Ministry of Health and Welfare of Japan. Report of the 4th National Survey of Cardiovascular Diseases (1990), 1993.

11. Division of Health Promotion and Nutrition, Ministry of Heath and Welfare of Japan. Report of National Nutrition Survey (1993), 1995.

12. Heath and Welfare Statistics Association of Japan. Trends in Public Health. 1991.

13. Tarui S. Study on etiology and pathophysiology of obesity in adults and children. Report of Sogo-Kenkyu, Ministry of Education and Culture of Japan, 1991.

14. Tokunaga K, Fujioka S, Matsuzawa Y. Ideal body weight estimated fom body mass index with lowest morbidity. Int J Obes 1991; 15:1.

15. Division of Health Promotion and Nutrition, Ministry of Health and Welfare of Japan. Report of Epidemiological Studies on Obesity (1994), 1995.

16. Yang MK. Childhood hyperlipidemia in Korea—a review. J Korean Pediatr Soc 1993; 36:1049–1058.

17. Cho KB, Park SB, Park SC, Lee DH, Lee SJ. The prevalence and trend of obesity in children and adolescents. J Korean Pediatr Soc 1989; 32:597–605.

18. Han BH, Kim DH, Park YK, Lee JH, Kim HS. Incidence and complications of obesity in pubescent school children. J Korean Pediatr Soc 1995; 38: 500–528.

19. Tanphaichitr V, Leelahagul P. Role of nutrition on healthy lifestyle. Intern Med (Bangkok) 1995; 11:34–40.

20. Sakai K, Ishikawa A, Okuyama H. Yearly change in quality and quantity of fat intaked in Japan. Abura-Kagaku (Oil Chemistry) 1990; 39:196–201.

21. Hirahara F. Yearly change in quality and quantity of dietary fat of Japanese. Fat Nutr 1995 (Toyama, Japan); 4:73–82.

22. Lands WE, Hamazaki T, Yamazaki K, Okuyama H, Sakai K, Goto Y, Hubbards VS. Changing dietary patterns. Am J Clin Nutr 1990; 51:991–993.

23. Ministry of Health and Social Affairs. Republic of Korea (1992) National Nutrition Survey Report, 1994.

24. Bang HO, Dyeberg J, Sinclair HM. The composition of the Eskimo food in northwestern Greenland. Am J Clin Nutr 1980; 33:3657–3661.

25. Kromhout D, Bosschieter EB, Coulander CDL. The inverse relation between fish consumption and 20-years mortality from coronary heart disease. New Engl J Med 1985; 312:1205–1209.

26. Burr ML, Fehily AM, Gilbert JF, Rogers S, Holliday RM, Sweetman PM, Elwood PC, Deadman NM. Effects of changes in fat, fish, and fiber intakes on death and myocardial infarction: diet and reinfarction trial (DART). Lancet 1989; ii:757–761.

27. Dolecek TA, Grandits G. Dietary polyunsaturated fatty acids and mortality in the mutiple risk factor intervention trial (MRFIT). World Rev Nutr Diet 1991; 66:205–216.

28. de Lorgeril M, Renaud S, Mamele N, Salen P, Martin J-L, Monjaud I, Guidollet J, Touboul P, Delaye J. Mediterranean alpha-linolenic acid-rich diet in secondary prevention of coronary heart disease. Lancet 1994; 343:1454–1459.

29. Yasugi T. Serum lipid level and incidences of ischemic arteriosclerotic diseases in Japanese population through the past 30 years with special reference on serum lipids and eicosapentaenoic acid levels. In: Atherosclerosis VII Frdge NH, Nestel PJ, eds, Amsterdam: Elsevier; 1986, pp 55–59.

30. Hirayama T. Fish consumption and health—the cause-specific death rate in reference to frequency of eating of fish. med Chugai (Tokyo) 1992; 46:157–162.

31. Hamazaki T, Urakaze M, Sawazaki S, Yamazaki K, Taki H, Yano S. Comparison of pulse wave velocity of the aorta between inhabitants of fishing and farming village in Japan. Atherosclerosis 1988; 73:157–160.

32. Yamaguchi T, Ishiki T, Nakamura M, Saeki F. Effect of fish oil on restenosis after PTCA. Atherosclerosis(Tokyo) 1990; 18:416.

33. Bairati I, Roy L, Meyer F. Double-blind, randomized, controlled trial of fish oil supplements in prevention of recurrence of stenosis after coronary angioplasty. Circulation 1992; 85:950–956.

34. Sakurai K, Tanabe T, Mishima Y, Sakaguchi S, Katsumura T, Kusaba A, Sakuma A. Clinical evaluation of MND-21 on chronic arterial occlusion—double-blind study in comparison with ticlopidine. Myakkan-gaku(Angiology)(Tokyo) 1988; 28:597–604.

35. Tanaka H, Date C, Yamaguchi M. Salt intake and hypertension. Igaku-no-Ayumi(Tokyo) 1994; 169:533–536.
36. Division of Health Promotion and Nutrition, Ministry of Health and Welfare of Japan. Recommended Dietary Allowance for the Japanese, 5th Revision, 1994.
37. Division of Health Promotion and Nutrition, Ministry of Health and Welfare of Japan. Recommended Dietary Allowance for the Japanese, 4th Revision, 1989.
38. Sakurai I, Miyakawa K, Komatsu A, Sawada T. Atherosclerosis in Japanese youth with reference to differences between each artery. Ann NY Acad Sci 1990; 598:410–417.
39. Tanaka K, Masuda J, Imamura T, Sueishi K, Nakashima T, Sakurai I, Shozawa T, Hosoda Y, Yoshida Y, Nishiyama Y, Yutani C, Hatano S. A nation-wide study of atherosclerosis in infants, children and young adults in Japan. Atherosclerosis 1988; 72:143–156.
40. Newman WP, Wattigney W, Berenson GS. Autopsy studies in the United States children and adolescents; relationship of risk factors to atherosclerotic lesion. In: Williams CL, Wynder EL, eds. Hyperlipidemia in children and the development of atherosclerosis. Ann NY Acad Sci 1991; 623:16–25.
41. The Korean Nutrition Society. Recommended Dietary Allowance for Koreans, 6th Revision, 1995.
42. Department of Health, Ministry of Public Health of Thailand. Recommended Daily Dietary Allowance and Dietary Guideline for Healthy Thais, 2nd Edition, 1989.

30 Goals for Preventive Nutrition in Developing Countries

Osman M. Galal and Gail G. Harrison

1. INTRODUCTION

Developing countries are increasingly facing the dilemma of dealing simultaneously with problems of persistent endemic malnutrition affecting primarily children and women of reproductive age and with increasing prevalences of obesity and of diet-related chronic diseases among adults. Unless this dilemma is squarely faced and rationally addressed, there is the real possibility that scarce preventive health and nutrition resources will be simply fragmented, resulting in deterioration rather than progress toward health for all. The health transition (and by implication, the nutrition transition) has widely different dynamics in different countries, but everywhere is bringing into focus the need to seriously reassess goals and objectives for disease control and for preventive nutrition.

2. THE HEALTH TRANSITION

Figure 1 shows the general relationships among the processes termed the "health transition," including both the "demographic transition" marked by declines in mortality and fertility and the "epidemiologic transition" in which as the population ages there is an emergence of adult chronic disease and a change in the major causes of mortality. In the original formulation by Omran (1), there were three proposed eras through which countries passed at different stages of socioeconomic development: the era of "pestilence and famine," in which life expectancy was low and the major causes death were those associated with malnutrition, infection, and reproduction; the era of "receding pandemics," in which life expectancy rises to 30–50 yr, morbidity is still dominated by nutritional and infectious causes, and major mortality fluctuations are less common; and finally the era of "degenerative and man-made diseases," with life expectancy over 50 yr and major causes of death including cardiovascular diseases, cancer, diabetes, and other chronic ailments. Acknowledging the heterogeneity of social and economic development among human societies, Omran suggested that there were at least three models of the transition: the traditional or Western model, an accelerated model (typified by Japan), and a delayed or contemporary model. The latter describes the incomplete transition that characterizes most developing countries today, in which pretransition and posttransition problems must be dealt with simultaneously (2).

Recently, Frank et al. (3) have elaborated the model, which they have termed "epidemiologic polarization," based on observations from several large, middle-income

From: *Preventive Nutrition: The Comprehensive Guide for Health Professionals*
Edited by A. Bendich and R. J. Deckelbaum Humana Press Inc., Totowa, NJ

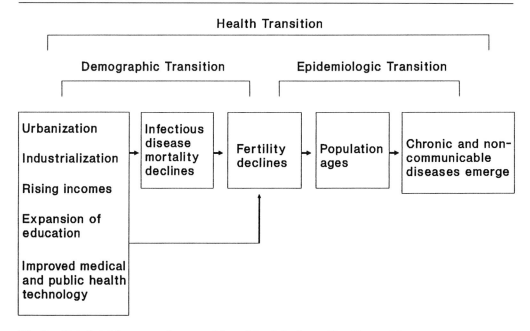

Fig. 1. Relationship among demographic, epidemiologic, and health transitions.

countries, to take account of widening within-country gaps in health status among so-cial classes and geographical regions. Features of this "protracted-polarized model" of health transition include recognition that the eras postulated by Omran are not necessar-ily sequential, but may overlap; that incomplete coverage of interventions to manage various health problems occurs; and the occurrence and persistence of major inequities in health status and even the reemergence of epidemic diseases that had been controlled or eradicated.

Table 1, from Jamison and Mosley *(4)*, shows one widely utilized summary by age group of the "unfinished agenda" of health problems associated with underdevelop-ment and those "neglected and emerging problems" that are increasingly coming to dominate the health agenda. The relative importance of the "emerging problems" on the health agenda is a function not only of socioeconomic development, but also of demo-graphic shifts. As populations age, adult problems become more important as causes of morbidity, mortality, disability, and health care costs. The elderly are becoming more numerous and more visible almost everywhere. Throughout the developing world, it has been estimated that populations over 65 yr of age will increase 134–164% between 1985 and 2015 *(4)*.

3. THE NUTRITION TRANSITION

Food consumption patterns, nutritional status, and diet-related morbidity and mortal-ity likewise show characteristic shifts with socioeconomic development, urbanization, education, and industrialization; these shifts have been most thoroughly articulated by Popkin *(5–7)*, who has postulated that the pace of dietary change seems to have recently accelerated to varying degrees in different regions of the world. The transition seems to converge on a rapid shift, when economic resources allow, to a dietary pattern charac-

Table 1
Important Health Problems in Developing Countries by Age Group[a]

Age group	Problems on the unfinished agenda	Neglected and emerging problems
Young children (0–4 yr)	Diarrheal disease Acute respiratory infection Measles, tetanus, polio Micronutrient deficiencies Malaria	Injury
School-age children (5–14 yr)	Schistosomiasis Geohelminth infections	Adolescent pregnancy Disability
Young adults (15–44 yr)	Maternal mortality Malaria Excess fertility	Tuberculosis Injury AIDS STDs Mental illness
Middle-aged (45–64 yr)		Cardiovascular disease Cancers COPD
Elderly (65+ yr)		Disability Depression

[a]Adapted from ref. 4.

terized by higher intakes of fat, animal products, sugar, and refined foods and lower intakes of fiber. The associated changes in nutritional status, often attributed to dietary changes because of their parallel in time, but also affected by changes in other risk factors, such as sanitation and physical activity patterns, include declines in general undernutrition and micronutrient deficiencies in children and increased prevalence of obesity and the chronic diseases for which obesity is a risk factor (cardiovascular disease and type II diabetes) among adults. It is evident, however, that the "polarization" noted by Frenk et al. *(3)* for general health status also applies to nutrition, with many countries facing the emergence of diet-related chronic diseases while still dealing with problems of undernutrition in children and among the poor *(see* Chapter 27).

Popkin *(8)* has pointed out several contrasting dynamics of the dietary transition; the "Western high-income model," characterized by the United States and a number of other countries, in which dietary transition occurred slowly; the "Japanese and Korean accelerated model," in which similar changes have occurred in < 30 yr, "emerging Asian models," epitomized by China and Thailand, in which urbanization and economic development have provoked very rapid dietary change among city dwellers and the higher socioeconomic classes; and the "Latin American pattern," which is similar to the US experience in occurring slowly and permeating the entire society, and in which obesity is as much or more a problem of the poor than of the well-to-do.

The pace of dietary change in many developing countries is very rapid, fueled largely by urbanization. It is estimated that 40% of the population of the developing world will live in cities by the year 2000, and 50% by 2015 *(9)*. Seven of the world's "megacities" (population more than 10 million) are in developing countries, and it is projected that six more will be added by the year 2000 *(4)*. The urban environment is generally more conducive to good nutritional status in children, but urbanization also brings disadvan-

Table 2
Proportion of Dietary Energy from Fat by Rural/Urban Residence
for Adults in China (China Health and Nutrition Survey, 1989)
and Egypt (Egypt Food Consumption Monitoring System, 1994)[a]

	Rural	Urban
Mean percent dietary energy from fat		
China	16.4	22.3
Egypt	22.8	27.5
Percent of adults with fat intakes		
<10% of energy		
China	26.4	8.5
Egypt	8.4	2.4
> 30% of energy		
China	8.9	21.1
Egypt	24.2	38.8

[a]Sources: Chinese data based on 3-d food intake from sample representative of
eight provinces, adults of both sexes ($N = 5891$), 1989; from ref. 15. Egyptian data
based on single 24-h recall, sampled over the calendar year 1994, on adult women in
representative sample in five of Egypt's 24 governorates ($N = 5680$); from ref. 16.

tages. Declines in breast-feeding rates and duration, household food insecurity linked to
the cash economy for very poor urban families, and increases in obesity associated with
sedentary lifestyles bring new nutritional risks that residents of the world's large cities
face in unprecedented numbers (10).

Table 2, constructed from large-sample surveys in China (1989) and Egypt (1994),
shows rural/urban contrasts in proportion of adult dietary energy intakes from fat, one
of the most sensitive and predictable changes in diet with urbanization. The increased
average proportion of energy from fat among urban dwellers in both countries substantially decreases the proportion of the population with very low fat intakes (<10% of energy) and increases the proportion with intakes of fat higher than optimal (>30% of energy). The Chinese data were analyzed additionally by income, showing a direct
relationship between household income and percent of dietary energy from fat in both
urban and rural households (11).

Nutritional status as judged by body mass index (BMI) in adults shows something of
the complexity of the relationships among income, diet, and body weight. Figure 2
shows an analysis of data on women's BMI as a function of family income in Brazil in
1989 (12). Among poor families, women's BMI increased linearly with household income, with the slope of the relationship steepest among the poorest families. Among the
30% of families with the highest household incomes, income showed no relationship to
women's BMI.

The prevalence of obesity is increasing in developing countries, and the associated
morbidities and mortality risks are emerging as public health problems (11,13–21).
Most of the literature comes from specific cohorts and localized community data, but
the available national surveys support the notion that the prevalence of obesity is increasing rapidly in many countries and that this phenomenon is taking place in the presence of continuing problems of undernutrition and micronutrient deficiencies in chil-

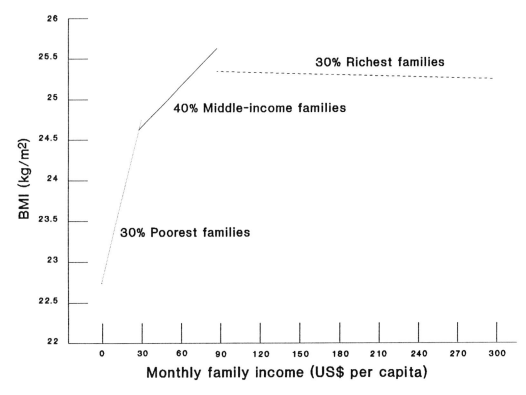

Fig. 2.   Women's body mass index regressed on family income in poor, middle, and rich families, Brazil, 1989.

dren. In the Egypt Food Consumption Monitoring Survey of 1994, the prevalence of obesity among adult women was shown to be high (>30%) even in the presence of continued endemic short stature and underweight in preschool children (31 and 11%, respectively). Risk of obesity was significantly higher for urban than for rural women *(22)*. The China Health and Nutrition Survey showed that the percentage of the population overweight increased between 1989 and 1991, and was greatest in the highest income groups *(23)*.

Whether early undernutrition might predispose to later adult obesity and associated conditions is a question with potentially important implications. In the United States, adult obesity shows no relationship to stature *(18)*. However, studies in the United States *(24)* and Norway *(25)* have demonstrated an inverse association between height and coronary heart disease (CHD), as well as other chronic disease causes of death, in adulthood.

Possible relationships between undernutrition early in life and later risk of obesity and related chronic disease has received recent attention largely as a result of the body of work published by Barker and colleagues from England *(26)*. Briefly, these investigators have observed that in the United Kingdom (as in the United States) obesity and related morbidity and mortality risks are more prevalent among the low socioeconomic portion of the population, as is the risk of low birthweight and poor postnatal growth. In a series of correlational studies, they have shown a relationship between low birth weight and risk in adult middle age of high blood pressure, noninsulin-dependent diabetes, and other risk factors for CHD. They hypothesize several possible mechanisms by which early undernutrition, either in utero or in early infancy, may "program" the individual for increased risk of adult chronic disease; these include modification of gene expression by the nutrient environment, modification of the endocrine milieu through permanent influences on endocrine structures or responses, reduced cell number and altered organ structure, and selection of clones of cells resulting in differences in proportions of different cell types.

Although intriguing, the hypotheses of Barker et al. require extensive examination in a variety of settings and designs. If correct, then part of what has been regarded as the genetic contribution to ischemic heart disease may in fact be the effect of the nutritional environment during early development *(27)*, the implications for developing countries are potentially great.

3.1. The Variety of Nutritional Patterns in Developing Countries

The differences among developing countries with regard to the distribution and prevalence of various nutrition problems and risks are at least as great as those between industrialized and less developed countries. The major determinants of the prevalence of various forms of malnutrition as well as other health problems are extremely variable. For example, the population of children under age 5 yr is expected to increase by only 2% in Latin America between 1985 and 2015, and 5% in Asia, but 38% in the Middle East and 70% in sub-Saharan Africa *(11)*. Some of the specific challenges facing public health nutrition planners in different economic contexts are highlighted below.

3.1.1. THE LOWEST-INCOME COUNTRIES: THE UNFINISHED AGENDA DOMINATES

It has been estimated that over the next decade perhaps 30–40 countries will remain in the lowest income bracket, in which health problems are dominated by infectious diseases of childhood, undernutrition, and high fertility *(4,28)*. The major problems continue to be diarrheal disease, acute respiratory illnesses in young children, measles, tetanus, polio, malaria, micronutrient deficiencies, parasitic diseases, and reproductive mortality. In these predominantly sub-Saharan and South Asian countries, the focus of nutrition goals must continue to be on establishing the basic primary health care infrastructure, breast-feeding, maternal nutrition, immunization against vaccine-preventable diseases, control of diarrheal disease, and family planning (*see* Chapter 18).

3.1.2. MIDDLE-INCOME COUNTRIES: SOCIAL POLARIZATION OF PRIORITIES

In a larger group of somewhat higher-income countries, predominantly in East Asia, Latin America, and the Middle East, the infectious disease, malnutrition, and reproductive health burdens remain substantial at the same time as rapid urbanization, industrialization, and economic development are leading to the emergence of new health problems, including injuries and preventable chronic diseases. Diet-related chronic disease emerges as a major priority quickly, since it affects first the higher-income, urban, educated segment of the population.

3.1.3. HIGH-INCOME COUNTRIES: THE CHALLENGE OF EQUITY

In high-income countries diet-related chronic diseases dominate the public health nutrition agenda. Problems of undernutrition and access to food affect mainly the lower income (and politically marginalized) segments of the population and generally have to fight for space on the political agenda and for resource allocation. Further, at least in the United States and the United Kingdom, obesity and its attendant problems also are most prevalent among low socioeconomic status segments of the population. So-called "diseases of affluence" are actually diseases of poverty in some of the richer countries. Policy makers often find it difficult to conceptualize the simultaneous occurrence of undernutrition and obesity, with the result that improvement of access to food and dietary quality often get a back seat to other priorities.

3.2. Industrialized Nonmarket Countries

The nations that comprise Eastern Europe and the former Soviet Union represent rather special cases; these have been categorized as "industrialized, non-market economies" *(29)*. Having long since passed through demographic, epidemiologic, and nutrition transitions, they have been recently undergoing an epidemic of excess mortality among relatively young adults from preventable causes *(30)*. These include trauma, poisoning, respiratory diseases (often secondary to smoking), and complications of pregnancy and childbirth *(31)*. Dietary and nutritional problems include high alcohol consumption, very high costs of food, limited dietary variety in terms of fruits and vegetables, micronutrient deficiencies in some groups, including iodine deficiency disease, and undernutrition, particularly in the elderly *(32)*.

3.3. The Challenge of Protecting the Nutritionally Vulnerable in the Course of Economic Adjustment Programs

The economic adjustment or "restructuring" programs that began in the 1980s and continue today resulted from a combination of pressures, including reduced foreign loans to governments of less developed countries, inability to generate internal monies through taxation or borrowing, and declines in real per capita income in a number of countries. Although the specifics vary, restructuring generally involves increased domestic savings, decreased government expenditures, increased economic efficiency, and contraction of public infrastructure.

In a number of countries, a major feature has been the elimination or drastic curtailment of untargeted or minimally targeted consumer subsidy programs. Without specific protection, one might expect such adjustments to have the greatest impact on the poorest consumers, with resultant increases in food insecurity and risk of undernutrition. Egypt is a major case in point *(22)*. Prior to 1990, a complex, but largely untargeted subsidy and price-control program made available to consumers at very minimal cost a basic and nutritionally adequate diet. The subsidy program has been largely dismantled except for wheat flour and local bread. The prices of basic food commodities, as well as other consumer goods and utilities, have increased three- to tenfold during the period 1990–1994, whereas real wages have only doubled. In 1994, two-thirds of households in a large survey of almost 7000 households reported having changed their food intake in the previous year as a result of rising food prices and almost half (48%) reported spending more than three-quarters of their household income on food. The prevalence of household food insecurity (measured by reporting spending >75% of household income on food plus giving a food response to an open-ended question about how any hypothetical additional household income would be used) ranged from 4–21% in various regions *(17)*. There is some suggestion that the prevalence of underweight children in preschools during the same period may have increased slightly, after several years of steady decrease.

Protecting the poorest consumers from the negative short-term impact of structural adjustment programs requires the formulation of explicit goals and strategies to redirect a portion of resources into direct targeted programs to protect and improve the situation of vulnerable groups, and to redirect economic and social policies to promote the availability and consumption of nutritionally adequate diets among low-income families and children. Examples are the integration of explicit food and nutrition objectives and programs into adjustment strategies and programs of assistance through World Bank loans in Venezuela, Mexico, El Salvador, Costa Rica, and Jamaica *(33)*.

4. GOALS FOR PREVENTIVE NUTRITION

4.1. Readiness to Take Advantage of New Information and Technology

Although nutritional improvements have generally paralleled economic development, there is far from a one-to-one or deterministic relationship between the two. Experience to date indicates that medical and public health interventions, per capita incomes, and behavior and lifestyle variables must all be taken into consideration. A few countries and regions have managed to improve nutritional status dramatically without major increases in per capita incomes, whereas others that have experienced large increases in income have not made concomitant strides in nutritional improvements. To cite a few extreme examples *(34)* Sri Lanka, China, and Vietnam, with per capita incomes in the range of US $330–420, have life expectancies between 66 and 71 yr, whereas Saudi Arabia, Libya, and Oman exhibit life expectancies of 61–64 yr against per capita incomes over US $5000.

Caldwell *(35)* has analyzed data on health and income, identifying 11 countries (plus the state of Kerala in India) with health achievements over and above what would be expected by per capita incomes and another 11 countries with the poorest performance. The areas that did best in achieving favorable health indicators were (in descending order) Kerala, Sri Lanka, China, Burma (now Myanmar), Jamaica, India, Zaire, Tanzania, Kenya, Costa Rica, Ghana, and Thailand. They averaged a life expectancy of 61 yr, infant mortality of 64/1000 live births, and a per capita income of $501. The countries that did worst in this analysis were (in order from the poorest performance) Oman, Saudi Arabia, Iran, Libya, Algeria, Iraq, Yemen AR, Morocco, Ivory Coast, Senegal, and Sierra Leone, with average per capita incomes of $4462, life expectancy 51 yr, and infant mortality rates 124/1000 live births. The analysis showed that the strongest relationships with improved health status at low cost were variables that reflected the education of women of reproductive age, the practice of family planning, and the education of men. Medical care variables were less strongly related to health indices, and income showed even weaker relationships (*see* Chapter 28).

These analyses strongly support the idea that societies that have an egalitarian tradition that includes relative independence for women and an emphasis on the value of education have been able to take advantage of advances in medical and public health knowledge and information to improve their situations. Those that have severe differentials between male and female educational opportunities, and for which other cultural and behavioral characteristics mitigate against reduced fertility, have done poorly with regard to health even with rapidly and drastically increased incomes.

4.1.1. THE IMPORTANCE OF SETTING GOALS

The explicit articulation of goals for protection and improvement of nutritional status has the effect of continuous reinforcement of the importance of nutrition to policy makers and program administrators. It also provides the basis for monitoring of progress. The incorporation of specific and measurable nutrition and dietary goals into national health policy plans has characterized some of the most successful national experiences, including those of Norway *(36)*, Costa Rica *(37)*, the United States *(38)*, Cuba *(39)*, and others.

The *World Declaration and Plan of Action for Nutrition*, agreed on at the International Conference on Nutrition (ICN) in Rome in December 1992, set an ambitious agenda before the year 2000 *(40)*. These included elimination of: famine and famine-related deaths; starvation and nutritional-deficiency diseases in communities affected by natural and man-made disasters; and iodine and vitamin A deficiencies. The goals also included substantial reduction by the year 2000 in starvation and widespread chronic hunger; undernutrition among children, women, and the aged; other important micronutrient deficiencies, including iron; diet-related communicable and noncommunicable diseases; social and other impediments to optimal breast-feeding; and inadequate sanitation and poor hygiene, including unsafe drinking water.

It has become clear that the goals of the ICN were unrealistic. At mid-decade, only 46% of participating countries and territories had finalized or drafted their national plans of action for nutrition; 29% had not yet begun. Progress toward reduction in protein-energy malnutrition, iodine deficiency disease, vitamin A deficiency, and other types of malnutrition is far, in every case, from the levels required if the goals are to be met *(41)*.

4.2. Primary Prevention vs Secondary Interventions and the Polarization of Priorities

Although the simultaneous existence of problems of deficit and excess are now generally acknowledged, the informed articulation of realistic goals for overall nutritional improvement in developing countries is far behind where it needs to be. As Popkin *(23)* has pointed out, a failure to acknowledge the role of nutrition in CHD, cancer, and other chronic diseases will lead to the domination of medical interventions in the allocation of resources. The experience of the industrialized countries to date argues that primary prevention strategies associated with lifestyle changes are the most effective strategies with regard to these posttransition health problems. The challenge will be to articulate goals for preventive nutrition clearly and to avoid the polarization that results from a conceptual framework that pits undernutrition and children and the poor against emerging problems associated with diets dense in energy and fat and with sedentary lifestyles. If the hypotheses of Barker et al. *(26)* prove to be correct, then the best weapon against chronic diseases of adulthood will prove to be protection and improvement of the nutritional status of mothers and children.

5. RECOMMENDATIONS

Our recommendations for policy makers and planners in developing countries are several:

1. Make explicit goals for reduction of malnutrition, undernutrition, and food insecurity in vulnerable population groups.
2. Allocate resources and direct policies to assure the achievement of these goals even in the face of overall economic stress.
3. Consider primary prevention strategies first for damming the flood of diet-related chronic diseases of adulthood.
4. Give priority to the development and maintenance of nutrition surveillance systems that will allow the tracking of the nutrition transition in specific circumstances.

On the research agenda, priority should be very high for efforts to better understand the relationships between early (in utero and early childhood) nutritional status and adult health, in a variety of contexts.

REFERENCES

1. Omran A. The epidemiologic transition: a theory of the epidemiology of population change. Milbank Memorial Fund 1971; 49:509–538.
2. Bobadilla JL, Frenk J, Lozano R, Frejka T, Stern C. The epidemiologic transition and health priorities. In: Disease Control Priorities in Developing Countries, Jamison DR, Mosley WH, Measham AR, Banadilla JL, eds., Oxford: Oxford University Press, 1993, pp. 51–63.
3. Frenk J, Bobadilla JL, Sepulveda J, Lopez-Cervantes M. Health transition in middle-income countries: new challenges for health care. Health Policy Plann 1987; 4:29–39.
4. Jamison DT, Mosley WH. Disease control priorities in developing countries: health policy responses to epidemiologic change. Am J Public Health 1991; 81:15–22.
5. Popkin B. Nutritional patterns and transitions. Popul Dev Rev 1993; 19:138–157.
6. Popkin B, Ge K, Zhai F, Guo X, Ma H, Zohoori N. The nutrition transition in China: a cross-sectional analysis. Eur J Clin Nutr 1993; 47:333–346.
7. Montiero CA, Mondini L, Medeiros de Souza AL, Popkin BM. The nutrition transition in Brazil. Eur J Clin Nutr 1995; 49:105–113.
8. Popkin B. The nutrition transition. SCN News No. 10, 1993. Geneva: Administrative Committee on Coordination: Subcommittee on Nutrition (ACC/SCN), United Nations, pp. 13–18.
9. Solomons NW, Gross R. Urban nutrition in developing countries. Nutr Rev 1995; 53:90–95.
10. Galal OM, Harrison GG. The crowded metropolis: health and nutrition in Cairo. In: Poverty, Population and Politics: Middle East Cities in Crisis Bonine M, ed, 1996; Gainesville, FL, University of Florida Press, 1996.
11. Popkin BM, Keyou G, Fengying Z, Guo X, Haijiang M, Zohoori N. The nutrition transition in China: a cross-sectional analysis. Eur J Clin Nutr 1993; 47:333–346.
12. Monteiro CA, Mondini L, Medeiors de Souza AL, Popkin BM. The nutrition transition in Brazil. Eur J Clin Nutr 1995; 49:105–113.
13. Billéwicz WZ, McGregor IA. A birth-to-maturity longitudinal study of heights and weights in two West African (Gambian) villages, 1951–1977. Ann Hum Biol 1992; 9:309–320.
14. Binhemd T, Larbi EB, Absoon D. Obesity in a primary health care center: a retrospective study. Ann Saudi Med 1991; 11:163–166.
15. Chinwe Okeke E, Nnanyelugo DO, Ngwu E. The prevalence of obesity in adults by age, sex and occupation in Anambra State, Nigeria. Growth 1983; 47:263–271.
16. Collins V, Dowse G, Zimmet P. Prevalence of obesity in Pacific and Indian Ocean populations. Diabetes Res Clin Pract 1990; 10(Suppl 1):29S–32S.
17. Dhurandhar NV, Kulkarni PR. Prevalence of obesity in Bombay. Int J Obes 1992; 16:367–375.
18. Gurney M, Gorstein J. The global prevalence of obesity: an initial overview of available data. World Health Statistics Q 1989; 41:251–254.

19. Lolio C, Latorre M. Prevalence of obesity in a county town of Sao Paulo State Brazil. Rev Saude Publica 1991; 25:33–36.
20. Norgan NG. Body mass index and body energy stores in developing countries. Eur Clin Nutr 1990; 44(Suppl 1):79–84.
21. Khan LK, Harrison GG, Galal OM, Ritenbaugh C, Shaheen FM, Kirksey A, Jerome NW. Prevalence and functional correlates of obesity in an Egyptian village. Ecology Food Nutr 1996; 34:311–325.
22. Khorshid A, Galal OM. Development of a food consumption monitoring system for Egypt. Final report to the US Department of Agriculture and the Ministry of Agriculture of Eygpt, September 1995.
23. Popkin BM. The nutrition transition. SCN News 1993; 10:13–15.
24. Palmer JR, Rosenberg L, Shapiro S. Stature and the risk of myocardial infarction in women. Am J Epidemiol 1990; 132:27–32.
25. Waaler HT. Height, weight and mortality. The Norwegian experience. Acata Med Scand (Suppl) 1984; 679:2–50.
26. Barker DJP. Mothers, Babies and Disease in Later Life. London: BMJ Publishing Group, 1994.
27. Barker DJP. Rise and fall of western diseases. Nature 1989; 338:371–372.
28. World Health Organization. Global Estimates for Health Situation Assessment and Projections, 1990. Geneva: WHO, 1990.
29. Lopez AD. Causes of death in industrial and developing countries: estimates for 1985–1990. In: Jamison DT, Mosley WH, Meashom AR, Bobodilla JL, eds, Disease Control Priorities in Developing Countries Oxford and New York: Oxford University Press for the World Bank, 1993.
30. Kinsella KG. Changes in life expectancy 1900–1990. Am J Clin Nutr 1992; 55:1196S–1202S.
31. Barr DA, Field MG. The current state of health care in the former Soviet Union: implications for health care policy and reform. Am J Public Health 1996; 86:307–312.
32. Tulchinsky TH, Varavikova EA. Addressing the epidemiologic transition in the former Soviet Union: strategies for health system and public health reform in Russia. Am J Public Health 1996; 86:313–320.
33. Selowsky M. Protecting nutrition status in adjustment programmes: recent World Bank activities and projects in Latin America. Food Nutr Bull 1991; 13:293–302.
34. Caldwell JC. Health transition: the cultural, social and behavioural determinants of health in the third world. Soc Sci Med 1993; 36:125–135.
35. Caldwell JC. Routes to low mortality in poor countries. Popul Dev Rev 1986; 12:171–220.
36. Oshaug A. Towards Nutrition Security. Country Paper for Norway for the International Conference on Nutrition. Oslo: University of Oslo Institute for Nutrition Research, 1992; pp. 1–99.
37. Mohs E. Health policies and strategies. In: The Nutrition and Health Transition of Democratic Costa Rica Monuz C, Scrimshaw NS, eds., Boston MA: International Foundation for Developing Countries, 1995.
38. US Department of Health and Human Services. Healthy people 2000: goals for the Health of the Nation. Washington DC: US Government Printing Office, 1990.
39. Amador M, Pena M. Nutrition and health issues in Cuba: strategies for a developing country. Food Nutr Bull 1991; 13:311–317.
40. FAO/WHO. World Declaration and Plan of Action for Nutrition. International Conference on Nutrition, 1992.
41. World Health Organization. Nutrition: highlights of recent activities in the context of the world declaration and plan of action for nutrition. 1995; Geneva: WHO Nutrition Programme, 1995.

PART VI
NUTRITION-RELATED RESOURCES

Books Related to Preventive Nutrition

1. 1993. *Fats and Oils in Human Nutrition: Report of a Joint Expert Consultation.* Rome: Food and Agriculture Organization of the United Nations and the World Health Organization.
2. Armstrong, D. (ed.) 1994. *Free Radicals in Diagnostic Medicine. A Systems Approach to Laboratory Technology, Clinical Correlations, and Antioxidant Therapy. Advances in Experimental Medicine and Biology,* Vol. 366. New York: Plenum Press.
3. Bailey, L. B. (ed.). 1994. *Folate in Health and Disease.* New York: Marcel Dekker.
4. Bendich, A., Butterworth, C. E. (eds.) 1991. *Micronutrients in Health and in Disease Prevention.* New York: Marcel Dekker.
5. Bendich, A., Phillips, M., Tengerdy, R. (eds.) 1990. *Antioxidant Nutrients and Immune Functions. Advances in Experimental Medicine and Biology,* Vol. 262. New York: Plenum Press.
6. Berger, H. 1988. *Vitamins and Minerals in Pregnancy and Lactation—Nestle Nutrition Workshop Series Vol. 16: Joint Symposium, Nestle-Hoffman-La Roche.* New York: Raven Press.
7. Blake, D., Winyard, P. G. (eds.) 1995. *Immunopharmacology of Free Radical Species.* London: Academic Press.
8. Bracco, U., Deckelbaum, R. J. (eds.) 1992. *Polyunsaturated Fatty Acids in Human Nutrition.* Nestle Nutrition Workshop Series.
9. Brag, G., Ryan, D. (eds) 1993. *Pennington Center Nutritional Series. Vol. 3: Vitamins and Cancer Prevention.* Louisiana: Baton Rouge University Press.
10. Burckhardt, P., Heaney, R. P. (eds.) 1995. *Nutritional Aspects of Osteoporosis '94. Challenges of Modern Medicine,* Vol. 7. Rome, Italy: Ares-Serono Symposia Publications.
11. Cadenas, E., Packer, L. (eds.) 1996. *Handbook of Antioxidants.* New York: Marcel Dekker.
12. Canfield, L. M., Krinsky, N. I., Olson, J. A. (eds.) 1993. *Carotenoids in Human Health,* Vol. 691. New York: Annals of the New York Academy of Sciences.
13. Cunningham-Rundles, S. (ed.) 1993. *Nutrient Modulation of the Immune Response.* New York: Marcel Dekker.
14. Dobbing, J. (ed.) 1993. *Lipids, Learning, and the Brain: Fats in Infant Formulas. Report of the 103rd Ross Conference on Pediatric Research.* Columbus, OH: Ross Laboratories.
15. Fomon, S. J. (ed.) 1993. *Nutrition of Normal Infants.* St. Louis: Mosby.
16. Frei, B. (ed.) 1994. *Natural Antioxidants in Human Health and Disease.* San Diego: Academic Press.
17. Gaby, S. K., Bendich, A., Singh, V. N., Machlin, L. J. (eds.) 1991. *Vitamin Intake and Health* New York: Marcel Dekker.
18. Galli, C., Simopoulos, A. P., Tremoli, E. (eds.) 1994. *Effects of Fatty Acids and Lipids in Health and Disease.* Basel: Karger.
19. Goldberg, I. (ed.) 1994. *Functional Foods. Designer Foods, Pharmufoods, Nutraceuticals.* London: Chapman & Hall.
20. Gutteridge, J. M. C., Halliwell, B. (eds.) 1994. *Antioxidants: Free Radicals in Nutrition, Health and Disease.* Oxford, UK: Oxford University Press.
21. Jacobs, M. M. (ed.) 1994. *Diet and Cancer: Markers, Prevention, and Treatment. Advances in Experimental Medicine and Biology,* Vol. 354. New York: Plenum Press.
22. Keen, C., Bendich, A., Willhite, C. (eds.). 1993. *Maternal Nutrition and Pregnancy Outcome,* Vol. 678. New York: Annals of the New York Academy of the Sciences.

23. Krinsky, N. I., Mathews-Roth, M. M., Taylor, R. F. (eds.) 1989. *Carotenoids: Chemistry and Biology. Based on 8th International Syposium on Carotenoids in Boston.* New York: Plenum Press.

24. Krishnamurti, Dakshinamurti (eds.) 1990. *Vitamin B6 Vol. 585 in the Arsenals of the New York Academy of Sciences.* New York: New York Academy of Sciences.

25. Kritchevsky, D., Carroll, K. (eds.) 1994. *Nutrition & Disease Update: Heart Disease.* Champaign, IL: AOCS Press.

26. Laidlaw, S., Swendseid, H. (eds.) 1991. *Vitamins and Cancer Prevention: Contemporary Issues in Clinical Nutrition,* Vol. 14. New York: J. Wiley and Sons.

27. Lees, R. S., Karel, M. (eds.) 1990. *Omega-3 Fatty Acids in Health and Disease.* New York: Marcel Dekker.

28. Litwack, G. (ed.) 1995. *Vitamins and Hormones: Advances in Research and Applications,* Vol. 50. San Diego, CA: Academic Press.

29. Louria, D. S. (ed.) 1992. *Your Healthy Body: Your Healthy Life: How to Take Control of Your Medical Destiny (Revised and Updated).* New York: Master Media Unlimited.

30. Machlin, L. J. (ed.). 1990. *Handbook of Vitamins.* New York: Marcel Dekker.

31. McCormick, D. B., Bier, D. M., Goodridge, A. G. (eds.) 1995. *Annual Review of Nutrition,* Vol. 15. Palo Alto, CA: Annual Reviews.

32. Morley, J. E., Glick, Z., Rubenstein, L. Z. (eds.) 1995. *Geriatric Nutrition. A Comprehensive Review.* New York: Raven Press.

33. National Institutes of Health (FISH), Office of Alternative Medicine (OAM). 1995. *Alternative Medicine: Expanding Medical Horizons. A Report to the National Institutes of Health on Alternative Medical Systems and Practices in the United States.* Washington, DC: Office of Alternative Medicine, NIH.

34. Nettleton, J. A. (ed.) 1995. *Omega-3 Fatty Acids and Health.* New York: Chapman & Hall.

35. Packer, L. (ed.) 1994. *Methods in Enzymology—Oxygen Radicals in Biological Systems,* Vol. 234. San Diego, CA: Academic Press.

36. Packer, L., Fuchs, J. (eds.) 1993. *Vitamin E in Health and Disease.* New York: Marcel Dekker.

37. Picciano, M. F., Stokstadt, E. L. R., Gregory, J. F. (eds.) 1990. *Folic Acid Metabolism in Health and Disease: Contemporary Issues in Clinical Nutrition,* Vol. 13. New York: Wiley Liss.

38. Romeyn, M. (ed.) 1995. *Nutrition and HIV.* San Francisco, CA: Jossey-Bass Publishers.

39. Saito, K. (ed.) 1994. *Dynamics of Trace Elements in Human Body and Diseases.* Sapporo, Japan: Hokkaido University School of Medicine.

40. Shahidi, F., Naczk, M. (eds.) 1995. *Food Phenolics: Sources, Chemistry, Effects, Applications.* Lancaster, PA: Technomic Publishing Company Inc.

41. Shils, M. E., Young, V. R. (eds) 1994. *Modern Nutrition in Health and Disease* [Vols. 1 & 2]. Philadelphia: Lea and Febiger.

42. Sirnonpoulos, A. P. (ed.) 1991. *Selected Vitamins, Minerals and Functional Consequences of Maternal Malnutrition (World Review of Nutrition and Dietetics).* Basel: Karger.

43. Spallholz, J. E. (ed.) 1995. *Journal of Nutritional Immunology.* Binghamton, New York: The Haworth Press, Inc.

44. Willett, W. (ed.) 1990. *Nutritional Epidemiology. Monographs in Epidemiology and Biostatistics,* Vol. 15. New York: Oxford University Press.

45. World Health Organization. 1996. *WHO Publication: Trace Elements in Human Nutrition and Health.* Albany, NY: WHO Publications Center USA.

46. Ziegler, E. E., Filer, L. J., Jr. (eds.). 1996. *Present Knowledge in Nutrition.* Washington, DC: ILSI Press.

Nutrition-Related Journals and Newsletters

American Journal of Cardiology
Editors: Dr. William C. Roberts, Judy Wagner
Publisher: Excerpta Medica, Inc.; Subsidiary of: Reed Elsevier Medical Group
105 Raider Blvd., Belle Mead, NJ 08502, Subscr. to: Box 10670, Riverton,
NJ 08076, Tel. 908-874-8550

American Journal of Clinical Nutrition; a journal reporting the practical application
of our world-wide knowledge of nutrition
Editor: Charles Halsted
Publisher: American Society for Clinical Nutrition, Inc.
9650 Rockville Pike, Rm. 2310, Bethesda, MD 20814-3998, Tel. 301-530-7026

American Journal of Epidemiology
Editor: Moyes Szklo
Sponsor: Society for Epidemiologic Research; **Publisher:** Johns Hopkins
University; School of Hygiene and Public Health
2007 E. Monument St., Baltimore, MD 21205, Tel. 410-955-3441

American Journal of Public Health
Editor: Dr. Michael Ibrahim
Publisher: American Public Health Association
1015 15th St., N.W., Washington, DC 20005, Tel. 202-789-5600

Arteriosclerosis, Thrombosis and Vascular Biology
Editor: Dr. Alan M. Fogelman
Publisher: American Heart Association
7272 Greenville Ave., Dallas, TX 75231-4596, Subscr. to: Box 843543,
Dallas, TX 75284-3543, Tel. 214-706-1426

Atherosclerosis; international journal for research and investigation on atherosclerosis
and related diseases
Sponsor: International Atherosclerosis Society; **Publisher**: Elsevier Science Ireland Ltd.
P.O. Box 85, Limerick, Ireland, Tel. 353-61-471944

British Journal of Nutrition
Editor: D.A.T. Southgate
Sponsor: Nutrition Society
Publisher: Cambridge University Press Edinburgh Bldg., Shaftesbury Rd., Cambridge CB2 2RU, England, Tel. 01223-312393

BMJ (British Medical Journal)
Editor: Richard Smith
Sponsor: British Medical Association; **Publisher:** BMJ Publishing Group B.M.A.
House, Tavistock Sq., London WC1H 9JR, England, Tel. 44-171-383-6270

551

Cancer
Editor: Dr. Robert V.P. Hutter
Sponsor: American Cancer Society, Inc.
Publisher: John Wiley & Sons, Inc.; Journals
605 Third Ave., New York, NY 10158, Tel. 212-850-6645

Cancer Causes & Control; an international journal of studies of cancer in human populations
Editor: Richard Monson
Publisher: Rapid Science Publishers
The Old Malthouse, Paradise St., Oxford OX1 1LD, England, Subscr. in US to: 115 Fifth Ave., 4th Fl., New York, NY 10003, Tel. 44-1865-790447

Cancer Epidemiology, Biomarkers & Prevention
Publisher: American Association for Cancer Research
Public Ledger Bldg., 150 S. Independence Mall West, Ste. 816, Philadelphia, PA 19106-3483, Subscr. to: Fulco, Box 3000, Denville, NJ 07843, Tel. 215-440-9300

Cancer Letters; an international journal providing a forum for original and pertinent contributions in cancer research
Publisher: Elsevier Science Ireland Ltd.
P.O. Box 85, Limerick, Ireland, Tel. 353-61-471944

Cancer Research
Editor: Carlo M. Croce
Publisher: American Association for Cancer Research
Public Ledger Bldg., 150 S. Independence Mall West, Ste. 816,
Philadelphia, PA 19106, Subscr. to: Fulco, Box 3000, Denville, NJ 07843, Tel. 215-440-9300

Chemical and Engineering News
Editor: Medelie Jacobs
Publisher: American Chemical Society
1155 16th St., N.W., Washington, DC 20036, Subscr. to: Membership and Subscription Services, Box 3337, Columbus, OH 43210, Tel. 202-872-4600

Circulation (Dallas)
Editor: James T. Willerson
Publisher: American Heart Association
7272 Greenville Ave., Dallas, TX 75231-4596, Subscr. to: Box 843543, Dallas, TX 75284-3543, Tel. 214-706-1310

Current Opinion in Lipidology
Editor: Dr. S. M. Grundy
Publisher: Rapid Science Publishers
2-6 Boundary Row, London SE1 8HN, England, Tel. 44-171-410-6600

Dairy Council Digest; an interpretive review of recent nutrition research
Publisher: National Dairy Council
O'Hare International Center, 10255 W. Higgins Rd., Ste. 900, IL 60018-5616, Tel. 708-803-2000

Diabetes
Ed. Bd.

Publisher: American Diabetes Association
1660 Duke St., Alexandria, VA 22314, Tel. 703-549-1500

Environmental Newsletter
Publisher: University of Newcastle; Board of Environmental Studies Newcastle,
N.S.W. 2308, Australia, Tel. 61-49-215093

European Journal of Clinical Nutrition
Publisher: Stockton Press; Subsidary of: Macmillan Press Ltd.
Houndmills, Basingstoke, Hampshire RG2 2XS, England, Tel. 01256-817245

FASEB Journal
Publisher: Federation of American Societies for Experimental Biology
9650 Rockville Pike, Bethesda, MD 20014

FDA Consumer
Publisher: Food and Drug Adminstration
5600 Fishers Lane, Rockviller, MD 20857

Food & Nutrition Research Briefs
Publisher: Agricultural Research Service, U.S. Department of Agriculture
6303 Ivy Lane, 4th Floor
Greenbelt, MD 20770

Food Product Design
Editor: Scott Hegenbart
Publisher: Weeks Publishing Co.
3400 Dundee Rd., Ste. 100, Northbrook, IL 60062-2333, Tel. 847-559-0385

Food Technology
Editor: John B. Klis
Publisher: Institute of Food Technologists
221 N. LaSalle St., Chicago, IL 60601, Tel. 312-782-8424

Free Radical Biology & Medicine
Publisher: Elsevier Science Inc.
655 Ave. of the Americas, New York, NY 10010, Subscr. to: Box 882,
Madison Sq. Sta., New York, NY 10159-0882, Tel. 212-989-5800

ILSI News
Editor: R. Gutman
Publisher: International Life Sciences Institute
1126 Sixteenth Street, N.W., Suite 300
Washington, DC 20036, Tel. 202-659-0074

Immunologist
Editor: J. B. Natvig
Sponsor: International Union of Immunological Societies
Publisher: Hogrefe & Huber Publishers
Box 2487, Kirkland, Canada, WA 98083-2487, Tel. 206-820-1500

International Clinical Nutrition Review
Publisher: Integrated Therapies Pty. Ltd.
P.O. Box 370, Manly, N.S.W. 2095, Australia, Tel. 61-2-99770771

International Journal of Cancer
Editor: N. Odartchenko
Sponsor: International Union Against Cancer (Union Internationale Contre le Cancer)
Publisher: John Wiley & Sons, Inc.; Journals
605 Third Ave., New York, NY 10158, Tel. 212-850-6645

International Journal for Vitamin and Nutrition Research
Editor: P. Walter
Publisher: Hogrefe & Huber Publishers
Box 2487, Kirkland, WA 98083, Tel. 206-820-1500

Investigative Ophthalmology & Visual Science
Editor: Dr. Harry A. Quigley
Sponsor: Association for Research in Vision and Ophthalmology
Publisher: Lippincott - Raven Publishers
227 E. Washington Sq., Philadelphia, PA 19106, Tel. 215-238-4200

JAMA: The Journal of the American Medical Association
Editor: Dr. George D. Lundberg
Publisher: American Medical Association
515 N. State St., Chicago, IL 60610, Tel. 312-464-5000

Johns Hopkins Medical Letter Health after 50
Sponsor: Johns Hopkins Medical Institutions
Publisher: Medletter Associates
632 Broadway, New York, NY 10012, Tel. 212-505-2255

Journal of Bone and Mineral Research
Sponsor: American Society for Bone and Mineral Research
Publisher: Blackwell Science Inc.
238 Main St., Cambridge, MA 02142, Tel. 617-876-7022

Journal of Immunology
Editor: Dr. Peter Lipsky
Publisher: American Association of Immunologists
9650 Rockville Pike, Bethesda, MD 20814, Subscr. to: Fulco, Box 3000,
Denville, NJ 07843, Tel. 301-530-7178

Journal of Lipid Research
Editor: Lewis I. Gidez
Publisher: Federation of American Societies for Experimental Biology
9650 Rockville Pike, Bethesda, MD 20814, Tel. 301-530-7100

Journal of Nutrition
Editor: Dr. Willard Visek
Publisher: American Institute of Nutrition
9650 Rockville Pike, Bethesda, MD 20814, Tel. 301-530-7027

Journal of Nutrition Education
Editor: Audrey N. Maretzki
Sponsor: Society for Nutrition Education
Publisher: Decker Periodicals
P.O. Box 620, LCD 1, Hamilton, ON L8N 3K7, Canada, U.S. addr.: Box 785,
Lewiston, NY 14092-0785, Tel. 905-522-7017

Journal of Nutritional Immunology
Editor: Jullian E. Spallholz
Publisher: Haworth Press, Inc.
10 Alice St., Binghamton, NY 13904, Tel. 607-722-5857

Journal American College of Nutrition
Editor: Dr. Fima Lifshitz
Publisher: American College of Nutrition
c/o Hospital for Joint Deseases, 301 E. 17th St., New York, NY 10003, Subscr. to: Fulco, Box 3000, Denville, NJ 07834, Tel. 718-283-7906

Journal of the National Cancer Institute
Editor: Dr. Barnett Kramer
Publisher: U.S. National Cancer Institute; Information Associates Program

Journal of Women's Health
Editor: Bernardine P. Healy
Publisher: Mary Ann Liebert, Inc.
2 Madison Avenue
Larchmont, NY 10538, Tel. 914-834-3100

Lancet, The
Editor: Dr. Richard Horton
Publisher: The Lancet Ltd.; Subsidiary of: Reed Elsevier group
42 Bedford Sq., London WC1B 3SL, England, Tel. 44-171-4364981

Medical Tribune
Editor: David Bronstein
Publisher: Medical Tribune, Inc.
100 Ave. of the Americas, 9th Fl., New York, NY 10013-1606, Tel. 212-674-8500

The Nation's Health
Editor: Kathryn Foxhall
Publisher: American Public Health Association
1015 15th St., N.W., Washington, DC 20005, Tel. 202-789-5600

New England Journal of Medicine
Editor: Jerome Kassirer
Publisher: Massachusetts Medical Society
1440 Main St., Waltham, MA 02154, Subscr. to: Box 1940, Waltham, MA 02254, Tel. 617-893-3800

Nutrition; the international journal of applied and basic nutritional sciences
Editor: Dr. Michael Meguid
Publisher: Elsevier Science Inc.
655 Ave. of the Americas, New York, NY 10010, Subscr. to: Box 882, Madison Sq. Sta., New York, NY 10159-0882, Tel. 212-989-5800

Nutrition & the M.D.; a continuing education service for physicians and nutritionists
Editor: Dr. Russell Merritt
Publisher: Quest Publishing Co., Inc.; A Division of Raven Press Ltd.; Subsidiary of: Wolters Kluwer N.V.
1351 Titan Way, Brea, CA 92621, Subscr. to: Raven Press, 1185 Ave. of the Americas, New York, NY 10036, Tel. 714-738-6400

Nutrition Action Healthletter
Editor: Stephen B. Schmidt
Publisher: Center for Science in the Public Interest
1875 Connecticut Ave., N.W., Ste. 300, Washington, DC 20009-5728, Tel. 202-332-9110

Nutrition and Cancer; an international journal
Editor: Dr. Gio B. Gori
Publisher: Lawrence Erlbaum Associates, Inc.
10 Industrial Dr., Mahwah, NJ 07430-2262, Tel. 201-236-9500

Nutrition Notes
Editor: Carolyn Berdanier
Publisher: American Institute of Nutrition
9650 Rockville Pike, Bethesda, MD 20814, Tel. 301-530-7050

Nutrition Research
Editor: Ranjit K. Chandra
Publisher: Elsevier Science Inc.
655 Ave. of the Americas, New York, NY 10010, Subscr. to: Box 882, Madison Sq. Sta., New York, NY 10159-0882, Tel. 212-989-5800

Nutrition Research Newsletter; a monthly update for food, nutrition, and health professionals
Editor: Lillian Langseth
Publisher: Lyda Associates, Inc.
Box 700, Palisades, NY 10964, Tel. 914-359-8282

Nutrition Reviews
Editor: Robert E. Olson
Sponsor: International Life Sciences Institute—Nutrition Foundation
Publisher: Allen Press, Inc.
Box 1897, Lawrence, KS 66044, Tel. 913-843-1234

Nutrition Week
Editor: Dominic Madigan
Publisher: Community Nutrition Institute
2001 S St., N.W., Washington, DC 20009, Tel. 202-776-0595

Nutrition Today
Editor: Helen A. Guthrie
Publisher: Williams and Wilkins
351 W. Camden St., Baltimore, MD 21201, Tel. 410-528-4000

Prepared Foods
Editor: Bob Swientek
Publisher: Cahners Publishing Company (Des Plaines)
Division of Reed Elsevier Inc., 1350 E. Touhy Ave., Box 5080, Des Plaines, IL 60018-5080, Tel. 847-635-8800

Prostaglandins, Leukotrienes and Essential Fatty Acids
Editor: Dr. David F. Horrobin
Publisher: Churchill Livingstone; Subsidiary of: Pearson Professional
Robert Stevenson House, 1-3 Baxter's Pl., Leith Walk, Edinburgh EH1 3AF, Scotland, Subscr. to: Pearson Professional Ltd., P.O. Box 77, Fourth Ave., Harlow, Essex CM19 5AA, England, Tel. 0131-556-2424

Science News; the weekly newsmagazine of science
Editor: Julie Ann Miller
Publisher: Science Service, Inc.
1719 N St., N.W., Washington, DC 20036, Subscr. to: 231 W. Center St., Box 1925, Marion, OH 43306-4025, Tel. 202-785-2255

Scientist, The; the newspaper for the life sciences professional
Editor: Eugene Garfield
Publisher: The Scientist, Inc.
3600 Market St., Philadelphia, PA 19104-2645, Subscr. to: The Scientist, Box 10525, Riverton, NJ 08076, Tel. 215-386-9601

Sciences, The
Editor: Peter Brown
Publisher: New York Academy of Sciences
2 E. 63rd St., New York, NY 10021

Science News; the weekly newsmagazine of science
Editor: Julie Ann Miller
Publisher: Science Service, Inc.
1719 N St., N.W., Washington, DC 20036, Subscr. to: 231 W. Center St., Box 1925, Marion, OH 43306-4025, Tel. 202-785-2255

Today's Chemist at Work
Publisher: American Chemical Society
1155 Sixteenth Street, N.W., Washington, DC 20036

Tufts University Diet and Nutrition Letter
Editor: Stanley N. Gershoff
53 Park Pl., 8th Fl., New York, NY 10007, Subscr. to: Box 57857, Boulder, CO 80322, Tel. 212-608-6515

University of California at Berkeley Wellness Letter; the newsletter of nutrition, fitness, and stress management
Editor: Michael Golden
Sponsor: University of California at Berkeley; School of Public Health
Publisher: Health Letter Associates
Box 412, Prince St. Sta., New York, NY 10012, Subscr. to: Box 420148, Palm Coast, FL 32142, Tel. 212-505-2255

INDEX

A

Acid ash residue, urinary loss of calcium, 294, 295

Adenocarcinoma,
  esophageal cancer, 38–40
  gastric cancer, 40
  histologic types, 40

Adhesion molecules, role of oxidants in expression, 307

Adipose tissue, indirect measures, 472

Adiposity, *see* Childhood obesity; Obesity

Aflatoxin B1, inhibition by naringin, 145

Aged, *see* Elderly

Age-Related Eye Disease Study, 262

Age-related macular degeneration (AMD),
  animal studies, 251, 259
  antioxidant theory, 246, 247, 255–258
    carotenoids, 249, 250
    metalloenzymes, 250
    oxidoreductase enzymes, 247, 248
    vitamins, 248, 249
  atherosclerotic theory, 247, 258, 259
  cardiovascular risk factors, 250, 251
  current and future studies, 262
  dietary fat, 247
  dietary recommendations, 262, 263
  epidemiological studies, 251, 255–259
  fruits and vegetables, 428, 429
  incidence and treatment, 245
  oxidized lipids, 251
  primary prevention, 245
  reactive oxygen species, 245, 246
  retinal pigment epithelium, 247

Aging, *see also* Elderly
  general changes in immunity, 317, 318, 322
  theories, 317
  thymus involution, 318
  T-lymphocyte functions, 318–321

Agriculture, in Chilean nutritional policy, 521

Alcohol,
  consumption, in preventive nutrition, 431
  DNA hypomethylation, 84

esophageal cancer, 33, 34, 39
  folate deficiency, 381, 382
  gastric cancer, 41
  lung cancer, 114

Allium compounds, anticarcinogenic activity, 64

Allyl compounds,
  anticarcinogenic activity, 137–140
  in garlic, 137–139
  hypercholesterolemia, 137

Alpha-linoleic acid,
  infant formula supplementation, 414, 415
  neurodevelopment, 407
  sources, 409

Alpha-tocopherol, *see* Vitamin E

Alpha-Tocopherol Beta-Carotene Cancer Prevention Study, 121, 126, 175

Aluminum, urinary loss of calcium, 295

AMD, *see* Age-related macular degeneration

Analytic studies, in breast cancer, 99

Anemia, in preterm delivery, 392

Animal studies,
  age-related macular degeneration, 251, 259
  coronary heart disease, 171, 172
  preventive nutrition, 423

Antacids, urinary loss of calcium, 295

Antibody responses, effect of vitamin A deficiency on, 341

Anticarcinogenic agents, *see also* Antioxidants
  allyl compounds, 137–140
  ellagic acid, 146
  flavanols, 143–145
  flavanones, 145
  flavones, 142, 143
  in fruits and vegetables, 62–65, 135, 136
  in garlic, 137–139
  glucosinolates and isothiocyanates, 140–146
  in green and black tea, 143–145
  indoles, 141, 142
  isoflavones, 145, 146

in onions, 139, 140
terpenes, 146, 147
Antioxidants,
    age-related macular degeneration, 246,
        247
    atherosclerosis, 425
    cancer and, 77, 78, 83, 175, 176, 310
        breast, 103, 104
        colon, 78–81
        esophageal, 37
    cataract, 270–279
    childhood leukemia, 28
    clinical trials, 83, 84
    colon polyps, 81–83
    coronary heart disease and, 190, 309
        animal studies, 171, 172
        descriptive studies, 172
        dietary recommendations, 178
        observational studies, 172–175
        randomized trials, 175–177
    degenerative disorders, 311
    glutathione peroxidase, 128
    metalloenzymes, 248, 250
    micronutrients, 77, 78
    mutation in germlines, 378–381
    oxidant-mediated disease, 310
    oxidative damage, 80
    oxidoreductase enzymes, 247, 248
    reactive oxygen species, 246, 247
    smoking-related diseases, 308–310
Apoprotein,
    B, effect of fish oil on, 236
    E, cholesterol absorption, 155, 156
Ascorbic acid, see Vitamin C
Asia,
    chronic disease in, 523, 524, 531–533
    hypercholesterolemia and hypertension
        in, 524–527
    incidence of atherosclerosis, 530, 531
    nutritional westernization, 529, 530
Astrocytic glioma, childhood,
    dietary factors, 26
    incidence, 22
    maternal diet, 23–25
Atherosclerosis,
    antioxidants, 425
    effect of fish oil on, 226
    fish consumption, 530, 531
    homocysteine, 215
    low density lipoprotein cholesterol, 171
    low density lipoprotein oxidation, 306,
        307

pathogenesis, 153
vitamin C, 172
vitamin E, 171, 172, 176, 177
Autopsy data, coronary heart disease, 189

B

Baltimore Longitudinal Study of Aging, 255
Barrett's esophagus,
    incidence, 38
    medications, 38, 39
B-cell lymphocytes, aging and, 321
Beaver Dam Eye Study, 258, 259, 262
Behavioral weight-loss intervention, in
        childhood obesity, 478
Beta-carotene,
    breast cancer, 103
    coronary heart disease, 173, 175–178, 309
    differences from vitamin A, 337
    effect on lymphocyte numbers, 341
    gastric cancer, 43
    immunity, 324–326
    lung cancer, 83, 118, 121
    prevention of oxidant-mediated disease,
        311, 312
    reactive oxygen, 78
    relation to neutrophil counts, 311, 312
    scavenger of phagocyte-derived oxidants,
        309
Beta-Carotene and Retinol Efficacy Trial
        (CARET), 118, 120, 175, 176
Bile acids,
    calcium, 69
    in cholesterol absorption, 156
    colon cancer, 58, 69
Birth defects, see also Congenital
        abnormalities; Neural tube defects
    folic acid, 2
    nutritional interventions, 366, 367
    paternal smoking, 375, 376
Bitot's spots, vitamin A deficiency, 342, 343
Black tea, anticarcinogenic activity, 143–
        145
Blindness, vitamin A deficiency, 340, 342,
        343, 344
Blood pressure, childhood obesity, 473
BMI, see Body mass index
Body mass index (BMI),
    childhood obesity, 472
    in developing countries, 540
    environmental influences, 475, 476
    genetic influences, 474, 475
    preterm delivery, 389

Body weight,
 dietary fat, 427, 428
 in preventive nutrition, 430, 431
Bone,
 age-related loss, 291–293
 calcium reserves, 285, 286
 cellular processes, 285
 mass,
  acquisition of genetic potential, 287–289
  conservation, 289, 290
  factors influencing, 285, 286
  gonadal hormone regulation, 290, 291
  interrelationship with bone strength, 286
  rate of accumulation in young adults, 289
 resorption, 288
 strength,
  factors influencing, 285, 286
  interrelationship with bone mass, 286
 vitamin K, 297, 298
Bone gla protein, *see* Osteocalcin
Brain tumors,
 adult, N-nitroso compounds and, 26, 27
 childhood,
  dietary factors, 25, 26
  histologic types, 22
  incidence, 17, 22
  maternal diet, 23–25
  micronutrient serum levels, 26
  N-nitroso compounds and, 21–28
Bran, intestinal absorption of calcium, 293
Brassica, anticarcinogenic agents, 140–143
Breast cancer,
 antioxidants, 103, 104
 cohort studies, 102–104
 dietary fat, 426
 dietary recommendations, 105
 energy balance, 426
 environmental risk factors, 97, 100
 epidemiological study types, 98, 99
 estrogen, 104
 fat intake, 99–103
 fiber, 104
 fruits and vegetables, 103
 future studies, 105
 hormonal markers, 97
 incidence, 97
 olive oil, 102, 103
 postmenopausal women, 101, 102
 red meat, 102, 103

Breast-feeding, in Chilean nutritional policy, 518
Bronchial squamous metaplasia, vitamin B12, 128
B vitamins,
 in homocysteine regulation, 194
 lung cancer, 128

C

CA, *see* Congenital abnormalities
Caffeic acid, anticarcinogenic activity, 146
Caffeine, intestinal absorption of calcium, 294
Calcium,
 absorption,
  age effect, 292
  efficiency, 287, 288
  estrogen effect, 290
  intestinal, 293, 294
 age-related bone loss, 291–293
 bile acids and, 69
 bone mass acquisition, 287–289
 colon cancer, 68–72
 contemporary US intake levels, 287
 daily loss, 287, 288
 dietary sources, 295, 296
 fortification, 296
 intake/retention relationship, 286–289
 interference with iron absorption, 296
 osteoporosis, 7
 phosphate absorption and, 295
 preterm delivery, 399, 400
 in preventive nutrition, 430
 recommended intakes, 299, 300
  postmenopausal women, 291
 reserves in bone, 285, 286
 supplements, 296
 urinary loss, 294, 295
 vegetarian diet, 295
 vitamin D, 296, 297
Caloric intake,
 in Chile, 492
 relationship to nutrition, 447
Cambridge Heart Antioxidant Study, 176, 177
Cancer, *see also* specific forms
 allyl compounds, 137–140
 antioxidants, 77, 78, 83, 175, 176, 310
 childhood,
  brain tumors, 22–27
  dietary factors, 21
  etiology, 17

incidence, 17
   leukemia, 27–29
   N-nitroso compounds, 21–28
   vitamin K, 29
cigarette smoking, 306
dietary factors, 6, 135, 136
dietary fat, 426, 427
fruits and vegetables in, 428
mortality rates, 4
oxidative damage, 76, 77
oxygen-derived free radicals, 76, 77
Carbohydrates,
   coronary heart disease, 157, 158
   hypertriglyceridemia, 232, 233
   noninsulin-dependent diabetes, 429
Carcinogens, oxidants, 305, 306
Cardiac arrhythmia, fish oil and, 238, 239
Cardiovascular birth defects,
      periconceptional multivitamin
      prevention, 358–360
Cardiovascular disease, *see* Coronary heart
      disease
CARET, *see* Beta-Carotene and Retinol
      Efficacy Trial
Carotenoids, *see also* Beta-carotene
   age-related macular degeneration, 249,
      250
   cataract, 275–278
   colon cancer, 79
   conversion to vitamin A, 337
   lung cancer, 120–124
Carrots, lung cancer and, 116
Case-control studies,
   breast cancer, 99
   cataract, 270
   coronary heart disease, 187–189
   lung cancer, 110
   in preventive nutrition, 423
Catalase, as antioxidant, 248
Cataract,
   carotenoids, 275–278
   clinical features, 268, 269
   formation, 267, 270
   fruits and vegetables, 428
   future studies, 280
   incidence, 267, 268
   intervention trials, 278, 279
   lens protein oxidation, 270
   public health issues, 267, 268
   smoking, 277
   vitamin C, 271–273, 277, 278
   vitamin E, 273–275, 277, 278

Catechins, in fresh tea leaf, 143
Cell cycle, calcium and, 69
Cell differentiation, calcium and, 69
Cell division, in germlines, 374
Cell proliferation kinetics, calcium and, 68–70
Cellular immunity, vitamin A deficiency,
      340, 341
Cereals, fortification, 445, 446
Cerebrovascular disease,
   dietary factors, 6
   homocysteine, 208, 209
   incidence in Asia, 524
   morbidity rates, 6
CHD, *see* Coronary heart disease
Childhood obesity,
   comorbidities, 473, 474
   environmental influences, 475, 476
   genetic influences, 474, 475
   health organizations, 471, 472
   inoculation versus environmental
      manipulation, 480
   mechanisms, 474–476
   prevalence, 472
   prevention, 476–478
      behavioral weight-loss interventions,
         478
      general recommendations, 481, 482
      primary, 477
      punitive vs nonpunitive approaches,
         480
      school-based interventions, 477, 478
      "shotgun" vs "rifle" approaches, 479,
         480
      timing of efforts, 480, 481
Children,
   homeless, in Chilean nutritional policy,
      519, 520
   Japanese serum cholesterol levels, 524–526
   Korean serum cholesterol levels, 526
   malnutrition, Chilean programs for
      treatment, 516–518
   vitamin A deficiency
      blindness, 342, 343
      diagnosis, 343, 344
      growth, 341, 342
      HIV transmission, 342
      mortality, 340, 344, 345
   vitamin A supplementation, 346
Chile,
   agriculture, 521
   breast-feeding, 518
   calorie consumption, 492

child malnutrition, 505
    treatment, 516–518
control and prevention of obesity, 500, 501
Council of Food and Nutrition, 514–521
diabetes, 496
food habits, 491, 492
health care, 511–513, 518
homeless children, 519, 520
hypertension, 497, 498
lipid disorders, 496, 497
nutritional policy, 514–521
    development, 509–511
nutrition education, 499, 500, 518
prevalence of conditions related to
    obesity, 496–498
primary education and school food
    programs, 519
sanitation, 520
targeted food and nutrition interventions,
    515
Chilean Nutrition Foundation (CONIN),
    516–518
Chinese Cancer Prevention Study, 175
Cholesterol, *see also* Low density
    lipoprotein cholesterol; Very low
    density lipoprotein cholesterol
dietary,
    coronary heart disease, 155, 156
    interaction with saturated fatty acids, 164
    lung cancer, 112–114
    reducing absorption of, 156
metabolism, 155, 156
serum,
    in Asian children, 524–526
    atherosclerosis, 153
    in Chile, 496, 497
    dietary fat, 156–158
    effect of fish oil on, 227–229, 231
    fatty acids, 153, 154, 157–159
    Keys-Hegsted equations, 159
    lung cancer, 113, 114
    polyunsaturated fatty acids, 159–161
    saturated fatty acids, 161–163
    triglycerides, 164, 165
Chronic disease,
    in Asia, 523, 524
    assessment of risk factors, 8, 9
    in Latin America, 487–489
Chylomicronemia,
    effect of fish oil on, 231
    syndrome, 227
Cigarette smoking, *see* Smoking

Cleft lip birth defects, periconceptional
    multivitamin prevention, 360, 361
Clinical trials, in immunity, 323–329
Cobalamin,
    deficiency, folic acid and, 219
    influence on homocysteine, 197–202
Coconut oil, serum cholesterol, 161
Cod liver oil, reduced risk of leukemia, 28
Cohort studies
    breast cancer, 99, 102–104
    coronary heart disease, 183–187
    lung cancer, 110
    transferrin saturation, 186
Collagenase, oxidant related tissue injury, 306
Colon cancer,
    antioxidants, 78–84
    bile acids, 69
    calcium, 67–73
    cooked food hypothesis, 58
    dietary fat, 426
    effect of fruits and vegetables on, 62–65
    epithelial cell proliferation, 68–70
    fat and meat risk factors, 57–60
    fiber, 60–62
    folate, 84
    intermediate endpoint trials, 80–83
    milk products, 73–76
    nutritional supplements, 86
    onions, 139
    oxidative damage, 76, 77
    paleolithic diet, 85, 86
    prevention, 68, 84–86
    red meat consumption, 426, 427
    reversibility, 84
    seafood, 60
    sucrose, 65–67
    total energy intake, 59
    vitamin D, 73
    vitamin E, 82
Colon crypt proliferative zone, 68
Colon polyps, antioxidants, 81–83
Colorectal epithelial cell proliferation,
    antioxidants, 80, 81
    in colon cancer prevention, 68
Complex carbohydrates, glycemic index, 429
Conception, periconceptional multivitamin
    supplementation, 356, 357
Congenital abnormalities (CA), *see also*
    Birth defects; Neural tube defects
    infant mortality, 364
    periconceptional multivitamin prevention
    of, 357–361

cardiovascular defects, 358–360
cleft lip, 361, 360
limb deficiency, 361
possible mechanisms, 362–364
pyloric stenosis, 361
urinary tract defects, 358
primary prevention, 365, 366
secondary prevention, 365
study of, 351
CONIN, see Chilean Nutrition Foundation
Conjuctival impression cytology, diagnosis
of vitamin A deficiency, 344
Consensus Development Conference on
Optimal Calcium Intake, 291
Controlled trials, in lung cancer, 111
Convenience foods, nutrient content, 443,
444
Cooked food, colon cancer and, 58
Copper,
osteoporosis, 298, 299
superoxide dismutase, 248, 250
Corn oil, effect on induced
hypertriglyceridemia, 233
Coronary heart disease (CHD),
antioxidants, 171–177, 190, 309
autopsy data, 189
beta-carotene, 173, 175–178, 309
carbohydrates, 157, 158
dietary cholesterol, 155, 156
dietary fat, 156–159, 424–426
dietary recommendations, 153, 165, 166,
178, 216, 240
diet therapy, 3, 4
epidemiological studies, 171–177, 181–
189
ferritin, 183–185, 187–189
fish oil, 238–240
folate, 209–213
folic acid, 216, 217
fortification, 217
fruits and vegetables, 428
history of in Norway, 455, 456
homocysteine, 202–207, 213, 215
hyperhomocyst(e)inemia, 213, 215
incidence in Asia, 523, 524
iron, 181, 184, 187, 189
LDL/HDL ratio, 154, 155, 424
leukocyte count as predictor, 311
lipoprotein lipase, 165
lipoproteins, 154, 155, 424–426
mortality rates, 3
Oslo study, 459

polyunsaturated fatty acids, 159–161
saturated fatty acids, 161–163, 425
selenium, 175
trans fatty acids, 163, 164, 425
transferrin saturation, 185, 186
triglycerides, 164, 165
vitamin A, 176
vitamin C, 173, 174, 177
vitamin E, 173–178, 309
Coumarins, anticarcinogenic activity, 62
Council for Food and Nutrition (Chile), 514–
521
Cross-sectional studies,
coronary heart disease, 187–189
lung cancer, 110
micronutrient nutrition and immunity,
323
Crypt cells, colonic, 68
Cryptoxanthin, lung cancer and, 121
Cystathionine β-synthase,
deficiency, 195
homocysteine formation, 194
Cytochrome P450, in anticarcinogenic
activity, 141

D

Dairy products, in preventive nutrition, 430
Dark adaptation, diagnosis of vitamin A
deficiency, 344
Degenerative disorders, effect of
antioxidants and phagocytes on, 311
Delayed hypersensitivity response, T-cell
aging, 320
Delayed hypersensitivity skin test (DHST),
morbidity/mortality predictor, 319,
322
Demographics, in developing countries, 536
Descriptive studies, in coronary heart
disease, 172
Developing countries,
body mass index and socioeconomic
level, 538
demographic shifts, 536
dietary changes, 536–538
economic adjustments and risk of
undernutrition, 541, 542
economic context of nutritional problems,
540, 541
goals for preventive nutrition, 542, 543
health transition, 535, 536
obesity, 540–542
DHA, see Docosahexaenoic acid

DHST, *see* Delayed hypersensitivity skin
  test
Diabetes,
  fish oil and, 237
  prevalence in Chile, 496
  type II,
    carbohydrates, 429
    dietary factors, 7
    morbidity rates, 6
Diallyl sulfide, anticarcinogenic activity,
  138, 139
Diet,
  correlation with cancer, 135, 136
  general recommendations, 433, 434
  paleolithic, 85, 86
Diffuse carcinomas, in adenocarcinoma
  classification, 40
Disease prevention,
  defined, 2
  recommendations for Latin America, 498,
    499
  strategies, 2, 3
Dithiolthiones, anticarcinogenic activity, 62
D-limonene, anticarcinogenic activity, 146, 147
DNA,
  antioxidant protein defense, 378–381
  hypomethylation, 84
  regulation, retinoic acid, 338
  repair, effect of garlic on, 137
Docosahexaenoic acid,
  effect on atherosclerosis, 226
  in fish oil, 225
  infant formula supplementation, 414, 415
  neurodevelopment, 407, 413
  retinal development, 412, 413
  visual development, 414, 415

E

Eating habits, contemporary, 443
Economic development, effect on health and
  nutrition, 508, 509
Egalitarian traditions, effect on nutritional
  policy in developing
countries, 542, 543
EGCG, *see* (-)-Epigallocatechin gallate
Egypt, economic adjustments and loss of
  food security, 543
Eicosapentaenoic fatty acid,
  effect on atherosclerosis, 226
  in fish oil, 225
Elastase, in oxidative inactivation of
  protease inhibitors, 306

Elderly, *see also* Aging
  bone loss, 291–293
  cataract, 267, 268
  delayed hypersensitivity skin test, 319
  health promotion, 9
  hip fractures, 299
  immunity, 322, 327–329
  increases of in developing countries, 538
  macular degeneration, 245
  multivitamin use, 327–329
  prevention of fragility fractures, 292
  preventive nutrition, 7, 8
  severity of infectious disease, 321
  "survivor" aspect, 321, 322
  undernutrition in, 322
  vitamin D status, 292, 296, 297
Ellagic acid, anticarcinogenic activity, 146
Endemic carcinomas, in adenocarcinoma
  classification, 40
Endothelial cells,
  desquamation, 215
  expression of adhesion molecules, 307
  proliferation, 145, 146
Environmental effects, in childhood obesity,
  475, 476
Environmental manipulations, in prevention
  strategies, 480
EPA, *see* Eicosapentaenoic acid
Epidemiological studies,
  coronary heart disease, 171–177, 181–
    189
  micronutrient nutrition and immunity,
    322–330
  types of breast cancer studies, 98, 99
  types of lung cancer studies, 109–111
(-)-Epigallocatechin gallate (EGCG),
  anticarcinogenic activity, 144, 145
Epipodophyllotoxins, in leukemia, 27
Epithelial cancers, cigarette smoking, 306
Epithelial cell proliferation, colorectal, 68–
  70
Esophageal cancer,
  adenocarcinoma, 38–40
  alcohol and tobacco risk factors, 33, 34,
    39
  Barrett's esophagus, 38, 39
  biochemical studies, 37
  chemoprevention studies, 37, 38
  dietary studies, 35–37
  obesity, 39, 40
  preventive measures, 49
  squamous cell carcinoma, 33–38

thermal irritation, 34, 35
vitamin supplements, 38
Esophageal dysplasia, micronutrient
    supplementation, 38
Esophageal reflux, medications, 38, 39
Esophagitis, thermal injury, 35
Esophagus, Barrett's, 38, 39
Estrogen,
    breast cancer, 104
    effect on calcium absorption and
        retention, 290
    isoflavones, 145
    regulation of bone mass, 290, 291
Exercise, effect on micronutrient/immunity
    relationship, 330
Experimental studies
    breast cancer, 98, 99
    lung cancer, 109, 110
Eye Disease Case-Control Study, 255, 258,
    259

F

Fabricated food, in food processing
    technology, 444
Family planning, in Chile, 512
Fast-food, in Latin America, 493
Fat,
    age-related macular degeneration, 247
    body weight, 427, 428
    cancer and, 426, 427
        breast, 99–104, 426
        colon, 57–60
        lung, 112–114
        prostate, 427
    coronary heart disease, 156–159, 424–
        426
    effect of urbanization on, 538
    lipoproteins, 158
    in preventive nutrition, 424–426
    recommended intakes in Asia, 533, 534
    recommended intakes in Norway, 450,
        465
    serum cholesterol, 156–158
Fatty acids, *see also* specific groups
    in fish oil, *see* Fish oil
    serum cholesterol, 153, 154, 157–159
Fenton reaction, 77
Ferritin,
    coronary heart disease, 183–185, 187–189
    measure of iron body stores, 182, 183
Fetal death, periconceptional multivitamin
    supplementation, 357

Fetal development, polyunsaturated fatty
    acids in, 411
Fetal growth, preterm delivery, 388, 389
Fiber,
    breast cancer, 104
    classifications, 60, 61
    colon cancer, 60–62
    intestinal absorption of calcium, 293, 294
Fish consumption, atherosclerosis and, 530,
    531
Fish oil,
    cardiac arrhythmia, 238, 239
    clinical trials, 240
    diabetes, 237
    dietary recommendations, 240
    experimental atherosclerosis, 226
    hyperlipidemia, 227–231
    hypertension, 237, 238
    lipoproteins, 226–231, 235, 236
    phytoplankton source, 225
    population studies, 239, 240
    preterm delivery, 400
    prevention of pre-eclampsia, 411
    preventive nutrition, 425
    serum cholesterol, 227–229, 231
    supplementation during pregnancy, 411
    thrombosis, 239
    triglycerides, 226–231
    very low density lipoprotein and
        in chylomicronemia, 231
        in hypertriglyceridemia, 227–233
        in normal subjects, 227
        synthesis and turnover, 234, 235
Flavanones, anticarcinogenic activity, 145
Flavones, anticarcinogenic activity, 142, 143
Flavonoids,
    anticarcinogenic activity, 62, 142–146
    classification, 142
    inhibition of topoisomerase II, 27
Flavonols,
    anticarcinogenic activity, 143–145
    in green and black tea, 143–145
Foam cells, formation, 307
Folate,
    colon cancer, 84
    coronary heart disease, 209–213
    deficiency, 381, 382
    increased need for during pregnancy, 363,
        364
    influence on homocysteine, 197–202, 216
    low birth weight, 399
    metabolism, 362

preterm delivery, 399
sperm DNA mutation, 381, 382
supplementation, 433
Folic acid,
    birth defect prevention, 2
    coronary heart disease, 216, 217
    dietary recommendations, 220
    dietary sources, 362
    fortification, 217, 219, 449, 450
    homocysteine, 197–202, 216, 217
    neural tube defects and, 219, 351, 352
        dosages, 366
        periconceptional supplementation,
           352–354
    pernicious anemia, 219
    supplementation, 431
    vitamin B12 deficiency masking, 450
Food distribution, in Chile, 512, 513
Food habits, in Latin America, 490–493
Food interventions, in Chilean nutritional
    policy, 515
Food preparation, nutrient losses, 445–447
Food processing,
    contemporary, 442
    divisions of food supply, 444
    history, 442
    nutrient losses, 445–447
Food regulations, history, 442
Formulated food, in food processing
    technology, 444
Fortification, see also Nutrient addition
    calcium, 296
    cereal-grain products, 445, 446
    concept of disease prevention, 447–451
    folic acid, 217, 219, 449, 450
    neural defects, 220
    policy in Norway, 456
    preventive medicine, 451
    of processed food, 446
    public health, 448, 449
    technology of, 448, 449
    vitamin A, 346
Fractures,
    in elderly, prevention, 292
    hip, 299
Free radicals, see Reactive oxygen species
Fruits,
    adult daily consumption, 135
    anticarcinogenic agents, 62–65, 135, 136
    brain tumors,
        adult diet, 26, 27
        maternal diet, 23, 24

breast cancer, 103
esophageal cancer, 35, 36
gastric cancer, 42, 43
human adaptation to, 64
lung cancer, 114–117, 135
in preventive nutrition, 428, 429

G
Gametes, oxidant damage, 374
Garlic, 64
    anticarcinogenic activity, 64, 137–139
    commercial preparations, 138, 139
    inhibition of platelet aggregation, 140
    interaction with selenium, 139
    modification of DNA repair, 137
    promotion of liver cell proliferation, 140
    sulfur compounds, 138, 139
Gastric cancer,
    alcohol and tobacco risk factors, 41, 42
    dietary risk factors, 42, 43
    garlic, 137
    Helicobacter pylori, 40, 41
    histologic types, 40
    micronutrients, 43, 49
    preventive measures, 49
Gelatinase, oxidant related tissue injury, 306
Genistein, anticarcinogenic activity, 145,
    146
Germline mutation,
    antioxidants, 378–381
    cigarette smoke, 377
    prevention, 381–383
Gestational weight gain,
    diet, 391
    preterm delivery, 389–391
Ginseng, esophageal cancer and, 36, 37
Glucose homeostasis, effect of fish oil on,
    237
Glucose intolerance, in childhood obesity,
    473
Glucosinolates, anticarcinogenic activity, 62,
    140–146
Glutathione, effect of garlic on, 138
Glutathione peroxidase,
    as antioxidant, 248
    selenium in, 128, 248, 250
Glutathione-S-transferase, effect of garlic
    on, 138
Glycemic index, complex carbohydrates
    and, 429
Grain products, fortification, 445, 446
Grapefruit, anticarcinogenic activity, 145

Grapes, ellagic acid in, 146
Green tea,
    anticarcinogenic activity, 143–145
    (-)-epigallocatechin gallate, 144, 145
    esophageal cancer, 36
Gross national product, life expectancy and,
    508
Growth, effect of vitamin A deficiency on,
    341, 342

H

HDL, *see* High density lipoprotein
Health,
    dietary fat, 427, 428
    general dietary recommendations, 433,
        434
    and socioeconomic development, 508, 509
Health care,
    annual expenditures, 11
    in Chile, 511–513, 518
    health promotion in, 10
    preventive nutrition in, 10, 12
Health policy,
    within political environments, 509–511
    primary health care in, 511–513
Health Professionals Follow-up Study, 173
Health promotion,
    defined, 2
    in health care, 10
    recommendations for in Latin America,
        498, 499
Heart disease, *see* Coronary heart disease
        (CHD)
Helicobacter pylori, in gastric cancer, 40, 41
Hematocrit levels, in preterm delivery, 392
Hematopoiesis, vitamin A deficiency, 342
Hematopoietic cancer, paternal smoking in,
    377
Hemoglobin levels, in preterm delivery, 392
Hepatic cholesterol synthesis, suppression
    of, 155
High density lipoprotein (HDL),
    coronary heart disease, 424–426
    dietary fat, 158
    LDL/HDL ratio in coronary heart disease,
        154, 155, 424
    saturated fatty acids, 161
High-income countries, nutritional problems,
    542, 543
Hip fractures, role of nutrition, 299
Histamine H2 receptor antagonists, in
    esophageal adenocarcinoma, 38, 39

HIV-1 infection, vitamin A deficiency, 340,
    342
Homeless children, in Chilean nutritional
    policy, 519, 520
Homocysteine,
    atherosclerotic mechanisms, 215
    cerebrovascular disease, 208, 209
    coronary heart disease, 202–207, 213, 215
        risk reduction, 207, 208, 215
    cystathionine β-synthase deficiency, 195
    folate intake, 197–202
    formation and metabolism, 193–195
    forms, 195
    homocystinuria, 195, 196
    hyperhomocyst(e)inemia, 195, 196, 203,
        206
    increasing folic acid intake, 216, 217
    measurement, 196, 197
    methylenetetrahydrofolate reductase
        deficiency, 195, 196
    neural tube defects, 363
    peripheral vascular disease and, 209
Homocystinuria, homocysteine metabolism
    and, 195, 196
Hot dogs, *see also* Nitrite-cured meat
    childhood leukemia, 28
Human milk,
    long-chain polyunsaturated fatty acids,
        408
    in neurodevelopment, 414, 415
    polyunsaturated fatty acids, 409
Human resources, protection and
    development, 509
Hungarian Optimal Family Planning
    Service, 355–357
Hydrogen peroxide,
    DNA-damaging effect, 306
    expression of adhesion molecules, 307
    in immunosuppression, 308
Hydroxycinnamic acids, anticarcinogenic
    activity, 146
Hypercholesterolemia,
    allyl compounds and, 137
    in Asia, 524–527
Hyperhomocyst(e)inemia,
    coronary heart disease, 213, 215
    homocysteine blood levels, 203, 206
    homocysteine metabolism, 195, 196
Hyperinsulinemia, in childhood obesity, 473
Hyperlipidemia,
    dietary recommendations, 240
    effect of fish oil on, 227–231

Hypertension,
  in Asia, 524–527
  effect of fish oil on, 237, 238
  prevalence in Chile, 497, 498
Hypertension Detection and Follow-up
    Program (HDFP), 121
Hypertriglyceridemia, effect of fish oil on,
    227–233
Hypochlorous acid,
  effect on DNA repair, 306
  immunosuppression, 308
  oxidative inactivation of protease
    inhibitors, 306

I

Idiopathic preterm labor, preterm delivery,
    387
Immunity,
  aging and,
    general changes, 317, 318
    nutrition, 322
    other immune system changes, 321, 322
    "survivor" aspect, 321, 322
    thymus involution, 318
    T-lymphocyte functions, 318–321
  delayed hypersensitivity skin test, 319
  dietary recommendations, 333
  effect of vitamin A deficiency on, 338–
    341
  micronutrient nutrition and,
    effect of excess body weight, 330, 331
    effect of exercise, 330
    effect of stress, 330
    epidemiological studies, 322–330
  RDA and, 331
Immunization, in Chile, 512
Immunosuppression, oxidants and, 308
Indoles, anticarcinogenic activity, 62, 141,
    142
Industrialized nonmarket countries,
    nutritional problems, 543
Infant formula, polyunsaturated fatty acids
    and, 410, 413–415, 417
Infant mortality,
  in Chile, 505
  in Latin America, 488
  preterm delivery, 387
Infants, polyunsaturated fatty acids in
    neurodevelopment, 411–414
Infectious disease,
  vitamin A deficiency, 338
  vitamin A supplementation, 345

Information and technology, use of in
    developing countries, 542, 543
Inoculation, in prevention strategies, 480
Inositol hexaphosphate, anticarcinogenic
    activity, 64
Intact food, in food processing technology, 444
Intake-effect relationship, calcium and, 286,
    287
Interleukins, aging and, 321
Intervention studies, in neural tube defects,
    352–354
Intestinal carcinomas, in adenocarcinoma
    classification, 40
Iowa Women's Health Study, 174
Iron,
  absorption, 296
  body stores, 182, 183
  colon cancer, 58
  coronary heart disease, 181, 184, 187, 189
  hepatic, 189
  overload disease, 189
  oxygen-derived free radicals, 77
  preterm delivery, 392, 393
  total iron binding capacity, 184
Iron-deficiency anemia, in preterm delivery,
    392, 393
Ischemic heart disease, incidence in Asia,
    523, 524
Isoflavones, anticarcinogenic activity, 63,
    64, 145, 146
Isothiocyanates, anticarcinogenic activity,
    62, 140–146

J

Japan,
  atherosclerosis and fish consumption,
    529, 530
  childhood hypercholesterolemia and
    hypertension, 524–526
  chronic disease, 523, 524
  dietary fat intake, 528, 531–533
  salt consumption, 531

K

Kaempferol, anticarcinogenic activity, 143
Keratomalacia, vitamin A deficiency, 340,
    342, 343
Keys-Hegsted equations, serum cholesterol
    and, 159
Korea,
  childhood hypercholesterolemia, 526
  chronic disease, 523, 524

dietary fat intake, 531–533
nutritional westernization, 528, 529
Kuopio Ischemic Heart Disease Risk Factor
    Study, 183, 184

L

Lactation, recommended polyunsaturated
    fatty acid intake, 416
Latin America,
    chronic disease, 487–489
    demographic characterization, 487, 488
    fast-food outlets, 493
    food habits, 490–493
        and socioeconomic level, 490, 491
    health promotion and disease prevention
        programs, 498, 499
    infant mortality rates, 488
    nutritional westernization, 487, 491
    obesity in, 493–498
        children, 495
        prevalence, 493, 494
        socioeconomic level and, 494, 495
        socioeconomic changes in, 489
LDL, see Low density lipoprotein
LDL-C, see Low density lipoprotein
    cholesterol
Lens,
    aging of, 267
    cataract formation, 270
    protein oxidation in, 270
    vitamin C, 271, 272, 277, 278
Leukemia,
    adult, dietary factors, 28, 29
    childhood,
        antioxidant serum levels, 28
        cod liver oil, 28
        incidence, 17, 27
        maternal factors, 27
        N-nitroso compounds, 27, 28
        topoisomerase II inhibitors, 27
Leukocytes,
    blood levels and recommended vitamin
        intake, 311, 312
    effect of cigarette smoking on, 304, 305
    predictors of degenerative disorders, 311
Life expectancy, in relation to gross national
    product, 508
Lifestyles, eating habits in, 443, 444
Limb deficiency birth defects,
        periconceptional multivitamin
        prevention, 361
Limonene, anticarcinogenic activity, 64

Linoleic acid,
    infant nutrition, 406
    long-chain polyunsaturated fatty acid
        supply, 408
    sources, 409
Lipid disorders, prevalence in Chile, 496,
    497
Lipid peroxidation,
    in sperm cells and seminal fluid, 381
    vitamin E and, 77
        antioxidative micronutrients, 80
        selenium, 248
Lipids,
    age-related macular degeneration, 251
    childhood obesity, 473
    plasma, see Triglycerides
Lipoprotein lipase, trans fatty acids and,
    163, 164
Lipoproteins, see also High density
        lipoprotein; Low density lipoprotein;
        Very low density lipoprotein
    childhood obesity, 473
    effect of fish oil on, 226–231, 235, 236
    LDL/HDL ratio in coronary heart disease,
        154, 155, 424
    saturated fatty acids, 161
Liver,
    cell proliferation, effect of sulfur
        compounds on, 140
    vitamin A storage, 338
Long-chain polyunsaturated fatty acids
    effect of linoleic acid on, 408
    human milk, 408
    industrial production, 410
    infant formula, 410, 413
    metabolic pathways, 407, 408
    structural role, 407
    supplementation during pregnancy, 411
Lovastatin, 172
Low birth weight,
    folate, 399
    preterm delivery, 387
    zinc, 393
Low density lipoprotein (LDL),
    atherosclerosis, 306, 307
    coronary heart disease, 424–426
    dietary fat, 158
    effect of fish oil on, 227, 228, 230, 231,
        235, 236
    formation of foam cells, 307
    LDL/HDL ratio in coronary heart disease,
        154, 155, 424

metabolism, 236
oxidation,
    antioxidant nutrient status, 309
    effect of cigarette smoking on, 306,
       307
    homocysteine, 215
    vitamin E, 425, 426
peroxidation, 153, 154
saturated fatty acids, 161
Low density lipoprotein cholesterol (LDL-C),
    dietary fat, 156–158
    effect of fish oil on, 228, 229
    oxidation, 171
Low density lipoprotein receptor, dietary
    cholesterol and, 155, 156
Low-income countries, nutritional problems
    in, 542
Lung cancer,
    alcohol, 114
    Alpha-tocopherol Beta-carotene Trial,
       121, 126
    β-carotene, 83, 118
    B vitamins, 128
    carotenoids, 120–124
    causes, 109
    cell-type classification, 109
    cholesterol, 112–114
    dietary recommendations, 130
    efforts at prevention, 4, 6
    epidemiological study types, 109–111
       sex in, 114, 116
       smoking in, 111, 112, 114, 116
    fat, 112–114
    fruits and vegetables, 114–117, 135
    onions, 139
    retinol, 117–120
    selenium, 128
    vitamin A, 117
    vitamin C, 126–128
    vitamin E, 124–126
    zinc, 128
Lung health,
    vitamin C, 308, 309
    vitamin E, 309
Lutein,
    age-related macular degeneration, 249, 250
    lung cancer, 121
Lycopene, in lung cancer, 121
Lymphocytes,
    effect of vitamin A and β-carotene
       supplementation on, 341
    subset changes in T-cell aging, 320, 321

M

Macrophages,
    effect of cigarette smoking on, 304
    in formation of foam cells, 307
Macula,
    lipids in, 251
    oxidative damage, 246
Magnesium, calcium absorption and, 298
Malnutrition
    in Chilean children, 505, 516–518
    neurodevelopment, 405, 406
    reduced immunity, 322
    socioeconomic conditions, 505
Manganese, as antioxidant, 248, 250
Maternal diet, childhood brain tumors and,
    23–25
Maternal serum α-fetoprotein (MS-AFP),
       detection of neural tube defects, 365
Measles, vitamin A supplementation, 345, 346
Meat, *see also* Nitrite-cured meat
    breast cancer, 102, 103
    childhood leukemia, 28
    colon cancer, 57–60, 426, 427
    in preventive nutrition, 430
Medulloblastoma, childhood,
    incidence, 22
    maternal diet, 23–25
Menhaden oil, effect on experimental
    atherosclerosis, 226
Menopause,
    osteoporosis, 290, 291
    recommended calcium intakes, 291
Menstruation, periconceptional multivitamin
    supplementation, 356
Metalloenzymes, in age-related macular
    degeneration, 250
Methionine,
    DNA hypomethylation, 84
    in homocysteine formation, 193–195
    neural tube defects, 363
Methylation cycle,
    fetal development, 364
    neural tube defects, 363
Methylenetetrahydrofolate reductase, in
    homocysteine metabolism, 195, 196
5,10-Methylene-THF reductase, in spina
    bifida, 363
Microbial growth, effect of garlic on, 137
Micronutrients,
    antioxidants, 77, 78, 80
    childhood brain tumors, 26

gastric cancer, 43, 49
immunity and,
    effect of excess body weight, 330, 331
    effect of exercise, 330
    effect of stress, 330
    epidemiological studies, 322–330
    future studies, 331, 332
    preterm delivery, 393, 399
Middle-income countries, nutritional
    problems in, 542
Milk, *see* Human milk
Milkfat, serum cholesterol, 161
Milk products, colon cancer and, 73–76
Minerals, loss of in food processing, 445
Modified relative dose response, diagnosis
    of vitamin A deficiency, 344
Monocytes, effect of cigarette smoking on,
    304
Monosaturated fatty acids,
    breast cancer, 100
    serum cholesterol, 153, 154
Morbidity,
    delayed hypersensitivity skin test and,
        319, 322
    diabetes type II, 6
    effect of vitamin A deficiency, 345, 346
    nutrition, 3–8
    osteoporosis, 7
    reduction, 10, 11
    stroke, 6
Morning sickness, periconceptional
    multivitamin supplementation, 357
Mortality, *see also* Infant mortality
    causes of and socioeconomic
        development, 537, 538
    childhood obesity, 474
    delayed hypersensitivity skin test and,
        319
    infant,
        in Latin America, 488
        preterm delivery, 387
    nutrition, 3–8
    vitamin A deficiency, 340, 344, 345
MS-AFP, *see* Maternal serum α-fetoprotein
Mucosal immunity, vitamin A deficiency,
    340
Multiple Risk Factor Intervention Trial
    (MRFIT), 121
Multivitamins,
    immunity, 327–329
    periconceptional, 356, 357
        neural tube defects, 352–354

Mutation, in germlines, 374
    antioxidants, 378–381
    cigarette smoke, 377
    prevention, 381–383
Myeloperoxidase, effect of cigarette
    smoking on, 304, 305

N

Naringin, anticarcinogenic activity, 145
National Health and Nutrition Examination
    Survey (NHANES), 173, 174, 211,
    213, 255
National Nutrition Council (Norway), 455–
    459, 466, 467
Neoplasms, inhibitory effect of garlic on, 139
Nested case-control studies, in lung cancer,
    110
Neural membranes, polyunsaturated fatty
    acids and, 408, 409
Neural tube defects (NTD)
    detection, 365
    environmental factors, 351, 352
    folic acid and, 219, 351, 352
        dosages, 366
        periconceptional supplementation,
            352–354
        possible mechanism, 362–364
    food fortification, 220
    fruits and vegetables, 428
    incidence, 351
    intervention studies, 352–354
    methylation cycle inhibition, 363
    nutritional interventions, 366, 367
    periconception care, 354, 355
    time of occurrence, 352
    vitamin B12 as risk factor, 365, 366
Neurodevelopment,
    docosahexaenoic acid, 413
    human milk, 414, 415
    linkage to somatic development, 405, 406
    nutrition, 406
    polyunsaturated fatty acids and, 408, 409
        long-term effects, 414, 415
        preterm infants, 411–414
        term infants, 414, 415
Neuroectodermal tumor, primitive, 22
Neutrophils,
    adherence to vascular endothelium, 307
    effect of cigarette smoking on, 304, 305
    granules, proteolytic enzymes in, 306
    plasma membrane viscosity and aging, 321
    predictors of degenenerative disorders, 311

N-3 fatty acids, *see* Fish oil
NHANES, *see* National Health and Nutrition Examination Survey
Nightblindness, vitamin A deficiency, 340, 342–344
Nitrite, in N-nitroso compounds, 21, 22
Nitrite-cured meat,
    brain tumors,
        adult diet, 26, 27
        childhood diet, 26
        maternal diet, 23–25
    childhood leukemia, 28
Nitrosamines,
    inhibitory effect of garlic, 137
    sources, 21
N-nitroso compounds (NOC),
    childhood cancer, 21–28
    effect of garlic on, 137
    endogenous synthesis, 21, 22
    gastric cancer, 42
    inhibitors, 22
N-nitrosoproline, garlic and, 137
Nobiletin, anticarcinogenic activity, 142, 143
NOC, *see* N-nitroso compounds
Nonpunitive approaches, in prevention strategies, 480
Nonshared environmental effects, in childhood obesity, 475, 476
Norwegian nutrition and food policy,
    dietary recommendations, 450, 465
    food production, 460
    goals, 457, 464–466
    history, 455–460
    implementation, 466, 467
    Oslo study, 459
    resistance to, 461
    results, 461–464
    strategy, 467, 468
Nurses' Health Study, 173, 262
Nutrient addition, *see also* Fortification
    future of, 451
    goals, 441
    history, 443
    public health goals and, 451, 452
Nutrients,
    divergent capacity, 10
    nonessential, cancer and, 136
Nutrition,
    in Chile, 514–521
        education, 499, 500, 518
    consumer interest, 11

medical education, 12
    within political environments, 509–511
    recommendations,
        convergence of, 10
        historical goals, 2
        public health policy, 1, 2
        sources, 1
    within socioeconomic development, 508, 509
Nutrition-disease relationship, assessment of, 8, 9
Nuts, ellagic acid in, 146

O

Obesity, *see also* Childhood obesity
    in Asia, 524–527
    in Chile, control and prevention, 500, 501
    in developing countries, 540–542
    esophageal cancer, 39, 40
    in Latin America, 493–498
        children, 495
        prevalence, 493, 494
        socioeconomic level, 494, 495
Observational studies,
    breast cancer, 99
    coronary heart disease, 172–175
    lung cancer, 110, 111
Olive oil,
    breast cancer, 102, 103
    serum cholesterol, 162, 163
Omega-3-fatty acids, *see also* Fish oil
    colon cancer, 60
    origins, 410
Onion oil, anticarcinogenic activity, 140
Onions,
    anticarcinogenic activity, 139, 140
    inhibition of platelet aggregation, 140
    promotion of liver cell proliferation, 140
    sulfur compounds in, 139
Oocytes, risk of heritable mutation in, 374
Organic radicals, in cigarette smoke, 304
Oslo study, 459
Osteocalcin, as indicator of bone turnover, 298
Osteoporosis,
    age-related bone loss, 291–293
    calcium, 7
    conservation of acquired bone mass, 289, 290
    dietary recommendations, 299, 300
    hip fractures, 299

magnesium and, 298
menopause, 290, 291
morbidity rates, 7
nutrition and bone processes, 285, 286
premenopausal women, 289, 290
primary prevention, 287–289
trace minerals in, 298, 299
vitamin D, 7, 297
vitamin K, 298
Oxalate, intestinal absorption of calcium,
    293, 294
Oxidant-mediated disease,
    antioxidant nutrient status, 310
    cigarette smoking, 303, 304
    exposure to pollution, 310
    lifestyle, 310
    oxidative stress, 303
    predictors, 310, 311
    prevention, 312
Oxidants,
    antioxidants, 80
    as carcinogens, 305, 306
    cellular damage, 373
    colon cancer, 76, 77
    damage to gametes, 374
    effect on DNA repair, 306
    immunosuppressive properties, 308
    proadhesive activity, 307, 308
    pro-atherogenic properties, 306, 307
    proteolytic activities, 306
    retinol, 118
Oxidative stress,
    cigarette smoking, 303–305
    environmental and lifestyle associations,
        303
Oxidoreductase enzymes, in age-related
    macular degeneration, 247, 248
Oxygen-derived free radicals, cancer and,
    76, 77

P

Paleolithic diet, colon cancer and, 85, 86
Palm oil, effect on serum cholesterol, 161–163
Parathyroid hormone, in bone resorption, 288
Parathyroid hormone (PTH), extracellular
    fluid calcium levels and, 286
Partitioned food, in food processing
    technology, 444
Pediatric obesity, see Childhood obesity
Periconception care,
    effect of multivitamin supplementation
        on, 356, 357

Hungarian Optimal Family Planning
    Service, 355–357
prevention of birth defects, 354, 355
Peripheral vascular disease, homocysteine
    and, 209
Pernicious anemia, folic acid and, 219
Peroxidation, of low density lipoproteins,
    153, 154
Phagocyte-derived reactive oxidants,
    DNA-damaging effect, 306
    DNA repair, 306
Phagocytes,
    effect of cigarette smoking on, 304
    predictors of degenerative disorders, 311
Phenols, anticarcinogenic activity, 62
Phosphorus,
    reserves in bone, 285, 286
    urinary loss of calcium, 295
Physicians' Health Study, 176
Phytate, intestinal absorption of calcium,
    293, 294
Phytoplankton, omega-3-fatty acid synthesis,
    225
Plasma lipids, see Triglycerides
Platelet aggregation, effect of garlic and
    onions on, 140
Politics, effect on nutrition and health
    policy, 509–511
Pollution, in oxidant-mediated disease, 310
Polyunsaturated fatty acids,
    breast cancer, 100–102
    in development, 406, 407
    dietary recommendations, 424
    dietary sources, 409, 410
    in fetal development, 411
    lipid peroxidation, 153, 154
    lung cancer, 112
    neural membrane function, 408, 409
    in neurodevelopment,
        long-term effect, 415
        preterm infants, 411–414
        term infants, 414, 415
    recommended intakes,
        formula-fed infants, 417
        pregnancy and lactation, 416
    serum cholesterol, 153, 154, 159–161
Post-communist countries, nutritional
    problems in, 543
Postmenopausal women, breast cancer and,
    101, 102
Postnatal development, periconceptional
    multivitamin supplementation, 357

Pre-eclampsia, prevention with fish oil, 411
Pregnancy,
  essential fatty acid supplementation, 411
  gestational weight gain, 389–391
  increased folate need, 363, 364
  periconception care, 354, 355
  periconception multivitamin
      supplementation, 356, 357
  recommended polyunsaturated fatty acid
      intake, 416
  vitamin A deficiency, 342
Pregravid body mass index, in preterm
    delivery, 389
Premature rupture of fetal membranes
    (PROM), preterm delivery and, 387,
    388
Preschool food programs, in Chilean
    nutritional policy, 519
Preterm delivery (PTD)
  calcium, 399, 400
  diet, 391
  dietary recommendations, 401
  fetal growth, 388, 389
  fish oil, 400
  folate, 399
  future studies, 400
  gestational weight gain, 389–391
  idiopathic preterm labor, 387
  infant mortality, 387
  iron, 392, 393
  low birth weight, 387
  maternal pregravid size, 389
  premature rupture of fetal membranes,
      387, 388
  zinc, 393
Preterm infants, polyunsaturated fatty acids
    in neurodevelopment, 411–414
Preventive medicine, food fortification and,
    451
Preventive nutrition,
  alcohol consumption, 431
  body weight, 430, 431
  calcium and dairy products, 430
  in developing countries
    egalitarian traditions and, 544, 545
    information and technology use, 544,
        545
    prioritizing interventions, 545
    setting goals, 545
  dietary fat, 424–426
  general dietary recommendations, 433,
      434

protein, 429
RDA, 423
reduction of salt and processed meats, 430
starches and complex carbohydrates, 429
types of studies, 423, 424
vegetables and fruits, 428, 429
vitamin supplements, 431–433
Primary education, in Chilean nutritional
    policy, 519
Primary health care,
  in Chile, 511–513
  in nutrition and health policy, 511–513
Primitive neuroectodermal tumor, in
    childhood, 22
Probucol, cholesterol lowering activity, 172
Processed food, fortification of, 446
PROM, see Premature rupture of fetal
    membranes
Prospective studies,
  cataract, 270
  coronary heart disease, 183–187
  lung cancer, 110, 111
  preventive nutrition, 423
  transferrin saturation, 186
Prostate cancer, dietary fat and, 427
Protease inhibitors, anticarcinogenic
    activity, 62
Protein,
  in preventive nutrition, 429
  urinary loss of calcium, 294
Proteinase 3, in oxidative inactivation of
    protease inhibitors, 306
Protein-calorie malnutrition, reduced
    immunity, 322
Protein energy malnutrition, in
    neurodevelopment, 405, 406
Proteolytic enzymes, neutrophil granules
    and, 306
Pseudogynecomastia, in childhood obesity,
    474
PTD, see Preterm delivery
Pteroylglutamic acid, see Folic acid
PTH, see Parathyroid hormone
Public health,
  annual costs and expenditures, 3–7
  cataract, 267, 268
  cigarette smoking, 303–305
  health promotion, 1
  nutrition recommendations, 1, 2
  vitamin A and,
    childhood mortality, 344–346
    deficiency prevention, 337, 346

infectious disease morbidity, 345, 346
  measles, 345
  supplementation in developing
    countries, 346
Punitive approaches, in prevention
  strategies, 480
Pyloric stenosis birth defects,
  periconceptional multivitamin
  prevention, 361
Pyridoxine,
  immunity, 324
  influence on homocysteine, 197–202

Q

Quercetin, anticarcinogenic activity, 143
Quinones, 143

R

RDA, *see* Recommended Dietary Allowance
Reactive oxygen species (ROS),
  age-related macular degeneration, 245, 246
  antioxidants, 246, 247
Recommended Dietary Allowance (RDA),
  calcium, 289
  determination of nutrient levels in, 447
  disease prevention, 447
  history of, 423
  inclusion of nonnutrients, 447, 448
Relative dose response, diagnosis of vitamin
  A deficiency, 344
Respiratory abnormalities, in childhood
  obesity, 473, 474
Retina,
  development, docosahexaenoic acid, 412,
    413
  lipids in, 251
  oxidative damage, 246
Retinal pigment epithelium, in age-related
  macular degeneration, 247
Retinoblastoma, childhood, 29
Retinoic acid, *see also* Vitamin A
  DNA regulation, 338
Retinol, *see also* Vitamin A
  breast cancer, 103
  carrier proteins, 338
  diagnosis of vitamin A deficiency, 343,
    344
  esophageal cancer, 37, 38
  lung cancer, 117–120
  receptors, 338
  repair of oxidative damage, 118
  as serum biomarker, 118

Rhabdomyosarcoma,
  childhood, 29
  paternal smoking and, 376
Riboflavin, esophageal cancer and, 37, 38
Risk factors, assessment of, 8, 9
ROS, *see* Reactive oxygen species
Rural health care, in Chilean nutritional
  policy, 518

S

S-adenosylmethionine, in homocysteine
  regulation, 194, 195
S-allyl cysteine, anticarcinogenic activity,
  138, 139
Salt,
  consumption, in Japan, 531
  gastric cancer, 42
  in preventive nutrition, 430
Sanitation, in Chilean nutritional policy, 520
Saponins, anticarcinogenic activity, 64
Saturated fatty acids,
  breast cancer, 100–102
  coronary heart disease, 161–163, 425
  interaction with dietary cholesterol, 164
  lipoproteins and, 161
  serum cholesterol and, 153, 154, 161–163
School-based interventions, in childhood
  obesity, 477, 478
School food programs, in Chilean nutritional
  policy, 519
Seafood, colon cancer and, 60
Selenium,
  colon cancer, 79, 80
  coronary heart disease, 175
  gastric cancer, 43
  glutathione peroxidase and, 128, 248, 250
  interaction with garlic, 139
  lipid peroxidation, 248
  lung cancer, 128
  oxygen-free radicals, 78
Seminal plasma,
  lipid peroxidation, 381
  vitamin C, 378–380
  vitamin E, 380, 381
Sexual activity, periconceptional
  multivitamin supplementation, 356
Shared environmental effects, in childhood
  obesity, 475, 476
Skinfold measures, assessment of body fat, 472
Skin tumors, effect of onion oil on, 140
Smoking,
  activation of proteolytic enzymes, 306
  atherosclerosis, 307

cataract, 277
depletion of seminal plasma vitamin C, 380
DNA-damaging effect, 305, 306
effect on antioxidants, 277
effect on LDL oxidation, 307
immunosuppression, 308
in lung cancer study design, 111, 112
mortality, 304
origins of oxidants in, 304
paternal,
    birth defects, 375, 376
    childhood tumors, 376, 377
    risk of mutation in germlines, 374–377
proinflammatory effect, 304, 305
public health, 303
Socioeconomic conditions,
    body mass index and, 540
    food habits and, 490–492
    in Latin America, 489–491
    lipid disorders and, 496, 497
    malnutrition, 505
Socioeconomic development,
    changes in mortality, 537, 538
    health and nutrition in, 508, 509
Sodium, urinary loss of calcium, 294
Somatic development, linkage to
    neurodevelopment, 405, 406
Soybean oil, tocopherols in, 425, 426
Soybeans, anticarcinogenic activity, 64, 145,
    146
Soy products, breast cancer and, 426
Spermatogenesis,
    nutritional requirements, 377, 378
    zinc, 382
Spermatozoa,
    lipid peroxidation, 381
    prevention of mutation, 381–383
    risk of heritable mutation, 374
Spina bifida, 5,10-methylene-THF reductase
    and, 363
Squamous cell carcinoma, in esophageal
    cancer, 33–38
Starches, in preventive nutrition, 429
Sterols, plant, 63
Stomach cancer, see Gastric cancer
Stress, effect on micronutrient/immunity
    relationship, 330
Stroke,
    dietary factors, 6
    homocysteine and, 208, 209
    incidence in Asia, 524
    morbidity rates, 6

Structural birth defects, see Birth defects;
    Congenital abnormalities
Sucrose, colon cancer and, 65–67
Superoxide, expression of adhesion
    molecules, 307
Superoxide dismutase,
    as antioxidant, 248
    copper in, 248, 250

T

Tangeretin, anticarcinogenic activity, 142,
    143
Tar,
    DNA-damaging effect, 305, 306
    organic radicals in, 304
T-cell lymphocytes, effect of vitamin A
    deficiency on, 341
Tea,
    anticarcinogenic activity, 143–145
    esophageal cancer, 34, 36
Teratology, history of, 351
Terpenes, anticarcinogenic activity, 146, 147
Testosterone, regulation of bone mass, 290
Tetrahydrofolate,
    in DNA and RNA synthesis, 363
    folic acid supplements, 362
    in methylation cycle, 363
Thailand,
    chronic disease in, 523, 524
    nutritional westernization, 530
    recommendations on dietary fat intake,
        533
    risk factors of chronic disease, 526, 527
Thiocyanates, anticarcinogenic activity, 62
Thrombosis,
    fish oil and, 239
    homocysteine and, 215
Thymus, involution of, 318
TIBC, see Total iron binding capacity
T-lymphocytes,
    aging and, 317–321
        antigen binding capacity, 321
        changing cell subsets, 320, 321
        delayed hypersensitivity skin test, 319
        lymphocyte proliferative response, 320
    maturation process, 318
Tobacco, see also Cigarettes
    esophageal cancer, 33, 34, 39
    gastric cancer, 41, 42
Tocopherols, see also Vitamin E
    cell proliferation studies, 80, 81
    colon cancer, 83

lung cancer, 124–126
    in soybean oil, 425, 426
Topoisomerase II, chilhood leukemia and, 27
Total iron binding capacity (TIBC),
    coronary heart disease, 184
    measure of iron body stores, 182, 183
Trans fatty acids,
    adverse effects, 163, 164
    coronary heart disease, 163, 164, 425
Transferrin saturation (TS),
    causes of mortality and, 186
    coronary heart disease, 185, 186
    measure of iron body stores, 182, 183
Triglycerides,
    effect of fish oil on, 226–231, 235, 236
    serum cholesterol, 164, 165
TS, *see* Transferrin saturation
Tumors, *see also* Brain tumors
    childhood, paternal smoking and, 376, 377
    effect of allyl sulfur compounds on, 138
    effect of onion oil on, 140
    induction by N-nitroso compounds, 22

U

Undernutrition, reduced immunity and, 322
Uracil, folate deficiency and, 381
Urbanization, dietary changes during, 540
Urinary tract birth defects, periconceptional
    multivitamin prevention, 358

V

Vascular endothelium, adherence of
    neutrophils, 307
Vegetables,
    adult daily consumption, 135
    anticarcinogenic agents, 62–65, 135, 136
    brain tumors and, maternal diet, 23, 24
    breast cancer, 103
    cruciferous, 62, 116, 140, 141
    esophageal cancer, 35, 36
    gastric cancer, 42, 43
    glucosinolates and isothiocyanates in,
        140–146
    human adaptation to, 64
    lung cancer, 114–117, 135
    in preventive nutrition, 428, 429
Vegetarian diet, calcium requirement and, 295
Ventricular fibrillation, fish oil and, 238, 239
Very low density lipoprotein (VLDL),
    effect of fish oil on,
        chylomicronmeia, 231
        hypertriglyceridemia, 227–233

normal subjects, 227
    synthesis and turnover, 234, 235
    metabolism, 236
Very low density lipoprotein cholesterol
    (VLDL-C), effect of fish oil on, 227–
    229, 235
Vision, vitamin A deficiency, 342, 343
Visual development,
    docosahexaenoic acid in, 414, 415
    long-term effect of polyunsaturated fatty
        acids, 415
Vitamin A, *see also* Retinoic acid; Retinol
    absorption, 337
    in age-related macular degeneration, 249
    breast cancer, 103
    coronary heart disease, 176
    deficiency,
        in children, 340–344
        diagnosis, 343, 344
        growth, 341, 342
        hematopoiesis, 342
        immunity, 338–341
        pregnancy and reproduction, 342
        prevention, 346
        vision, 340, 342, 343
    in fortification, 446, 447
    immunity, 326
    lung cancer, 117
    metabolism, 337, 338
    public health intervention, 344–346
    recommendations, 347
    storage and transport, 338
    supplementation, 433
        in developing countries, 346
Vitamin B12,
    bronchial squamous metaplasia, 128
    dietary recommendations, 220
    folic acid and, 450
    homocysteine levels, 202
    as neural tube defect risk factor, 365, 366
Vitamin B6, immunity and, 324
Vitamin C,
    age-related macular degeneration, 248
    atherosclerosis, 172
    brain tumors and, maternal diet, 24, 25
    breast cancer, 103, 104
    cataract, 271–273, 277, 278
    colon cancer, 79, 80
    coronary heart disease, 173, 174, 177
    esophageal cancer, 35, 36
    in fortification, 446
    gastric cancer, 43, 49

immunity, 323–326
impact of cigarette smoking on, 308, 309
inhibition of N-nitroso compounds, 22
LDL oxidation and, 309
in lens, 271, 272, 277, 278
lung cancer, 126–128
male fertility, 380
oxygen-free radicals, 78
prevention of germline mutations, 378–380
prevention of oxidant-mediated disease, 311, 312
pulmonary functioning, 308, 309
relation to leukocyte counts, 311, 312
in serum, 126
supplementation, 432
Vitamin D,
calcium, 296, 297
colon cancer, 73
in elderly, 292
in fortification, 446, 447
osteoporosis, 7, 297
Vitamin E, *see also* Tocopherols
age-related macular degeneration, 248, 249
atherosclerosis, 171, 172, 176, 177
cataract, 273–275, 277, 278
colon cancer, 79, 80, 82
coronary heart disease, 173–178, 309
gastric cancer, 43
immunity, 324–326
lung cancer, 124–126
oxidation of low density lipoproteins, 425, 426
oxygen-free radicals, 77, 78
prevention of germline mutations, 380, 381
prevention of oxidant-mediated disease, 311, 312
in pulmonary functioning, 309
regulation of neutrophil-activated oxidants, 309
supplementation, 431, 432

Vitamin K,
administration to newborns, 29
bone health, 297, 298
Vitamins,
age-related macular degeneration, 248, 249
loss of in food processing, 445
Vitamin supplements,
brain tumors and,
childhood diet, 26
maternal diet, 24, 25
cataract, 278, 279
colon cancer, 86
esophageal cancer, 38
harmful effects, 433
in preventive nutrition, 431–433
VLDL, *see* Very low density lipoprotein
VLDL-C, *see* Very low density lipoprotein cholesterol

W

Weight loss, effect on micronutrient/immunity relationship, 330, 331
Wheat bran, intestinal absorption of calcium, 293

X

Xerophthalmia,
vitamin A deficiency, 342, 343
vitamin A supplementation, 346

Z

Zeaxanthin,
age-related macular degeneration, 249, 250
lung cancer, 121
Zinc,
esophageal cancer, 37, 38
functions, 250
gastric cancer, 43
immunity, 325
lung cancer, 128
osteoporosis, 298
spermatogenesis, 382

Robert R. Williams Professor of Nutrition and Professor of Pediatrics, **Dr. Richard Deckelbaum** serves as Director of the Institute of Human Nutrition and Director of Pediatric Gastroenterology and Nutrition at Columbia University. Dr. Deckelbaum's research programs are supported by the National Institutes of Health and other agencies. In addition to his own basic laboratory work delineating cellular pathways of lipid metabolism, Dr. Deckelbaum has made important contributions defining the role of nutrition in promoting health and decreasing disease risk. Dr. Deckelbaum has published over 180 research papers and reviews. He has served on national and international task forces (e.g., the National Heart, Blood and Lung Institute's National Cholesterol Education Program, the Nutrition Committee of the American Heart Association, and the International Task Force for Prevention of Coronary Heart Disease) promoting nutrition as a key modality for disease prevention.

Dr. Adrianne Bendich is an internationally recognized authority on the importance of vitamins for optimal health. She is best known for her reseach regarding antioxidants and improvements in immune function, her expertise in vitamin safety issues, and her pioneering efforts to assure the daily use of multivitamins containing folic acid for all women of childbearing potential. Dr. Bendich co-chaired two New York Academy of Sciences conferences: "Micronutrients and Immune Responses" and "Maternal Nutrition and Pregnancy Outcome." Dr. Bendich is an editor of the *Journal of Nutritional Immunology*, a member of the Editorial Board of the *Journal of Free Radical Biology and Medicine*, and past member of the editorial board of the *Journal of Nutrition*. She also served as an advsior to NIH, the New York Academy of Sciences, and numerous committees for international organizations, including the WHO and US AID. Dr. Bendich has also given expert testimony to Federal Congressional Subcommittees, State Legislative Committees, and the FDA. She has over 100 reviewed publications and is the editor of five other books, including *Micronutrients in Health and Disease Prevention*. Dr. Bendich was awarded the Roche Research Prize in 1992 and the Tribute to Women in Industry Award in 1995, and was recognized by the Spina Bifida Association of America in 1996.